Veterinary Viral Diseases: Diagnosis and Treatment

Veterinary Viral Diseases: Diagnosis and Treatment

Edited by Zoe Lucas

MURPHY & MOORE
www.murphy-moorepublishing.com

Published by Murphy & Moore Publishing,
1 Rockefeller Plaza,
New York City, NY 10020, USA
www.murphy-moorepublishing.com

Veterinary Viral Diseases: Diagnosis and Treatment
Edited by Zoe Lucas

International Standard Book Number: 978-1-63987-566-5 (Hardback)

Cataloging-in-Publication Data

Veterinary viral diseases : diagnosis and treatment / edited by Zoe Lucas.
p. cm.
Includes bibliographical references and index.
ISBN 978-1-63987-566-5
1. Veterinary virology. 2. Virus diseases. 3. Virus diseases--Diagnosis. 4. Virus diseases--Treatment.
5. Veterinary medicine. I. Lucas, Zoe.
SF780.4 .V48 2022
636.089 601 94--dc23

TABLE OF CONTENTS

PREFACE

Over the recent decade, advancements and applications have progressed exponentially. This has led to the increased interest in this field and projects are being conducted to enhance knowledge. The main objective of this book is to present some of the critical challenges and provide insights into possible solutions. This book will answer the varied questions that arise in the field and also provide an increased scope for furthering studies.

A viral disease or infection is an infectious disease which occurs due to the invasion and proliferation of infectious viruses. Identification and control of these viruses that cause diseases in domesticated and wild animal represent continuous challenges to animal and human welfare. A lot of diagnostic techniques like biochemical tests and behavioral tests are used for the detection of viral diseases. Discovery of new techniques and technologies in this field has resulted in accurate understanding of diseases in less time with high accuracy and efficiency. The treatment of veterinary viral diseases depends upon the nature and uniqueness of the virus. The treatment usually follows the medical advice of veterinarians and the use of veterinary drugs specific to viruses and animals. This book provides comprehensive insights into the field of veterinary viral diseases. It discusses the fundamentals as well as modern approaches of diagnosis and treatment of veterinary viral diseases. Researchers and students in this field will be assisted by this book.

I hope that this book, with its visionary approach, will be a valuable addition and will promote interest among readers. Each of the authors has provided their extraordinary competence in their specific fields by providing different perspectives as they come from diverse nations and regions. I thank them for their contributions.

Editor

1

Construction of a camelid VHH yeast two-hybrid library and the selection of VHH against haemagglutinin-neuraminidase protein of the Newcastle disease virus

Xiaolong Gao[†], Xiangyun Hu[†], Lina Tong, Dandan Liu, Xudong Chang, Haixin Wang, Ruyi Dang, Xinglong Wang, Sa Xiao, Enqi Du[*] and Zengqi Yang[*]

Abstract

Background: Newcastle disease (ND), which is caused by the Newcastle disease virus (NDV), is one of the most important avian diseases in poultry. Since its discovery in 1926, ND has caused great economic losses to the world poultry industry and remains a threat to chickens and wild birds. Although a stringent vaccination policy is widely adopted to control ND, ND outbreaks still occur, and virulent NDV is sporadically isolated from chickens and wild birds. To study the pathogenesis of ND and provide tools to prevent its prevalence, novel antibody fragments should be developed. The variable domains of the heavy chain of the heavy-chain antibodies (VHH) are the smallest naturally occurring antibodies derived from camelid heavy-chain antibodies. The comparatively small size, high affinity, high solubility, low immunogenicity and ability to bind epitopes inaccessible to conventional antibodies of VHH make them ideal candidates for a considerable number of therapeutic and biotechnological applications. However, an anti-NDV VHH has not been reported to date.

Results: In this study, a VHH yeast two-hybrid library was constructed from NDV vaccine immunized *C. bactrianus,* and seven VHH fragments to the haemagglutinin-neuraminidase (HN) protein of NDV were successfully screened and characterized for the first time. These selected VHH clones were all expressed as soluble protein in *E. coli*. ELISA, dot blot, immunocytochemistry and pull down results showed that the screened VHHs could interact with NDV virion, among which five had neutralizing activity. In addition, the seven VHHs could inhibit the haemagglutination activity of different NDV strains.

Conclusions: We constructed an NDV-immunized VHH yeast two-hybrid library and screened and characterized seven VHHs targeting NDV HN protein for the first time. The seven VHHs may have great potential for NDV diagnosis, pathogenesis and therapeutics.

Keywords: Newcastle disease virus, VHH, HN protein, Yeast two-hybrid

* Correspondence: duenqi227@126.com; yzq1106@nwsuaf.edu.cn; 15191415891@163.com
[†]Equal contributors
College of Veterinary Medicine, Northwest A & F University, Yangling, Shaanxi Province 712100, P. R. China

Background

Newcastle disease (ND), which is caused by the Newcastle disease virus (NDV), is one of the most serious avian diseases. NDV belongs to the family *Paramyxoviridae* and genus *Avulavirus.* NDV can infect a wide range of domestic and wild bird species and cause great economic losses to the poultry industry [1, 2]. It is an enveloped, single-stranded, non-segmented, negative-sense RNA virus with a genome length of approximately 15 kb nucleotides that contain six genes encoding for six structural proteins and two additional proteins [3]. Haemagglutinin-neuraminidase (HN) protein is one of the major glycoproteins. It forms spike-like structures on the outer surface of the virion and mediates the attachment of the virus to the sialic acid-containing receptors [4]. The HN protein is also an important target of host immune responses and a major protective antigen. Monoclonal antibodies of the HN protein were found to neutralize NDV infectivity [5]. Therefore, the HN protein is considered the most predominant antigen in the control of NDV.

In the past decades, ND epidemics were effectively controlled because of widespread vaccination. However, recent ND outbreaks in vaccinated flocks still caused damage to the poultry industry, and virulent NDV is continually isolated from vaccinated chickens [6–9]. A considerable number of studies indicated that current vaccines and therapeutic antibody-like biological agents could not completely stop the transmission of virulent NDVs [10–12]. Therefore, the development of novel methods for ND control is necessary.

The variable domains of camelid heavy-chain antibodies (VHH) are the smallest naturally occurring functional antibody fragments that maintain the antigen-binding capacity [13, 14]. Their comparatively small size, monomeric behavior, high stability, high solubility, powerful penetrability, low immunogenicity, and ability to bind epitopes inaccessible to conventional antibodies make VHHs ideal candidates for many therapeutic and biotechnological applications [15]. Therefore, the screening and characterization of VHH against NDV have great importance in ND control, discovery of potential epitopes, and antigenic variation research.

In this study, a VHH yeast two-hybrid library was successfully constructed from inactivated NDV vaccine-immunized *C. bactrianus*, and seven HN-targeted VHHs were obtained after screening. Deduced amino acid sequence alignment results indicated that the residues at position 37, 44, 45 and 47 of the amino acids sequence of the seven VHHs were also characteristic of a previously reported VHH, except VHH7. Using prokaryotic expression vector pHSIE, seven VHHs were expressed as a soluble recombinant protein fused with 6 × His-SUMO tag in *E. coli.* ELISA, dot blot and immnunocytochemistry results showed that the selected VHHs could specifically interact with the NDV. Haemagglutination inhibition assay (HI) showed that the seven selected VHHs could inhibit the haemagglutinin activity (HA) of NDV. Furthermore, five VHHs showed neutralizing activity against virulent NDV. The selected HN-targeted VHHs have potential for developing of NDV therapeutic and diagnostic reagents.

Methods

Viruses

La Sota and F48E9 strains of the NDV were used in this study. The La Sota is a widely used genotype II lentogenic vaccine strain. While the F48E9 is a standard genotype IX velogenic strain in China. These two strains were propagated in the allantoic cavity of 9–11 day-old specific pathogen-free embryonated chicken eggs. Allantoic fluid was harvested from embryonated chicken eggs and stored at −70 °C until use.

Cells, yeast strains, and plasmids

DF-1 cells and HEK 293 T cells were maintained in Dulbecco's modified Eagle's medium (DMEM) supplemented with 10 % fetal bovine serum (FBS), 100 U/mL penicillin, and 0.1 mg/mL streptomycin. Plasmid pHSIE was kindly provided by Yi Zheng of the Shenzhen Key Lab of Gene and Antibody Therapy, Tsinghua University. Y2HGold yeast strain, Y187 yeast strain, pGADT7-Rec (cloning vector), pGBKT7 (cloning vector), pGADT7-T (control vector), pGBKT7-Lam (control vector), and pGBKT7-53 (control vector) were purchased from Clontech (Japan).

Animal and vaccination

A six-month-old female *C. bactrianus* was immunized with a combination of inactivated NDV (La Sota) and subtype H9 avian influenza (Strain F) vaccine (Qingdao Yebio Bioengineering Co., Ltd, China) five times at two-weeks intervals. The administrated dose was based on the weight ratio between chicken and *C. bactrianus.* After vaccination, the humoral immune response was monitored by HI assay in V-bottom microtiter plates as previously described [16]. The animal with a strong response was bled 20 day after the last immunization.

RNA isolation and VHH amplification

Approximately 70 mL immunized animal blood was collected 20 day after the last immunization. Lymphocytes were isolated with Ficoll-Paque PLUS and stored at −70 °C until use. Total RNA was extracted from approximately 10^7 lymphocytes using the RNeasy Plus Mini Kit (Qiagen, Germany), and the first-strand cDNA was synthesized using the HiScript 1st Strand cDNA Synthesis Kit (Vazyme, China) with Oligo-dT primers.

The first round of polymerase chain reaction (PCR) was performed with synthesized cDNA as a template using the primers V-F and V-R (Table 1) to amplify a 900 bp fragment encoding VH-CH1-CH2 and a 600 bp fragment encoding VHH-CH2. The 400 bp fragment of VHH was amplified through a second round of PCR using the gel-purified 600 bp fragment from the first round of PCR as a template with primers VHH-F and VHH-R (Table 1). The 400 bp VHH fragment was excised from the gel and purified using a gel extraction kit (OMEGA, USA).

Yeast two-hybrid library construction and quality evaluation

Y187 yeast competent cells were prepared using the Yeastmaker Yeast Transformation System 2 kit according to the user manual. About 20 μL of VHH fragments (4–5 μg) and 3 μg of linearized pGADT7-Rec were co-transformed into Y187 yeast cells to construct the VHH Y2H library according to the Make Your Own "Mate & Plate™" Library System User Manual (Clontech, Japan). To determine the complexity of the library, 100 μL of 1/10, 1/100 and 1/1000 dilutions of transformed cells was spread on SD/–Leu (synthetically defined medium lacking leucine) 100 mm agar plates. After incubation at 30 °C for 3 –4 days, numbers of independent colonies that appeared on the dilution plates were counted to calculate library capacity. To determine the titer of the constructed VHH yeast two-hybrid library, 100 μL of library aliquot was taken out and serially diluted to 1/100, 1/1000, 1/10000, and 1/100000. The library titer was calculated according to the colonies appearing.

Simultaneously, 47 random clones were picked for insertion diversity identification by PCR using the universal primers 3'AD and T7 (Table 1). Ten positive clones produced a PCR product of approximately 400 bp were chosen randomly for gel-purification and sequencing. The sequence results were analyzed using the NCBI BLASTP program to verify the signature of the VHH insertions.

Table 1 Primers used in this study

Primer name	Sequence[a] (5'-3')
V-F	GTCCTGGCTGCTCTTCTACAAGG
V-R	GGTACGTGCTGTTGAACTGTTCC
VHH-F	***TTCCACCCAAGCAGTGGTATCAACGCAGAGTGG***GAGTCTGGRGGAGG
VHH-R	***GTATCGATGCCCACCCTCTAGAGGCCGAGGCGGCCGAC***ATGGAGACGGTGACCWGGGT
T7	TAATACGACTCACTATAGGG
3'AD	AGATGGTGCACGATGCACAG
HN-F	CGGGATCCGTGGGGCTAGCACACCTAGCGAT
HN-R	GCGTCGACCTAGCCAGACCTGGCTTCTC
VHH-EF	CGGGATCCCAGGTGCAGCTGGTGGAGTCTGGRGGAGG
VHH-ER	GCGTCGACTTAGCTGGAGACGGTGACCWGGGT

[a]Letters in bold italics is the homologous arms
Underlined nucleotides in primers representing the restriction enzyme sites

Yeast two-hybrid screen

To obtain HN protein targeting VHH antibodies from yeast two-hybrid library, the bait protein with truncate coding sequences of HN (49–577 aa) from La Sota strain was cloned into the *BamH* I and *Sal* I sites of pGBKT7 and expressed as a fusion to the yeast GAL4 DNA-BD. Before screening, the bait protein was tested against the autoactivity and toxicity of HN. Then, a concentrated Y2HGold (pBD-HN) culture with 1 mL of Y187 (pAD-VHHs) yeast two-hybrid library aliquot was mixed for mating according to the Matchmaker™ Gold Yeast Two-Hybrid protocol (Clontech, Japan). Seventy 150 mm DDO/X/A (double dropout medium lacking tryptophan and leucine and supplemented with X-α-Gal and Aureobasidin A) plates were used to screen the clones after mating for 3–5 days. All blue colonies that appeared on DDO/X/A plates were then patched out and allowed to grow on QDO/X/A (quadruple dropout medium lacking adenine, histidine, tryptophan and leucine and supplemented with X-α-Gal and Aureobasidin A) plates. The blue colonies were screened twice on QDO/X/A plates to rescue the additional library plasmids and eliminate the false positives. The bait plasmid (pBD-HN) and rescued prey plasmid (pAD-VHH)s were co-transformed into Y2HGold yeast strain to confirm the interactions in yeast cells. The bait plasmid (pGBKT7-53 or pGBKT7-Lam) was co-transformed into Y2HGold with the prey plasmid (pGADT7-T) to serve as positive and negative controls, respectively. The rescued genuine positive AD/library VHH inserts were further sequenced and aligned using the NCBI BLASTP program.

Expression and purification of VHH

The screened VHH fragments were amplified with the primers VHH-EF and VHH-ER (Table 1) and cloned into plasmid pHSIE using the *Bam*H I and *Sal* I restriction enzyme sites for fusion with the 6 × His-SUMO tag at the N-terminus. After sequencing, the recombinant expression plasmids were transformed into *E. coli* Rosetta (Novagen) and incubated at 37 °C overnight. Subsequently, 1 mL of an overnight culture of cell was inoculated into 100 mL LB ampicillin broth and further incubated at 37 °C for 3–4 h (OD_{600} reached 0.4–0.6). The culture was induced by 0.5 mM isopropyl-D-thiogalactopyranoside (IPTG) at 30 °C for 5 h. The cell pellets were collected to check the expression of VHH antibodies by 12 % sodium dodecyl sulfate polyacrylamide gel electrophoresis (SDS-PAGE). The VHH antibodies were further purified using Talon Metal Affinity Resins (Clontech) according to the user manual and eluted with phosphate-buffered saline (PBS) containing 250 mM imidazole.

HI assay

The specific interaction between purified VHH and HN was tested using HI assay as previously described [16]. Briefly, 25 μL of PBS containing 4 HA units of antigen was incubated in a V-bottom 96-well plate with 25 μL of twofold serially diluted VHHs at room temperature for 40 min. Subsequently, 50 μL of 1 % suspension of chicken erythrocytes was added. The mixture was incubated at room temperature for 30 min. The purified bacterial lysate of bacteria transformed with an empty pHSIE vector or an anti-NDV positive serum were used as negative and positive controls, respectively. Agglutination of erythrocyte in the plate was scored. HI assay was performed using different strains. Titers were calculated as the highest reciprocal dilutions that completely inhibited haemagglutination. All tests were performed twice.

ELISA

To verify the interaction between the selected VHH and NDV, the NDV La Sota strain was coated onto Maxisorp 96-well plates (Nunc) in Na_2CO_3 (0.05 M, pH 9.6) overnight at 4 °C with 100 μL/well. The purified 6 × His-SUMO tag and anti-NDV negative serum served as the negative control, and the anti-NDV positive serum (kept by our laboratory) served as the positive control. In the following, the plates were blocked with 5 % skimmed milk–PBS with 0.05 % Tween 20 (PBST) for 1 h at 37 °C. After rinsing for five times with PBST, 100 μL diluted VHH (200 μg/mL) was added into each well for 2 h further incubation at 37 °C in triplicate. Subsequently, the wells were rinsed five times with PBST, and 100 μL of horseradish peroxidase (HRP)-conjugated Anti His-Tag Mouse Monoclonal Antibody (CWBIO, Beijing) was added at a 1:3000 dilution for 1 h at 37 °C. whereas, the positive control wells were treated with HRP-conjugated goat anti-chicken antibody (Bioss, Beijing). After washing with PBST for five times, the reaction was developed by adding 100 μL tetramethylbenzidine (TMB) and stopped by adding 50 μL 2 N H_2SO_4 after 20 min of incubation at room temperature. The absorbance was read using a microplate reader at 450 nm (Bio-Rad).

Dot blot analysis

Dot blots were performed according to western blot protocols, except that sucrose-gradient centrifugation purified NDV were spotted on a polyvinylidene fluoride membrane (0.45 μm, Millipore, USA) without preceding gel electrophoresis. The membrane was blocked with 5 % skimmed milk for 2 h at room temperature and then washed twice with TBST (Tris buffered saline containing 0.5 % Tween 20). The purified VHHs (200 μg/mL) were applied at 1:100 dilution. After 2 h incubation at 37 °C, the membrane was washed four times and incubated with HRP-conjugated anti His-Tag mAb (1:5000 dilution) for 1 h at 37 °C. After four further washes with TBST, the immunoreactive was visualized with cECL Plus Western blotting detection reagent (CWBIO). The anti-NDV positive serum and negative serum were used as positive and negative controls.

Pull down

To determine the interaction between VHH and HN protein, HEK 293 T cells were seeded in a 6 wells plate. The next day, 293 T cells were transfected with pCAGGS-HN plasmid or pCAGGS empty plasmid using lipofectamine 2000 reagent (invitrogen). Cells were put on ice 36 h post transfection, washed once with PBS and subsequently lysised with 150 μL/well RIPA buffer for 10 min. The lysate was centrifugated for 5 min at 13000 rpm to remove cell debris. The supernatant was used as cell derived HN protein.

1000 μL of the 293 T-HN lysate was incubated with 80 μg VHH, 500 μL talon Metal affinity resin (Clontech) and 4 mL PBS for 2 h at 4 °C. Talon matrix was washed twice with 4 mL PBS. 300 μL sample buffer was added, boiled for 10 min and separated with SDS-PAGE. The gel was blotted and the membrane was immunolabeled with guinea pigs anti-HN polyclonal antibody (prepared by our lab), HRP goat anti-Guinea pig IgG (ABclonal) and HRP-conjugated anti His-Tag mAb (CWBIO).

Neutralizing assay

Virus neutralization (VN) assay was conducted to confirm the neutralizing activities of the selected VHH. Briefly, 50 μL of the purified VHH (200 μg/mL) was twofold serially diluted and then incubated for 1 h at 37 °C with 100 $TCID_{50}$ of the NDV F48E9 strain in DMEM. After incubation, the DF-1 monolayer of cells grown in 96-well tissue culture plates was infected with the virus-VHH mixture. After absorption at 37 °C for 1 h, the cell cultures were washed twice with PBS. Fresh DMEM with 2 % FBS was subsequently added. The cell cultures were further incubated for 36 h at 37 °C. Syncytium formation of the infected cells was observed in each well. Virus- and mock-infected cells were used as controls. Anti-NDV positive and negative serum were also included as positive and negative controls, respectively. Neutralizing activity was primarily confirmed by the absence of syncytium formation.

To further quantify the neutralization activity, supernatants of cell cultures were harvested at 36 h post inoculation, serially diluted, and assayed for virus titer using Reed-Muench method [17].

Immunocytochemistry assay

To verify the specific intracellular binding activity between selected VHHs and NDV virus, LaSota-infected DF-1 cells and mock control were grown on 24-well dishes for the immunoperoxidase assay. After 48 h, the cells were fixed with 4 % paraformaldehyde on 24-well dishes and were permeabilized with PBS-0.5 % Triton X-100. The fixed cells were incubated with blocking solution (2 % BSA) followed by the VHH for 2 h at 37 °C. Subsequently, the treated cells were incubated with horseradish peroxidase (HRP)-Conjugated Anti His-Tag Mouse Monoclonal Antibody (CWBIO, Beijing) at a 1:4000 dilution for 1 h at 37 °C. The detection of the antigen was carried out using DAB Kits (CWBIO). At last, the nuclear of cells were stained by hematoxylin. The results were examined under an inverted light microscope.

Statistical analysis

Statistically significant differences in HI assay and ELISA assay among VHHs were evaluated using Student's *t* test with the Prism 5.0 (Graph Pad Software, Inc., San Diego, CA). The calculated P values of < 0.05 were considered statistically different.

Ethics statement

C. bactrianus was grown in a farm of the Gobi Desert, northwest of China, with feed and water administrated *ad libitum.* The inactivated vaccine immunizations and jugular vein blood sampling were performed in strict accordance with the Animal Ethics Procedures and Guidelines of the People's Republic of China. The study was approved by the Animal Ethics Committee of Northwest A&F University, Shaanxi Province, China. In this study, the owner of the *C. bactrianus* gave us permission to experiment on the animal, which was returned to the owner after the completion of the experiment. We unequivocally state that this work did not involve any ethical issues.

Results

Anti-NDV specific HI antibody titer of camel serum

Approximately 5 mL blood of was aseptically collected from the immunized animal 14 day after second and fifth immunization to evaluate the humoral response. The blood was allowed to clot to extract the serum. Then, the serum was used for HI assay with 4 HA units of La Sota strain as the antigen, as described in the OIE manual [16]. The anti-NDV HI antibody titer was 10 log2 (Additional file 1: Table S1).

VHH amplification and yeast two-hybrid library construction

As shown in Additional file 1: Figure S1A, a 900 bp fragment and a 600 bp fragment were successfully amplified with the primers V-F and V-R in the first round of PCR. Then, the 400 bp VHH fragment was amplified using the gel-purified 600 bp fragment from the first round of PCR as the template with the primers VHH-F and VHH-R through a nest PCR (Additional file 1: Figure S1B).

During the library construction, 4.4 μg gel-purified VHH fragment was co-transformed with 3 μg *Sma* I linearized pGADT7-Rec plasmid into Y187 competent cells for recombination. Three parameters were used to evaluate the quality of the yeast two-hybrid library: library capacity, library titer, and percentage of library clones that contain insertions. Results of the calculations were as follows: the library capacity was 1.25×10^7(Additional file 1: Figure S3A), and the library titer was 3.45×10^8 cfu/mL(Additional file 1: Figure S3B). A total of 45 clones in 47 randomly selected clones had 400 bp VHH bands after PCR identification with primers T7 and 3'AD (Additional file 1: Figure S2); thus, the percentage of library insertion rate was approximately 96 %. Ten PCR positive clones were chosen randomly for sequencing. The results showed that these clones were all unique sequences, indicating diversity of the library (Additional file 1: Figure S4). Thus, the quality of the VHH yeast two-hybrid library met the demand for screening.

Bait construction

The truncate HN gene was amplified from the cDNA of the La Sota strain using the primers HN-F and HN-R. The amplified products were approximately 1600 bp (Additional file 1: Figure S5A). Subsequently, the amplified fragments were subcloned into vector pGBKT7 by *BamH* I and *Sal* I digestion and ligation (Additional file 1: Figure S5B). Clones were verified by sequencing. Finally, the pGBKT7-HN was transformed into Y2HGold yeast strain as a bait.

Selection of HN-specific VHH antibody fragments

Before screening, no autoactivator activity of the BD-HN was confirmed in yeast (Lane A, Fig. 1). When zygotes formed after mating the Y2H Gold (pBD-HN) and the Y187 yeast library (pAD-VHHs), the mating products were spread on the DDO/X/A plates for incubation at 30 °C for 3–5 days. Hundreds of blue yeast colonies were selected. However, only seven clones were recovered after two rounds of screening on the QDO/X/A plates. To verify the positive interactions between VHHs and HN protein in yeast, the prey plasmid isolated from the seven clones were co-transformed with the bait plasmid (pBD-HN) or the pGBKT7 empty vector. The co-transformation results showed that all the seven clones

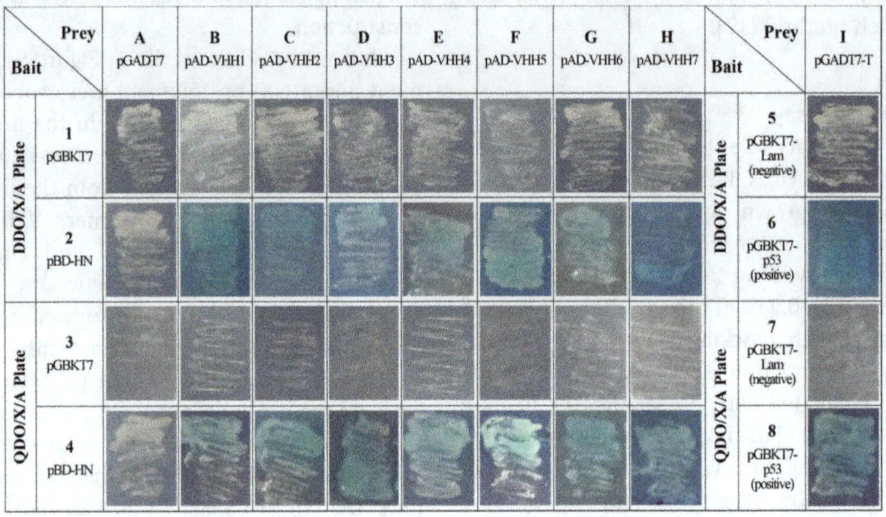

Fig. 1 Interaction between HN and VHH in yeast. The white clones in lane A showed that the bait(pBD-HN) has no autoactivator activity in yeast. When pBD-HN and 7 positive pAD-VHH were cotransformed into Y2HGold yeast strain, all cotransformants turned blue on DDO/X/A and QDO/X/A plates after incubation. At the same time, the pGBKT7-p53 and pGADT7-T co-transformants was used as positive control, whereas pGBKT7-Lam and pGADT7-T co-transformants was used as negative control

rescued from the QDO/X/A plates were genuine positive clones (Lanes B–H, Fig. 1). The sequencing results showed that the seven positive clones were of different clone origins and that the insertions were homologous to the properties of camel VHH, except VHH7 (Fig. 2).

Expression and purification of VHH

Seven VHH fragments were cloned into pHSIE using the *BamH* I and *Sal* I restriction enzyme sites for expression and purification (Additional file 1: Figure S6). As 6 × His-SUMO tag was fused with the VHH fragments at the N-terminus, the recombinant VHHs were purified using Talon Metal Affinity Resin (Clontech). After electrophoresis on a 12 % SDS-PAGE, the 6 × His-SUMO-VHHs fusion proteins exhibited bands that were approximately 30 kDa (Lanes 1–7, Fig. 3). All VHH fragments were solubly expressed.

HI titer of VHH

The HI assay is an important and convenient method widely used for antibody detection. As shown in Table 2, all selected VHHs shared an HI titer ≥ 4 log2 except VHH2, and the HI titer of the VHH was significantly lower than that of the positive serum. The HI titers, which were tested using different NDV strains as 4 HAU, were slightly different.

ELISA

Indirect ELISA was conducted to verify the specific interaction between the VHH and the NDV. For the plate coated with the NDV La Sota ($TCID_{50} = 10^{-8.17}/0.1$ mL), the optimized coated concentration was 1:20. ELISA results showed that all the selected VHHs could react with the NDV virions (Fig. 4). The OD_{450} of the seven VHHs were significantly stronger than the negative controls ($P < 0.05$; Fig. 4). The reaction in the wells of the negative control was very weak ($OD_{450} < 0.10$). All tests were performed three times.

Dot blot

The seven VHHs and positive serum could bind native NDV virion (Fig. 5, a-g and p). While the positive serum

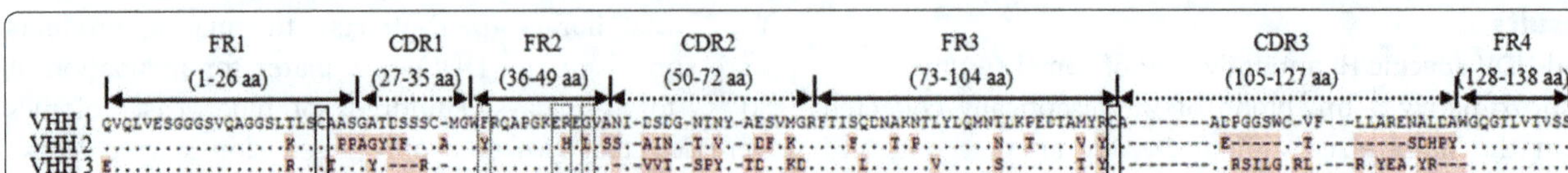

Fig. 2 Deduced amino acid alignment of 7 selected anti-HN VHH. Deduced amino acid sequences were analyzed according to the Kabat numbering [54]. The dots indicate the same sequences compared with VHH1. Differences in the sequences are pinked, and the dash represent the missing sequences. Two hallmark Cys residues are labeled by the thick-line boxes. The four conservative hallmark residues of VHH in FR2 are labeled by the dotted line boxes

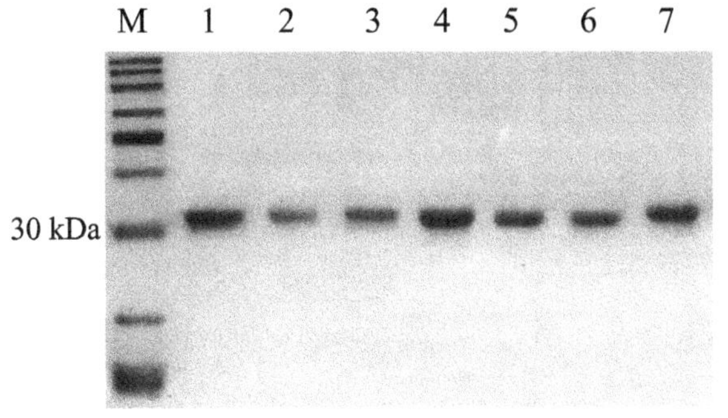

Fig. 3 SDS-PAGE of purified VHH. All seven purified VHH were separated on 12 % SDS-PAGE gels. And the gel was stained with coomassie blue. Lane 1 to 7 represent VHH 1 to VHH 7, respectively. The molecular weight of the 6 × His-SUMO-VHH fusion proteins were about 33 kDa in size

and VHHs could not bind allantoic fluids without NDV (Fig. 5, n1 and n2). This result suggested that the VHHs could recognize NDV.

Pull down

Using VHH6 as model, the interaction between VHH and HN protein was detected by His-tag Pull down assay. As shown in Fig. 6, VHH6 were able to pull down the HN protein from a HN transfected 293 T cell lysate and not from a pCAGGS empty vector transfected 293 T control cell lysate. The result indicated that these VHH6 could interact with HN protein.

Neutralizing assay

Neutralizing assay was performed to evaluate the neutralization ability of the VHHs against F48E9 infection. As shown in Fig. 7, the five VHHs (VHH3, VHH4, VHH5, VHH6, and VHH7) had neutralizing activity to inhibit the replication of F48E9 on the DF-1 cell as there was no syncytia appeared at 24 h post-inoculation, although the neutralizing titer was significantly lower than the positive control (VHH $\leq 2^2$,positive serum $> 2^7$). However, some syncytia can be observed on cells at 36–72 h post-inoculation in experiment wells, while positive serum can effectively inhibit the infection of virus. The negative control showed no neutralizing activity.

VHH6 was picked out as an example to quantify neutralization activity. Thirty-six hour post-inoculation, supernatants were harvested and tested for virus titer. Results indicated that virus propagation was significantly inhibited by the VHH6 (Fig. 8).

Detection of NDV-infected cells by immunocytochemistry

Using VHH6 as model, the intracellular specificity and binding affinity of selected VHHs were further detected by immunocytochemistry. As shown in Fig. 9, the strong cytoplasm brownish staining was specifically appeared in NDV-infected DF-1 cells (0.01 MOI) group but not in the mock control. These results indicated the feasibility of detection intracellular NDV antigen by using selected VHHs.

Discussion

The HN protein, which is an important multifunctional surface glycoprotein consists of a cytoplasmic domain, a transmembrane region, a stalk region and a globular head, possesses both HA and NA activities and all the antigenic sites [18]. HN protein binds to the sialic acid receptor mediating virus attachment to cells and promotes the fusion activity of the F protein, allowing the virus to penetrate the cell surface, and receptor-destroying activity to facilitate virus budding. The polyclonal or monoclonal antibody targeting HN protein has been reported to neutralize the infectivity of the NDV. Therefore, the HN protein is an ideal target for NDV treatment and many therapeutic reagents have been developed against HN protein, including hyper-immune sera, egg yolk antibody, and monoclonal antibodies [19–23]. However, anti-HN VHH have not been reported yet.

A phage display library is widely used to select scFv and VHH from a considerable number of interested targets, such as Influenza A virus M2 ion channel, chemokine receptor CXCR4, and murine ADP-ribosyltransferase C2 [24–26]. Acquiring pure antigen is the premise to panning a phage library. However, not all antigens are easy to prepare, and the process is usually time consuming and laborious. Yeast two-hybrid technology is a useful tool to study protein-protein interactions, including

Table 2 HI titer of selected VHH

Strain	Origin	Genotype	HI titer (X Log2)								
			VHH1	VHH2	VHH3	VHH4	VHH5	VHH6	VHH7	Posivtive[a]	Negative[b]
F48E9	Chicken	IX	4	1	5	5	5	5	4	9	0
LaSota	Chicken	II	4	2	4	6	6	4	4	8	0
YuLin	Chicken	IX	4	1	5	5	5	5	5	8	0
Dove	Chicken	IX	4	1	4	4	4	5	4	6	0
W2	Chicken	VII	6	1	5	4	4	5	4	6	0

[a]Represent anti-NDV positive serum
[b]Represent sumo-tag

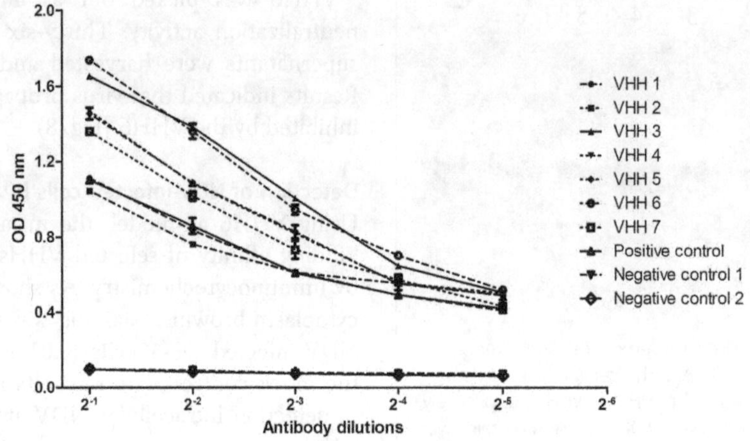

Fig. 4 Detection of interaction between selected VHH and NDV virion by ELISA. Microplates were coated with NDV La Sota virion ($TCID_{50}$ $10^{-8.17}$/ 0.1 mL, 1:20 dilution). The 7 selected VHH (200 μg/mL) were diluted at different concentrations, and anti-NDV positive serum (Positive control), negative serum (Negative control 1) and 6 × His SUMO tag (Negative control 2) were used as positive and negative control. The value of absorbance at 450 nm indicate the reactivity between VHH and NDV. And the data represents the average of 3 wells

antibody-antigen interaction. A previous study reported the feasibility of using yeast two-hybrid to screen high affinity VHH against the targeted protein *in vivo*, which avoid the time-consuming antigen preparation [27]. In the present study, in order to avoid HN protein preparation, the truncate HN gene was cloned into bait plasmid for fusion expression with binding domain (BD) of Gal4. Then the autoactivity and toxicity of the bait protein were assessed, result showed that HN-BD had no autoactivity and toxicity. Whereas, the expression level of HN-BD in yeast Y2H Gold cells was relatively low (Additional file 1: Figure S7). The low expression level may be ascribed to the following reasons. On the one hand, HN protein contains 12 cysteines, the Y2H yeast strain might have problems in the production of proteins with multiple cysteine bridges. On the other hand, the host yeast cells, although a eukaryote, is distant from human, mamalian, and higher eukaryotic organisms. So, sometimes the conditions in yeast cells may not allow the proper folding or posttranslational modifications required for some proteins. Although in a low expression level, after screening the VHH yeast two-hybrid library with the truncate HN bait protein, seven VHHs were successfully obtained for the first time. HI assay, dot blot, ELISA, immunocytochemistry and pull down results indicated that the purified VHHs could react with the NDV virions or HN protein.

The VHH is generated from a V-D-JH gene rearrangement using a specific set of V gene segments, which exist in the germline of the camelid genome [28]. At least four distinct VHH subfamilies have been defined, but they all share several crucial amino acid substitutions in the framework 2 region, namely, Val37-Phe/Tyr, Gly44-Glu/Gln, Leu45-Arg, and Trp47-Gly/Phe/Leu (Kabat numbering), which increase the hydrophilicity of the VHH. These VHH hallmark residues compensate for the possible instability, hydrophobicity, and aggregation tendency of VHH because

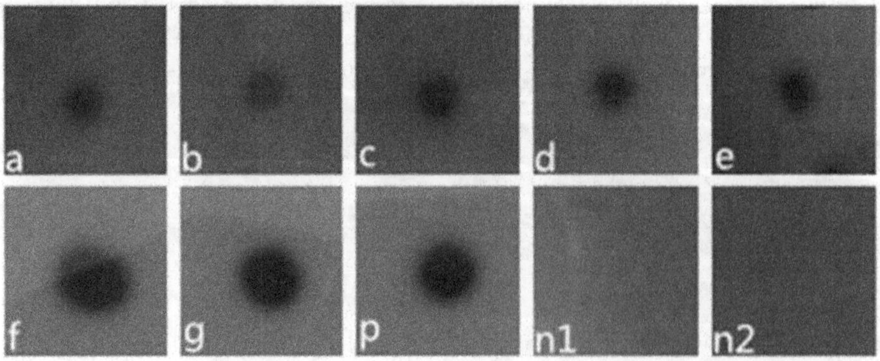

Fig. 5 Detection of interaction between VHH and NDV virion by Dot blot. Purified NDV (a-p) or allantoic fluid (n1 and n2) were spotted on a PVDF membrane for blot. VHHs binding were visualized using HRP labeled anti-His Mabs While positive serum was visualized using HRP labeled anti-chicken antibody. a-g represent VHH1-VHH7; p represent positive serum; n1 represent VHHs (VHH 1 to VHH 7); n2 represent positive serum

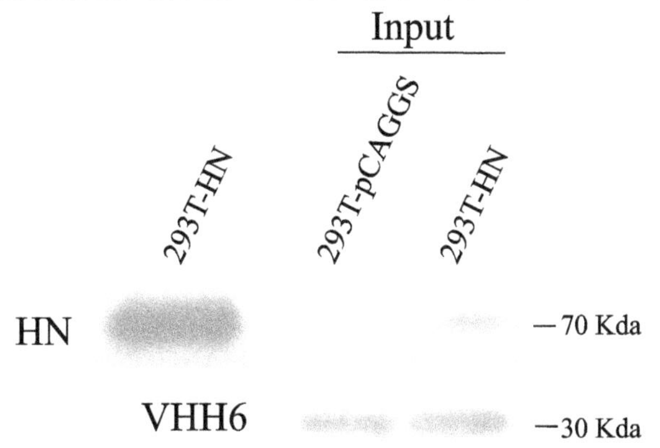

Fig. 6 Validation of VHH against cell derived HN protein. Pull down of cell derived HN protein from pCAGGS-HN transfected 293 T cells lysate or pCAGGS empty vector transfected 293 T cells lysate using VHH6 with talon metal affinity resin. Western blot with anti-HN polyclonal antibodies and anti-his tag mAb

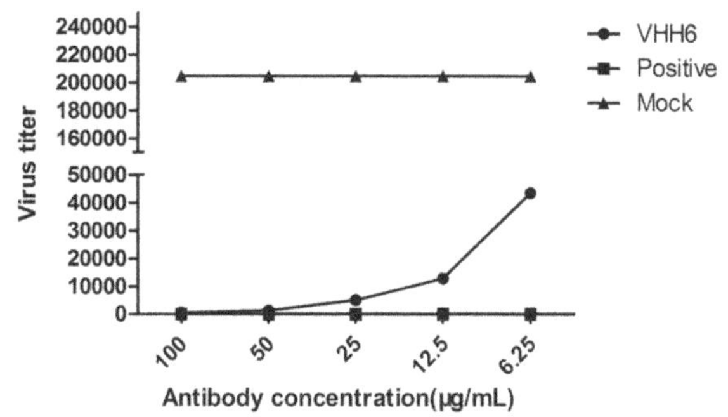

Fig. 8 The determination of the effects of VHH on the virus production. Virus titer in the culture supernatants was measured at different VHH concentration by Reed-Muench method

of the lack of VL domains [13, 29, 30]. The variable domains of antibody consist of four framework regions (FRs) and three complementary determining region (CDRs) [31, 32]. The amino acid sequences of the FR are generally constant and not easily changed. The amino acid sequences of the CDR are highly variable, and they determine the antibody specificity and diversity [33]. In this work, we screened seven VHH antibodies from *C. bactrianus* for the first time. The sequence alignment results showed that the four conservative hallmark residues of the VHH in FR2 were in accordance with previous reports [34], except for VHH7. By analyzing the alignment results we also found that the sequence differences of these VHHs were mainly localized in the CDRs as others reported [28, 30].

To avoid VH contamination in VHH library, usually two rounds PCRs are performed. The first is used to discriminate VH (VH-CH1-hinge-CH2) from VHH (VHH-hinge-CH2) based on amplicon sizes which differ by 300 bp in length. The second is used to amplified VHH from the short amplicons (VHH-hinge-CH2) with primers annealing at the codons of FR1 and FR4. Afterward VHH fragments are cloned for library construction and selection. In the present study, two successive PCRs were performed during Ilama VHH library construction to select for VHH sequence rather than VH. After screening, seven positive clones were obtained. However, sequence alignment result showed that especially VHH7 did not contain the hallmark residues in FR2 that are typical of VHHs as described in previous reports [34]. The presence of variable single domains that seem to originated from VH have been repeatedly identified together with canonical VHHs in immune libraries [35, 36]. Monegal reported that single domains antibodies with VH hallmarks could be positively

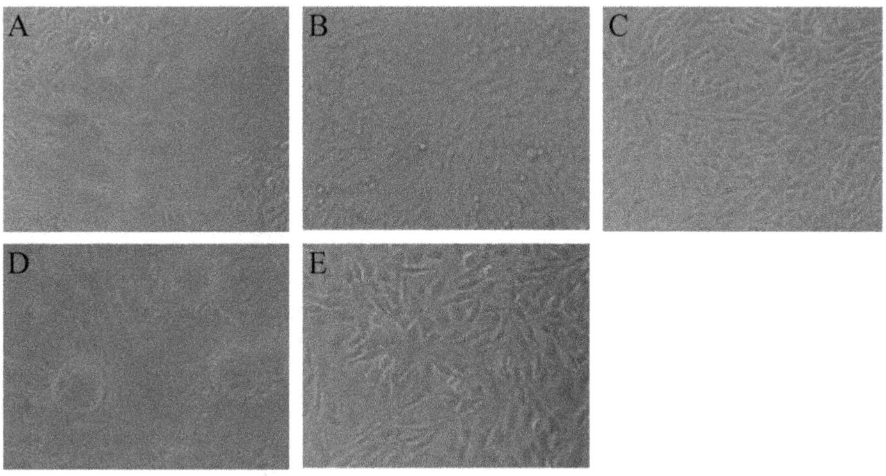

Fig. 7 Syncytium formation of DF-1 cell treated with anti-HN VHH. Virus neutralizing assay was performed on DF-1 cells. Syncytium formation was observed under a microscope 36 h post inoculation. **a** 6 × His-SUMO tag treated. **b** VHH treated. **c** Anti-NDV positive serum treated. **d** Negative serum treated. **e** Mock

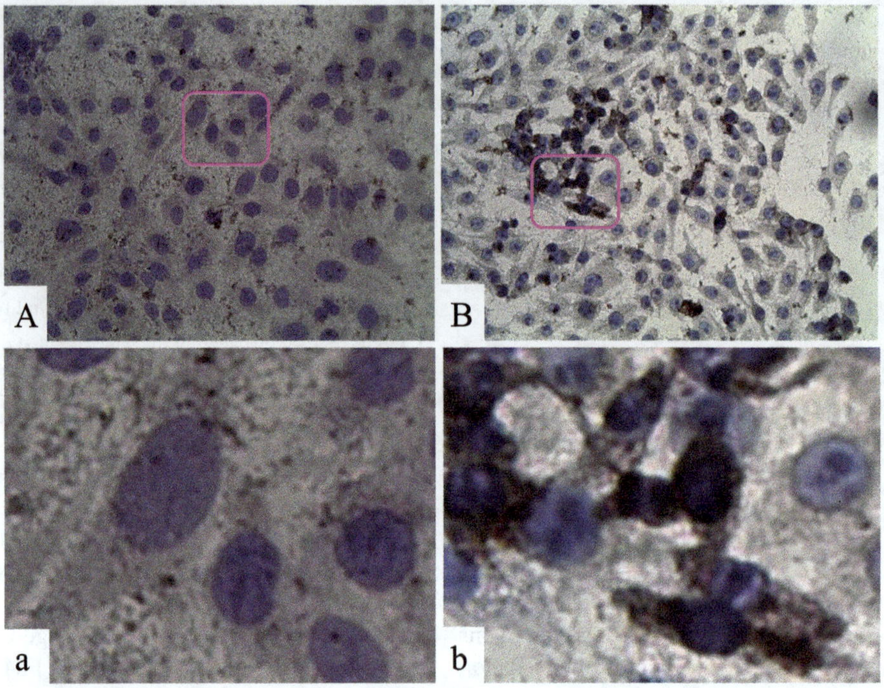

Fig. 9 Immunocytochemistry analysis with VHH6. A and a, mock-infected DF-1 cells; B and b, LaSota infected DF-1 cells. All cells were examined under an inverted light microscope (40×). The expression of NDV HN glycoprotein is visualized as a brown color in the cytoplasm, and cell nuclei stained with hematoxylin are shown in blue in the DF-1 cells

selected during panning of VHH libraries [37]. These unexpected VH sequences could result from PCR crossover between VHH and VH fragments or re-arrangement of classical VH domains to IgG2 or IgG3 constant regions [38].

To investigate the reactivity of the selected VHHs with the NDV, ELISA, HI, dot blot and immunocytochemistry were performed. As shown in Fig. 4, all the selected VHHs could specifically interact with the NDV La Sota strain, and the reactivity were significantly stronger than negative controls ($P < 0.05$). The ELISA results suggested that all the selected VHHs could interact with NDV virions. HI assay is a convenient method widely used for the detection of interactivity between antibody and HN protein. As shown in Table 2, all VHHs could inhibit the HA activity of different strains, but they shared different HI titers against different strains. The different HI titers indicated that antigenic variations exists among different NDV strains, which is consistent with previously reported [39–41]. Whereas, the HI titers of VHHs were significantly lower than that of the positive serum. Previously, it has been demonstrated that HA activity was determined by multiple sites on HN protein [42–45]. Therefore, the lower HI titer of the VHH compared with the positive serum may be attributed to the fact that each selected VHH only recognized a limited number of epitopes associated with the HA activity. Moreover, the small size of the VHH may not be sufficient to form a steric hindrance that will completely block the active site involved in HA activity when binding on the HN. Multimerization or polyvalence of the VHH may be a promising method to enhance its function in the future.

Using monoclonal antibodies, seven antigenic sites have been identified in the HN glycoprotein and formed a linked continuum, in the order of sites 4-14-1-12-1-23-3 [5, 46]. And most of the HN epitopes were conformational epitopes, only one linear epitope was revealed (residues 345 to 353 aa) [5]. In the present study, we proved that all the selected VHHs could interact with NDV through dot blot, ELISA, and HI. At the same time, the VHH were also able to pull down HN protein from cell lysate. However, the reactivity were not detected using western blot (data not shown). These results suggested the VHHs might recognize conformational eipitopes rather than linear epitopes. The findings are in accordance with Iorio's that most of the selected monoclonal antibodies bind to HN, but only when it has been neither reduced nor boiled [47]. Which epitopes are recognized by our VHHs and do the epitopes different from previously reported need further investigation.

The NDV HN antibodies can be separated into two groups with respect to their mechanism of neutralization, namely, those that prevent receptor recognition and those that do not [46]. And evidence for a multiple-antibody mechanism of neutralization has been gathered in several systems with both polyclonal and monoclonal antibodies

[48]. In the present study, as shown in Fig. 7, five of the seven VHHs displayed neutralizing activity against the virulent NDV F48E9, but the neutralizing titers were significantly lower than that of positive serum. Some syncytia could be observed on cells at 36–72 h post-infection (data not shown). Iorio reported that complete neutralization of NDV required monoclonal antibodies to different sites of HN glycoprotein [49]. So the neutralizing activity of a single VHH may be limited. Apart from the above reason, the following aspects might be also account for the relatively poor neutralizing activity: 1) Antigenic difference exist between LaSota strain and F48E9 strain (Table 2) lead to the low antibody binding activity. 2) The epitopes recognized by these VHH were not the crucial region for the blockage of virus. Therefore, we will attempt to identify the epitopes recognized by these selected VHHs in our future work. 3) The antibodies targeting fusion protein (F protein) are reportedly more effective in preventing virus infection than the antibodies targeting the HN protein [50–53]. So the screening of the VHH targeting F protein or other viral proteins is an alternative way. 4) As mentioned previously, we presume that the smaller size of the VHH could enhance its tissue penetration and make it bind some cryptic epitopes. However, on the contrary, the smaller size may be unable to fully occupy the targeting site or form a steric hindrance to prevent virus infection. The multimerization of the selected VHHs may be a mechanism to enhance their function.

Conclusions

In this study, we constructed a VHH yeast two-hybrid library. After two rounds of screening, seven VHHs targeted to HN protein were selected and characterized for the first time. These selected VHHs can specifically interact with the HN protein and inhibit the HA activity of the NDV. Most VHHs also showed a neutralizing activity. These VHHs have great potential for application in NDV diagnosis, therapy, and pathogenesis. Moreover, the VHHs screened on the basis of the yeast two-hybrid may be an effective tool to examine the mechanism of ND pathogenesis and vaccination.

Additional file

Additional file 1: Table S1. Humoral immune response after immunization. Sera from llama was collected, two-fold diluted and tested by HI using LaSota as antigen. Figure S1 Amplification of VHH through a nested PCR. (A) First round PCR to separate VH from VHH. The upper 900 bp bands represent the VH-CH1-Hinge-CH2 of conventional Abs (lane 1–8). The lower 600 bp bands represent the VHH-Hinge-CH2 of HCAbs (lane 1–8). (B) VHH amplified through nested PCR using 600 bp fragment recovered from first round PCR as template (lane 1–4). M in A and B was the DL2000 DNA marker. C in A and B represent the negative control. Figure S2 PCR identification of inserted VHH. 47 clones were randomly picked to determine the library functional diversity by PCR using universal primers T7 and 3'AD (Table 1). Meanwhile, Sterile water was used as negative controls. 45 clones have amplified the 500 bp VHH fragments (lane 1–47), while negative templates control haven't amplified any bands (lane C). M indicated the DL2000 DNA marker. Figure S3 Detection of library capacity and library titer. (A) 10^{-3} dilution plating of the transformed cells calculated a library capacity of 1.25×10^7 independent clones. (B) 10^{-5} dilution plating of the cultured library indicated a library titer of 3.45×10^8 cfu/mL. Figure S4 Deduced amino acid aligment of 10 random picked VHH. Deduced amino acid sequences were analyzed according to the Kabat numbering. Differences in the sequences are pinked, and the dash represent the missing sequences. Two hallmark Cys residues are labeled by the thick-line boxes. The four conservative hallmark residues of VHH in FR2 are labeled by the dotted line boxes. Figure S5 pGBKT7-HN bait plasmid construction. (A) PCR was carried out to amplify a truncate HN gene (without transmembrane region) from La Sota strain. M, 5000 DNA marker. 1, Truncate HN. C, Negative control. (B) A truncate HN was cloned into pGBKT7 through *BamH* I and *Sal* I. M, 5000 DNA marker. 1, Double restriction enzyme digestion of pGBKT7-HN. Figure S6 pHSIE-VHH plasmid construction. (A) 7 positive VHH fragment were amplified from recovered positive clones containing pGADT7-VHH by PCR. M, 5000 DNA marker. 1–7, VHH 1–7. C, Negative control. (B) Double restriction enzyme digestion of pHSIE-VHHs. M, 5000 DNA marker. 1–7, pHSIE-VHH 1–7. Figure S7 Western blot analysis of bait protein expression. 2 mL of Y2HGold(pGBKT7-HN) culture liquid was extracted using yeast protein extraction reagent (Takara). c-Myc tag monoclonal antibody (1:4000 dilution) was used as first antibody and HRP-labeled goat anti-mouse antibody (1:5000) was used as second antibody. The immunoreactive was visualized with cECL Plus Western blotting detection reagent (CWBIO). (DOC 1129 kb)

Abbreviations

ND: Newcastle disease; NDV: Newcastle disease virus; VHH: Variable domain of heavy chain of the heavy-chain antibody; HA: Haemagglutinin activity; HN: Haemagglutinin-neuraminidase protein; HI: Haemagglutination inhibition; SUMO: Small ubiquitin-related modifier; Y2H: Yeast two-hybrid; SD/-Leu: Synthetically defined medium lacking leucine; DDO/X/A: Double dropout medium lacking tryptophan and leucine and supplemented with X-α-Gal and Aureobasidin A; QDO/X/A: Quadruple dropout medium lacking adenine, histidine, tryptophan and leucine and supplemented with X-α-Gal and Aureobasidin A; PBS: Phosphate-buffered saline; IPTG: Isopropyl-D-thiogalactopyranoside; TMB: Tetramethylbenzidine; VN: Virus neutralization assay; CDR: Complementary determining region; FR: Framework region.

Competing interests

The authors declare that they have no competing interests.

Authors' contributions

XG and XH designed the study, carried out the experiments, analyzed data and wrote the manuscript. LT, DL, XC and HW helped perform the experiments. RD and XW helped in provide reagents and materials. SX helped revised the manuscript. ED and ZY designed the study and draft the manuscript. All authors read and approved the final manuscript.

Acknowledgments

This work was supported by the Basic Research Foundation for Dr. Enqi Du in Northwest A & F University, National Natural Science Foundations of China (No.31101803, No.31272578).

References

1. Alexander DJ. Newcastle diseases in the European Union 2000 to 2009. Avian Pathol. 2011;40(6):547–58.
2. Alexander DJ. Gordon memorial lecture. Newcastle disease. Br Poult Sci. 2001;42(1):5–22.
3. Alexander DJ, Senne DA. Newcastle disease, other avian paramyxoviruses, and pneumovirus infections. In: Saif YM, Fadly AM, Glisson JR, McDougald LR, Nolan K, Swayne DE, editors. Diseases of poultry. 11th ed. Ames: Iowa State University Press; 2008. p. 75–116.
4. Lamb R, Parks G. Paramyxoviridae: the viruses and their replication. In: Knipe DM et al., editors. Fields virology. 5th ed. Philadelphia: Lippincott Williams & Wilkins; 2007. p. 1449–96.

5. Iorio RM, Syddall RJ, Sheehan JP, Bratt MA, Glickman RL, Riel AM. Neutralization map of the Hemagglutinin-Neuraminidase glycoprotein of NDV: Domains recognized by Monoclonal antibodies that prevent receptor recognition. J Virol. 1991;65(9):4999–5006.
6. Rui Z, Juan P, Jingliang S, Jixun Z, Xiaoting W, Shouping Z, et al. Phylogenetic characterization of Newcastle disease virus isolated in the mainland of China during 2001–2009. Vet Microbiol. 2010;141(3–4):246–57.
7. Lien YY, Lee JW, Su HY, Tsai HJ, Tsai MC, Hsieh CY, et al. Phylogenetic characterization of Newcastle disease viruses isolated in Taiwan during 2003–2006. Vet Microbiol. 2007;123(1–3):194–202.
8. Cho SH, Kim SJ, Kwon HJ. Genomic sequence of an antigenic variant Newcastle disease virus isolated in Korea. Virus Genes. 2007;35(2):293–302.
9. Diel DG, Susta L, Garcia SC, Killian ML, Brown CC, Miller PJ, et al. Complete genome and clinicopathological characterization of a virulent Newcastle disease virus isolate from South America. J Clin Microbiol. 2012;50(2):378–87.
10. Miller PJ, Estevez C, Yu Q, Suarez DL, King DK. Comparison of viral shedding following vaccination with inactivated and live Newcastle disease vaccines formulated with wild-type and recombinant viruses. Avian Dis. 2009;53(1):39–49.
11. Hu SL, Ma HL, Wu YT, Liu WB, Wang XQ, Liu YL, et al. A vaccine candidate of attenuated genotype VII Newcastle disease virus generated by reverse genetics. Vaccine. 2009;27(6):904–10.
12. Xiao S, Nayak B, Samuel A, Paldurai A, Kanabagattebasavaraiappa M, Prajitno TY, et al. Generation by reverse genetics of an effective, stable, live-attenuated Newcastle disease virus vaccine based on a currently circulation, highly virulent indonesian strain. PloS One. 2012;7(12):1–15.
13. Hamers-Casterman C, Atarhouch T, Muyldermans S, Robinson G, Hamers C, Songa EB, et al. Naturally occurring antibodies devoid of light chains. Nature. 1993;363(6428):446–8.
14. Holliger P, Hudson PJ. Engineered antibody fragments and the rise of single domains. Nat Biotechnol. 2005;23:1126–36.
15. Vanlandschoot P, Stortelers C, Beirnaert E, Ibanez IL, Schepens B, Depla E, et al. Nanobodies: New ammunition to battle viruses. Antiviral Res. 2011;92:389–407.
16. OIE. Manual of diagnostic tests and vaccines for terrestrial animals: mammals, birds and bees. Paris: Biological Standards Commission. World Organization for Animal Health; 2012. p. 1–19.
17. Reed J, Muench H. A simple method of estimating fifty percent endpoint. Am J Hyg. 1938;27:493–7.
18. Peeters BP, de Leeuw OS, Verstegen I, Koch G, Gielkens AL. Generation of a recombinant chimeric Newcastle disease virus vaccine that allows serological differentiation between vaccinated and infected animals. Vaccine. 2001;19:1616–27.
19. Stedman RA, Singleton L, Box PG. Purification of Newcastle disease virus antibody from the egg yolk of the hen. J Comp Pathol. 1969;79(4):507–16.
20. Dorn P, Seidi H, Wessling E. Comparative studies on the determination of antibodies against Newcastle disease in the serum and egg yolk of laying hens. Berl Munch Tierarztl Wochenschr. 1973;86(18):349–50.
21. Box PG, Stedman RA, Singleton L. Newcastle disease I. The use of egg yolk derived antibody for passive immunisation of chickens. J Comp Pathol. 1969;79(4):495–506.
22. Wills FK, Luginbuhi RE. The use of egg yolk for passive immunization of chickens against Newcastle disease. Avian Dis. 1963;7(1):5–12.
23. Borzemska WB. Effect of neutralizing and hemagglutination inhibiting antibodies on the course of Newcastle disease infection in chickens. Pol Arch Weter. 1972;15(3):495–512.
24. Wei GW, Meng W, Guo H, Pan W, Liu J, Peng T, et al. Potent neutralization of influenza A virus by a single-domain antibody blocking M2 ion channel protein. PLoS One. 2011;6(12):1–11.
25. Jahnichen S, Blanchetot C, Maussang D, Gonzalez-Pajuelo M, Chow KY, Bosch L, et al. CXCR4 nanobodies potently inhibit chemotaxis and HIV-1 replication and mobilize stem cells. Proc Natl Acad Sci USA. 2010;107(47):20565–70.
26. Menzel S, Rissiek B, Haag F, Goldbaum FA, Koch NF. The art of blocking ADP-ribosyltransferases (ARTs): nanobodies as experimental and therapeutic tools to block mammalian and toxin ARTs. FEBS J. 2013;280(15):3543–50.
27. Fu XJ, Gao XL, He SF, Huang D, Zhang P, Wang XL, et al. Design and selection of a camelid single-chain antibody yeast two-hybrid library produced de novo for the Cap protein of Porcine Circoviru Type 2 (PCV2). PLoS One. 2013;8(3):1–11.
28. Harmsen MM, Ruuls RC, Nijman IJ, Niewold TA, Frenken LG, de Geus B. Llama heavy-chain V regions consist of at least four distinct subfamilies revealing novel sequence features. Mol Immunol. 2000;37(10):579–90.
29. Muyldermans S, Atarhouch T, Saldanha J, Barbosa JA, Hamers R. Sequence and structure of VH domain from naturally occurring camel heavy chain immunoglobulins lacking light chains. Protein Eng. 1994;7(9):1129–35.
30. Vu KB, Ghahroudi MA, Wyns L, Muyldermans S. Comparison of llama VH sequences from conventional and heavy chain antibodies. Mol Immunol. 1997;34(16–17):1121–31.
31. McCormack WT, Tjoelker LW, Thompson CB. Immunoglobulin gene diversification by gene conversion. Prog Nucleic Acid Res Mol Biol. 1993;45:27–45.
32. Refega S, Cluzeaud M, Pery P, Labbe M, Girard-Misguich F. Production of a functional chicken single-chain variable fragment antibody derived from caecal tonsils B lymphocytes against macrogamonts of Eimeria tenella. Vet Immunol Immunopathol. 2004;97:219–30.
33. Magari M, Kanehiro Y, Todo K, Ikeda M, Kanayama N, Ohmori H. Enhancement of hypermutation frequency in the chicken B cell line DT40 for efficient diversification of the antibody repertoire. Biochem Biophys Res Commun. 2010;396:353–8.
34. van der Linden R, de Geus B, Stok W, Bos W, van Wassenaar D, Verrips T, et al. Induction of immune responses and molecular cloning of the heavy chain antibody repertoire of Lama glama. J Immunol Methods. 2000;240(1–2):185–95.
35. Saerens D, Kinne J, Bosmans E, Wernery U, Muyldermans S, Conrath K. Single domain antibodies derived from dromedary lymph node and peripheral blood lymphocytes sensing conformational variants of prostate-specific antigen. J Biol Chem. 2004;279:51965–72.
36. Harmsen MM, De Haard HJ. Properties, production, and applications of camelid single-domain antibody fragments. Appl Microbiol Biotechnol. 2007;77:13–22.
37. Monegal A, Olichon A, Bery N, Filleron T, Favre G, de Marco A. Single domain antibodies with VH hallmark are positively selected during panning of llama naive libraries. Dev Comp Immunol. 2012;36(1):150–6.
38. Sinkora M, Sun J, Butler JE. Antibody repertoire development in fetal and neonatal piglets. V. VDJ gene chimeras resembling gene conversion products are generated at high frequency by PCR in vitro. Mol Immunol. 2000;37(17):1025–34.
39. Collins MS, Franklin S, Strong I, Meulemans G, Alexander DJ. Antigenic variation of Newcastle disease virus strains detected by monoclonal antibodies. Avian Pathol. 1998;27(1):90–6.
40. Meulemans G, Gonze M, Carlier MC, Petit P, Burny A, Le Long. Evaluation of the use of monoclonal antibodies to hemagglutinin and fusion glycoproteins of Newcastle disease virus for virus identification and strain differentiation purposes. Arch Virol. 1987;92(1–2):55–62.
41. Chen WF, Tsaur NJ, Lai CY, Lai CY, Lai CK, Tserng HB. Monoclonal antibodies against Newcastle disease virus. J Chin Soc Vet Sci. 1992;18:1–6.
42. Morrison TG, Portner A. Structure, function, and intracellular processing of the glycoproteins of Paramyxoviridae. In d.w. Kingsbury (ed.), The paramyxoviruses. Plenum Press. 1991:347–382.
43. Connaris H, Takimoto T, Russell R, Crennell S, Moustafa I, Portner A, et al. Probing the sialic acid binding site of the hemagglutinin-neuraminidase of Newcastle disease virus: identification of key amino acids involved in cell binding, catalysis, and fusion. J Virol. 2002;76(4):1816–24.
44. Iorio RM, Field GM, Sauvron JM, Mirza AM, Deng R, Mahon PJ, et al. Structural and functional relationship between the receptor recognition and neuraminidase activities of the Newcastle disease virus hemagglutinin-neuraminidase protein: receptor recognition is dependent on neuraminidase activity. J Virol. 2001;75(4):1918–27.
45. Zaitsev V, von Itzstein M, Groves D, Kiefel M, Takimoto T, Portner A, et al. Second sialic acid binding site in Newcastle disease virus hemagglutinin-neuraminidase: Implications for fusion. J Virol. 2004;78(7):3733–41.
46. Iorio RM, Glickman RL, Riel AM, Sheehan JP, Bratt MA. Functional and neutralization profile of seven overlapping antigenic sites on the HN glycoprotein of Newcastle disease virus: monoclonal antibodies to some sites prevent viral attachment. Virus Res. 1989;13(3):245–62.
47. Iorio RM, Bratt MA. Monoclonal antibodies to newcastle disease virus: delineation of four epitopes on the HN glycoprotein. J Virol. 1983;48(2):440–50.
48. Della-Porta AJ, Westaway EG. A multi-hit model for the neutralization of animal viruses. J Gen Virol. 1978;38:1–19.
49. Iorio RM, Bratt MA. Neutralization of Newcastle disease virus by monoclonal antibodies to the hemagglutinin-neuraminidase glycoprotein: requirement for antibodies to four sites for complete neutralization. J Virol. 1984;51(2):445–51.
50. Zhao Y, Hammond RW. Development of a candidate vaccine for Newcastle disease virus by epitope display in the Cucumber mosaic virus capsid protein. Biotechnol Lett. 2005;27(6):375–82.

51. Panshin A, Shihmanter E, Weisman Y, Orvell C, Lipkind M. Variability of antigenic epitope of the fusion protein of Newcastle disease virus. Comp Immunol Microbiol Infec Dis. 1998;21(1):51–63.
52. Umino Y, Kohama T, Sato TA, Sugiura A. Protective effect of monoclonal antibodies to NDV in passive immunization. J Gen Virol. 1990;71(5):1199–203.
53. Umino Y, Kohama T, Kohase M, Sugiura A, Klenk HD, Rott R. Protective effect of antibodies to two viral envelope glycoproteins on lethal infection with Newcastle disease virus. Arch Virol. 1987;94(1–2):97–107.
54. Kabat E, Wu TT, Perry HM, Gottesman KS, Foeller C. Sequences of immunological interest. 5th ed. Washington DC: US Department of Health and Human Services; 1999.

2

Detection of rabbit Haemorrhagic disease virus 2 during the wild rabbit (*Oryctolagus cuniculus*) eradication

F.A. Abade dos Santos[1,5*†], C. Carvalho[2†], Oliveira Nuno[3], J. J. Correia[1], M. Henriques[4], M. C. Peleteiro[1], M. Fevereiro[4] and M. D. Duarte[4]

Abstract

Background: In the regular wildlife monitoring action carried out in the summer of the past few years at the Berlenga Island, wild rabbits (*Oryctolagus cuniculus*) have been repeatedly found dead. However, the origin of those deaths was never investigated. Our aim was to investigate the cause of death of 11 rabbits collected between April and May 2016.

Results: While screening samples from rabbit carcasses for the major viral rabbit pathogens, five tested positive to RHDV2 but all were negative for RHDV and myxoma virus (MYXV). For six RHDV2-negative specimens, emaciation and parasitism were considered the most probable cause of death. Lesions identified in the RHDV2-positive rabbits included non-suppurative diffuse hepatic necrosis and pulmonary lesions varying from congestion and oedema of the lungs to interstitial pneumonia. Sequencing analysis of the *vp60* gene obtained from two specimens showed identical *vp60* sequences. Comparison with other known RHDV2 strains from public databases through BLAST analysis revealed a closer similarity with strains from Alentejo collected during 2013. Maximum Likelihood and Bayesian phylogenetic analysis showed that the 2016 strains from the archipelago have a higher resemblance with a group of strains mostly collected in the South of Portugal between 2013 and 2014.

Conclusion: The results suggest that RHDV2 may have been introduced on the Berlenga Island a few years ago, having evolved separately from mainland strains due to insularity.

Keywords: Rabbit haemorrhagic disease virus, RHDV2, Wild rabbit, *Oryctolagus cuniculus*, Berlengas, Berlenga Island, UNESCO

Background

The Berlengas (Fig. 1) is a small archipelago located 5.5 nautical miles (about 10 km) west off Peniche, a fishing town in the Portuguese Atlantic coast. It encompasses the Berlenga Island (1500 by 800 m long with a surface area of 80 ha), a group of small surrounding islets as well as two other more distant groups of islets (Estelas and Farilhões), being designated as Natural Reserve since 1981.

Berlenga is the only island that receives tourists, holding only a small group of houses used seasonally by local fishermen. During the fifteenth century, this island was a popular hunting royal province, probably due to the high population of European rabbits (*Oryctolagus cunniculus*), which exceptional abundance was reported already in 1465 [5].

Presently, Berlenga is the only Island from this archipelago where wild rabbits are present, with a population size estimated at 38 to 133 individuals, calculated through several transects performed over 2015 and 2016 (Fig. 2) (Oliveira N, *unpublished data*). It is assumed that rabbits of

* Correspondence: fabio.santos@campus.ul.pt
†Equal contributors
[1]Centro de Investigação Interdisciplinar em Sanidade Animal (CIISA), Faculdade de Medicina Veterinária, Universidade de Lisboa. Av. da Universidade Técnica, 1300-477 Lisbon, Portugal
[5]Rua Quinta do Pinto N°5 3°D, 2660-067 Loures, Frielas, Portugal
Full list of author information is available at the end of the article

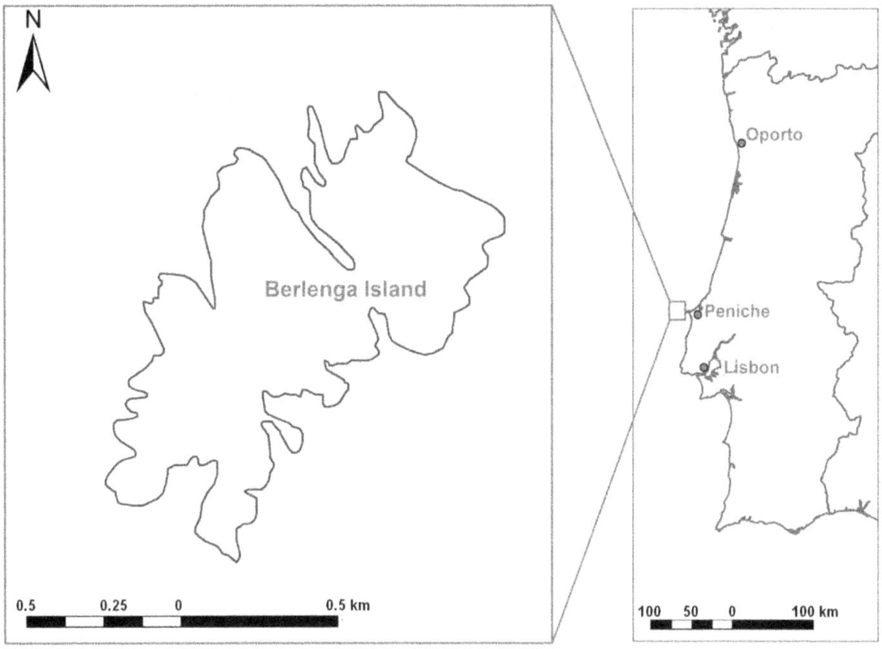

Fig. 1 Berlengas Island, the major island of the Berlengas' archipelago, located in the Portuguese maritime coast, and Peniche municipality (Portugal mainland) are marked on the map

unknown origin were brought onto this island for the first time during the fifteenth century [5]. Lighthouse keepers are known to have taken domestic rabbits into the island for backyard farming, on different occasions during the last two centuries. Those animals eventually escaped and mixed together with the remaining population [5]. Recent molecular data analysis has proved the presence of domestic genome on Berlenga Island's rabbits (Oliveira N, *unpublished data*). Over the last six centuries, rabbits have deeply changed the soil dynamics thereby speeding up erosion due to their digging behaviour [5]. Also, the detrimental impact of *Rattus rattus* (Linneaus 1758) on

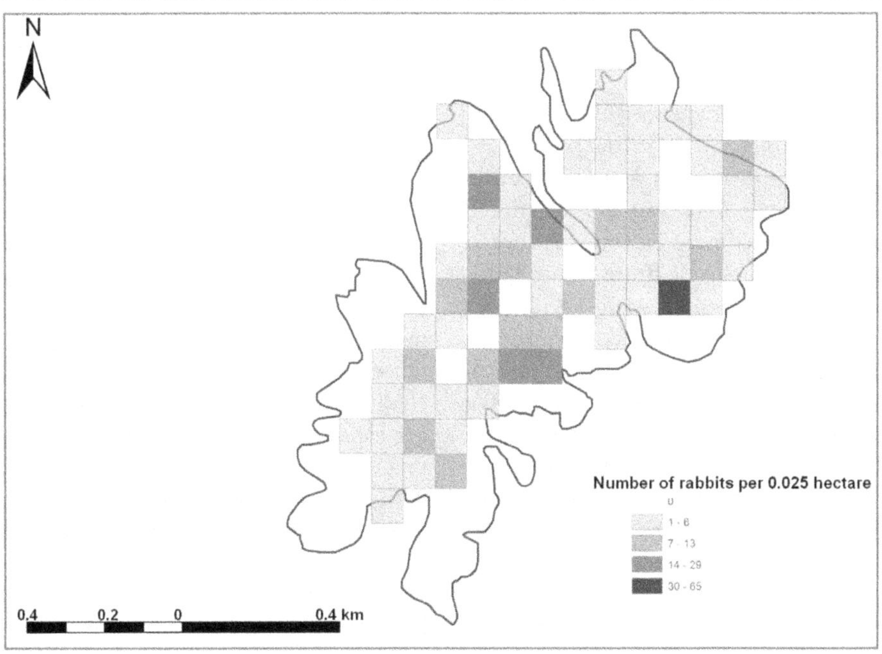

Fig. 2 Density of the wild rabbit population in the Berlengas Natural Reserve calculated through several transects performed over 2015 and 2016

the Berlengas ecosystem was recognized [5]. Those reasons are leading a current process to eradicate rabbit and black rat populations from the Berlenga Island.

In the last couple of years, an abnormal mortality of rabbits has been observed on the island by marine biologists that are regular visitors (Oliveira N, *personal communication*). However, neither infectious pathogens nor toxicological agents were ever investigated to determine the origin of those deaths. Furthermore, to the best of our knowledge, no serological or pathogen surveys have been conducted in the past on the rabbit population of the island. The only available data originates from a study on the ecology of rabbits and black rats (*Rattus rattus*) ectoparasites [54].

Among the pathogens that most severely affect rabbit, myxoma virus (MYXV) [6, 28, 57] and rabbit haemorrhagic disease virus (RHDV) [40] assume a major relevance and their rate of transmission in the wild is affected by fluctuations in the wild rabbits' population density [30, 32].

Myxoma virus (MYXV), a large dsDNA virus, is a member of the *Leporipoxvirus* genus of the family *Poxviridae,* subfamily *Chordopoxvirinae,* [35]. It appears to be passively transmitted to European and American rabbits (*Sylvilagus brasiliensis* and *S. bachmani*) as well as to hares (*Lepus europaeus*) through the biting of insects that act as mechanical vectors, once the virus adheres to their mouthparts [35, 34, 12]. In its natural host (*S. brasiliensis*) and in hares, MYXV rarely causes disease [35], but European domestic and wild rabbits may develop a rapid systemic infection causing death in few days [35].

Rabbit haemorrhagic disease (RHD) is a highly contagious infectious disease of the European wild and domestic rabbits, caused by a virus of the *Lagovirus* genus, family Caliciviridae. RHD is characterised by high morbidity and mortality: 70–90% for RHDV/RHDVa and 5–70% for RHDV2 [52]. The disease was first identified in 1984 in China [40]. In Europe, RHD was first diagnosed in Italy in 1986 [15], soon becoming endemic in several countries [2]. In the Iberian Peninsula, from where European rabbits originated and where they are key species of the ecosystem [21], the first outbreaks occurred in 1988 in Spain [7] and in the following year in Portugal (Anonymous, 1989)[2], causing severe reduction of the wild rabbit populations (Villafuerte et al., 1995)[2] and considerable economic losses in the rabbit industry [7]. Despite the low level of genetic variation found, the molecular characterization of RHDV strains allowed the distinction of six well-defined phylogenetic genogroups (G1 to G6) [51, 36].

In 2010, a new virus designated RHDV2 emerged with a distinct genetic and antigenic profile [38]. It was first identified in France in 2010 [38], and rapidly spread to several European countries including Italy [37], Spain [20], Portugal [1], the United Kingdom [64] and Scotland [9]. Outside the European continent, RHDV2 was first detected between late 2014 and early 2015, in the Azores archipelago [22]. More recently, RHDV2 was also reported in Australia [31], Finland (http://www.oie.int/wahis_2/public/wahid.php/Countryinformation/Countryreports) and North of Africa [44].

RHDV2 differs from RHDV in the clinical characteristics of the induced disease in terms of duration, mortality rates and the more frequent occurrence of subacute/chronic forms [37]. Furthermore, RHDV2 also affects young rabbits with less than two months old, often before they leave the burrows, as well as RHDV vaccinated rabbits that, although protected against classical strains, are susceptible to RHDV2 infection [38, 20, 37]. In addition, RHDV2 is also able to infect hosts other than rabbits as the virus was detected in cape hares (*Lepus capensis*) [55] as well as Italian hares (*Lepus corsicanus*) [14].

In Portugal, since RHDV2 cases were found [1], the former circulating classical RHDV genogroups, mostly G1-related strains in mainland [49, 3] and G5 in Azores [25], were no longer identified, suggesting that RHDV2 replaced the classical RHDV strains probably due to a selective advantage of this new virus by overcoming the existing immunity to older strains [41].

In this study, we aimed to investigate the cause of death of wild rabbits on the Berlenga Island, occurring in the spring of 2016.

Methods

Sample collection

The rabbits used in this study were collected on the Berlenga Island, Portugal, between April and May 2016, within the scope of the LIFE Berlengas project ("Conserving threatened habitats and species in Berlengas SPA through sustainable management", LIFE13 NAT/PT/000458).

Eleven cadavers, consisting of seven females (64%) and four males (26%), were selected from a larger group, based upon their good preservation status. All collected specimens were weighed. Age was estimated upon tarsus and skull length (occipitonasal length), measured with a micrometre. Skull length was defined as the highest distance from the cranial extremity of the premaxillae (excluding the incisors) to the rear of the occipital crest. This age estimation was determined according to the equation first used by Southern [60] and revised by Dunnet (1956) [27]. Prior to freezing, liver samples were collected. All cadavers were then frozen at −20 °C until necropsy.

Virological examination

At the National Reference Laboratory (INIAV), rabbit pathogens associated with high mortality rates, namely RHDV, RHDV2 and MYXV, were investigated. Liver samples from the 11 specimens were homogenised with phosphate buffered saline (PBS) and clarified at 3000 g for 5 min. DNA and RNA were extracted from 200 μl of the clarified supernatant, corresponding to approximately 50 mg of tissue, in a BioSprint 96 nucleic acid extractor (Qiagen, Hilden, Germany) according to the manufacturer's instructions. Samples were tested for RHDV2 by a specific RT-qPCR [23]. Screening for RHDV [62] was performed by sequencing of the amplicons obtained with primers RC9F and RC10R [62]. Conventional RT-PCR and RT-qPCR were performed with the One Step RT-PCR kit (Qiagen, Hilden, Germany).

The presence of myxoma virus was investigated by qPCR [26], using the FastStart TaqMan Probe Master Kit (Roche, Roche Diagnostics GmbH, Manheim, Germany).

For the real-time PCR systems described, undetectable Cq or Cq values >40 were considered negative.

Nucleotide sequencing analysis

Amplification of the complete *vp60* sequences of RHDV2 strains was accomplished with two pairs of primers, 27F (5′-CCATGCCAGACTTGCGTCCC-3′) and 986R (5′-AACCATCTGGAGCAATTTGGG-3′), 717F (5′-CGCA GATCTCCTCACAACCC-3′) [24], and RC10R [62] enabling the obtainment of two overlapping fragments. Both 717F and 986R are specific for RHDV2. The One Step (Qiagen, Hilden, Germany) kit was used, under the manufacturers' recommendations. Sequencing was accomplished using the BigDyeTM Terminator cycle sequencing kit (Applied Biosystems, Foster City, CA, USA).

The complete *vp60* nucleotide sequences of two RHDV2 strains (GenBank accession numbers KY247124 and KY247125) were determined on an automated 3130 Genetic Analyzer system (Applied Biosystems, Foster City, CA, USA).

Phylogenetic analysis

The phylogenetic relationships between two RHDV2 *vp60* sequences from the Berlenga Island with other RHDV2 sequences originated in Portugal mainland, Azores and worldwide, were investigated. Sequence KC345614 (from a classical RHDV strain belonging to genogroup G5) was chosen as outgroup to root the trees.

Multiple alignments of the nucleotide sequences were generated by CLUSTAL Omega [58].

Phylogenetic inference was performed by Maximum Likelihood (ML) and Bayesian methods. For ML analysis, the appropriated substitution model was determined resourcing to R software (R Development Core Team, 2011). The GTR model [61] with gamma-distributed rate variation across sites (GTR + G) showed the lowest BIC and AICc values and was subsequently used to infer phylogenetic relationships. Robustness of the tree nodes was assessed by bootstrapping 1000 times.

For the Bayesian analysis, the CLUSTAL Omega results were converted to the NEXUS format using Mesquite software [42] The phylogenetic tree was obtained with a Bayesian inference of phylogeny throughout the MrBayes version 3.1.2 software that uses the Markov chain Monte Carlo simulation technique to approximate the posterior probabilities (pp) of trees [33, 56]. MrBayes analysis was performed using the GTR model (nst = 6) with gamma-shaped rate variation with a proportion of invariable sites (rates = invgamma). The analysis was run for 10^6 generations (ngen = 10^6) with four chains of temperature (nchains = 4), and each chain was sampled every 10th generations (samplefreq = 10).

The graphical representation and edition of the phylogenetic trees were performed with FigTree v1.3.1 (http://tree.bio.ed.ac.uk/software/figtree/).

Necropsy and histopathological examination

Necropsy and histopathological examination was carried out the Pathology Laboratory of the Faculty of Veterinary Medicine of the University of Lisbon.

Organs collected from necropsy (liver and lungs) were submitted to fixation in 10% buffered formalin and processed for routine histopathological analysis. Sections were stained with H&E and Pearls Blue and microphotographs were obtained with a DP23 Olympus digital camera.

Results

Morphometric data

Weight of the 11 selected rabbits varied between 330 and 600 g (10 g sensitive scale). Mean tarsus and skull length was 44 mm and 75 mm, respectively corresponding to an estimated age of 43 to 83 days. All RHDV2-positive rabbits were less than six months old.

Virological examination

Six liver samples were negative to RHDV2 and RHDV. The other five tested positively to RHDV2 by RT-qPCR [23]. None of the eleven rabbits showed cutaneous myxomas or were positive to myxoma virus by qPCR.

Sequencing of the complete *vp60* gene obtained from two specimens confirmed the presence of RHDV2 circulating in the island. These *vp60* sequences (KY247124 and KY247125) are identical (100% similarity).

Phylogenetic analysis

Blast analysis of the Berlengas' *vp60* sequence showed higher similarity (99%) with strains from the South of Portugal mainland, in particularly with strains from Barrancos obtained in 2013.

ML (Fig. 3) and Bayesian (*not* shown) trees were consistent, showing that the strains from the Berlenga Island are most closely related (Bootstrap value of 75) with a major group of strains originated mostly in the South

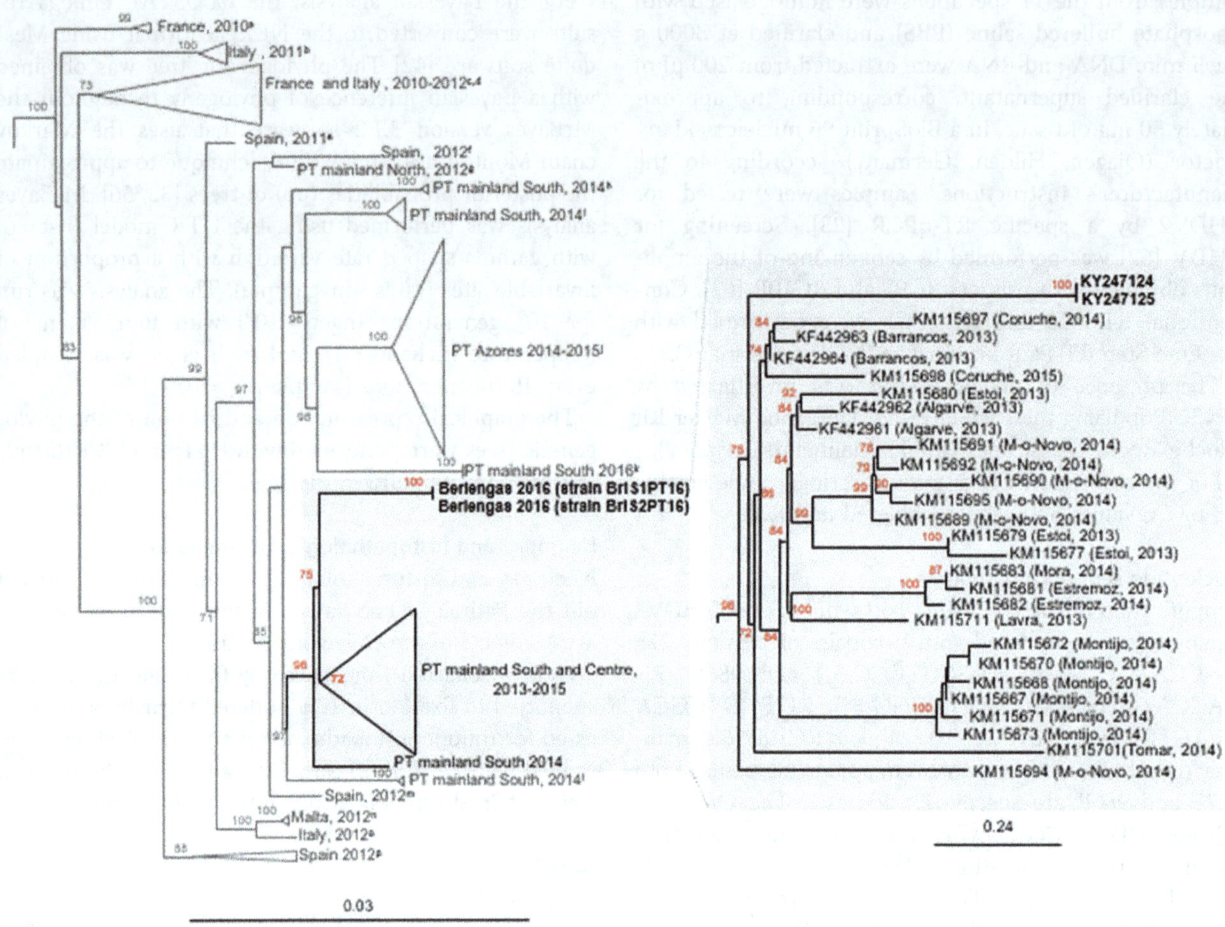

Fig. 3 Maximum Likelihood (ML) phylogenetic tree of the RHDV2 *vp60* complete nucleotide sequences from the Berlenga island (2016) and others originated in Portugal mainland, Azores, Spain, France, Italy and Malta, available in Genbank. Bootstrap values (BS) are shown next to the nodes if equal or greater than 70. Sequence KC345614 (*not displayed*) was chosen as outgroup to root the tree. In the left side tree, the major groups are collapsed to facilitate visualization. a-HE800531, HE819400; b-JX106023, KC345611–12; c-HE800529, HE800530, HE800532 and FR819781; d-JQ929052, KC907712 and JX106022; e-KM87868; f-KP129395; g-KM979445; h-KM115675–76; i-KM115712–13; j-KT000295, KT000303, KT000308, KT000311, KT000316–319, KT000322–325 KT000327, KT000329–330, KT000332–333, KT000336, KT000339 and KT000341–343; k-KX132812 and KX132813; l-KM115684–5; m-KP129396; n-KJ957809 and KJ957810; o-KC741409; p-KP129397 and KP129399. "M-o-Novo" refers to the municipality of Montemor-o-Novo. A close-up of the RHDV2 strains more closely related with the strains from the Berlenga Island is shown in the right side of the figure

between 2013 and 2014. No clear resemblance was noticed with any strain collected more recently.

Necropsy and histopathological examination

The six RHDV2-negative rabbits, all aged less than six months, showed severe emaciation with reduced fat stores and muscle mass. The hair coat was in poor condition (rude and dull) and faecal material was adherent to the perineum. At necropsy, macroscopic lesions were neither observed in the liver nor in any of the other organs except for the small intestines that were distended, with inflammation and oedema of the jejunum and ileum. No bleedings or mucosal ulcerations were however found. In the fecal smear of the jejunum and ileum contents *Eimeria* spp. oocysts were observed (*results not shown*).

Four of the five RHDV2-positive rabbits showed low body condition (score 1 in the 1 to 5 in body condition scoring for rabbits, according to [53]). In all these specimens the noses were soiled by bloody discharge, and in three rabbits fluid faecal material in the perianal region was present. Organ preservation was considered good enough to assure lesions identification. Changes were mostly restricted to the respiratory apparatus and liver. Respiratory lesions, present in all rabbits, included congestion of the trachea, which contained serohaemorrhagic fluid, and congestion of the lungs. No signs of overt haemorrhage were detected. In all cases, there was discoloration and diminished consistency of the liver. Three rabbits, the same with soiled perianal region, showed distended caeca and had unsolidified faecal material in the colon. The fresh faecal smear analysis of the jejunum and ileum revealed the presence of *Eimeria* spp. oocysts.

Histology analysis of the liver showed diffuse hepatocyte coagulation necrosis with no pattern distribution, supporting a diagnosis of diffuse non-suppurative acute hepatic necrosis. Most hepatocytes were karyolytic and only very few displayed karyorrhexis or pyknosis (Fig. 4a and b). In one case, the necrotic hepatic cells revealed vacuolated profile. Iron pigment deposition in Kuppfer cells was regularly seen. Lung lesions varied from congestion and alveolar oedema ($n = 2$) to inflammatory infiltrates in the alveolar septa by mononuclear cells with atelectasia and inflammatory cells in the alveolar lumen, consistent with interstitial pneumonia ($n = 3$) (Fig. 5a and b).

Discussion

Notwithstanding rabbit mortality at the Berlenga Island had not been investigated in previous years, our study clearly shows that RHDV2 was circulating in the island, at least since May 2016, and caused the death of five of the eleven rabbits investigated that died during the last spring. It is known that limited food availability and predation by dogs are also a cause for rabbit mortality in the island. Also, given the scarcity of fresh water in the island, the rabbit population of the Berlenga is highly dependent on the rainfall regime, with the mortality rate increasing during the dry months [63]. Despite no detailed parasitological examination was carried out during this study, the five RHDV2-negative young found in April, presented signs of intestinal coccidiosis along with emaciation that could have contributed to their deaths. Also, apart from those findings, no lesions were found in the liver and lungs that could suggest haemorrhagic disease. The impact of coccidiosis, caused by *Eimeria* spp., in the European rabbit populations of the Iberian Peninsula was recently evaluated in two ecological regions of Spain, estimating the coccidian prevalence by the mean oocyst excretion levels detected in faeces. Although in both areas the oocyst per gram of faeces was generally low, six *Eimeria* species were identified [59]. Among those (*E. coecicola, E. perforans, E media, E. magna, E. irresidua and E. flavescens*), *E. flavescens* is considered highly pathogenic for rabbits [39]. Curiously, the abundance and loads of Coccidia and nematodes in reintroduced rabbit populations in Spain showed no clear pattern with rabbit haemorrhagic disease prevalence [10]. Nonetheless, the impact of coccidea infection on morbidity and mortality of wild rabbit populations of the Berlenga Island was never investigated.

Myxoma virus-DNA was not detected in any of the 11 rabbits tested. Furthermore, none of these animals exhibited skin lesions, oedema or signs of conjunctivitis suggestive of nodular myxomatosis disease. Also, the qPCR developed by Duarte et al. [26] has allowed to detect MYXV-DNA in several organs of wild rabbits (*results not published*, Duarte et al.), which increases the confidence on the MYXV-PCR negative results obtained in the liver samples during this study.

RHDV2 infection was the cause of death of five rabbits from Berlenga Island collected in May 2016. However, given the reduced size of our sample, the positivity percentage of 45.5% (5/11 animals) is, most likely, merely indicative of the true mortality induced during the outbreak.

The characterization of RHDV2 induced lesions is still limited compared with that regarding RHDV. Post-mortem examination of RHDV2-infected rabbits revealed macroscopic lesions consistent with haemorrhages in several organs including heart, trachea, thymus, lungs, liver, kidneys, and gut, as well as jaundice [20, 24]. The liver appearance was described as soft and pale [24]. Histopathologic descriptions refer to haemorrhagic pneumonia and tracheitis, congestion of the liver and diffuse necrotizing hepatitis. Areas of focal necrosis were also described in the intestinal villi in the small intestine [20].

In the present report, lung lesions varied from simple congestion and alveolar oedema, indicating an acute evolution, to interstitial pneumonia suggesting a longer disease process. Haemorrhagic lesions were neither identified in the lungs nor in other organs, although rabbits consistently showed soiled noses, probably by blood tinged

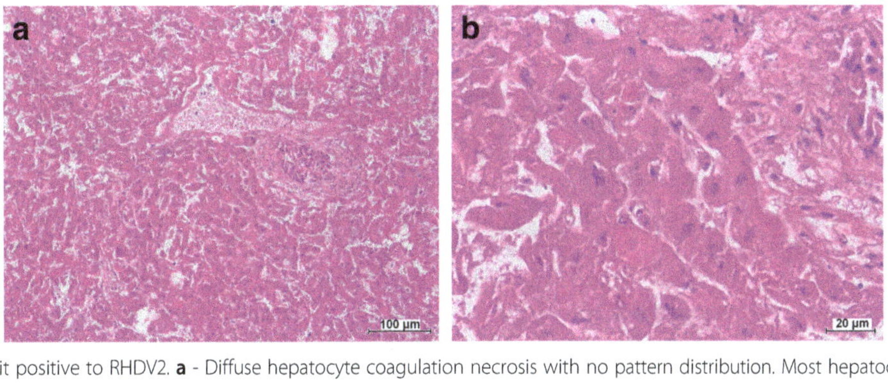

Fig. 4 Liver of rabbit positive to RHDV2. **a** - Diffuse hepatocyte coagulation necrosis with no pattern distribution. Most hepatocytes are karyolytic and only very few display karyorrhexis or pyknosis. **b** – Detail of A showing necrotic hepatic cells dysplaing karyorrhexis and pyknosis (H&E)

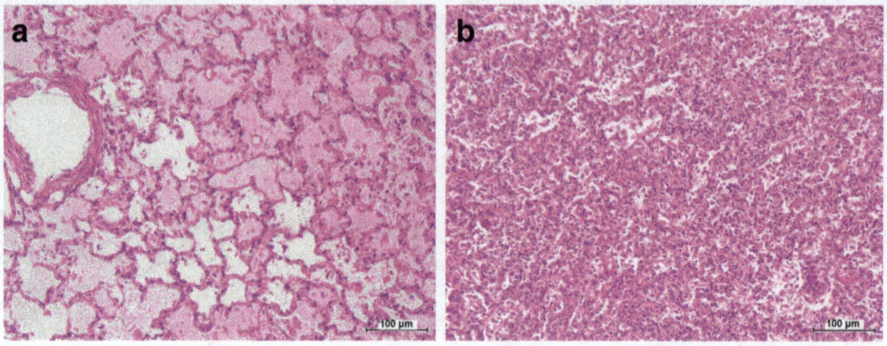

Fig. 5 Lung of rabbits positive to RHDV2. **a** – Alveolar congestion and oedema. **b**-Interstitial pneumonia with inflammatory infiltrates in the alveolar septa by mononuclear cells, which are also present in the alveolar lumen (H&E)

oedematous lung fluid. Interstitial pneumonia observed in three out of five rabbits have not been reported before in the post-mortem examination of RHDV or RHDV2 infected rabbits [43, 46, 24, 41]. It is possible that pneumonia could have eventually be due to a longer disease evolution or to bacterial infections occurring prior to the contact with the RHDV2. Inflammatory infiltrates by mononuclear cells are quite compatible with viral infection (Fig. 5b).

In fact, the diffuse coagulation necrosis registered in the liver of all rabbits is only compatible with an acute or hyperacute course the disease possibly favoured by the low body condition of the rabbits. The type of necrosis with most of the cells karyolitic and without a defined pattern distribution is more in agreement with the lesions described in European Brown Hare Syndrome (EBHS) [43], although the reports of RHDV and RDHV2 infected rabbits consistently refer to severe necrotic liver lesions [43, 46, 24, 41].

In summary, death of the infected rabbits analysed in this study must have been due to acute hepatic failure with lung congestion and oedema occurring closer to death. The relevance of the interstitial pneumonia remains unclarified as no other infectious agents were investigated apart from the aforementioned leporid-specific viruses. The fact that the cadavers were not fresh limited the confidence and significance in any bacterial identification.

The phylogenetic results revealed that the 2016 strains from the Berlenga Island formed an independent cluster in closer proximity with a group of sequences obtained between 2013 and 2014, mainly in the South of Portugal mainland. The higher resemblance with a group of older strains may suggest that RHDV2 was not introduced recently in the Island. Instead, and with accordance with the mortalities observed in the last years, RHDV2 introduction may have taken place a few years ago, circulating since then in the island. Because no intermediate strains between the Barrancos 2013 and Berlengas 2016 strains were found until the moment (*results not shown*), this possibility remains only hypothetical. Yet, the island geographic location may well have provided the necessary isolation for the Berlenga Island strains to evolve apart from other haplotypes that have been characterized in the latest years in Portugal mainland [1] [16] and in Azores [24, 4]. Due to the advanced stage of rabbit eradication at the time samples were collected, no serologic study could be carried out which may have allowed to clarify if RHDV2 was introduced on the island prior the 2016 outbreak.

Given the island eco-geographic particularities, RHDV2 introduction may have occurred by several routes. Beside human means and mechanical action of arthropod vectors [8, 19, 45], black rat may also have accounted for the viral introduction. Native from the Indian peninsula [50], the black rat is worldwide distributed [11] and is the only rodent species found on the island [5]. Although never demonstrated, similarly to *Apodemus silvaticus* and *Mus spretus* [48], black rats from RHDV2 infected areas may have carried the virus to the rabbit population of Berlengas after being inadvertently transported by the boats that arrive at the island. Other possibilities concern resident birds of prey such as the Common Kestrel (*Falco tinnunculus*) and the Peregrine Falcon (*Falco peregrinus*) or vagrant birds as the Common Buzzard (*Buteo buteo*), that may also have carried contaminated leftovers from RHDV2 infected rabbits from Portugal mainland. Furthermore, Berlenga Island holds a large population of Yellow-legged Gulls (*Larus michahellis*), estimated near 13,150 individuals [47], which daily feed on waste treatment plants, farms and aviaries on the surrounding grounds of the Peniche municipality (located in mainland and which also includes the Berlengas archipelago) [18]. No reliable data could be gathered regarding the occurrence of haemorrhagic disease in domestic rabbits in Peniche. However, abnormal mortality rates have been observed in wild rabbits from local game reserves, Atouguia da Baleia, Ferrel and Serra d'el-Rei, during the last years.

RHDV2 infections have been demonstrated in most of the national territory since its introduction in 2012, drastically reducing the wild rabbit population in particular areas [1, 4, 24, 41]. Therefore, it is highly likely that the three Peniche neighbouring parishes were the game reserves are sited may have also been affected. The Berlenga Island location near the coast, support the hypothesis that the virus strains found in the island may have been introduced from the nearby RHDV2 affected geographical area. Direct contact with rabbit contaminated materials is therefore likely to have occurred since Yellow-legged Gulls are commonly seen transporting dead corpses of several animals into the island including parts of rabbits (Oliveira N., *personal communication*).

The exceptional terrestrial insular ecosystem of Berlengas encompasses unique characteristics [17]. The archipelago provides nesting conditions for seabird species from the families *Procellariidae, Hydrobatidae, Phalacrocoracidae,* and *Laridae,* such as the Cory's Shearwater (*Calonectris borealis),* the Band-rumped storm-petrel (*Hydrobates castro)* only present in Farilhões, the European Shag (*Phalacrocorax aristotelis),* the Yellow-legged Gull and the Lesser Black-backed Gull (*Larus fuscus*) [17]. Cory's Shearwater, Band-rumped Storm-petrel and European Shag are classified as vulnerable by the Portuguese RedList Book [13]. The role of rabbits on deviation of the original ecology of the Berlenga Island is controversial. Besides the effect of rabbits, it is known that the decline of the unique endemic vegetation such as the *Armeria berlengensi, Herniaria berlengiana, Pulicaria microcephala* as well as the *Lobularia maritime,* and *Frankenia laevis,* is also a consequence of the acid excrements of the overpopulated Yellow-legged Gull and competition by Ice plant (*Carpobrotus edulis*), an invasive plant native to South Africa brought into the island in the 1980's and which threatens its natural vegetation biodiversity [29].

The current conservation policy of the Berlengas archipelago biological heritage, classified as of high interest, is due to its protected habitats and vulnerable surrounding marine ecosystem, one of the richest Portuguese seawaters for which it was considered Nature Reserve by UNESCO since 2010. Aiming to guarantee the survival of several endangered species, a national plan to eradicate the rabbit and black rat population from Berlenga is in course. If successful, this study may have been the last opportunity to trace the RHDV2 passage through the Berlengas archipelago.

Conclusions

Our results showed that the mortality observed in wild rabbits from the Berlenga Island during the spring of 2016 was due, at least in part, to RHDV2. Despite marine biologists working in the island have observed rabbit mortality in the last years, this study provides the first evidence of the circulation of RHDV2 in the Berlengas archipelago. Phylogenetic analysis showed that the RHDV2 strain circulating in Berlenga in 2016 is distinct from mainland Portugal strains, possibly due to geo-segregation, and more closely related with strains from the South of the country.

Abbreviations

BLAST: Basic local alignment search tool; cq : Quantification cycle; DNA: Deoxyribonucleic acid; GTR: General time reversible; H&E: Hematoxylin and eosin; INIAV: Instituto Nacional de Investigação Agrária e Veterinária; ML: Maximum likelihood; MYXV: Myxoma virus; PBS: Phosphate buffered saline; RHD: Rabbit haemorrhagic disease; RHDV: Rabbit haemorrhagic disease virus; RHDV2: Rabbit haemorrhagic disease virus 2; RNA: Ribonucleic acid; RT-PCR: Reverse transcription polymerase chain reaction; RT-qPCR: Quantitative reverse transcription PCR; vp60: Major capsid protein

Acknowledgements

We are thankful to João Teixeira, Fátima Cordeiro, Sandra Carvalho and Rosário Luís for excellent technical assistance. We also present our acknowledgments to Berlengas Natural Reserve guards (Paulo Crisóstomo, Eduardo Mourato, Filipe Correia, Tiago Menino and António Figueiredo), all volunteers and SPEA staff (namely Isabel Fagundes and Pedro Luís Geraldes) who supported the entire field work. Thanks to the National Maritime Authority and Peniche Captaincy for the transport to and from the Berlenga Island. Finally, thank you to the Instituto de Conservação da Natureza e das Florestas, namely to Maria de Jesus Fernandes and Maria de Lurdes Morais for their full support to this study.

Funding

Most of the field and laboratory work refered to in this manuscript was supported by the Interdisciplinary Research Centre on Animal Health, Faculty of Veterinary Medicine, University of Lisbon (CIISA, FMV, UL) (Portugal) (Project UID/CVT/00276/2013).

Molecular analysis was partially funded by the Fundação para a Ciência e Tecnologia (FCT) (grant SFRH/79225/2011) and and Instituto de Ciências Agrárias e Ambientais Mediterrânicas (ICAAM) (Project UID/AGR/00115/2013).

Field work was partially supported by the LIFE + Berlengas (LIFE13 NAT/PT/000458), a contribution of the LIFE financial instrument of the European Union and the "Fundo de Biodiversidade" funded from the Portuguese Government.

Funding bodies played no direct role in the design or conclusion of the study.

Authors' contributions

Drafted the manuscript: FAS; Conceived and designed the experiments: FAS, CC, CP and MD. Collected the samples: FAS, NO. Performed the experiments: FAS, CC, MH, JC and CP. Analysed the data: MD, CP, CC. Wrote the manuscript: FAS, CC, NO, CP and MD. Revised the manuscript: CC, NO, CP, MF, MD. All authors read and approved the final manuscript.

Consent for publication

Not applicable.

Competing interests

The authors declare that they have no competing interests. All permissions to handling animals and collect rabbit samples were obtained from the national authorities.

Author details
[1]Centro de Investigação Interdisciplinar em Sanidade Animal (CIISA), Faculdade de Medicina Veterinária, Universidade de Lisboa. Av. da Universidade Técnica, 1300-477 Lisbon, Portugal. [2]Instituto de Ciências Agrárias e Ambientais Mediterrânicas (ICAAM); Instituto de Investigação e Formação Avançada (IIFA), Universidade de Évora. Núcleo da Mitra, 7000 Évora, Portugal. [3]Sociedade Portuguesa para o Estudo das Aves (SPEA), Av. Columbano Bordalo Pinheiro, 87, 3º Andar, 1070-062 Lisboa, Portugal. [4]Instituto Nacional de Investigação Agrária e Veterinária (INIAV), Laboratório de Virologia. Av. da República, Quinta do Marquês, 2780-157 Oeiras, Portugal. [5]Rua Quinta do Pinto Nº5 3ºD, 2660-067 Loures, Frielas, Portugal.

References

1. Abrantes J, Lopes AM, Dalton KP, Melo P, Correia JJ, Ramada M, Alves PC, Parra F, Esteves PJ. New variant of rabbit hemorrhagic disease virus, Portugal, 2012-2013. Emerg Infect Dis. 2013;19:1900–2. https://doi.org/10.3201/eid1911.130908.
2. Abrantes J, van der Loo W, Le Pendu J, Esteves PJ. Rabbit haemorrhagic disease (RHD) and rabbit haemorrhagic disease virus (RHDV): a review. Vet Res. 2012;43:12. https://doi.org/10.1186/1297-9716-43-12.
3. Alda F, Gaitero T, Suárez M, Merchán T, Rocha G, Doadrio I. Evolutionary history and molecular epidemiology of rabbit haemorrhagic disease virus in the Iberian peninsula and Western Europe. BMC Evol Biol. 2010;10:347. https://doi.org/10.1186/1471-2148-10-347.
4. Almeida T, Lopes AM, Magalhães MJ, Neves F, Pinheiro A, Gonçalves D, Leitão M, Esteves PJ, Abrantes J. Tracking the evolution of the G1/RHDVb recombinant strains introduced from the Iberian peninsula to the Azores islands. Portugal Infect Genet Evol. 2015;34:307–13. https://doi.org/10.1016/j.meegid.2015.07.010.
5. Amado, A.; Gafeira, C.; Teixeira, A.; Preto, A. Relatório do Plano de Ordenamento da Reserva Natural das Berlengas. (2007) Instituto de Conservação da Natureza e Florestas, (in Portuguese).
6. Aragão HB. Myxoma of rabbits. Mem. Inst. Oswaldo Cruz. 1927;20:237–47.
7. Argüello Villares J, Llanos Pellitero A, Pérez-Ordoyo Garcia L. Enfermedad vírica hemorragica canejo en España. Rev Med Vet. 1988;5:645–50.
8. Asgari S, Hardy JR, Sinclair RG, Cooke BD. Field evidence for mechanical transmission of rabbit haemorrhagic disease virus (RHDV) by flies (Diptera: Calliphoridae) among wild rabbits in Australia. Virus Res. 1998;54:123–32.
9. Baily JL, Dagleish MP, Graham M, Maley M, Rocchi MS. RHDV variant 2 presence detected in Scotland. Vet. Rec. 2014;174:411–1. https://doi.org/10.1136/vr.g2781.
10. Bertó-Moran A, Pacios I, Serrano E, Moreno S, Rouco C. Coccidian and nematode infections influence prevalence of antibody to MYXOMA and rabbit hemorrhagic disease viruses in European rabbits. J Wildl Dis. 2013;49:10–7. https://doi.org/10.7589/2011-12-343.
11. Brouat C, Tollenaere C, Estoup A, Loiseau A, Sommer S, Soanandrasana R, Rahalison L, Rajerison M, Piry S, Goodman SM, Duplantier J-M. Invasion genetics of a human commensal rodent: the black rat *Rattus rattus* in Madagascar. Mol Ecol. 2014;23:4153–67. https://doi.org/10.1111/mec.12848.
12. Brugman VA, Hernández-Triana LM, Prosser SWJ, Weland C, Westcott DG, Fooks AR, Johnson N. Molecular species identification, host preference and detection of myxoma virus in the Anopheles Maculipennis Complex (Diptera: Culicidae) in southern England. UK Parasit Vectors. 2015;8:421. https://doi.org/10.1186/s13071-015-1034-8.
13. Cabral, M.J. (coord.); J. Almeida, P.R. Almeida, T. Delliger, N. Ferrand de Almeida, M.E. Oliveira, J.M. Palmeirim, A.I. Queirós, L. Rogado, M. Santos-Reis (eds.) (2005). Livro Vermelho dos Vertebrados de Portugal. Instituto da Conservação da Natureza. Lisboa. 659p. https://dspace.uevora.pt/rdpc/handle/10174/6006?locale=pt.
14. Camarda A, Pugliese N, Cavadini P, Circella E, Capucci L, Caroli A, Legretto M, Mallia E, Lavazza A. Detection of the new emerging rabbit haemorrhagic disease type 2 virus (RHDV2) in Sicily from rabbit (Oryctolagus Cuniculus) and Italian hare (Lepus Corsicanus). Res Vet Sci. 2014;97:642–5. https://doi.org/10.1016/j.rvsc.2014.10.008.
15. Cancellotti FM, Renzi M. Epidemiology and current situation of viral haemorrhagic disease of rabbits and the European brown hare syndrome in Italy. Rev Sci Tech. 1991;10:409–22.
16. Carvalho CL, Rodeia J, Branco S, Monteiro M, Duarte EL, Melo P, Santos PT, Henriques AM, Barros SS, Ramos F, Fagulha T, Fevereiro M, Duarte MD. Tracking the origin of a rabbit Haemorrhagic virus 2 outbreak in a wild rabbit breeding Centre in Portugal; epidemiological and genetic investigation. J Emerg Infect Dis. 2016;1:114. https://doi.org/10.4172/24724998.1000114.
17. Catry P, Costa H, Elias G, Matias R. Aves de Portugal, Ornitologia do Território Continental. Lisboa: Assírio e Alvim; 2010.
18. Ceia F, Paiva V, Fidalgo V, Morais L, Baeta A, Crisóstomo P, Mourato E, Garthe S, Marques J, Ramos J. Annual and seasonal consistency in the feeding ecology of an opportunistic species, the yellow-legged gull Larus Michahellis. Mar Ecol Prog Ser. 2014;497:273–84. https://doi.org/10.3354/meps10586.
19. Cooke BD. Rabbit haemorrhagic disease: field epidemiology and the management of wild rabbit populations. Rev Sci Tech. 2002;21:347–58.
20. Dalton KP, Nicieza I, Balseiro A, Muguerza MA, Rosell JM, Casais R, Álvarez ÁL, Parra F. Variant rabbit hemorrhagic disease virus in young rabbits. Spain Emerg Infect Dis. 2012;18:2009–12. https://doi.org/10.3201/eid1812.120341.
21. Delibes-Mateos M, Delibes M, Ferreras P, Villafuerte R. Key role of European rabbits in the conservation of the western Mediterranean basin hotspot. Conserv Biol. 2008;22:1106–17. https://doi.org/10.1111/j.1523-1739.2008.00993.x.
22. Duarte M, Henriques M, Barros SC, Fagulha T, Ramos F, Luís T, Fevereiro M, Benevides S, Flor L, Barros SV, Bernardo S. Detection of RHDV variant 2 in the Azores. Vet Rec. 2015a;176:130. https://doi.org/10.1136/vr.h497.
23. Duarte MD, Carvalho CL, Barros SC, Henriques AM, Ramos F, Fagulha T, Luís T, Duarte EL, Fevereiro M. A real time Taqman RT-PCR for the detection of rabbit hemorrhagic disease virus 2 (RHDV2). J Virol Methods. 2015b;219:90–5. https://doi.org/10.1016/j.jviromet.2015.03.017.
24. Duarte M, Carvalho C, Bernardo S, Barros SV, Benevides S, Flor L, Monteiro M, Marques I, Henriques M, Barros SC, Fagulha T, Ramos F, Luís T, Fevereiro M. Rabbit haemorrhagic disease virus 2 (RHDV2) outbreak in Azores: disclosure of common genetic markers and phylogenetic segregation within the European strains. Infect Genet Evol. 2015c;35:163–71. https://doi.org/10.1016/j.meegid.2015.08.005.
25. Duarte MD, Henriques AM, Barros S, Luís T, Fagulha T, Ramos F, Fevereiro M. New insight into the epidemiology of rabbit hemorrhagic disease viruses in Portugal: retrospective study reveals the circulation of genogroup 5 (G5) in Azores and discloses the circulation of G1 and G6 strains in mainland until 2008. Infect Genet Evol. 2014a;27:149–55. https://doi.org/10.1016/j.meegid.2014.07.017.
26. Duarte MD, Barros SC, Henriques AM, Fagulha MT, Ramos F, Luís T, Fevereiro M. Development and validation of a real time PCR for the detection of myxoma virus based on the diploid gene M000.5L/R. J Virol Methods. 2014b;196:219–24. https://doi.org/10.1016/j.jviromet.2013.11.014.
27. Dunnet, G., Dunnet, G., 1956. Growth rate of young rabbits, Oryctolagus Cuniculus (L.). CSIRO Wildl. Res. 1, 66. doi:https://doi.org/10.1071/CWR9560066.
28. Fenner F, Ratcliffe FN. Myxomatosis. London: Cambridge University Press; 1965.
29. Gomes C.T, Draper D., Marques I., Rosello-Graell A., 2004. Componente Vegetal do Plano de Ordenamento da Reserva Natural das Berlengas: Flora e vegetação do arquipélago das Berlengas. Unpublished report.
30. Gonçalves H, Alves PC, Rocha A, Gonçalves H, Alves PC, Rocha A. Seasonal variation in the reproductive activity of the wild rabbit (Oryctolagus Cuniculus Algirus) in a Mediterranean ecosystem. Wildl Res. 2002;29:165. https://doi.org/10.1071/WR00048.
31. Hall RN, Mahar JE, Haboury S, Stevens V, Holmes EC, Strive T. Emerging rabbit hemorrhagic disease virus 2 (RHDVb). Australia Emerg Infect Dis. 2015;21:2276–8. https://doi.org/10.3201/eid2112.151210.
32. Henning J, Meers J, Davies PR, Morris RS. Survival of rabbit haemorrhagic disease virus (RHDV) in the environment. Epidemiol Infect. 2005;133:719–30.
33. Huelsenbeck JP, Ronquist F, Nielsen R, Bollback JP. Bayesian inference of phylogeny and its impact on evolutionary biology. Science. 2001;294:2310–4. https://doi.org/10.1126/science.1065889.
34. Kerr PJ. Myxomatosis in Australia and Europe: a model for emerging infectious diseases. Antivir Res. 2012;93:387–415. https://doi.org/10.1016/j.antiviral.2012.01.009.
35. Kerr PJ, Liu J, Cattadori I, Ghedin E, Read AF, Holmes EC. Myxoma virus and the Leporipoxviruses: an evolutionary paradigm. Viruses. 2015;7:1020–61. https://doi.org/10.3390/v7031020.
36. Le Gall G, Arnauld C, Boilletot E, Morisse JP, Rasschaert D. Molecular epidemiology of rabbit haemorrhagic disease virus outbreaks in France during 1988 to 1995. J Gen Virol. 1998;79(Pt 1):11–6. https://doi.org/10.1099/0022-1317-79-1-11.
37. Le Gall-Reculé G, Lavazza A, Marchandeau S, Bertagnoli S, Zwingelstein F, Cavadini P, Martinelli N, Lombardi G, Guérin J-L, Lemaitre E, Decors A, Boucher S, Le Normand B, Capucci L. Emergence of a new lagovirus related

37. Le Gall-Reculé G, Lavazza A, Marchandeau S, Bertagnoli S, Zwingelstein F, Cavadini P, Martinelli N, Lombardi G, Guérin J-L, Lemaitre E, Decors A, Boucher S, Le Normand B, Capucci L. Emergence of a new lagovirus related to rabbit Haemorrhagic disease virus. Vet Res. 2013;44:81. https://doi.org/10.1186/1297-9716-44-81.
38. Le Gall-Reculé G, Zwingelstein F, Boucher S, Le Normand B, Plassiart G, Portejoie Y, Decors A, Bertagnoli S, Guérin J-L, Marchandeau S. Detection of a new variant of rabbit haemorrhagic disease virus in France. Vet. Rec. 2011; 168:137–8. https://doi.org/10.1136/vr.d697.
39. Licois D. Domestic rabbit enteropathies, in: proc. 8th world rabbit congress. Mexico: Puebla; 2004. p. 385–403.
40. Liu S.J., Xue H.P., Pu B.Q., Qian N.H., 1984. A new viral disease of rabbits. Animal husbandry vet med.16, 253-255.
41. Lopes AM, Correia J, Abrantes J, Melo P, Ramada M, Magalhães MJ, Alves PC, Esteves PJ. Is the new variant RHDV replacing genogroup 1 in Portuguese wild rabbit populations? Viruses. 2015;7:27–36. https://doi.org/10.3390/v7010027.
42. Maddison WP, Maddison DR. Mesquite: a modular system for evolutionary analysis. Version 2.72. 2009. http://mesquiteproject.org.
43. Marcato PS, Benazzi C, Vecchi G, Galeotti M, Della Salda L, Sarli G, Lucidi P. Clinical and pathological features of viral haemorrhagic disease of rabbits and the European brown hare syndrome. Rev Sci Tech. 1991;10:371–92.
44. Martin-Alonso A, Martin-Carrillo N, Garcia-Livia K, Valladares B, Foronda P. Emerging rabbit haemorrhagic disease virus 2 (RHDV2) at the gates of the African continent. Infect Genet Evol. 2016;44:46–50. https://doi.org/10.1016/j.meegid.2016.06.034.
45. McColl KA, Merchant JC, Hardy J, Cooke BD, Robinson A, Westbury HA. Evidence for insect transmission of rabbit haemorrhagic disease virus. Epidemiol Infect. 2002;129:655–63.
46. McIntosh MT, Behan SC, Mohamed FM, Lu Z, Moran KE, Burrage TG, Neilan JG, Ward GB, Botti G, Capucci L, Metwally SA. A pandemic strain of calicivirus threatens rabbit industries in the Americas. Virol J. 2007;4:96. https://doi.org/10.1186/1743-422X-4-96.
47. Meirinho A, Barros N, Oliveira N, Catry P, Lecoq M, Paiva V, Geraldes P, Granadeiro JP, Ramírez I & Andrade J (2014). Atlas das Aves Marinhas de Portugal. Sociedade Portuguesa para o Estudo das Aves.
48. Merchán T, Rocha G, Alda F, Silva E, Thompson G, de Trucios SH, Pagés A. Detection of rabbit haemorrhagic disease virus (RHDV) in nonspecific vertebrate hosts sympatric to the European wild rabbit (Oryctolagus Cuniculus). Infect Genet Evol. 2011;11:1469–74. https://doi.org/10.1016/j.meegid.2011.05.001.
49. Muller A, Freitas J, Silva E, Le Gall-Reculé G, Zwingelstein F, Abrantes J, Esteves PJ, Alves PC, van der Loo W, Kolodziejek J, Nowotny N, Thompson G. Evolution of rabbit haemorrhagic disease virus (RHDV) in the European rabbit (Oryctolagus Cuniculus) from the Iberian peninsula. Vet Microbiol. 2009;135:368–73. https://doi.org/10.1016/j.vetmic.2008.09.057.
50. Musser GG, Carlton MD. Superfamily Muroidea. In: Wilson DE, Reeder DM, editors. Mammal species of the world. 3rd ed. Baltimore, MD: The Johns Hopkins University Press; 2005. p. 894–1531.
51. Nowotny N, Bascuñana CR, Ballagi-Pordány A, Gavier-Widén D, Uhlén M, Belák S. Phylogenetic analysis of rabbit haemorrhagic disease and European brown hare syndrome viruses by comparison of sequences from the capsid protein gene. Arch Virol. 1997;142:657–73.
52. OIE. 2016. Terrestrial manual. Chapter 2.6.2. Rabbit haemorrhagic disease. http://www.oie.int/fileadmin/Home/eng/Health_standards/tahm/2.06.02_RHD.pdf.
53. PFMA (Pet Food Manufacturers Association. (2012). Rabbit Size-O-Meter. https://research.unc.edu/files/2012/11/Body-Condition-Scoring-Rabbit.pdf.
54. Pinto, Gabriela A., 1995- Contribuição para o Estudo Bioecológico dos Ectoparasitas do Coelho (*Oryctolagus cuniculus* L. 1758) e do Rato-preto (*Rattus rattus* L. 1758) na Reserva Natural da Berlenga. Relatório entregue ao Instituto da Conservação da Natureza, 15pp.
55. Puggioni G, Cavadini P, Maestrale C, Scivoli R, Botti G, Ligios C, Le Gall-Reculé G, Lavazza A, Capucci L. The new French 2010 rabbit hemorrhagic disease virus causes an RHD-like disease in the Sardinian cape hare (Lepus Capensis Mediterraneus). Vet Res. 2013;44:96. https://doi.org/10.1186/1297-9716-44-96.
56. Ronquist F, Huelsenbeck JP. MrBayes 3: Bayesian phylogenetic inference under mixed models. Bioinformatics. 2003;19:1572–4.
57. Sanarelli, G., 1898. Das myxomatogene Virus. Beitrag zum Stadium der Krankheit-serreger ausserhalbdes Sichtbaren Zbl Bakt 23, 865–873.
58. Sievers F, Wilm A, Dineen D, Gibson TJ, Karplus K, Li W, Lopez R, McWilliam H, Remmert M, Söding J, Thompson JD, Higgins DG. Fast, scalable generation of high-quality protein multiple sequence alignments using Clustal omega. Mol Syst Biol. 2011;7:539. https://doi.org/10.1038/msb.2011.75.
59. Silva SM, Ferreira C, Paupério J, Silva RM, Alves PC, Lemos A. Coccidiosis in European rabbit (Oryctolagus Cuniculus Algirus) populations in the Iberian peninsula. Acta Parasitol. 2015;60:350–5. https://doi.org/10.1515/ap-2015-0049.
60. Southern HN. THE ECOLOGY AND POPULATION DYNAMICS OF THE WILD RABBIT (ORYCTOLAGUS CUNICULUS). Ann Appl Biol. 1940;27:509–26. https://doi.org/10.1111/j.1744-7348.1940.tb07522.x.
61. Tavaré, S., 1986. Some probabilistic and statistical problems in the anal- ysis of DNA sequences. In: Miura R. M., (Ed). Lectures on math- ematics in the life sciences. Volume 17. Providence (RI):American Mathematical Society. Pp. 57–86.
62. Tham KM, Barnes SM, Hunter SN. Polymerase chain reaction amplification and gene sequence analysis of a calicivirus from a feral rabbit. Virus Genes. 1999;18:235–42.
63. Vicente, L. A., 1989- Sobre a História Natural dos Répteis da Ilha Berlenga – A síndrome de Insularidade. Dissertação de Doutoramento. Faculdade de Ciências, Universidade de Lisboa, 487pp.
64. Westcott DG, Frossard J-P, Everest D, Dastjerdi A, Duff JP, Choudhury B. Incursion of RHDV2-like variant in great Britain. Vet. Rec. 2014;174:333–3. https://doi.org/10.1136/vr.g2345.

3

Evidence of Aujeszky's disease in wild boar

V. Milicevic[1*], S. Radojicic[2], M. Valcic[2], V. Ivovic[3] and V. Radosavljevic[4]

Abstract

Background: Aujeszky's disease is a viral disease of suids caused by *Suid Herpesvirus 1*. The disease has worldwide distribution with significant economic impact. In Serbia, there is neither an Aujeszky's disease eradication nor national vaccination programme of domestic pigs.

Since clinical symptoms of Aujeszky's disease are not specific, it is important to establish a link between clinical signs and presence of ADV active infection in wild boars. The aim of this study was to investigate the possibility of active infection within wild boar showing signs of ADV and also to examine relationship between isolates from domestic pigs and wild boar. Having in mind that virus has not been previously isolated from wild boars in Serbia, we report the first isolation of *Suid Herpesvirus 1* from this species in Serbia.

Results: Tissue and serum samples from 40 wild boars from eastern Serbia were examined for evidence of Aujeszky's disease (AD). *Suid Herpesvirus 1* (SHV1), the cause of AD was isolated on PK15 cell line from three tissue samples, inducing cytopathic effect (CPE) with syncytia forming, and viral genome was detected by polymerase chain reaction (PCR) in eight samples. Genetic analysis of us4, us9 and ul49.5 partial sequences showed high homology between ADV isolates from wild boars and between isolates from wild boars and domestic animals. Neutralizing antibodies were not detected by virus neutralisation test (VNT) in sera from four out of eight PCR positive wild boars suggesting recent infection in those animals.

Conclusions: This is the first demonstration of Aujeszky's disease virus (ADV) in the wild boar population in Serbia although seroconversion has been detected previously.

Keywords: Aujeszky's disease virus, PCR, Virus isolation, Virus neutralization test, Wild boar

Background

Aujeszky's disease (AD) is a viral disease of suids caused by *Suid Herpesvirus 1* (SHV1) [1], also referred to as Aujeszky's disease virus (ADV). The virus belongs to the genus Varicellovirus, subfamily Alphaherpesvirinae, family Herpesviridae. It has a double-stranded DNA genome composed of 143461 nucleotides with more than 70 open reading frames homologues to related Alphaherpesviruses [2]. Based on restriction fragment length polymorphism (RFLP) analysis patterns, ADV can be divided into four major genotypes [3]. But according to partial gC (ul44) coding region, it is possible to divide ADV into five genotypes that appear to be unspecific to countries or continents [4].

AD is also named pseudorabies (PR) and the virus Pseudorabies Virus (PRV), because carnivores and pigs may display neurological signs which can be similar to rabies.

Wild boar (*Sus scrofa*) are the natural host, but a wide range of species can be infected with SHV1 [5]. Wild boars are known as reservoirs for many important infectious diseases in domestic animals, such as classical swine fever, brucellosis and trichinellosis. Also, they can play a role of reservoirs for zoonotic diseases such as hepatitis E, tuberculosis, leptospirosis and trichinellosis [6]. Worldwide distribution, great potential of adaptation, fast reproductive rate and complex social behaviour make wild boar almost ideal reservoir species [7].

However, some diseases, like AD can sporadically occur in free living wild boars under natural conditions. Occurrence of these diseases is facilitated by social stress, age related change from passive to active immunity,

* Correspondence: mvekac@yahoo.com
[1]Virology department, Institute of Veterinary Medicine of Serbia, Vojvode Toze 14, 11000 Belgrade, Serbia
Full list of author information is available at the end of the article

individual susceptibility to ADV infection and environmental conditions [8].

AD has worldwide distribution [9]. The economic impact of AD is significant, consequently many developed countries (Belgium, Czech Republic, Denmark, Germany, Ireland, Cyprus, Luxembourg, Netherlands, Austria, Slovenia, Slovakia, Finland, Sweden, UK) have eradicated, or are in the process of eradication of the infection from domestic pigs[1]. AD may also be controlled nationally by a vaccination programme. In Serbia, there is neither an AD eradication nor national vaccination programme of domestic pigs. Vaccination is conducted on individual voluntary basis only. Only in commercial farms, pigs are regularly vaccinated to reduce potential losses due to AD and therefore AD has rarely been reported in swine.

In Serbia, intensive pig production is located in the north part of the country, in the Autonomous Province of Vojvodina. In this area AD has moderate impact on intensive pig production, with the 32.8 % ADV seroprevalence in unvaccinated breeding pigs [10]. Pusic et al. [10] demonstrated that the swine population in Vojvodina region, the most developed region in Serbia with the biosecurity measures most applied, was enzootically infected with ADV and that vaccination was only performed on large commercial farms. Those farms were usually surrounded by small backyard holdings with occasionally vaccinated animals, which presented a potential source of infection. Due to vaccination with attenuated vaccine of Bartha strain, which is not a marker vaccine, seroprevalence attributed to the natural infection is difficult to estimate. The sampling has been done in this region where the virus can be transferred from wild to domestic pigs since it is separated from Vojvodina only by the river Danube.

Clinical AD in wild boar has rarely been seen, although Gortazar et al. [11] described an outbreak in wild boar in Spain. It has been demonstrated that the virus could be successfully isolated from latently infected wild boars [12]. Serosurveillance studies have demonstrated that the prevalence of AD could be high within the European wild boar population, indicating a potentially significant wildlife reservoir of ADV [13]. Seroprevalence ranges from 0 % in the Netherlands and Sweden [14, 15] to more than 50 % in Croatia [16] and central Italy [17] and 100 % in Spain, on local level [18]. As documented in Germany, continuous parallel increase of both AD seroprevalence and wild boar population density implies the correlation of these two parameters [19].

Within the Classical Swine Fever (CSF) monitoring programme in Serbia, 20 % of wild boars tested annually for CSF were also tested for ADV antibodies. The Monitoring is issued annually by The Ministry of Agriculture and Environmental protection and prescribes the number of samples to be collected for each district. Hunting season in Serbia lasts from April 15th to February 28th for boars and young wild boars up to 60 kg and from July 1st to December 31st for sows, although hunting is the most intensive from November to February. Specified percent of wild boars were subjected to AD serology tests, either VNT or ELISA. ADV seroprevalence in different regions varies with the highest percentage found in the east - 83 % as average for the last three years (unpublished data).

Until 2011, vaccination of wild boar against classical swine fever has been performed in hunting grounds in Serbia. Wild boars have been trapped, vaccinated, ear tagged and released back in the nature. Classical swine fever vaccine used for wild boar vaccination was produced by local company and composed of CSF C strain and attenuated ADV Bartha strain viruses. Therefore, unintentionally, some wild boars had been vaccinated against AD. The wild boar population in Serbia is estimated at around 20000 animals, with density of 0.2 - 1.38 animals/km[2].

Natural transmission of *Suid Herpesvirus 1* requires close contact between animals such as during coitus, licking, or nuzzling. Although, in high density commercial farms, sneezing and short distance droplet spreads are major routes of transmission [20].

The clinical presentation of ADV infection depends on the virulence and initial dose of virus; and also the age, immunological and reproductive status of the host [21]. Within wild boar, Gortazar et al. [11] reported that young animals were mostly affected, between four and eight months of age, with 14 % mortality. Although there is no evidence of any different susceptibility and disease course between wild and domestic pigs, it has been shown that strains from free-living wild boars differed genetically from those isolated from domestic pigs, but that both might have had a common origin [1, 22].

An important mechanism of ADV persistence, characteristic of all Alphaherpesviruses, is lifelong latency within the peripheral nervous system.

Diagnosis of Aujeszky's disease can be achieved using various tests including viral isolation, molecular biology (PCR) and serology.

Since clinical symptoms of Aujeszky's disease are not specific, it is important to establish a link between clinical signs and presence of ADV active infection in wild boars. The aim of this study was to investigate the possibility of active infection within wild boar showing signs of ADV and also to examine relationship between isolates from domestic pigs and wild boar. Having in mind that virus has not been previously isolated from wild boars in Serbia, we report the first isolation of *Suid Herpesvirus 1* from this species in Serbia.

Methods

Samples

Fourty samples were received from Eastern Serbia (44° 22′1.417″N, 21°44′28.524″E) during the period November 2014 – January 2015, collected by hunters, for classical swine fever monitoring which was compulsory for each hunting ground. During that period, hunts were organised by local hunting associations every Sunday, and samples from each hunt were independently sent to the laboratory. According to the CSF monitoring plan, each sample set consisted of spleen, kidney, blood and, if possible, tonsils. Commonly used practice was that hunters at spot took samples and therefore, due to difficult sampling, tonsils were rarely submitted. Hunters were requested to fill in the form for each shot wild boar, specifying age, gender, previous vaccinations and a reason for hunt (injured, ill, sport). The hunters reported signs of illness as the reason for the kill of 18 wild boars, in independent hunts during the mentioned period. That high frequency of reported illness led to examinations for other viral diseases after CSF was excluded. Bearing in mind high AD seroprevalence in that region, samples were initially screened for ADV, first by PCR and then by virus isolation on PCR positive samples. Serum samples were tested for ADV antibodies by VNT.

The samples were also tested for *Porcine Circovirus 2* (PCV2), *Porcine Parvovirus* (PPV), *Swine Influenza Virus* (SIV), *Porcine Respiratory Corona virus* (PRCV) and *Porcine Reproductive and Respiratory Syndrome Virus* (PRRSV) by serological and molecular methods. For antibody detection, commercial ELISA kits were used for PCV2 (Ingezim Circovirus IgG/IgM, ING1.1.PCV.K.2, Ingenasa, Spain), SIV (Ingezim Influenza A, ING 1.0.FKU.K.3, Ingenasa, Spain), PRCV (Ingezim Corona Diferencial 2.0, 11.DIF.K3, Ingenasa, Spain) and PRRS (Ingezim PRRS Universal, ING 1.1PRU.K1, Ingenasa, Spain). Hemagglutination inhibition test was used for PPV antibody detection using reference strain NADL-2 (ATCC® VR-742) at 4HU. Genome detection of those viruses was performed following previously published protocols [23–25].

DNA extraction and ADV PCR

DNA was extracted from pools of spleen and kidney tissues respectively using QIAamp DNA Mini Kit (Qiagen; Hilden, Germany), following the recommended tissue protocol.

The ul4 gene was amplified using previously published primers [26]. The PCR reaction was carried out in a total volume of 50 μL using HotStarTaq Master Mix Kit (Qiagen; Hilden, Germany) and 0.4 μM concentration of primers. The thermal profile for the PCR was 95 °C for 15 min, followed by 35 cycles of 95 °C for 1 min, 60 °C for 45 s and 72 °C for 1 min. The final extension step was performed at 72 °C for 5 min.

The amplified products were analysed by electrophoresis through 1.5 % agarose gel containing 0.5 mg/mL ethidium bromide. Each PCR run included positive and negative controls.

DNA sequencing and sequence analysis

Eight PCR positive tissue samples from wild boars and three ADV isolates from domestic pigs were amplified with primers for us4, used in screening PCR, us9 and ul49.5 following a previously published protocol [27]. Amplified products were purified with MinElute PCR Purification Kit (Qiagen; Hilden, Germany) and sequenced by Macrogen Europe (Amsterdam, The Netherlands). For phylogenetic analysis, MEGA software version 6, Basic Local Alignment Searching Tool (BLAST) (http://blast.ncbi.nlm.nih.gov/Blast.cgi) and ADV sequences available in GeneBank (NCBI) were used.

Newly described ADV us4, us9 and ul49.5 sequences are available from GenBank under accession numbers KT187309-KT187326, KT273927-KT273941.

Within this study, three ADV strains isolated during the last 6 years from domestic animals - domestic pig/2009 (KT187312, KT187318, KT187324), dog/2010 (KT187313, KT187319, KT187325), domestic pig/2014 (KT187314, KT187320, KT187326) were submitted to the GenBank and used for genetic comparison with isolates from wild boars.

Virus isolation and neutralisation

Positive PCR samples were prepared for virus isolation following the method described in OIE Terrestrial Manual (2012). Briefly, spleen and renal tissues were homogenized together in minimal essential medium with Earle's salts and L glutamine (MEM, Gibco BRL, USA) with addition of antibiotics. Homogenates were centrifuged at 900 g for 10 minutes and supernatants were used for inoculation in 24 well plates (Sarstedt, Germany) with 80-100 % confluent monolayer of PK15 (BS CL 72, IZS, Brescia, Italy) cells maintained with 5 % newborn bovine serum (Gibco BRL, USA) and 5 % CO_2 in air.

The cells were incubated at 37 °C and observed daily for CPE. In the samples where no CPE was observed, blind passage was performed by transferring of supernatant and inoculated tissue culture cells which were not demonstrating CPE to another plate containing fresh cells; in order to dilute out possible inhibitors and/or allow possible early viral replication due to low concentration of virus particles to progress to detectable CPE. If no CPE was evident after the second passage, the sample was considered negative.

To confirm the identity of the isolated virus, the cell culture supernatants were used in the neutralisation test with PRV S1 antiserum (CVI, Wageningen, Lelystad, Netherlands). The first aliquot was pre-incubated with PRV antiserum while the second aliquot was pre-incubated with a non-related serum of swine origin previously tested negative on VNT and ELISA test. Following pre-incubation at 37 °C for 1 h, the mixtures were inoculated into cell cultures. The virus isolate was considered to be ADV when the CPE was inhibited by the antiserum.

Virus neutralisation test (VNT)

Before the performance of virus neutralisation test the serum samples were heat-inactivated at 56 °C for 30 minutes. PK15 (BS CL 72, IZS, Brescia, Italy) cells used for VNT were maintained in the minimum essential medium (MEM; Gibco BRL, USA) containing 5 % fetal bovine serum (Gibco BRL, USA), with the addition of antibiotics and antimycotics. The ADV used for the VNT was NIA3 strain (CVI, Wageningen, Lelystad, The Netherlands). The VNT was carried out in 96-well microplates. Each serum sample was serially diluted by two folds and each dilution mixed with 100 $TCID_{50}$/50 μL of the virus. After 60 min of incubation at 37 °C, 100 μL of PK15 cells suspension was added to each well. Positive and negative control sera were included and tested the same way. VNT titre was determined after the plates had been incubated for 72 h at 37 °C. The antibody titres of serum samples were expressed as the reciprocal of the highest serum dilution completely inhibiting CPE in the wells. Serum samples neutralising the virus at any dilution were considered to be positive.

Statistical analysis

Ninety-five per cent confidence intervals (CI) for the standard errors (SE) were estimated from the expression se95% CI = 1 · 96(p [1−p])/n1/2.

To test for significant differences in seroprevalence and also virus-prevalence between gender and age groups, Z-test for two proportions was used. The level of significance was established at 5 %. Statistical analysis was performed using Social Science Statistics website[2].

Results

Wild boars were divided by age, determined by hunters, into three groups depending on number of permanent molars according to SCHEDA Ecological Associates, inc. (one molar 6–18 months, two molars 1.5-2.5 year, three molars over 2.5 years of age). The age group 6–18 months old wild boar consisted of 28 animals (females, $n = 13$; males, $n = 15$), the group 1.5-2.5 years old of five wild boars (females, $n = 3$; males, $n = 2$) and the group of animals older than 2.5 years of seven wild boars (females, $n = 3$; males, $n = 4$).

The majority of ill animals belonged to the age group 6–18 months old wild boar (females, $n = 6$; males, $n = 7$). Three wild boars belonged to the group 1.5-2.5 years old animals (females, $n = 1$; males, $n = 2$) and two to older than 2.5 years group (females, $n = 1$; males, $n = 1$). The most common symptoms described by hunters for the 18 ill wild boars were depression, dyspnea, slow movement, and no fear of humans. There was no evidence of any previous vaccination. Among 18 ill wild boars, there were 9 males (6–18 months old, $n = 7$; 1.5-2.5 years old, $n = 1$; older than 2.5 years, $n = 1$) and 9 females (6–18 months old, $n = 6$; 1.5-2.5 years old $n = 2$; older than 2.5 years, $n = 1$) (Fig. 1).

AD virus genome was detected in 8 of 40 samples (20 %). All PCR positive ($n = 8$) wild boars were reported to be ill and belonged to the group 6–18 months old wild boar (females, $n = 3$; males, $n = 5$) (Table 1). Based on partial us4, us9 and ul49.5 sequences, which are submitted to and available from NCBI GeneBank under accession numbers: KT187309, KT187310, KT187311, KT187315, KT187316, KT187317, KT187321, KT187322, KT187323, KT273927, KT273928, KT273929, KT273930, KT273931, KT273932, KT273933, KT273934, KT273935, KT273936, KT273937, KT273938, KT273939, KT273940, KT273941, and other available sequences for the same regions, wild boar and domestic animals ADV strains showed high similarity (Figs. 2, 3 and 4). The greatest distance between isolates from wild and domestic animals was observed for us9 gene (3 %), followed by ul49.5 (1 %). There was no distance between those groups of isolates for us4 gene. Comparing isolates from Serbian wild boars and other sequences used for phylogenetic analysis, 32 % distance was determined for us 9gene, 26 % for ul49.5 and 4 % for us4 gene. Certain distance, but highest for ul49.5 gene (6 %), was obvious between wild boar isolates and Bartha vaccine strain. However, no distance was observed between wild boar isolates based on any of three examined sequences.

ADV was isolated on PK 15 cells from 3 of 8 PCR positive samples. All isolates originated from pool of organs (kidney and spleen) from young (6–18 months old) male wild boars which were serologically negative. CPE was evident after 24 hours of incubation for one sample, and after 72 hours for the other two samples. Observed syncytia, different in size, were well developed. In the neutralisation test, all isolates were inhibited with antiserum, confirming the recovered viruses were ADV. No further virus isolations were obtained from negative samples by further blind passage.

Twenty-three out of 40 (57.5 %) serum samples had neutralising antibodies in the VNT against ADV.

Eight ill wild boars were negative by VNT, out of which four were PCR positive.

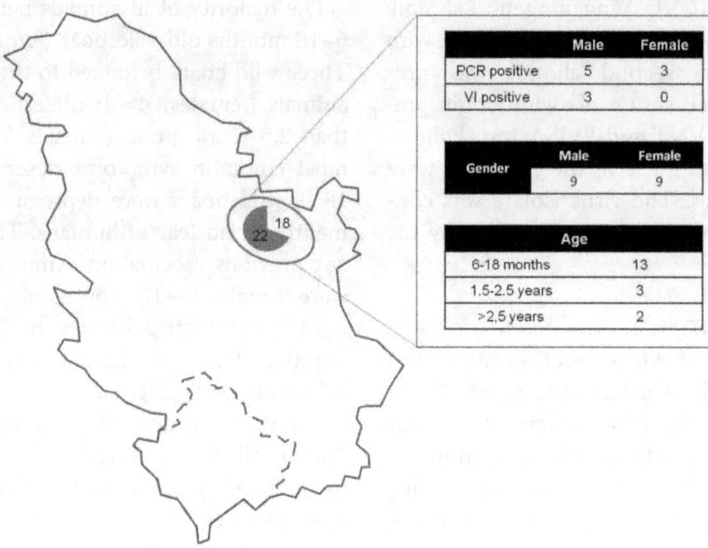

Fig. 1 Summarized results of ADV investigations in wild boar from Eastern Serbia where 18 ill wild boars were hunted

The other four PCR positive animals were seropositive by VNT, two at a titre of 1:8, and one each at titres of 1:16 and 1:64 (Fig. 5). The rest of ill animals had titres 1:64 ($n = 1$), 1:128 ($n = 3$), 1:256 ($n = 1$) and 1:512 ($n = 1$). Out of 9 ill males, 5 were negative by VNT, two had titre 1:8, and one each 1:64 and 1:256. Out of 9 ill females, 3 were negative by VNT and 6 had certain VN titre (1:16, $n = 1$; 1:64, $n = 1$; 1:128, $n = 3$; 1:512, $n = 1$)

Thirteen of 22 healthy wild boars were seropositive (Table 1), three at titre 1:8 (6–18 months old, $n = 3$), three at titre 1:16 (6–18 months old, $n = 2$; older than 2.5 years, $n = 1$), four at titre 1:64 (6–18 months old, $n = 2$, 1.5-2.5 year old, $n = 1$; older than 2.5 years, $n = 1$).

However, the results of this study did not show any statistically significant difference between neither genders nor age categories ($P > 0.05$)

PRRSV, PCV2, SIV, PRCV and PPV were not detected by molecular methods in samples from the 18 ill wild boars. Anti-PPV2 antibodies were detected in 11 of 18 serum samples (61.1 %). No antibodies to other viruses were detected.

No PRRSV, PCV2, SIV, PRCV, PPV and ADV were detected by molecular tests on samples from the 22 clinically healthy wild boars. Seroprevalence for ADV and PPV in that group were 59.1 % ($n = 13/22$) and 63.6 % ($n = 14/22$) respectively. No antibodies to other viruses were detected.

Discussion

Previous serological surveys conducted in wild boar in Serbia were limited but suggested a relatively high AD seroprevalence [28]. Lazic et al. (2014) [28] reported the mean prevalence of 38.21 % with the highest percentage among population older than 2.5 years - 46.86 %. However, neither virus nor clinical disease were reported in wild boar in Serbia[3].

Nasal swabs, oropharyngeal fluids and tonsil biopsies were reported as the samples of choice to be collected from live animals, and brain, tonsils [29], spleen and lung[4] from dead animals. Also, virus could be successfully isolated from vaginal secretions, ejaculates, milk, urine, rectal swab, even before the onset of clinical symptoms [20]. In this study, ADV was isolated from spleen and renal tissue samples, reported to be virus positive during active infection [29]. Wittnamm et al. [30] showed that, after experimental infection in piglets, the virus could not be detected in spleen, liver, and mediastinal lymph nodes; but could be demonstrated in kidneys, CNS and peripheral lymph nodes. Since we used samples already submitted for Classical Swine Fever monitoring, other tissue samples were not available. In this study, ADV was isolated on cell culture from 3 out of 8 PCR positive samples. Those 3 samples originated from seronegative wild boars. ADV was not isolated from one more seronegative but PCR positive animal. The discrepancy between results of virus isolation and PCR occurred due to the characteristics of the applied tests, their limitations and advantages. Presence of antigen-antibody complexes, cytotoxic substances, storage and transport conditions could significantly affect virus isolation requiring viable viruses in sample, in contrast with molecular tests detecting only genome fragments. Bearing in mind the characteristics of the applied tests, we presume that virus isolation failed in seropositive animals due to presence of antibodies, and in one sample from seronegative animal due to dependence

Table 1 Results of serological and molecular tests on spleen and renal samples to demonstrate AD in wild boar *(Sus Scrofa)* in Serbia by detecting anti-ADV antibodies and viral DNA

	Serology results										PCR results			
			Total		VN titre								Total	
Age group	Female	Male	No (%)	95 % CI	1:8	1:16	1:64	1:128	1:256	1:512	Female	Male	No (%)	95 % CI
	No (%)	No (%)			No (%)	No (%)	No (%)	No (%)	No (%)	No (%)	No (%)	No (%)		
6 - 18 months	7/13 (53,8)	7/15 (46,7)	14/28(50)	31,48-68,52	5/14(35,7)	3/14(21,4)	3/14(21,4)	3/14(21,4)	0/14(0)	0/14(0)	3/13(23,1)	5/15(33,3)	8/28(28,6)	11,86-45,34
1.5 - 2.5 years	2/3 (66,7)	2/2 (100)	4/5 (80)	44,94-115,06	0/4(0)	0/4(0)	1/4(25)	1/4(25)	1/4(25)	1/4(25)	0/3 (0)	0/3 (0)	0/6 (0)	0
>2,5 years	2/3 (66,7)	3/4 (75)	5/7(71,4)	37,92-104,88	0/5(0)	1/5(20)	2/5(40)	0/5(0)	2/5(40)	0/5(0)	0/3 (0)	0/3 (0)	0/6 (0)	0
Total	11/19 (57,9)	12/21 (57,1)	23/40(57,5)	42,18-72,82	5/23 (21,7)	4/23(17,4)	6/23(26,1)	4/23(17,4)	3/23(13)	1/23(4,3)	3/19 (15,8)	5/21(23,8)	8/40 (20)	7,6-32,4

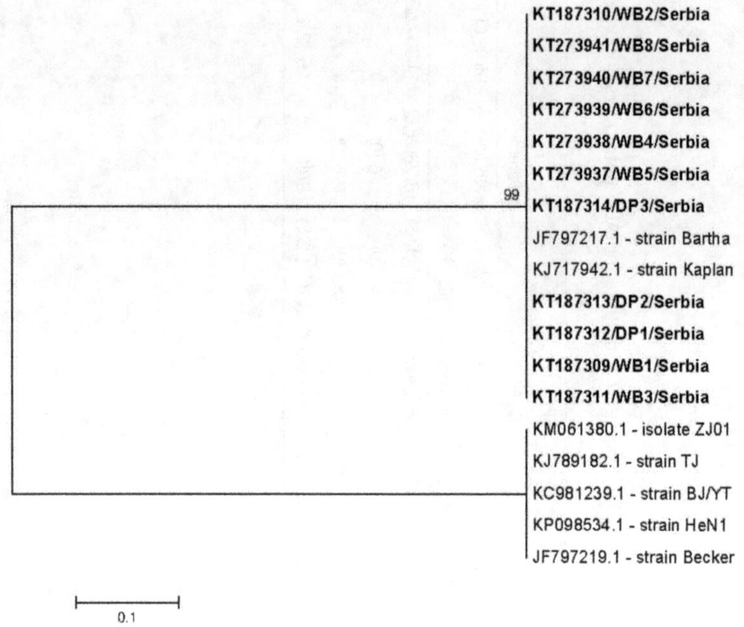

Fig. 2 Phylogenetic tree based on us4 sequence constructed using Maximum Parsimony Test. The analysis involved 18 nucleotide sequences. Codon positions included were 1st + 2nd + 3rd + Noncoding. All positions containing gaps and missing data were eliminated. Evolutionary analyses were conducted in MEGA6. Serbian sequences are in bold typewriting, identified by GenBank accession number/species/country. Numbers along the branches represent percentages of 1000 bootstrap iterations. WB: wild boar. DP1: domestic pig, DP2: dog, DP3: domestic pig

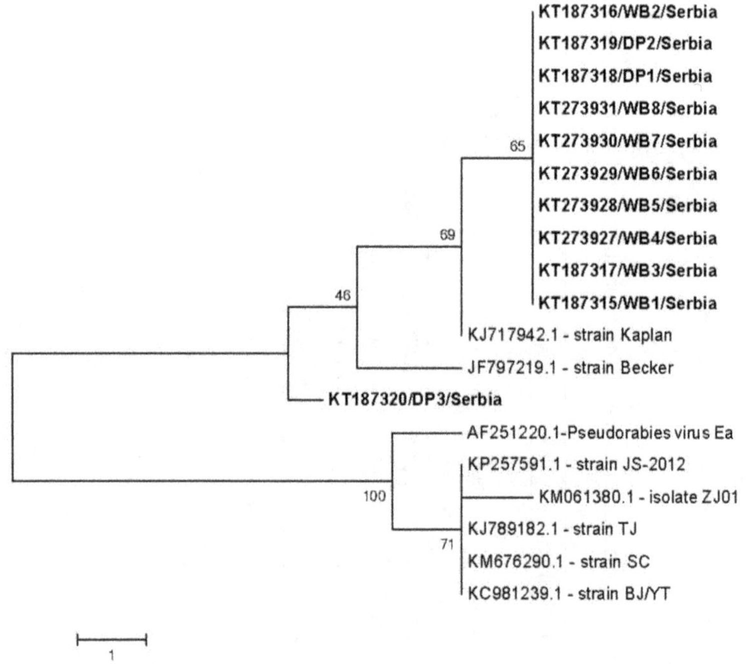

Fig. 3 Phylogenetic tree based on us9 sequence constructed using Maximum Parsimony Test. The analysis involved 19 nucleotide sequences. Codon positions included were 1st + 2nd + 3rd + Noncoding. All positions containing gaps and missing data were eliminated. Evolutionary analyses were conducted in MEGA6. Serbian sequences are in bold typewriting, identified by GenBank accession number/species/country. Numbers along the branches represent percentages of 1000 bootstrap iterations. WB: wild boar. DP1: domestic pig, DP2: dog, DP3: domestic pig

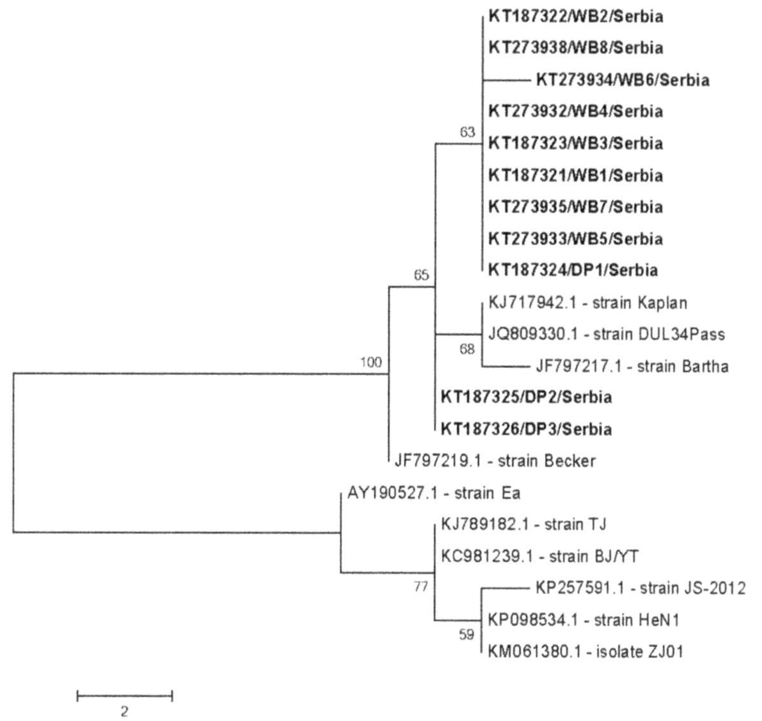

Fig. 4 Phylogenetic tree based on ul49.5 sequence constructed using Maximum Parsimony Test. The analysis involved 21 nucleotide sequences. Codon positions included were 1st + 2nd + 3rd + Noncoding. All positions containing gaps and missing data were eliminated. Evolutionary analyses were conducted in MEGA6. Serbian sequences are in bold typewriting, identified by GenBank accession number/species/country. Numbers along the branches represent percentages of 1000 bootstrap iterations. WB: wild boar. DP1: domestic pig, DP2: dog, DP3: domestic pig

of virus isolation on sample quality. The isolation of ADV from spleen and renal tissues and low serum antibody titres indicated those were cases of active ADV infection. Virus isolation was performed on the PK15 cell line where the virus induced syncytia, previously associated with virus pathogenicity [25]. Bitsch et al. [25] concluded that such isolates were highly pathogenic for pigs and cattle, although conversely lack of syncytia formation was not considered as an indicator of attenuation.

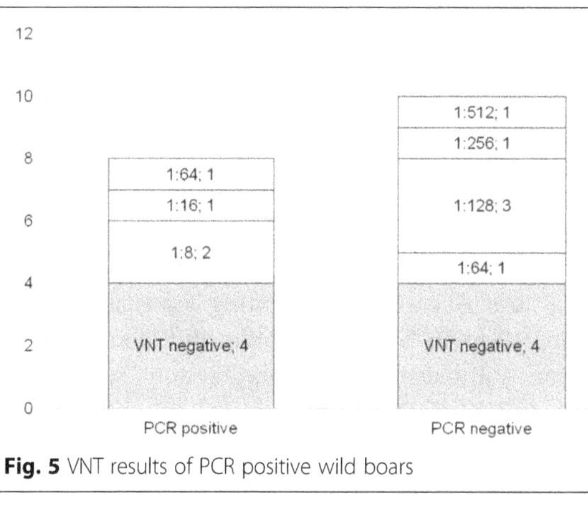

Fig. 5 VNT results of PCR positive wild boars

The highly developed syncytia observed in the study supported the conclusion the cause of the depression and other symptoms reported by the hunters was active AD.

The herpesvirus genome is highly conserved and most genes are not sufficiently variable for high–resolution phylogenetic analysis. With ADV slow rate of genetic evolution, genetic diversity within a population may be primarily caused by a high prevalence of infection [27].

According to partial ul44 gene, 5 groups of ADV could be distinguished, A-E. Strains isolated from feral pigs belonged to groups A and C, strains isolated from domestic pigs belonged to B and D groups. Group E was formed mainly of strains from Eastern regions, primarily China [4]. Fonseca et al. (2014) [26] found, analysing other genes, two clusters forming which separated viral isolates from East and West.

In this study, three partial sequences, (us4, us9 and ul49.5) were analized in order to increase the probability of detecting variation between the isolates from wild and domestic animals. However, the overall distance between isolates (eight wild boars, three domestic animals) as well as between viruses detected in the wild and domestic animals was negligible. This finding was consequence of the insufficient number of samples and a short sampling period, along with limited number of available sequences for those three regions in GeneBank. The biggest differences were observed for the us9 gene which encoded 11 kDa protein responsible for axonal transport, followed by ul49.5 gene encoding gN, involved in viral morphogenesis and membrane fusion. Analysis of gG sequence from Serbian wild boar and domestic animals isolates showed that the gene was highest conserved among examined genes. However, certain distance between isolates from wild and domestic animals indicated different origin of those strains, but no difference between isolates from wild boar, based on three genome sequences. The low genetic diversity, which is characteristic of herpesviruses, is also responsible for the low bootstrap values observed in the constructed trees.

Similar findings were reported by Keros et al., [31]. The authors reported that genetically identical viral strains belonging to Clade A were circulating in Croatia in wild boar and domestic pigs, according to the gC sequences derived from six domestic pigs and one wild boar. Furthermore, sequencing the gC genome fragment of ADV isolated from two hunting dogs confirmed the presence of Clade A genotype, similar to strains derived previously from domestic pigs and wild boars in Croatia [32].

Experimental infections showed that wild boar ADV isolates could be species adapted, leading to a different clinical and immunological response than in domestic pigs [1].

Manifested clinical symptoms are a product of virus virulence and dose, age of host animal and its reproductive and immunological status. They are the most observed in piglets and sows. The most affected age category in our study was young wild boars, 6–18 months old. Clinical signs expected in that category caused by ADV were rather nonspecific, i.e. depression, appetite loss, fever, cough etc. Pathomorphological signs were not typical or were absent. Such observations were reported by the hunters, but could not be linked to any specific disease.

Numerous reports have suggested that females have been more frequently infected with ADV [33–35]. Females are considered to be at higher risk of infection with ADV due to their different behaviour. Females live in groups in which contacts between animals are more frequent than among solitary males. Additionally, older and socially more active adults are at a higher risk of infection [36]. However, the results of this study did not show that there was any statistically significant difference between genders or age categories ($P > 0.05$). However, all ADV positive animals in this study were 6–18 months of age and it was consistent with the results from the outbreak in Spain where most affected animals were 4–8 months old [11]. Sample bias could not be excluded due to the majority of samples (70 %) being acquired from that age class.

Serological results showed that 50 % of wild boars 6–18 months of age were ADV antibody positive. High VN titres, higher than 1:128, which were seen in the age groups 1.5-2.5 years and more than 2.5 years, might be due to the higher stimulation of the immune system by a putative reactivated latency. Low VN titres in young animals and no neutralising antibodies in ADV positive animals indicated that this was a recent infection rather than latent virus reactivation. Verin et al. [37] demonstrated that serology tests could be negative in recently infected animals. Up to 45 % of animals with the virus in tonsils could be seronegative [34].

All PCR positive animals were hunted in one hunting ground (area of 44349 ha) with a total number of wild boars estimated at 100, leading to an estimated morbidity of 18 %. The seroprevalence in that hunting ground was 57.5 %, and in a previous survey 57 % (unpublished data). The seroprevalence in Spain affected by an outbreak in wild boar was also above 50 % [11].

ADV transmission depends on a direct contact between animals [20] but since the outbreak occurred in the less-inhabited area of Serbia, there was a low probability of contact between wild and domestic pigs, and consequently a low risk of ADV transmission to domestic pigs. So although feral pigs and wild boars were recognised as reservoirs of ADV [13, 38], the detection of active ADV infection within wild boar did not indicate they were a likely source of infection for domestic pigs. Nonetheless, the findings were supported that wild boar species was able to maintain infection without the presence of domestic pigs [35] and with no discernible effect on the population structure [37].

ADV infection affects the reproduction and health status of wild boars, particularly in piglets and the higher presence of viral genome in piglets and genital swabs also indicating both vertical and venereal transmission [37].

Nevertheless, a relatively low risk of transmission to domestic pigs still exists since there is evidence that ADV was spontaneously shed in the nasal secretion of a sow after parturition 19 months post infection with no clinical signs [39]. Additionally, daily migrations and frequent contacts with different subjects plays significant role in virus spreading [35].

There are many reports suggesting increase of population of wild boar in Europe, causing significant damage to agriculture. According to hunting associations, wild boar population in Serbia is stable. But domestic pigs production, still based on back yard system, with low or no biosecurity measures applied, is the critical place where the virus can enter domestic pig population and further on into intensive production systems.

The accurate diagnosis of AD can also be affected by previous vaccination of domestic pigs. There is evidence that the viruses from modified live vaccine (MLV) can be shed from the oronasal cavity [40], but Terpstra and Pol [41] showed that vaccination with MLV vaccines was not likely to interfere with the laboratory diagnosis of ADV field strains. However, since the attenuated virus replicates in the body and can be excreted, transmission to other animals, reverse mutations and genetic recombination with field strains cannot be excluded [42]. The most commonly used AD vaccine in Serbia for domestic pig vaccination is made using the attenuated Bartha strain, which minimizes field virus excretion comparing to inactivated vaccines [43]. Though, Gielkens at al. [44] reported two cases where the ADV field isolate, recovered from diseased pigs, was suspected to be of attenuated vaccine virus origin, they also did not exclude the possibility that the disease was caused by a virulent virus present in the herd before vaccination. Due to the long term vaccination of wild boars in Serbia, it was interesting to compare genome sequences between wild boar isolates and Bartha strain. Greatest distance of 6 % has been shown for ul49.5 gene, where Bartha strain, along with Kaplan and DUL34-pass strain, forms separated cluster.

Conclusions

Successful isolation of AD virus from tissues of wild boars showing signs of illness (depression, dyspnoea, slow movement) indicates that an AD outbreak did occur in Eastern Serbia during the winter 2014–2015. The hypothesis that this was a recent infection is supported by serological results showing low VN titre or no titre in virus positive animals. Furthermore, other viral diseases that could affect the health status of wild boar were excluded.

Genetic analysis based on three partial sequences showed that isolates from both domestic pigs and wild boars from East Serbia were very close to each other. Nevertheless, we presume that due to the different status and management between wild boar and domestic pigs, ADV can evolve but to follow this process genes, that exhibit evidence of positive selection, should be selected.

Endnotes

[1]See: Official Journal of the European Union: http://eur-lex.europa.eu/legal-content/EN/TXT/PDF/?uri=CELEX:32008D0185&from=EN (accessed March 2015)

[2]See: http://www.socscistatistics.com/pvalues/normaldistribution.aspx (accessed March 2015)

[3]See: World Animal Health Information Database (WAHID): http://www.oie.int/wahis_2/public/wahid.php/Diseaseinformation/Immsummary (accessed March 2015)

[4]See: The Merck Veterinary Manual: http://www.merckvetmanual.com/mvm/nervous_system/pseudorabies/overview_of_pseudorabies.html (accessed March 2015)

Abbreviations

AD, Aujeszky's disease; ADV, Aujeszky's disease virus; CI, confidence intervals; CPE, cytopatic effect; CSF, Classical Swine Fever; DNA, deoxyribonucleic acid; ELISA, enzyme-linked immunosorbent assay; NCBI, National Centre for Biotechnology Information; OIE, World Organisation for Animal Health; PCR, Polymerase Chain Reaction ; PCV2, *Porcine Circovirus2* ; PPV, *Porcine Parvovirus*; PR, Pseudorabies; PRCV, *Porcine Respiratory Corona virus*; PRRSV, *Porcine reproductive and respiratory syndrome virus*; PRV, Pseudorabies virus; SE, standard error; SHV1, *Suid Herpesvirus 1*; SIV, *Swine Influenza Virus*; TCID, tissue culture infective dose; UK, United Kingdom; VNT, virus neutralisation test; WAHID, World Animal Health Information System

Acknowledgements

This work was supported by the Ministry of Education, Science and Technological Development, Republic of Serbia (grant numbers TR31088, TR 31075).

Funding

This study has been funded by the Institute of Veterinary Medicine of Serbia.

Authors' contributions

VM carried out serological and molecular tests and drafted the manuscript. SR designed and coordinated the study. MV participated in sequence analysis and performed descriptive epidemiology. VI participated in sequence analysis and carried out phylogenetic trees. VR performed virus isolation and statistical analysis. All authors read and approved the final version of the manuscript.

Competing interests

The authors declare that they have no competing interests.

Consent for publication

Not applicable.

Ethics approval and consent to participate

In Serbia, this kind of study does not require formal ethical approval, since the samples originated from wild boars shot during the regular hunting seasons which were organized by Hunting Associations according to the Law on Hunting ("Sl. glasnik RS", br. 18/2010). Also, these samples were initially tested on Classical Swine Fever according to the Monitoring plan issued by the Ministry of Agriculture and Environmental protection (No 323-02-6816/2014-05 from 27.11.2014).

Author details

[1]Virology department, Institute of Veterinary Medicine of Serbia, Vojvode Toze 14, 11000 Belgrade, Serbia. [2]Infectious Animals Diseases and Diseases of Bees, Faculty of Veterinary Medicine, Bulevar oslobodjenja 18, 11000 Belgrade, Serbia. [3]Department of Biodiversity, University of Primorska, Faculty of Mathematics, Natural Sciences and Information Technologies, Glagoljaska 8, SI-6000 Koper, Slovenia. [4]Institute of Veterinary Medicine of Serbia, Vojvode Toze 14, 11000 Belgrade, Serbia.

References

1. Muller TF, Teuffert J, Zellmer R, Conraths FJ. Experimental infection of European wild boars and domestic pigs with pseudorabies viruses with differing virulence. Am J Vet Res. 2001;62:252–58.
2. Klupp BG, Hengartner CJ, Mettenleiter TC, Enquist LW. Complete, annotated sequence of the pseudorabies virus genome. J Virol. 2004;78:424–40.

3. Herrmann G, Heppner B, Ludwig H. Pseudorabies viruses from clinical outbreaks and latent infections group into four genome types. In: Wittmann G, Gaskell RM, Rziha HJ, editors. Latent herpesvirus infections in veterinary medicine. Dordrecht: Martinus Nijhoff; 1984. p. 387–401.
4. Fonseca A, Camargos MF, Sales ML, Heinemann MB, Leite RC, Reis JKP. Pseudorabies virus can be classified into five genotypes using partial sequences of UL44. Braz J Microbiol. 2012;43:1632–40.
5. Schollum L. Aujeszky's disease: epidemiology. Surveill. 1987;14:16–21.
6. Meng XJ, Lindsay DS, Sriranganathan N. Wild boars as sources for infectious diseases in livestock and humans. Philos Trans Royal Society B: Biol Sci. 2009;364:2697–707.
7. Ruiz-Fons F, Segalés J, Gortázar CA. A review of viral diseases of the European wild boar: effects of population dynamics and reservoir role. Vet J. 2008;176:158–69.
8. Schulze C, Hlinak A, Wohlsein P, Kutzer P, Muller T. Spontaneous Aujeszky's disease (pseudorabies) in European wild boars (Sus scrofa) in the federal state of Brandenburg, Germany. Berl Munch Tierarztl Wochenschr. 2010;123:359–64.
9. Kluge JP, Beran GW, Hill HT, Platt KB. Pseudorabies (Aujeszky's disease). In: Straw BE, D'Allaire S, Mengeling WL, Taylor DJ, editors. Diseases of Swine. 8th ed. Ames: Iowa State University Press; 1999. p. 233–46.
10. Pusic I, Prodanov-Radulovic J, Dosen R, Stojanov I, Stojanovic D, Petrovic T. Epizootical characteristics of Aujeszky's disease in Vojvodina region and biosecurity concernes. Biotechnol Anim Husbandry. 2011;27:875–82.
11. Gortazar C, Vicente J, Fierro Y, Leon L, Cubero MJ, Gonzalez M. Natural Aujeszky's disease in a Spanish wild boar population. Ann N Y Acad Sci. 2002;969:210–12.
12. Muller T, Klupp B, Zellmer R, Teuffert J, Ziedler K, Possardt C, Mewes L, Dresenkamp B, Conraths FJ, Mettenleiter TC. Characterisation of pseudorabies virus isolated from wild boar (*Sus scrofa*). Vet Rec. 1998;143:337–40.
13. Lipowski A. European wild boar (*Sus scrofa L.*) as a reservoir of infectious diseases for domestic pigs. Med Weterynaryja. 2003;59:861–63.
14. Elbers ARW, Dekkers LJM, Van Der Giessen JWB. Sero-surveillance of wild boar in the Netherlands, 1996–1999. Rev Sci Tech. 2000;19:848–54.
15. Anon. Surveillance of zoonotic and other animal disease agents in Sweden 2010, The National Veterinary Institute (SVA). Uppsala: SVA:s rapportserie 22 ISSN; 2010. p. 1654–7098.
16. Zupancic Z, Jukic B, Lojkic M, Cac Z, Jemersic L, Staresina V. Prevalence of antibodies to classical swine fever, Aujeszky's disease, porcine reproductive and respiratory syndrome, and bovine viral diarrhoea viruses in wild boars in Croatia. J Vet Med B Infect Dis Vet Public Health. 2002;49:253–6.
17. Lari A, Lorenzi D, Nigrelli D, Brocchi E, Faccini S, Poli A. Pseudorabies virus in European wild boar from central Italy. J Wildl Dis. 2006;42:319–24.
18. Boadella M, Vicente J, Ruiz-Fons F, de la Fuente J, Gortazar C. Effects of culling Eurasian wild boar on the prevalence of mycobacterium bovis and Aujeszky's disease virus. Prev Vet Med. 2012;107:214–21.
19. Pannwitz G et al. A longterm serological survey on Aujeszky's disease virus infections in wild boar in East Germany. Epidemiol Infect. 2012;140:348–58.
20. Murphy AF, Gibbs EPJ, Horzinek CM, Studdert JM. Veterinary virology. Thirdth ed. London: Academic Press, UK; 1999. p. 312–14.
21. Pesjak ZK, Truszczynsky M. Aujeszky's disease (Pseudorabies). In: Straw BE, Zimmerman JJ, D'Allaire S, Taylor DJ, editors. Diseases of swine. 9th ed. Oxford: Blackwell Science, UK; 2006. p. 419–33.
22. Capua I, Casaccia C, Calzetta G, Caporale V. Characterization of Aujeszky's disease viruses isolated from domestic animals and from a wild boar (*Sus scrofa*) in Italy between 1972 and 1995. Vet Microbiolgy. 1997;51:143–49.
23. Huang C, Hung JJ, Wu CY, Chien MS. Multiplex PCR for rapid detection of pseudorabies virus, porcine parvovirus and porcine circoviruses. Vet Microbiol. 2004;101:209–14.
24. Song DS et al. Multiplex reverse transcription-PCR for rapid differential detection of porcine epidemic diarrhea virus, transmissible gastroenteritis virus, and porcine group a rotavirus. J Vet Diagn Investig. 2006;18:278–81.
25. Kim J, Han DU, Choi C, Chae C. Simultaneous detection and differentiation between porcine circovirus and porcine parvovirus in boar semen by miltiplex seminested polymerase chain reaction. J Vet Med Sci. 2003;65:741–4.
26. Hermann JR, Hoff SJ, Yoon KJ, Burkhardt AC, Evans RB, Zimmerman JJ. Optimization of a sampling system for recovery and detection of airborne porcine reproductive and respiratory syndrome virus and swine influenza virus. Appl Environ Microbiol. 2006;72:4811–8.
27. Fonseca AA, Sales EB, Heinemann MB, Jenner KP, Reis JKP. Molecular Phylogeny of Suid Herpesvirus 1. ISRN Virology. 2014. doi:10.1155/2014/463173.
28. Lazic S, Plavsic B, Polacek V, Lupulovic D, Milicevic V, Veljovic L, Lazic G, Prodanov-Radulovic J, Bugarski D, Petrovic T. Testing the presence of Aujeszky disease among wild boars in Republic of Serbia. In: Petrovic T, editor. Book of abstracts of the XVII epozootiology and epidemiology symposium. Subotica: Serbian Veterinary Society: Section for Zoonoses; 2015. p. 70–1.
29. Spickler AR. Emerging and Exotic Diseases of Animals, Fourth Ed. Ames: CFSPH Iowa State University, USA. 2010.p.329.
30. Wittmann G, Jakubik J, Ahl R. Multiplication and distribution of Aujeszky's disease (pseudorabies) virus in vaccinated and non-vaccinated pigs after intranasal infection. Arch Virol. 1980;66:227–40.
31. Keros T, Brnic D, Prpic J, Dezdek D, Jemersic L, Roic B, Bedekovic T. Characterisation of pseudorabies virus in domestic pigs and wild boars in Croatia. Acta Vet Hung. 2014;62:512–19.
32. Keros T, Jemersic L, Brnic D, Prpic J, Dezdek D. Pseudorabies in hunting dogs in Croatia with phylogenetic analysis of detected strains. Vet Rec Case Rep. 2015;3:1 e000181. doi:10.1136/vetreccr-2015-000181.
33. Vicente J, Ruiz-Fons F, Vidal D, Hofle U, Acevedo P, Villanúa D, Fernandez-de-Mera G, Martín MP, Gortazar C. Serosurvey of Aujeszky's disease virus infection in European wild boar in Spain. Vet Rec. 2005;156:408–12.
34. Ruiz-Fons F, Vidal D, Hofle U, Vicente J, Gortazar C. Aujeszky's disease virus infection patterns in European wild boar. Vet Microbiol. 2007;120:241–50.
35. Ruiz-Fons F. Aujeszky's Disease, or Preudorabies. In: Gavier-Widen D, Meredith A, Daff JP, editors. Infectious Diseases of Wild Mammals and Birds in Europe. Oxford: Wiley-Blackwel, 2012. p. 1–36.
36. Van der Leek ML, Becker HN, Pirtle EC, Humphrey P, Adams CL, All BP, Erickson A, Belden RC, Frankenberger, WB, Gibbs EP. Prevalence of pseudorabies (Aujeszky's disease) virus antibodies in feral swine in Florida. J Wildl Dis. 1993;29:403–9.
37. Verin R, Varuzza P, Mazzei M, Poli A. Serologic, molecular, and pathologic survey of pseudorabies virus infection in hunted wild boars (*Sus scrofa*) in Italy. J Wildl Dis. 2014;50:559–65.
38. Lee JYS, Wilson MR. A review of pseudorabies (Aujeszky's disease) in pigs. Can Vet J. 1979;20:65–6.
39. Wittmann G, Rziha HJ, Doller PC. Occurence of clinical Aujeszky's disease in immunosupressed latently infected pigs. Curr Top Vet Med Anim Sci. 1982;7:211–9.
40. De Leeuw PW, Tiessink JWA. Evaluation of Aujeszky's Disease Virus Vaccine. In: Nielsen NC, Hogh P, Bille N, editors. Proceedings of International Pig Veterinary Society, Copenhagen, Denmark: International Pig Veterinary Society, 1980. p.112.
41. Terpstra C, Pol JMA. Influence of vaccination with modified live vaccine on the laboratory diagnosis of Aujeszky's disease. In: Witman G, Hall SA, editors. Current topics in veterinary medicine and animal science. Germany.: Tubingen; 1981. p. 57–65.
42. Wittmann G. Aujeszky's disease: factors important for epizootiology and control. Sci Tech Rev Off Int des Epizooties (Paris). 1985;4:5–20.
43. Nauwynck HJ, Zonnekeyn V, Pensaert MB. Virological protection of sows upon challenge with Aujeszky's disease virus after multiple vaccinations with attenuated or inactivated vaccines. Zentralbl Veterinarmed B. 1997;44:609–15.
44. Gielkens JA, Van Oirschot JT, Berns AJM. Genome differences among field isolates and vaccine strains of pseudorabies virus. J Gen Virol. 1985;66:69–82.

4

New isolations of the rabies-related Mokola virus

Jessica Coertse[1], Wanda Markotter[1], Kevin le Roux[2], Daniel Stewart[3], Claude T. Sabeta[4] and Louis H. Nel[5*]

Abstract

Background: Mokola virus (MOKV) is a rabies-related lyssavirus and appears to be exclusive to the African continent. Only 24 cases of MOKV, which includes two human cases, have been reported since its identification in 1968. MOKV has an unknown reservoir host and current commercial vaccines do not confer protection against MOKV.

Results: We describe three new isolations of MOKV from domestic cats in South Africa. Two cases were retrospectively identified from 2012 and an additional one in 2014.

Conclusions: These cases emphasize the generally poor surveillance for rabies-related lyssaviruses and our inadequate comprehension of the epidemiology and ecology of *Mokola lyssavirus* per se.

Keywords: Mokola virus, Lyssavirus, Rabies-related, South Africa

Background

The *Lyssavirus* genus currently consists of 14 recognized species all capable of causing rabies, a fatal encephalitic disease. The prototype species of this genus is *Rabies lyssavirus* and the rest are known as the rabies-related lyssaviruses [1]. Mokola virus (MOKV), a rabies-related lyssavirus, was first isolated from shrews in the Mokola forest in Nigeria in the late 1960s [2, 3]. Shortly thereafter, MOKV was reported as the causative agent of a neurological disease in two children from Nigeria [4, 5]. However, these reports remain controversial for a variety of reasons. The first isolation was made from the cerebrospinal fluid of a 3.5-year-old girl in 1968. The girl recovered without any neurological sequelae while no virus neutralizing antibodies (VNAs) were detected [4]. This is unexpected as reports of patients surviving rabies are exceptionally rare. In the majority of survivor cases the patient is burdened with moderate to severe neurological sequelae [6, 7] with VNAs regarded as a primary mechanism of viral clearance [6, 8]. The second human isolate was obtained from the brain tissue of a 6-year-old girl in 1971 that died from suspected meningitis or encephalitis. In both these human cases clinical symptoms were atypical for classical rabies virus (RABV) infection [5]. It is doubtful that these isolates are still in existence and no genetic information is available [9].

Up until 2013, only 18 confirmed MOKV isolations, from a variety of mammalian host species including shrews, cats, dogs and a rodent (*Lophuromys sikapusi*), were known to exist [9]. MOKV was first encountered in South Africa in 1970, when the virus was isolated from a domestic cat in the KwaZulu-Natal (KZN) province [10]. In 1981, it became evident that the available rabies vaccines did not confer protection against MOKV when this virus was isolated from vaccinated cats and a dog in Zimbabwe [11]. It appears that MOKV is exclusive to the African continent and all isolations for the last 20 years have been made from southern Africa. Little is known about the epidemiology of this lyssavirus and the problem is compounded by an unknown reservoir and limited surveillance throughout the continent. In the few instances where rabies diagnostic facilities are available and operational in Africa, only the fluorescent antibody test (FAT) is used. The FAT relies on the use of a polyclonal fluorescein isothiocyanate conjugated anti-lyssavirus globulin that is capable of detecting all known lyssavirus species but cannot distinguish between them. As a result, positive cases are reported as rabies but the actual causative lyssavirus species is rarely identified. In South Africa, where molecular characterization of FAT-positive samples is frequently done, the majority of MOKV isolations have been from the KZN (n=4) and

* Correspondence: louis.nel@up.ac.za
[5]Department of Microbiology and Plant Pathology, Faculty of Natural and Agricultural Sciences, University of Pretoria, Pretoria 0001, South Africa
Full list of author information is available at the end of the article

Eastern Cape (EC) provinces (n=5) with a single isolation reported from the Mpumalanga province. These isolates differ by between 0–5.7% and 0–2% at the nucleotide and amino acid levels of the nucleoprotein (N) gene. However, comparison of the N-gene of all known MOKV isolates demonstrated variations of up to 15% and 6.4% on the nucleotide and amino acids levels respectively [9].

Rabies virus (RABV) vaccines do not protect against MOKV [9, 11, 12] and it should be appreciated that the domestic cat is the most commonly MOKV-infected host species. The frequent contact between cats and their owners suggests a potential risk of spill-over infection to humans. Considering this situation, it is clear that a better understanding of the incidence and ecology of MOKV ecology is of utmost importance. Here we report the isolation and characterization of three MOKV isolations from cats from KZN, South Africa, 4 years after the last isolation of this virus in 2008 from South Africa. The first case was identified in January 2014 and subsequently a small retrospective study on selected samples was undertaken, identifying an additional two cases from 2012.

Methods

The study

In January 2014, a private veterinarian submitted brain material from a domestic cat that had died of suspected rabies in Pietermaritzburg, KZN, South Africa (laboratory reference number: 14/024) to the Allerton Provincial Veterinary Laboratory. The FAT was performed by staining acetone-fixed impression smears of the brain material with a polyclonal fluorescein isothiocyanate conjugated anti-lyssavirus globulin (OIE Rabies Reference Laboratory of the Agricultural Research Council-Onderstepoort Veterinary Institute (ARC-OVI), South Africa) [13]. Lyssavirus antigen was observed, but in this specific case the staining was of dull fluorescence clearly atypical of rabies virus positive samples. Such atypical staining which has previously been noted in MOKV infections prompted further investigation of this case. The positive FAT result was confirmed at the OIE Rabies Reference Laboratory at Onderstepoort (ARC-OVI, South Africa) and the sample genetically characterized at the University of Pretoria. Following the subsequent identification of sample 14/024 as MOKV, it was decided to investigate and molecularly characterize other FAT positive rabies samples from domestic animals from throughout KZN. Selected archived samples (n=36), were characterized by nucleotide sequencing resulting in the identification of an additional two MOKV cases.

RNA extraction, RT-PCR and phylogenetic analysis

Total RNA was isolated from brain material using Trizol reagent (Invitrogen) according to the manufacturer's instructions. The complete N-, phosphoprotein- (P), matrix protein- (M) and glycoprotein (G) genes were sequenced using different primer combinations and cycling conditions (Additional file 1: Table S1) for all MOKV samples. Briefly, reverse transcription was performed for all samples using the following protocol: 10 pmol of forward primer was added to 5 μl total RNA and incubated at 94 °C for 1 min. These reactions were cooled on ice for 5 min followed by reverse transcription for 90 min at 42 °C in a final volume of 20 μl containing 1 x reverse transcriptase buffer (containing 250 mM Tris-HCl, 40 mM $MgCl_2$, 150 mM KCl, 5 mM dithiothreithol, Roche), 2.2 μl dNTP mix (10 mM, Promega), 8 U Avian myeloblastosis virus reverse transcriptase (Roche) and 16 U Recombinant RNasin Ribonuclease inhibitor (Promega). The genes were subsequently amplified using 20 μl cDNA in a final volume of 100 μl containing 1 x DreamTaq Buffer (containing KCl, $(NH4)_2SO_4$ and 20 mM $MgCl_2$, Thermo Scientific), 10 pmol of forward primer (Additional file 1: Table S1), 12.5 pmol reverse primer (Additional file 1: Table S1) and 1.25 U DreamTaq DNA polymerase (Thermo Scientific). Analysis and sequencing of PCR products were performed as described previously [14]. Nucleotide sequences were edited and assembled using BioEdit Sequence Alignment Editor Version 7 [15]. The partial N-gene for RABV sequences (Additional file 2: Table S2) or concatenated and individual genes for MOKV sequences (Additional file 3: Table S3) was analyzed with jModeltest 2 [16] for each dataset to determine the most appropriate substitution model. Data was analyzed using BEAST v.1.8 [17] using a random starting tree with a strict clock for each dataset and assuming an exponential population growth with Markov Chain Monte Carlo (MCMC) chains of 50 million generations.

Virus isolation

Virus was isolated from MOKV samples on murine neuroblastoma cells as described previously [18].

Results

The partial N-gene sequences (using primers 001lys/550B, Additional file 1: Table S1) [19] of the 36 samples were determined and subsequent to the analyses two more MOKV cases were identified i.e. 12/458 and 12/604 (Table 1). Based on partial N-gene sequences, the remaining 33 archival samples were determined to be the canid variant of RABV. Bayesian analysis indicated that all new RABV sequences group with other RABV sequences from the same time period (Fig. 1).

Table 1 Information of domestic animals from the KwaZulu-Natal province submitted for molecular characterization

Laboratory reference number	Host	Collection area	Date	Genbank accession number (gene)
07/30	*Felis catus* (feline)	Empangeni	11/01/2007	KP994621
07/76	*Felis catus* (feline)	Melmoth	29/01/2007	KP994616
08/105	*Felis catus* (feline)	Kwadukuza	18/02/2008	KP994617
08/426	*Felis catus* (feline)	Jozini	03/07/2008	KP994618
08/642	*Felis catus* (feline)	Exodondakukuska	15/10/2008	KP994619
09/353	*Felis catus* (feline)	Nkambanana	07/08/2009	KP994620
10/268	*Canis familiaris* (canine)	Umdoni	20/05/2010	KJ744302
10/274	*Canis familiaris* (canine)	Hibiscus coast	24/05/2010	KJ744308
10/387	*Canis familiaris* (canine)	Umzumbe	23/08/2010	KJ744303
10/458	*Capra aegagrus hircus* (goat)	Umzimkulu	29/09/2010	KJ744309
10/509	*Canis familiaris* (canine)	Mkhambathini	22/10/2010	KJ744304
10/598	*Felis catus* (feline)	Dundee	16/11/2010	KP994606
11/28	*Canis familiaris* (canine)	Richmond	14/01/2011	KP994597
11/185	*Canis familiaris* (canine)	Mkahambathini	24/03/2011	KJ744305
11/195	*Canis familiaris* (canine)	Mkhambathini	28/03/2011	KP944598
11/217	*Canis familiaris* (canine)	Umdoni	12/04/2011	KJ744310
11/300	*Canis familiaris* (canine)	Richmond	30/05/2011	KJ744307
11/419	*Felis catus* (feline)	Ethekweni	16/08/2011	KP994607
12/069	*Felis catus* (feline)	Okhalamba	31/01/2012	KP994610
12/458	*Felis catus* (feline)	Durban	13/06/2012	KP899610(N), KP899619(P), KP899613(M), KP899616(G)
12/604	*Felis catus* (feline)	Durban	08/07/2012	KP899611(N), KP899620(P), KP899614(M), KP899617(G)
12/696	*Felis catus* (feline)	Ethekweni	27/07/2012	KP994608
12/903	*Felis catus* (feline)	Okhahlamba	02/10/2013	KP994609
13/058	*Felis catus* (feline)	Ethekweni	25/01/2013	KP994611
13/079	*Canis familiaris* (canine)	Umlazi	01/02/2013	KP994601
13/104	*Canis familiaris* (canine)	Amanzimtoti	14/02/2013	KP994599
13/107	*Canis familiaris* (canine)	Westville	18/02/2013	KP994602
13/167	*Canis familiaris* (canine)	Adams mission	18/03/2013	KP994612
13/256	*Canis familiaris* (canine)	Amanzimtoti	09/05/2013	KP994613
13/310	*Canis familiaris* (canine)	Umkomaas	10/06/2013	KP994603
13/339	*Canis familiaris* (canine)	Umlazi	21/06/2013	KP994614
13/355	*Canis familiaris* (canine)	Amanzimtoti	28/06/2013	KP994615
13/522	*Canis familiaris* (canine)	Athlone Park	27/09/2013	KP994604
13/525	*Canis familiaris* (canine)	Lewis Drive	30/09/2013	KP994605
13/589	*Canis familiaris* (canine)	Uthukela	29/10/2013	KP994600
14/024	*Felis catus* (feline)	Pietermaritzburg	09/01/2014	KP899612(N), KP899621(P), KP899615(M), KP899618(G)

Details and clinical history of the cats that tested positive for MOKV are summarized in Table 2. For all the MOKV cases, the complete sequences of four structural genes (i.e. N-, P-, M- and G genes) were determined.

For all the MOKV cases, the complete coding region sequence of four structural genes (i.e. N-, P-, M-, and G-genes) were determined. Each dataset (concatenated or individual genes) were analysed using a Bayesian approach. The tree topology (Fig. 2) observed was similar irrespective of the gene used for analysis (Additional file 4: Figure S1, Additional file 5: Figure S2, Additional file 6: Figure S3, Additional file 7: Figure S4) with the exception

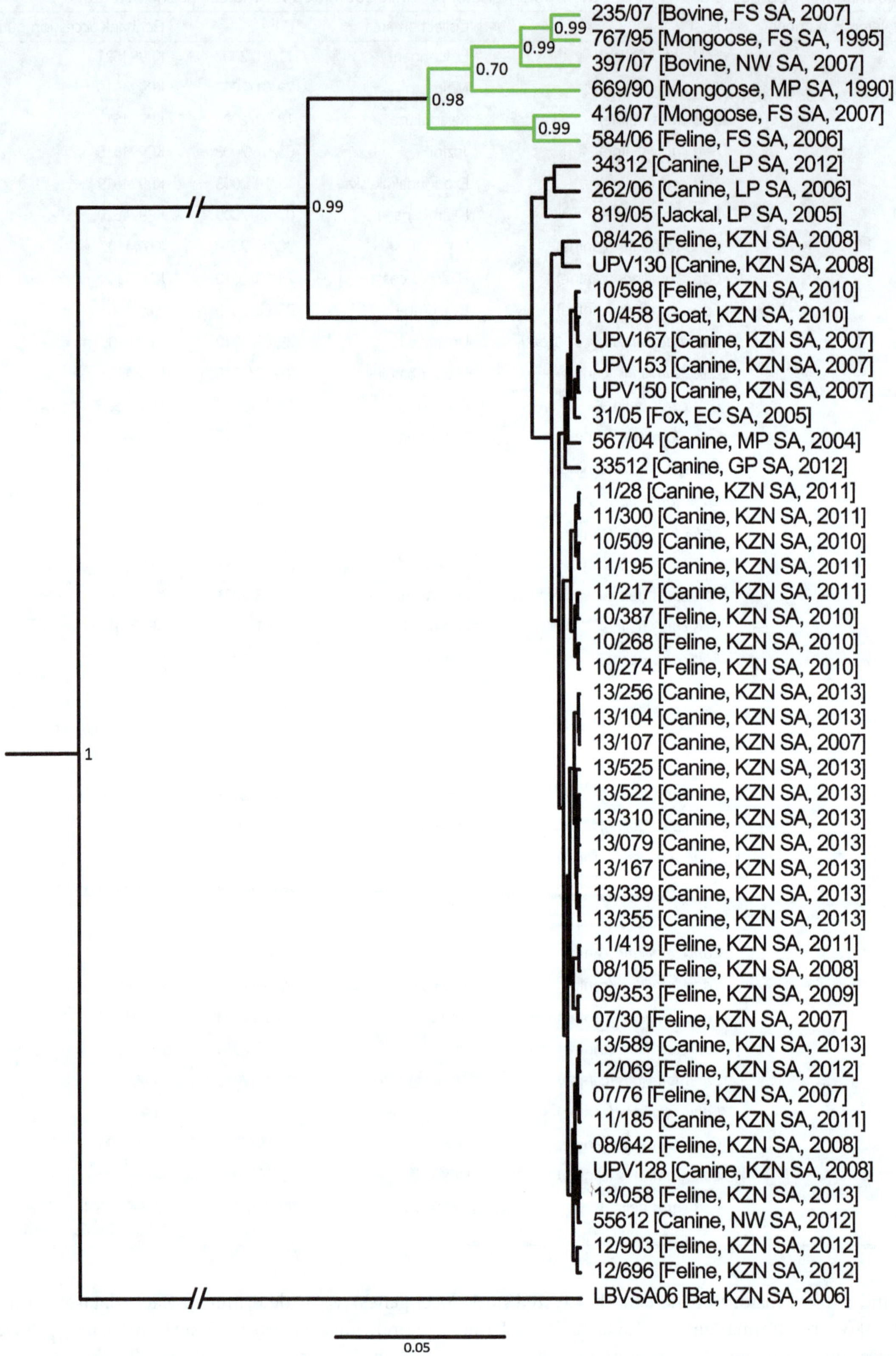

Fig. 1 (See legend on next page.)

(See figure on previous page.)

Fig. 1 Bayesian analysis of the partial N-gene sequences (540 bp) of the 33 archival samples and other rabies virus sequences from South Africa (Additional file 2: Table S2) applying the general time reversible substitution model with gamma distribution. Laboratory reference numbers are shown for all sequences, followed by the host species, country of origin (EC SA: Eastern Cape province, South Africa; FS SA: Free State province, South Africa; GP SA: Gauteng province, South Africa; KZN SA: Kwa-Zulu Natal province, South Africa; LP SA: Limpopo province, South Africa; MP SA: Mpumalanga province, South Africa; NW SA: North West province, South Africa) and year. All rabies virus sequences determined in this study are indicated in blue

of the M-gene. For the M-gene dataset (Additional file 6: Figure S3), isolate RV4 (from Nigeria) grouped with an isolate from Zimbabwe (posterior probability = 0.8144) and not with the isolate from the Central African Republic as observed for the other datasets. This support findings from previous studies that MOKV phylogeny is strongly influenced by geographical derivation [9]. For the isolates from South Africa, two separate clusters were found to represent isolates from the two provinces viz. KZN and EC. Within the KZN cluster, the new MOKV isolates form a well-supported new clade. Nucleotide divergence of all known MOKV isolates (Additional file 8: Table S4, Additional file 9: Table S5, Additional file 10: Table S6 and Additional file 11: Table S7) ranged from 0.1-13.9%, 0-25.2%, 0-17.8% and 0.2-19.6% for the N-, P-, M- and G-genes respectively.

Discussion

There is no active surveillance for rabies-related lyssaviruses in Africa and subsequently the epidemiology of these viruses remains obscure. Rabies, caused by RABV, is endemic in KZN, South Africa and has been tackled through mass vaccination campaigns [20]. As a result, the annual number of suspected and confirmed rabies cases in dogs has decreased due to an enhanced awareness about the disease. This in turn has led to veterinary laboratories and veterinarians identifying unusual cases of animals displaying rabies symptoms. More cases (and isolations) of rabies-related lyssaviruses should occur in future – like the cases described here. Identification of infections caused by rabies-related viruses is important and any additional information may improve our understanding of the epidemiology of these viruses. However, the recommended diagnostic technique for rabies, the FAT, cannot distinguish between the lyssavirus species. A broad-spectrum polyclonal fluorescein isothiocyanate conjugated anti-lyssavirus globulin, capable of detecting all lyssavirus species, is used in countries with laboratory diagnostics. In some MOKV cases atypical staining, i.e. the inclusions stain less intensely than is usually seen with rabies virus, has been observed [21]; as described for sample 14/024. The identification of a MOKV infection prompted a small retrospective study to determine if other MOKV cases, which did not produce atypical staining with the FAT, were overlooked. Subsequently, 35 samples collected over a 7 year period were tested and two additional MOKV cases from 2012 were identified. The remaining 33 samples were shown to belong to the canid variant of RABV.

In southern Africa, two variants of RABV circulate i.e. the canid variant infecting members of the *Canidae* family and the mongoose variant infecting members of the *Herpestidae* [22]. The conserved N-gene used in the Bayesian analysis is not ideally suited to distinguish between closely related viral variants. Nevertheless, the RABV sequences determined in this study all grouped with other canid variant RABV sequences from the same time period which is indicative of the continued rabies epidemical cycle in domestic dogs that was established in 1976 [23].

Bayesian analysis including all known MOKV isolates demonstrated a pattern of grouping of viruses according to geographical origin, irrespective of the gene(s) used; in agreement with previous reports [9]. The South African isolates grouped according to province – KZN and EC cluster. All previous isolates from KZN collected over a 28 year period (1970–1998) displayed a variation of 2.3% and 0.7% at the nucleotide and amino acid levels of the N-gene respectively. When comparing the new isolates from 2012–2014 (14 years after the last isolation

Table 2 Details and clinical history of cats from the KwaZulu-Natal province, South Africa that tested positive for Mokola virus

	Laboratory reference number		
	14/024	12/458	12/604
Location	Pietermaritzburg	Durban	Durban
Host details	Male, 4-year-old	Female, 1-year-old	Female, 1-year-old
Clinical signs	Fever (>40 °C), ataxia convulsions	Fever (39.6 °C), ataxia, decreased appetite	Growling, aggression, ataxia
Clinical duration	8-9 January 2014	10-13 June 2012	6-8 July 2012
Clinical outcome	Died of the disease	Euthanized after collapsing and being non-responsive	Euthanized after being non-responsive

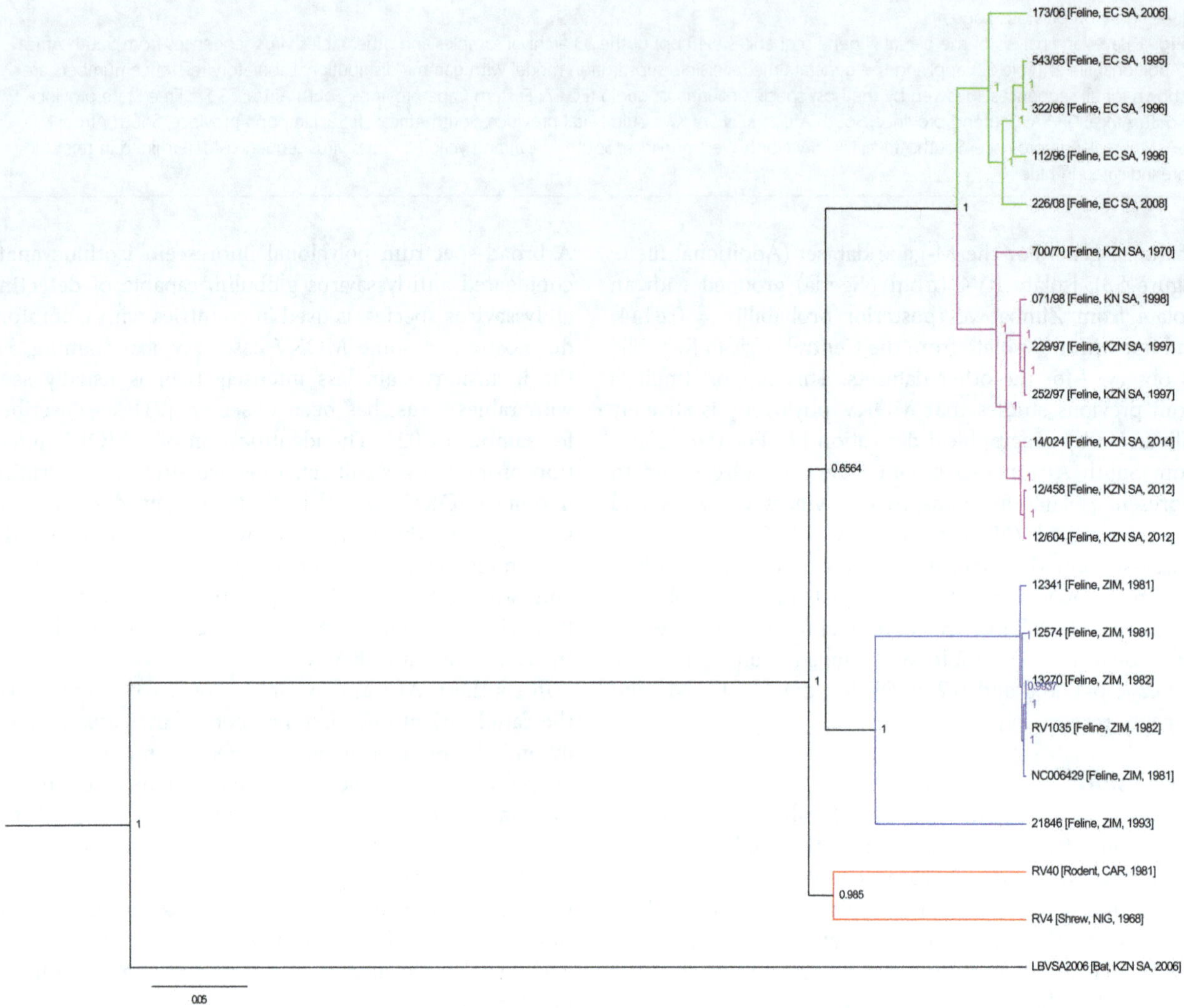

Fig. 2 Bayesian analysis of the concatenated coding region of the N-, P-, M- and G-genes of all Mokola virus isolates (Additional file 3: Table S3) applying the general time reversible substitution model with gamma distribution and invariable sites. Laboratory reference numbers are shown for all sequences, followed by the host species, country of origin (KZN SA: KwaZulu-Natal province, South Africa; EC SA: Eastern Cape province South Africa; ZIM: Zimbabwe; CAR: Central African Republic; NIG: Nigeria) and year of isolation

from KZN) to the previous isolates from KZN, variation of 3% and 1.1% is observed at the nucleotide and amino acid levels of the N-gene respectively. Although the monophyletic grouping of South African MOKV isolates is indicative of the continual presence and stability of MOKV [9], the new isolates form a unique and well-supported clade (posterior probability = 1) within the KZN cluster. These new cases provide yet further confirmation that MOKV cycles are well established and that cases are underreported given the lack of capability/capacity to routinely characterize rabies positive samples and the lack of rabies surveillance in most developing countries. While the majority of MOKV cases are reported in cats, the identity of the reservoir species is unknown. It has been suggested that the reservoir might be a species that interacts with cats [9, 21], but there is little evidence to support this notion. MOKV has been isolated from shrews on three occasions and once from a rodent (*Lophuromys sikapusi*) and in conjunction with limited pathogenicity studies demonstrating significant amounts of virus in the saliva of shrews and rodents sufficient for transmission, invite speculation that these animals could be possible reservoir hosts [12, 24]. The majority of the lyssaviruses have a strong association with bats, with the exceptions of MOKV and Ikoma lyssavirus [25]. Given the diversity observed for bat lyssaviruses, it has been suggested that bats constitute the main evolutionary hosts [26]. Although MOKV has never been isolated from bats, the possibility of an African bat(s) reservoir cannot be excluded. Nevertheless, the identity of the reservoir host(s) for MOKV remains speculative. The close association of humans with domestic cats, an unknown reservoir and the lack of MOKV-protective vaccines [9, 11, 12] collectively support the argument that more research into the epidemiological aspects of MOKV is warranted.

Conclusion

Considering the close contact of domestic cats with humans and the lack of protection from RABV based commercial vaccines, the risk to public and veterinary health is highlighted. These cases emphasize the lack of surveillance for rabies-related lyssaviruses and as such, the true incidence may be underestimated and is a major contributor to our incomplete understanding of the epidemiology and ecology of MOKV.

Additional files

Additional file 1: Table S1. Primers and PCR conditions for amplification of the Nucleoprotein-, Phosphoprotein-, Matrix protein- and Glycoprotein genes of Mokola virus isolates. (XLSX 12 kb)

Additional file 2: Table S2. Details of sequences used for the Bayesian analysis of the rabies virus positive samples. (XLSX 11 kb)

Additional file 3: Table S3. Details of sequences used for the Bayesian analysis of the new Mokola virus isolates. (XLSX 11 kb)

Additional file 4: Figure S1. Bayesian analysis of the coding region of the Nucleoprotein gene (1353 bp) of all Mokola virus isolates (Additional file 3: Table S3) applying the general time reversible substitution model with invariable sites. Laboratory reference numbers are shown for all sequences, followed by the host species, country of origin (KZN SA: KwaZulu-Natal province, South Africa; EC SA: Eastern Cape province South Africa; ZIM: Zimbabwe; CAR: Central African Republic; NIG: Nigeria) and year of isolation. (TIFF 248 kb)

Additional file 5: Figure S2. Bayesian analysis of the coding region of the Phosphoprotein gene (913 bp) applying the general time reversible substitution model with gamma distribution. Laboratory reference numbers are shown for all sequences, followed by the host species, country of origin (KZN SA: KwaZulu-Natal province, South Africa; EC SA: Eastern Cape province South Africa; ZIM: Zimbabwe; CAR: Central African Republic; NIG: Nigeria) and year of isolation. (TIFF 222 kb)

Additional file 6: Figure S3. Bayesian analysis of the coding region of the Matrix protein gene (609 bp) applying the general time reversible substitution model with gamma distribution. Laboratory reference numbers are shown for all sequences, followed by the host species, country of origin (KZN SA: KwaZulu-Natal province, South Africa; EC SA: Eastern Cape province South Africa; ZIM: Zimbabwe; CAR: Central African Republic; NIG: Nigeria) and year of isolation. (TIFF 140 kb)

Additional file 7: Figure S4. Bayesian analysis of the coding region of the Glycoprotein gene (1569 bp) applying the general time reversible substitution model with gamma distribution and invariable sites. Laboratory reference numbers are shown for all sequences, followed by the host species, country of origin (KZN SA: KwaZulu-Natal province, South Africa; EC SA: Eastern Cape province South Africa; ZIM: Zimbabwe; CAR: Central African Republic; NIG: Nigeria) and year of isolation. (TIFF 218 kb)

Additional file 8: Table S4. Nucleotide identity of the Nucleoprotein gene of all Mokola virus isolates. (XLSX 10 kb)

Additional file 9: Table S5. Nucleotide identity of the Phosphoprotein gene of all Mokola virus isolates. (XLSX 10 kb)

Additional file 10: Table S6. Nucleotide identity of the Matrix protein gene of all Mokola virus isolates. (XLSX 10 kb)

Additional file 11: Table S7. Nucleotide identity of the Glycoprotein gene of all Mokola virus isolates. (XLSX 10 kb)

Abbreviations

ARC-OVI: Agricultural research council-onderstepoort veterinary institute; EC: Eastern Cape province; FAT: Fluorescent antibody test; G-gene: Glycoprotein gene; KZN: KwaZulu-Natal province; MCMC: Markov Chain Monte Carlo; M-gene: Matrix protein gene; MOKV: Mokola virus; N-gene: Nucleoprotein gene; P-gene: Phosphoprotein gene; RABV: Rabies virus; VNAs: Virus neutralizing antibodies

Acknowledgments

Not applicable.

Funding

This work was partially funded by the National Research Foundation (Grant UID 92524 & RISP grant UID78566), the Poliomyelitis Research Foundation (Grant no. 10/40, 12/14) and the Animal and Zoonotic Diseases Institutional Research Theme of the University of Pretoria. The funding sponsors had no role in the design of the study; in the collection, analyses, or interpretation of data; in the writing of the manuscript, and in the decision to publish the results.

Authors' contributions

J.C., W.M. and L.H.N. conceived and designed the experiments, K.L.R. and D.S. collected samples for molecular characterization and compiled case histories, C.T.S. confirmed FAT results and assisted in obtaining samples for molecular characterization, J.C. performed the experiments and analyzed the data, J.C., W.M., and L.H.N. wrote the paper. All authors read and approved the final manuscript.

Competing interests

The authors declare that they have no competing interests.

Consent for publication

Not applicable. Rabies is a controlled animal disease in South Africa. According to legislature all suspected rabies cases must be reported and investigated. Therefore, veterinarians are legally obligated to notify the responsible authorities and collect and submit samples for laboratory investigation.

Author details

[1]Center for Viral Zoonoses, Department of Medical Virology, School of Medicine, Faculty of Health Sciences, University of Pretoria, Pretoria 0001, South Africa. [2]Allerton Provincial Veterinary Laboratory, Pietermaritzburg, KwaZulu-Natal 3200, South Africa. [3]Department of Agriculture and Environmental Affairs, KwaZulu-Natal Rabies Project, Pietermaritzburg, KwaZulu-Natal, South Africa. [4]Agricultural Research Council-Onderstepoort Veterinary Institute (ARC-OVI), Pretoria 0110, South Africa. [5]Department of Microbiology and Plant Pathology, Faculty of Natural and Agricultural Sciences, University of Pretoria, Pretoria 0001, South Africa.

References

1. Afonso CL, Amarasinghe GK, Bányai K, Bào Y, Basler CF, Bavari S, et al. Taxonomy of the order *Mononegavirales*: update 2016. Arch Virol. In Press.
2. Shope RE, Murphy FA, Harrison AK, Causey OR, Kemp GE, Simpson DIH, Moore DL. Two African viruses serologically and morphologically related to rabies virus. J Virol. 1970;6:690–2.
3. Kemp GE, Causey OR, Moore DL, Odelola A, Fabiyi A. Mokola virus: Further studies on IbAn 27377, a new rabies-related etiological agent of zoonosis in Nigeria. Am J Trop Hyg. 1972;21:356–9.
4. Familusi JB, Moore DL. Isolation of a rabies-related virus from the cerebrospinal fluid of a child with aseptic meningitis. Afr J Med Sci. 1972;3:93–6.

5. Familusi JB, Osunkoya BO, Moore DL, Kemp GE, Fabiyi A. A fatal human infection with Mokola virus. Am J Trop Med Hyg. 1972;21:959–63.
6. Jackson AC. Current and future approaches to the therapy of human rabies. Antiviral Res. 2013;99:61–7.
7. Weyer J, Msimang-Dermaux V, Paweska JT, le Roux K, Govender P, Coertse J, et al. A case of human survival of rabies, South Africa. S Afr J Infect Dis. 2016. doi:10.1080/23120053.2016.1128151.
8. Johnson N, Cunningham AF, Fooks AR. The immune response to rabies virus infection and vaccination. Vaccine. 2010;28:3896–901.
9. Kgaladi J, Wright N, Coertse J, Markotter W, Marston D, Fooks AR, et al. Diversity and epidemiology of Mokola virus. PLoS Negl Trop Dis. 2013;7:e2511.
10. Meredith CD, Nel LH, Von Teichman BF. Further isolation of Mokola virus in South Africa. Vet Record. 1996;138:119–20.
11. Foggin CM. Atypical rabies virus in cats and a dog in Zimbabwe. Vet Record. 1982;110:338.
12. Foggin CM. Rabies and rabies-related viruses in Zimbabwe: Historical, virological and ecological aspects, PhD thesis. Harare: University of Zimbabwe; 1988.
13. Dean DJ, Abelseth MK, Atansiu P. The fluorescent antibody test. In: Meslin FC, Kaplan MM, Koprowski H, editors. Laboratory techniques in rabies. 4th ed. Geneva: World Health Organization; 1996. p. 88–95.
14. Coertse J, Weyer J, Nel LH, Markotter W. Improved PCR methods for detection of African rabies and rabies-related lyssaviruses. J Clin Microbiol. 2010;48:3949–55.
15. Hall TA. BioEdit: a user-friendly biological sequence alignment editor and analysis program for Windows 95/98/NT. Nucleic Acids Sym Ser. 1999;41:95–8.
16. Darriba D, Taboada GL, Doallo R, Posada D. jModelTest2: more models, new heuristics and high-performance computing. Nat Methods. 2012;9(8):772.
17. Drummond AJ, Suchard MA, Xie D, Rambaut A. Bayesian phylogenetics with BEUTi and the BEAST 1.7. Mol Biol Evol. 2012;29(8):1969–73.
18. Webster WA, Casey GA. Virus isolation in neuroblastoma cell culture. In: Meslin FC, Kaplan MM, Koprowski H, editors. Laboratory techniques in rabies. 4th ed. Geneva: World Health Organization; 1996. p. 96–103.
19. Markotter W, Kuzmin I, Rupprecht CE, Randles J, Sabeta CT, Wandeler AI, et al. Isolation of Lagos bat virus from water mongoose. Emerg Infect Dis. 2006;12:1913–8.
20. Nel LH. Factors impacting the control of rabies. Microbiol Spec. 2013. doi:10.1128/microbiolspec.OH-0006-2012.
21. Von Teichman BF, de Koker WC, Bosch SJE, Bishop GC, Meredith CD, Bingham J. Mokola virus infection: description of recent South African cases and a review of the virus epidemiology. S Afr Vet Assoc. 1998;69:169–71.
22. Von Teichman BF, Thomson GR, Meredith CD, Nel LH. Molecular epidemiology of rabies virus in South Africa: evidence for two distinct virus groups. J Gen Virol. 1995;76:73–82.
23. Coetzee P, Nel LH. Emerging epidemic dog rabies in coastal South Africa: A molecular epidemiological analysis. Virus Res. 2007;126:186–95.
24. Kemp GE, Moore DL, Isoun TT, Fabiyi A. Mokola virus: Experimental infection and transmission studies with the shrew, a natural host. Arch Gesamte Virusforsch. 1973;43:242–50.
25. Banyard AC, Evans JS, Luo TR, Fooks AR. Lyssaviruses and bats: Emergence and zoonotic threat. Viruses. 2014;6:2974–90.
26. Rupprecht CE, Turmelle A, Kuzmin IV. A perspective on lyssavirus emergence and perpetuation. Curr Opin Virol. 2011;1:1–9.

Serological and virological surveillance of avian influenza virus in domestic ducks of the north-east region

Rahul Deb Sarker[1], Mohammad Giasuddin[2], Emdadul Haque Chowdhury[1] and Mohammad Rafiqul Islam[1*]

Abstract

Background: Wild waterfowl are considered as the natural reservoir for avian influenza (AI) viruses. Bangladesh has been experiencing highly pathogenic avian influenza (HPAI) outbreaks since 2007, mostly in chickens and occasionally in ducks. Ducks play an important role in the persistence and genetic recombination of AI viruses. This paper presents the results of serological and virological monitoring of AI in domestic ducks in 2013 in the north-east region of Bangladesh.

Results: A total of 871 and 662 serum samples and 909 and 302 pairs of cloacal and oropharyngeal swabs from domestic ducks of Mymensingh and Sylhet division, respectively, were analysed. Antibodies to type A influenza virus were detected by blocking ELISA in 60.73 and 47.73% serum samples of Mymensingh and Sylhet division, respectively. On haemagglutination-inhibition (HI) test 17.5% of ELISA positive serum samples were found to be seropositive to H5 avian influenza virus. Five cloacal swabs and one oropharyngeal swab were positive for M gene of type A influenza virus by real time RT-PCR (rRT-PCR), but all of them were negative for H5 influenza virus. Three of the six viruses were successfully characterized as H1N5, H2N5 and H7N5 subtype of AI virus, the other three remained uncharacterized. On sequencing and phylogenetic analysis the HA and NA genes were found to be of Eurasian avian lineage. The H7 virus had cleavage site motif of low pathogenic virus.

Conclusions: Low pathogenic avian influenza viruses were detected from apparently healthy domestic ducks. A small proportion of domestic ducks were found seropositive to H5 AI virus.

Keywords: Avian influenza virus, Ducks, Seroprevalence, Molecular characterization, Phylogenetic analysis

Background

Wild waterfowl serve as the natural reservoir for Type A influenza viruses and play an important role in the persistence and transmission of these viruses among birds and other mammalian species. Influenza A viruses are classified into subtypes based on two surface proteins, the hemagglutinin (HA) and neuraminidase (NA). At least 16 hemagglutinins (H1 to H16) and 9 neuraminidases (N1 to N9) have been found in AI viruses from birds [1], while two additional HA and NA types have been identified only in bats [2]. Influenza viruses in birds are classified as either low pathogenic avian influenza (LPAI) or highly pathogenic avian influenza (HPAI) viruses. The HPAI viruses that produce acute clinical disease in chickens, turkeys and other birds belong to either H5 and H7 subtypes. Many different subtypes of AI viruses resulting from the combination of the 16 HA and 9 NA antigens have been found in wild waterfowl [3]. Low pathogenic AI viruses of H5 or H7 subtypes also may persist in wild ducks, which may evolve into HPAI viruses. The ancestor of the currently circulating H5N1 HPAI viruses was first detected in bar-headed goose in Guangdong province, China in 1996. Following some genetic recombinations, the global dissemination of this H5N1 virus began in 2003 with devastating consequences for the poultry industry [4]. In Bangladesh H5N1 HPAI virus was first detected in 2007 [5, 6] and 550 outbreaks have been reported to OIE until now [7]. Most of the outbreaks were in chickens, but clinical disease also has been observed in quails, crows, ducks

* Correspondence: mrislam_bau@yahoo.com
[1]Department of Pathology, Bangladesh Agricultural University, Mymensingh, Bangladesh
Full list of author information is available at the end of the article

and geese [8–10]. Three different genetic clades of HPAI H5N1 virus, namely clade 2.2, 2.3.4 and 2.3.2.1 were detected [8, 11, 12]. As of 19 July 2016, 8 human cases of H5N1 AI virus with one case fatality have been reported from Bangladesh [13]. In addition to H5N1 HPAI, low pathogenic H9N2 influenza virus also has been circulating in poultry [14–16].

Total population of domestic ducks (*Anas platyrhynchos*) in Bangladesh is 48.86 million [17]. Ducks are reared either in scavenging or semi-intensive system. In scavenging system chickens and ducks are usually reared in the same household. In semi-intensive system ducks are brought to the rivers and lakes for feeding, where they get a chance to mingle with the wild waterfowl. Thus AI viruses can transmit from wild waterfowl to domestic ducks. The present paper reports on the serosurveillance and molecular detection and characterization of AI viruses from domestic ducks in north-eastern districts of Bangladesh.

Methods

Sample collection

An AI surveillance programme was conducted by the Department of Livestock Services (DLS), Bangladesh in collaboration with several national laboratories with assistance from the Food and Agriculture Organisation (FAO) of the United Nations in 2013. The samples we used in this study were collected through this surveillance platform. This surveillance program targeted ducks and swine population of the country. Samples collected by DLS veterinarians from different regions of the country were sent to the nearby national laboratories. Our laboratory was entrusted with the responsibility of analyzing samples from the north-western region of Bangladesh including Mymensingh division (Jamalpur, Sherpur, Tangail, Mymensingh, Netrokona and Kishoreganj districs) and Sylhet division (Sunamganj, Hobiganj, Sylhet and Moulvibazar districts) (Fig. 1). Duck rearing is popular in this region because of the presence of many natural waterbodies. With the exception of Netrokona district there was no clinical outbreak of AI in ducks during the period from 2007 to 2013. Serum samples and cloacal and oropharyngeal swabs of 909 and 671 domestic scavenging or semi-scavenging ducks of more than 8 weeks of age from the Mymensingh and Sylhet division, respectively, were collected during the period from January to August 2013. Cloacal and oropharyngeal swabs were placed individually in cryovials containing virus transport medium. The transport medium was prepared with Dulbecco's modified Eagle Medium supplemented with HEPES (20 mM), L-glutamine (2 mM), gentamycin (250 μg/ml), sulfamethoxazole (200 μg/ml), ofloxacin (60 μg/ml), polymyxin B (2000 IU/ml), amphotericin B (2 μg/ml) and bovine serum albumin (2.5%). The samples were shipped to the laboratory either in a cooler with ice pack or in liquid nitrogen, depending on the time required for transportation. Blood samples were also collected from the wing vein of the ducks. The blood was allowed to clot and the serum was separated by centrifugation using a portable centrifuge, and shipped to the laboratory maintening the cool chain as mentioned above.

Detection of antibodies to influenza virus

A blocking ELISA kit (IDEXX AI Multi S-Screen ELISA kit, IDEXX Laboratories, USA) was used to measure antibodies to Type A influenza virus in all the duck serum samples according to manufacturer's instruction. Positive and negative control samples provided with the test kit were included on each plate. Serum samples with a sample-to-negative control (S/N) absorbance ratio less than 0.50 were considered positive.

A total of 80 serum samples out of 845 ELISA-positive samples were randomly selected. The selected samples had a wide range of ELISA values; S/N absorbance ratio 0.10–0.19 (n = 27), 0.20–0.29 (n = 16), 0.30–0.39 (n = 24) and 0.40–0.49 (n = 13). These samples were tested for antibodies to H5 avian influenza virus by haemagglutination-inhibition (HI) test. The H5 antigen (inactivated allantoic fluid containing H5N1 avian influenza virus of clade 2.3.2.1a virus) was obtained from the National Reference Laboratory for Avian Influenza, Bangladesh Livestock Research Institute, Savar, Dhaka. The HI test was performed as described in OIE manual [18].

Molecular detection of avian influenza virus

Viral RNA was extracted from swab samples with KingFisher ML automated RNA extraction machine (Thermo Scientific, USA) using Ambion MagMAX Viral RNA Isolation Kit (Life Technologies, USA). Extraction protocol provided by the kit manufacturer was adapted to KingFisher ML automated RNA extraction machine.

All samples were first screened for the presence of Type A influenza virus by Taqman real time RT-PCR for M gene [19]. The real time RT-PCR was performed on AB 7500 Fast Real Time PCR machine (Applied Biosystems Inc., USA). The reaction was performed in MicroAmp Optical 96 Well Fast PCR plates using AgPath-ID™ One Step RT-PCR kit (Life Technologies, USA) following manufacturer's instruction. The primer and probe sequences are given in Table 1.

All M gene positive samples were then tested for H5 avian influenza virus by conventional RT-PCR for H5 gene [20]. The one step RT-PCR was performed on Eppendorf Mastercycler Gradient thermocycler (Eppendorf, Germany) using SuperScript® III One-Step RT-PCR System with Platinum® Taq DNA polymerase (life Technologies, USA)

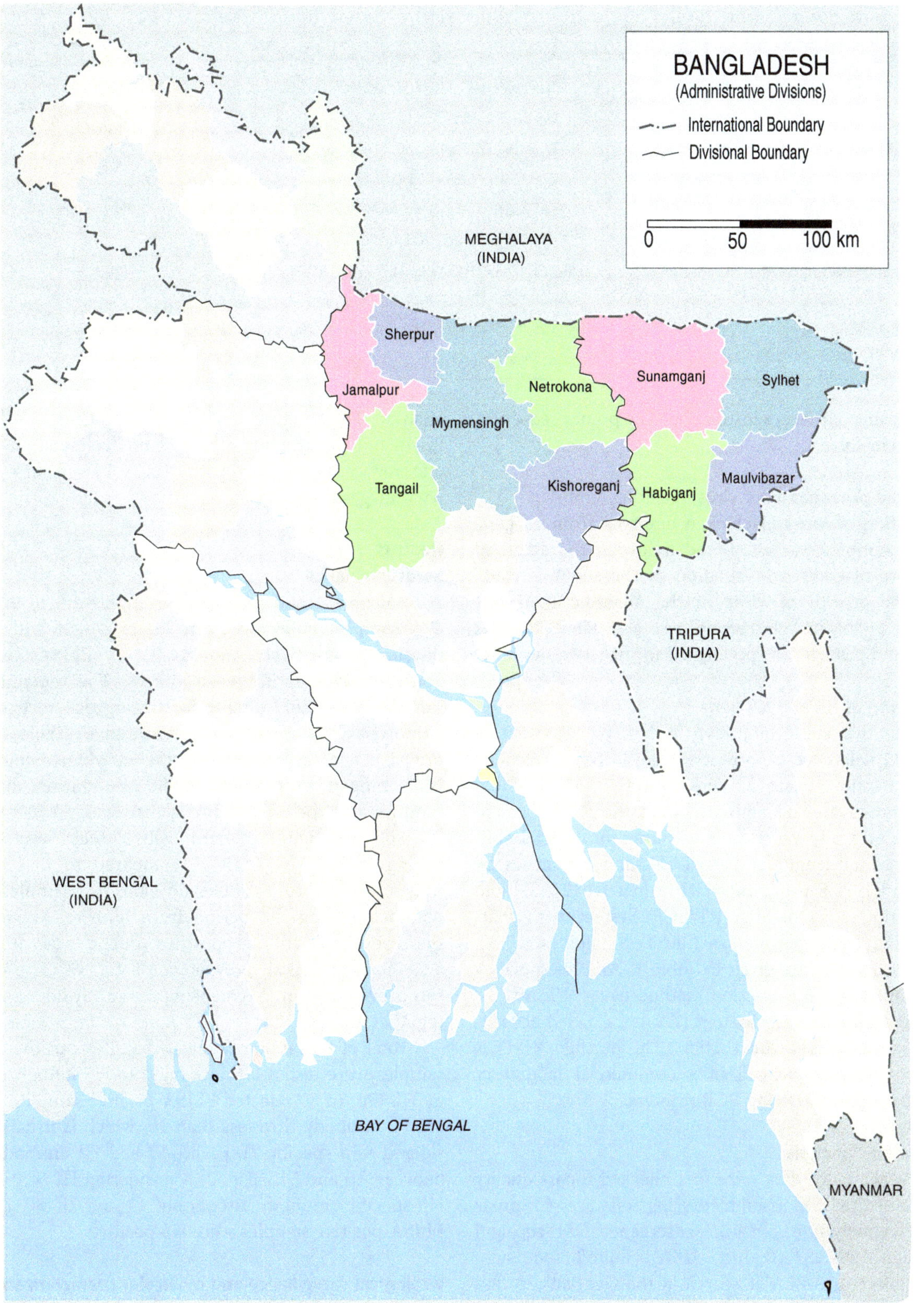

Fig. 1 The *map of Bangladesh* showing the areas of sample collection (*shaded and labelled*). (Map template source: https://commons.wikimedia.org/wiki/File:BD_Map_admin.svg)

Table 1 Oligonucleotide primers and probes used in RT-PCR

Target Gene	Primer/Probe Name	Sequence	Product size(bp)	Reference
M gene (Type A AIV) (TaqMan Real time RT-PCR)	M + 25P F	5′-AGA TGA GTC TTC TAA CCG AGG TCG-3′	100 bp	[20]
	M-124 R	5′-TGC AAA AAC ATC TTC AAG TCT CTG-3′		
	M + 64 Probe	[FAM] 5′-TCA GGC CCC CTC AAA GCC GA-3′ [BHQ1]		
HA gene (H5 AIV)	H5–155 F	5′-ACA CAT GCY CAR GAC ATA CT-3′	545 bp	[21]
	H5-699R	5′-CTY TGR TTY AGT GTT GAT GT-3′		
HA gene, full-length (All Type A AIV)	Bm-HA-1F	5′-TATTCGTCTCAGGGAGCAAAAGCAGGGG-3′	1778 + 29 bp	[22]
	Bm-NS-890 (HA) F	5′-ATA TCG TCT CGT ATT AGT AGA AAC AAG GGT GTT TT-3′		
HA gene, partial (All Type A AIV)	HA-1134F	5′-GGR ATG RTH GAY GGN TGG TAY GG-3′	640 bp	[23]
	Bm-NS-890 (HA) R	5′-ATA TCG TCT CGT ATT AGT AGA AAC AAG GGT GTT TT-3′		[22]
NA gene, full-length (All Type A AIV)	Ba-NA-1F	5′-TAT TGG TCT CAG GGA GCA AAA GCA GGA GT-3′	1413 + 29 bp	[22]
	Ba-NA-1413R	5′-ATATGGTCTCGTATTAGTAGAAACAAGGAGTTTTTT-3′		

following manufacturer's instruction. The primer sequences are given in Table 1.

Attempted propagation of virus in chicken embryos

Propagation of virus in chicken embryos from M gene positive samples was attempted following the standard procedure of embryo inoculation by the allantoic route [18]. The growth of virus in the allantoic fluid was checked by haemagglutination test and RT-PCR. One more blind passage was performed for negative samples.

Sequencing of HA and NA gene

The virus that could be grown in embryos was sent to OIE-FAO Reference Laboratory, Padova, Italy for genetic characterization. If any M gene posititive sample could not be propagated in embryos, then the RNA isolated from the original swab sample was used for direct amplification of full-length or partial HA and NA genes by one step RT-PCR using universal primer set [21, 22] and SuperScript® III One-Step RT-PCR System with Platinum® Taq DNA polymerase (life Technologies, USA). Primer sequences are given in Table 1. Amplified cDNA was cleaned by gel extraction method using Wizard® SV Gel and PCR Clean-Up System (Promega, USA) according to manufacturer's instruction. The purified RT-PCR products were sequenced in a commercial laboratory (1st Base, Malaysia) using PCR primers.

Phylogenetic analysis

The raw sequence data were first checked for its quality and then edited and assembled using softwares Chromas (http://technelysium.com.au), Lasergene EditSeq and MegAlign (DNASTAR Inc., USA). Edited sequences were subjected to BLAST search in the GenBank to find the sequences closely related to the sequences established in the present study. HA and NA sequences of the same subtype representing different genetic lineages were downloaded from the GenBank and used in phylogenetic analysis. The multiple alignment using Clustal W algorithym and construction of maximum likelihood phylogenetic tree were performed with MEGA 5.1 software (http://www.megasoftware.net).

Results

Serosurveillance

A total of 871 and 662 serum samples out of 909 and 671 samples collected from Mymensingh and Sylhet division, respectively, were tested by ELISA for antibodies to type A influenza viruses. The remaining 47 samples were not suitable for testing due to excessive hemolysis. The results are presented in Table 2. The prevalence of seropositive ducks in Mymensingh division ranged from 41.48 to 86.24% during different months and the overall prevalence was 60.73% (Table 2). The prevalence of seropositive ducks was higher during January to April as compared to that during May to July. From Sylhet division the samples were obtained during the period from June to August and the prevalence of seropositive ducks was 40.41 to 52.94%, with overall prevalence of 47.73%. The overall seroprevalence in Mymensingh and Sylhet divisions together was 55.12%.

A total of 80 randomly selected ELISA-positive serum samples were tested for antibodies to H5 influenza virus by HI. Out of 80 selected ELISA-positive samples 32 had H5 HI antibody titre less than 16, which is usually considered non-specific [18], and 48 had HI antibody titre between 16 and 512 (Fig. 2). Considering HI titre >32 as H5-specific antibody titre, only 14 out of 80 (17.5%) ELISA positive samples were H5 positive.

Virological surveillance and molecular characterization of the virus

For virological surveillance all the 909 pairs of oropharyngeal and cloacal swabs from ducks of Mymensingh division and 302 pairs (out of 671 pairs) of oropharyngeal

Table 2 Seroprevalence of type A influenza virus in ducks of Mymensingh and Sylhet divisions during January to July 2013

Month	No. of samples tested	No. of samples positive	% of sample positive
Mymensingh division			
January 2013	78	61	78.20%
February 2013	174	105	60.34%
March 2013	134	111	82.83%
April 2013	109	94	86.23%
May 2013	112	60	53.57%
June 2013	170	59	34.70%
July 2013	94	39	41.48%
Total	871	529	60.73%
Sylhet division			
June 2013	146	59	40.41%
July 2013	125	50	44.00%
August 2013	391	207	52.94%
Total	662	316	47.73%
Overall	1533	845	55.12%

and cloacal swabs from ducks of Sylhet division were tested for M gene of type A influenza virus by rRT-PCR. The remaing 369 pairs of samples from Sylhet division could not be tested due to shortage of reagents. Only six samples (0.5%) including one oropharyngeal swab and 5 cloacal swabs were positive for type A influenza virus; all the positive samples were from Mymensingh division. However, all the 6 M gene positive samples were negative for H5 gene on RT-PCR.

Out of 6 M gene positive samples, only one (22-C) could be successfully propagated in chicken embryos. This sample was characctecterized as H7N5 virus at OIE-FAO Reference Laboratory for Avian Influenza, Padova, Italy. The laboratory has made the HA gene sequence of this isolate publicly available in the GenBank (accession no. KM267817). Examination of the deduced amino acid sequence reveals that this H7N5 virus is a low pathogenic one with cleavage site sequence PELPKGR*GLF. The HA gene sequence of this isolate was downloaded from the GenBank and included in phylogenetic analysis in the present study.

For the remaining 5 samples, which were positive for M gene in rRT-PCR but could not be propagated in embryos, molecular characterization was attempted from the RNA extracted from the original swab samples. We were successful in amplifying nearly full-length NA gene (1413+ bp) and partial HA gene (640 bp) from two samples (18-C and 33-O) by RT-PCR (Fig. 3). Nucleotide sequence of the amplified RT-PCR products were established and submitted to GenBank (Accession No. KX185879, KX185880, KX185881, KX185882). Amplification of full-length HA gene was not successful. The amplified 640 bp fragment of the HA gene was from the 3′ end and that did not cover the cleavage site. BLAST search for homology in the GenBank revealed that the virus from the sample 18-C and 33-O belonged to H1N5 and H2N5 subtype of avian influenza virus, respectively. The summary results of molecular characterization of the viruses are presented in Table 3.

Phylogenetic analysis

The partial H1 gene sequence of the sample 18-C [A/duck/Bangladesh/18-C/2013(H1N5)], H2 gene sequence of the sample 33-O [A/duck/Bangladesh/33-O/2013(H2N5)]

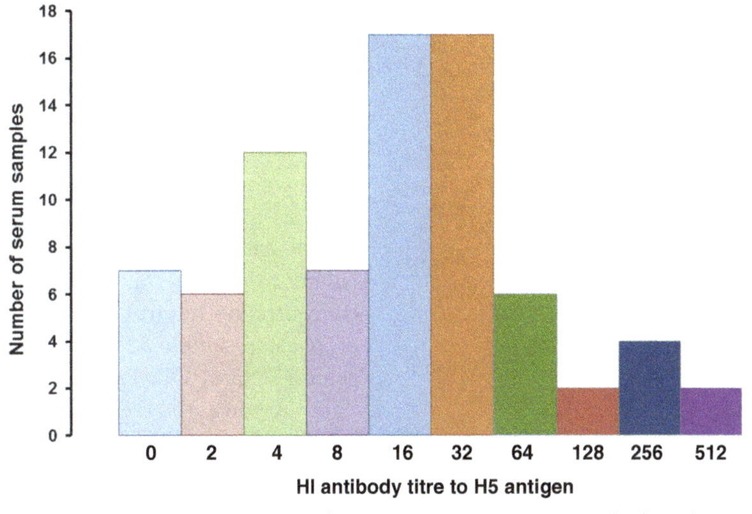

Fig. 2 HI antibody titre against H5 antigen among Type A avian influenza ELISA-positive serum samples from domestic ducks

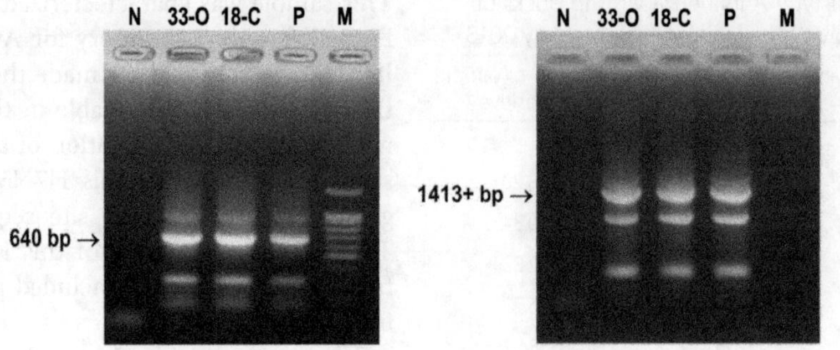

Fig. 3 Amplification of HA (left) and NA (*right*) gene of avian influenza virus by RT-PCR for sequencing. (M = marker, P = positive control, N = water control, 330 and 18C are two samples)

and H7 gene sequence of the sample 22-C [(A/duck/Bangladesh/14VIR1121–1/2013(H7N5)], as well as N5 sequences of the sample 18-C and 33-O were subjected to phylogenetic analysis along with downloaded sequences representing different genetic lineages. The phylogenetic tree revealed that the HA gene segments of 18-C (H1N5), 33-O (H2N5) and 22-C or 14VIR1121–1 (H7N5) virus belonged to Eurasian Avian H1 lineage, Eurasian Avian H2 lineage and Eurasian H7 lineage, respectively (Figs. 4, 5 and 6). The H7 sequence of the present strain was different from that of influenza A(H7N9) virus, which caused human infection in China. The NA gene segment of 18-C and 33-O viruses are quite similar and belonged to Eurasian N5 lineage (Fig. 7).

Discussion

Wild aquatic birds are the natural reservoir of all influenza A viruses [3]. Domestic ducks also have been shown to harbour many subtypes of avian influenza viruses and allow their reassortments [23]. The present study revealed a widespread seroconversion of domestic ducks to Type A influenza virus with an overall seroprevalence of 60.73% in Mymensingh and 47.73% in Sylhet division in 2013. Another study reported 39.76% seroprevalence of type A avian influenza virus in semi-scavenging ducks of Sylhet Hakaluki Haor and Jahangirnagar University Lake areas during winter months of 2009 to 2012 [24]. On further investigation of selected serum samples by HI test for H5 antibodies only 17.5% of ELISA-positive samples were positive for H5 antibodies using HI titre >32 as the cut-off titre for H5-specific antibodies. In West Bengal of India 2.2% ducks were found to be seropositive in HI test for H5 AI considering >40 as the cut-off titre [25].

On virological surveillance only one oropharyngeal swab and five cloacal swabs out of 909 sampled ducks from Mymensingh division were found positive for type A influenza virus M gene by rRT-PCR. No positive sample was found from Sylhet division. This prevalence rate of type A influenza virus in domestic ducks is quite low (0.50%) as compared to that reported by others in domestic ducks of Bangladesh, such as 5.9% [26], 22.05% [24] and 16 out of 39 (41.03%) [27]. This variation might be due to the different time period of sampling. In the present study the samples were collected during January to August, 2013, where as in the previous studies the samples were collected during the period from 2007 to 2012.

All of the 6 M gene positive samples of the present study were negative for H5. Attempted propagation of these M gene positive samples in embryos was not successful with the exception of one sample (22-C). This failure to isolate the virus could be due to very low concentration of virus in the samples. The only embryo-propagated sample 22-C was characterized as low pathogenic H7N5 at OIE-FAO Reference Laboratory, Padova, Italy. Among the remaining 5 M gene-positive but culture-negative swab samples, it was possible to amplify a 640 bp fragment of HA gene and nearly full-length (1413+ bp) NA gene from two samples (18-C and 33-O). The sample 18-C was characterized as subtype H1N5

Table 3 Molecular characterization of avian influenza viruses detected from apparently healthy domestic ducks of Mymensingh division in 2013

Sample ID	Sample type	C_T value in rRT-PCR for Type A influenza virus M gene	Propagation in chicken embryos	Subtyping result
18-C	Cloacal swab	26	- [a]	H1N5
122-C	Cloacal swab	35	-	-
22-C	Cloacal swab	35	Yes	H7N5
23-C	Cloacal swab	35	-	-
25-C	Cloacal swab	35	-	-
33-O	Oropharyngeal swab	34	-	H2N5

[a]Not successful

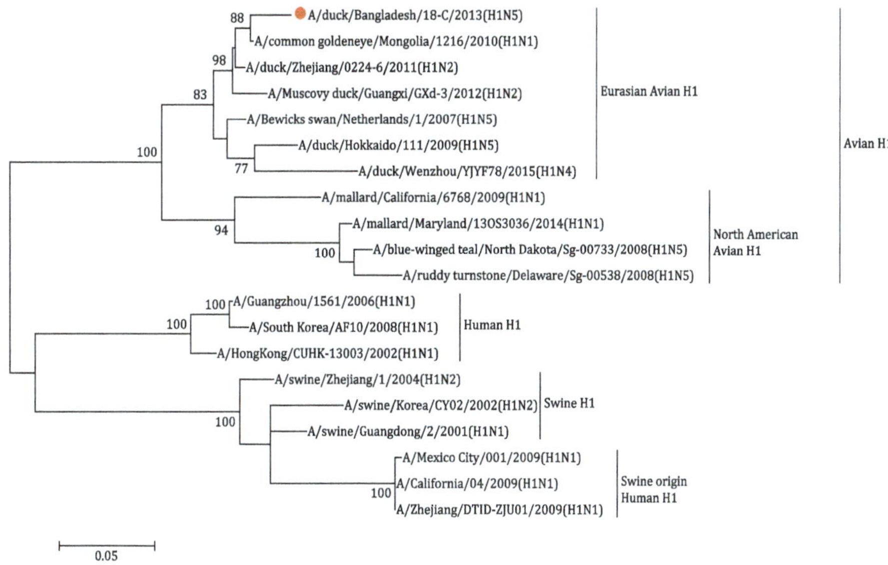

Fig. 4 The Maximum Likelihood (ML) phylogenetic tree based on the partial H1 gene sequences (600 bp) of H1N5 virus of the present study and representative H1 viruses of different genetic lineages. The *scale* indicates the number of substitutions per site. The H1N5 sequence of the present study is indicated with a closed *circle symbol*

and the sample 33-O as subtype H2N5. Aquatic birds are known to harbour a wide variety of avian influenza viruses. So the detection of viruses of three different subtypes (H7N5, H1N5 and H2N5) is not surprising. In an earlier study 14 different subtypes of LPAI viruses including H1N1, H1N3, H2N4, H3N2, H3N6, H3N8, H4N2, H4N6, H5N2, H6N1, H6N7, H7N9, H9N2 and H11N3 were identified from domestic ducks of Bangladesh [27]. Isolation of H1N1, H1N2 and H1N3 viruses have been reported from wild and domestic ducks in Korea [28], H1N3 and H1N9 viruses from free-range ducks in Thailand [29] and H2N7 and H2N2 virus from domestic ducks in China [30, 31]. It was interesting that the N gene component of all of the three viruses (H1N5, H2N5 and H7N5) detected in the present study was N5. However, in the previous study [27] all the different N subtypes except N5 were detected in domestic ducks of Bangladesh. Taken together, the findings of these two studies reveal that all the 9 N genes are present in domestic ducks of Bangladesh. Phylogenetically the HA gene of H1N5, H2N5 and H7N5 viruses

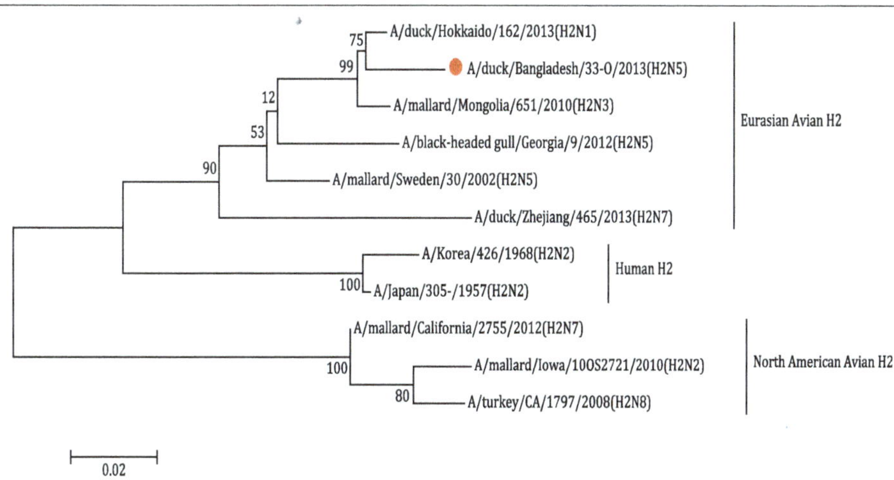

Fig. 5 The Maximum Likelihood (ML) phylogenetic tree based on the partial H2 gene sequences (600 bp) of H2N5 virus of the present study and representative H2 viruses of different genetic lineages. The *scale* indicates the number of substitutions per site. The H2N5 sequence of the present study is indicated with a closed *circle symbol*

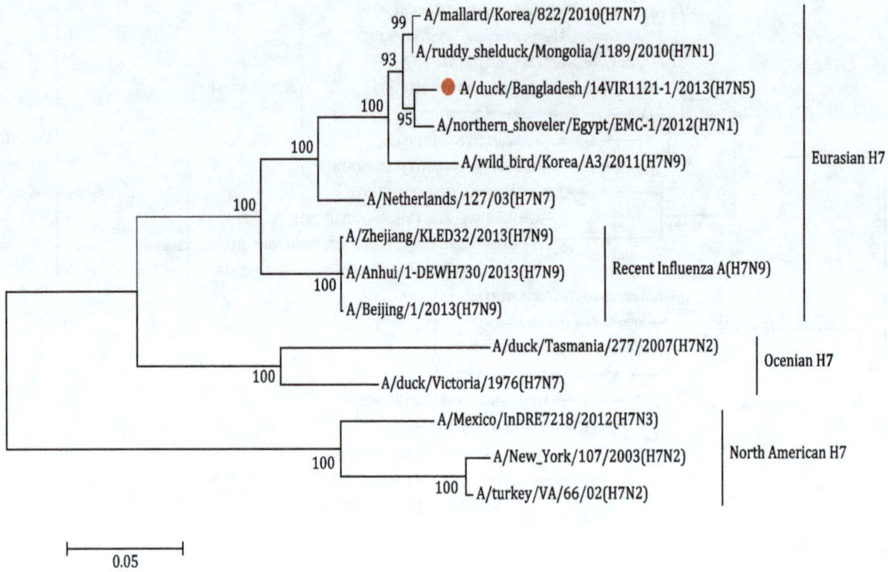

Fig. 6 The Maximum Likelihood (ML) phylogenetic tree based on the H7 gene sequences of H7N5 virus of the present study and representative H7 viruses of different genetic lineages. The *scale* indicates the number of substitutions per site. The H7N5 sequence of the present study is indicated with a closed *circle symbol*

belonged to Eurasian avian lineages as observed in the previous study [27]. The HA gene of H7N5 was distinct from the HA gene of the newly emerged Influenza A(H7N9) virus. The N5 gene of H1N5 and H2N5 viruses were very similar and also belonged to Eurasian lineage; the NA gene sequence of H7N5 virus was not available.

Conclusions

Present study shows that 55.12% of the ducks were seropositive for antibodies to Type A influenza virus and a small proportion of Type A influenza virus positive ducks (14 out of 80 randomly selected samples) had previous exposure to H5 subtype viruses, probably H5N1 HPAI or H5N2 LPAI viruses. Active shedding of AI virus at the time of the study was very limited (0.5%). Three viruses were characterized as H1N5, H2N5 and H7N5 subtypes and no H5N1 virus was detected. Findings of the present study warrant further detailed surveillance on avain influenza virus in ducks for better understanding of the ecology of avian influenza viruses in domestic duck population.

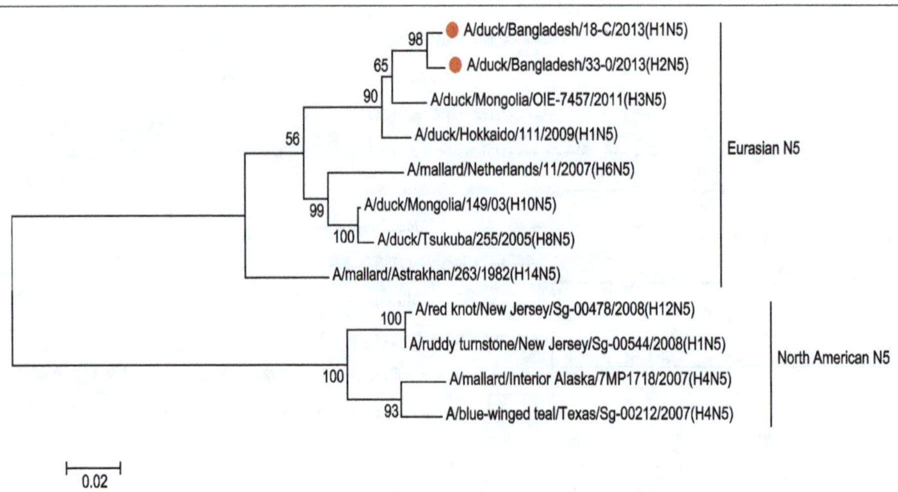

Fig. 7 The Maximum Likelihood (ML) phylogenetic tree based on the N5 gene sequences of H1N5 and H2N5 viruses of the present study and representative N5 viruses of different genetic lineages. The *scale* indicates the number of substitutions per site. The H1N5 and H2N5 sequences of the present study are indicated with closed *circle symbols*

Abbreviations
AI: Avian influenza; ELISA: Enzyme-linked immunosorbent assay; FAO: Food and Agriculture Organization; HA: Haemagglutinin; HI: Haemagglutination inhibition; HPAI: Highly pathogenic; LPAI: Low pathogenic avian influenza; NA: Neuraminidase; OIE: Office international des epizooties; rRT-PCR: Real time Reverse transcription- polymerase chain reaction; RT-PCR: Reverse transcription- polymerase chain reaction; S/N: Sample - negative; WOAH: World Organization for Animal Health

Funding
The study was supported by FAO, Bangladesh.

Authors' contributions
RDS and MG contributed to acquisition of data, analysis and interpretation of data; RDS drafted the manuscripts; EHC and MRI conceived and designed the study, supervised the research work and approved the manuscript.

Competing interests
The authors declare that they have no competing interests.

Consent for publication
Not applicable.

Author details
[1]Department of Pathology, Bangladesh Agricultural University, Mymensingh, Bangladesh. [2]National Reference Laboratory for Avian Influenza, Bangladesh Livestock Research Institute, Savar, Dhaka, Bangladesh.

References
1. Fouchier RA, Munster V, Wallensten A, Bestebroer TM, Herfst S, Smith D, et al. Characterization of a novel influenza a virus hemagglutinin subtype (H16) obtained from black-headed gulls. J Virol. 2005;79:2814–22.
2. Tong S, Zhu X, Li Y, Shi M, Zhang J, Bourgeois M, et al. New world bats harbor diverse influenza a viruses. Plos Pathog. 2013;9:e1003657.
3. Krauss S, Obert CA, Franks J, Walker D, Jones K, Seiler P, et al. Influenza in migratory birds and evidence of limited intercontinental virus exchange. Plos Pathog. 2007;3:e167.
4. Sonnberg S, Webby RJ, Webster RG. Natural history of highly pathogenic avian influenza H5N1. Virus Res. 2013;178:63–77.
5. Islam MR, Baqi MA, Giasuddin M, Samad MA. Molecular characterization and phylogenetic analysis of highly pathogenic H5N1 avian influenza virus of chickens of Bangladesh. Proceedings of the Bangkok International Conference on Avian Influenza 2008: Integration from Knowledge to Control. Bangkok: 2008.
6. Biswas PK, Christensen JP, Ahmed SSU, Barua H, Das A, Rahman MH, et al. Avian influenza outbreaks in chickens, Bangladesh. Emerg Infect Dis. 2008; 14:1909–12.
7. OIE: World Animal Health Information Database (WAHID) Interface. Disease information. Available at http://www.oie.int/wahis_2/public/wahid.php/ Diseaseinformation/Immsummary. Accessed 8 Sept 2016.
8. Islam MR, Haque ME, Giasuddin M, Chowdhury EH, Samad MA, Parvin R, et al. New introduction of clade 2.3.2.1 avian influenza virus (H5N1) into Bangladesh. Transbound Emerg Dis. 2012;59:460–3.
9. Khan SU, Berman L, Haider N, Gerloff N, Rahman MZ, Shu B, et al. Investigating a crow die-off in January-February 2011 during the introduction of a new clade of highly pathogenic avian influenza virus H5N1 into Bangladesh. Arch Virol. 2014;159:509–18.
10. Haider N, Sturm-Ramirez K, Khan SU, Rahman MZ, Sarkar S, Poh MK, Shivaprasad HL, Kalam MA, Paul SK, Karmakar PC, Balish A,Chakraborty A, Mamun AA, Mikolon AB, Davis CT, Rahman M, Donis RO, Heffelfinger JD, Luby SP, Zeidner N. Unusually High Mortality in Waterfowl Caused by Highly Pathogenic Avian Influenza A (H5N1) in Bangladesh. Transboun Emerg Dis. 2015. doi:10.1111/tbed.12354. Epub ahead of print.
11. Marinova-Petkova A, Feeroz MM, Rabiul Alam SM, Kamrul Hasan M, Akhtar S, Jones-Engel L, et al. Multiple introductions of highly pathogenic avian influenza H5N1 viruses into Bangladesh. Emerg Microbe Infect. 2014;3:e11. doi:10.1038/emi.
12. Haque ME, Giasuddin M, Chowdhury EH, Islam MR. Molecular evolution of H5N1 highly pathogenic avian influenza viruses in Bangladesh between 2007 and 2012. Avian Pathol. 2014;43:183–94.
13. WHO. Cumulative number of confirmed human cases for avian influenza A(H5N1) reported to WHO, 2003–2015. Available at http://www.who.int/ influenza/human_animal_interface/2016_01_20_tableH5N1.pdf?ua=1. Accessed 8 Sept 2016.
14. Negovetich NJ, Feeroz MM, Jones-Engel L, Walker D, Alam SMR, Hasan K, et al. Live bird markets of Bangladesh: H9N2 viruses and the near absence of highly pathogenic H5N1 influenza. Plos One. 6:e19311. doi:10.1371/ journal.pone.0019311.
15. Jannat N, Chowdhury EH, Parvin R, Begum JA, Giasuddin M, MAHNA K, et al. Investigation of an outbreak of low pathogenic avian influenza in poultry in Bangladesh. Intl J Livestock Res. 2013;3:21–32.
16. Parvin R, Heenemann K, Halami MY, Chowdhury EH, Islam MR, Vahlenkamp TW. Full-genome analysis of avian influenza virus H9N2 from Bangladesh reveals internal gene reassortments with two distinct highly pathogenic avian influenza viruses. Arch Virol. 2014;159:1651–61.
17. FAOSTAT: Live animals_Bangladesh_Stock_Ducks_2014. Available at http:// fenix.fao.org/faostat/beta/en/#data/QA. Accessed 8 Sept 2016.
18. OIE: Manual of Diagnostic Tests and Vaccines for Terrestrial Animals 2016. Chapter 2.3.4. Avian influenza (infection with avian influenza viruses). Available at http://www.oie.int/fileadmin/Home/eng/Health_standards/ tahm/2.03.04_AI.pdf. Accessed 8 Sept 2016.
19. Spackman E, Senne DA, Myers TJ, Bulaga LL, Garber LP, Perdue ML, et al. Development of a real-time reverse transcriptase PCR assay for type a influenza virus and the avian H5 and H7 Hemagglutinin subtypes. J Clin Microbiol. 2002;40:3256–60.
20. Lee MS, Chang PC, Shien JH, Cheng MC, Shieh HK. Identification and subtyping of avian influenza viruses by reverse transcription-PCR. J Virol Methods. 2001;97:13–22.
21. Hoffmann E, Stech J, Guan Y, Webster RG, Perez DR. Universal primer set for the full-length amplification of all influenza a viruses. Arch Virol. 2001;146: 2275–89.
22. Lindsay LL, Kelly TR, Plancarte M, Schobel S, Lin X, Dugan VG, et al. Avian influenza: mixed infections and missing viruses. Viruses. 2013;5:1964–77.
23. Deng G, Tan D, Shi J, Cui P, Jiang Y, Liu L, et al. Complex reassortment of multiple subtypes of avian influenza viruses in domestic ducks at the Dongting Lake region of China. J Virol. 2013;87:9452–62.
24. Khatun A, Giasuddin M, Islam KM, Hanom S, Samad MA, Islam MR, et al. Surveillance of avian influenza virus type a in semi-scavenging ducks in Bangladesh. BMC Vet Res. 2013;9:196.
25. Pawar SD, Kale SD, Rawankar AS, Koratkar SS, Raut CG, Pande SA, et al. Avian influenza surveillance reveals presence of low pathogenic avian influenza viruses in poultry during 2009–2011 in the West Bengal state, India. Virol J. 2012;9:151.
26. Annon. Avian influenza virus surveillance at live bird markets in Bangladesh, 2007-2012. ICDDR,B Health Sci Bull. 2012;11:8–16.
27. Gerloff NA, Khan SU, Zanders N, Balish A, Haider N, Islam A, et al. Genetically diverse low pathogenicity avian influenza a virus subtypes co-circulate among poultry in Bangladesh. Plos One. 2016;11:e0152131.
28. Jeong OM, Kim YJ, Choi JG, Kang HM, Kim MC, Kwon JH, et al. Genetic characterization of H1 avian influenza viruses isolated from migratory birds and domestic ducks in Korea. Virus Genes. 2011;42:55–63.
29. Chaiyawong S, Boonyapisitsopa S, Jairak W, Nonthabenjawan N, Tangwangvivat R, Bunpapong N, et al. Genetic characterization of influenza a virus subtypes H1N3 and H1N9 isolated from free-grazing ducks in Thailand. Arch Virol. 2016;161:2819–24.
30. Peng X, Wu H, Jin C, Yao H, Lu X, Cheng L, et al. Sequence and phylogenetic analysis of H2N7 avian influenza viruses isolated from domestic ducks in Zhejiang Province, eastern China, 2013. Virus Genes. 2014;48:391–6.

6

Evaluation of serological cross-reactivity and cross-neutralization between the United States porcine epidemic diarrhea virus prototype and S-INDEL-variant strains

Qi Chen[1], Joseph T. Thomas[1], Luis G. Giménez-Lirola[1], John M. Hardham[2], Qinshan Gao[2], Priscilla F. Gerber[3], Tanja Opriessnig[1,3], Ying Zheng[1], Ganwu Li[1], Phillip C. Gauger[1], Darin M. Madson[1], Drew R. Magstadt[1] and Jianqiang Zhang[1*]

Abstract

Background: At least two genetically different porcine epidemic diarrhea virus (PEDV) strains have been identified in the United States (U.S. PEDV prototype and S-INDEL-variant strains). The current serological assays offered at veterinary diagnostic laboratories for detection of PEDV-specific antibody are based on the U.S. PEDV prototype strain. The objectives of this study were: 1) isolate the U.S. PEDV S-INDEL-variant strain in cell culture; 2) generate antisera against the U.S. PEDV prototype and S-INDEL-variant strains by experimentally infecting weaned pigs; 3) determine if the various PEDV serological assays could detect antibodies against the U.S. PEDV S-INDEL-variant strain and vice versa.

Results: A U.S. PEDV S-INDEL-variant strain was isolated in cell culture in this study. Three groups of PEDV-negative, 3-week-old pigs (five pigs per group) were inoculated orally with a U.S. PEDV prototype isolate (previously isolated in our lab), an S-INDEL-variant isolate or virus-negative culture medium. Serum samples collected at 0, 7, 14, 21 and 28 days post inoculation were evaluated by the following PEDV serological assays: 1) indirect fluorescent antibody (IFA) assays using the prototype and S-INDEL-variant strains as indicator viruses; 2) virus neutralization (VN) tests against the prototype and S-INDEL-variant viruses; 3) PEDV prototype strain whole virus based ELISA; 4) PEDV prototype strain S1-based ELISA; and 5) PEDV S-INDEL-variant strain S1-based ELISA. The positive antisera against the prototype strain reacted to and neutralized both prototype and S-INDEL-variant viruses, and the positive antisera against the S-INDEL-variant strain also reacted to and neutralized both prototype and S-INDEL-variant viruses, as examined by IFA antibody assays and VN tests. Antibodies against the two PEDV strains could be detected by all three ELISAs although detection rates varied to some degree.

Conclusions: These data indicate that the antibodies against U.S. PEDV prototype and S-INDEL-variant strains cross-reacted and cross-neutralized both strains in vitro. The current serological assays based on U.S. PEDV prototype strain can detect antibodies against both U.S. PEDV strains.

Keywords: Porcine epidemic diarrhea virus, PEDV, Prototype, S-INDEL, Variant, IFA, Virus neutralization, ELISA

* Correspondence: jqzhang@iastate.edu
[1]Department of Veterinary Diagnostic and Production Animal Medicine, College of Veterinary Medicine, Iowa State University, 1800 Christensen Drive, Ames, IA 50011, USA
Full list of author information is available at the end of the article

Background

Porcine epidemic diarrhea (PED), caused by porcine epidemic diarrhea virus (PEDV), was first recorded in England in the early 1970s and has since spread to other European and Asian countries [1]. In North America, PEDV was detected for the first time in the United States (U.S.) in April 2013 [2] and subsequently PEDV was reported in Canada [3] and Mexico [4]. PEDV is an enveloped, single-stranded, positive-sense RNA virus belonging to the order *Nidovirales*, the family *Coronaviridae*, subfamily *Coronavirinae*, genus *Alphacoronavirus* [5]. The PEDV genome is approximately 28 kb in length and includes ORF1a and ORF1b encoding the replicase polyproteins and other opening reading frames (ORFs) encoding four structural proteins [spike (S), envelope (E), membrane (M), and nucleocapsid (N)] and one nonstructural protein NS3B (encoded by ORF3) [1].

In the U.S., a highly virulent PEDV strain (U.S. PEDV prototype strain) was identified during the initial PED outbreaks [2, 6, 7]. Lately, a PEDV variant strain having insertions and deletions (INDEL) in the spike gene compared to the U.S. prototype strain was identified in U.S. swine with mild clinical signs based on field observations [8]. This U.S. PEDV variant strain, also known as S INDEL strain [4], formed a distinct phylogenetic cluster compared to U.S. PEDV prototype strains [4, 8, 9]. One PEDV isolate (PC177) having a 197-aa deletion in the N-terminal S protein was discovered during PEDV isolation in cell culture; however, this PEDV isolate still phylogenetically clustered with the U.S. PEDV prototype strains and was not considered as one of the S-INDEL-variant strains [10]. Marthaler et al [11] reported a 'third' strain of PEDV (Minnesota188) in U.S. swine that had 6 nucleotide deletions (2 amino acid deletions) in the spike gene (different from the U.S. S-INDEL-variant strains). However, the PEDV Minnesota188 was genetically very closely related to the U.S. PEDV prototype strains and it is arguable whether it should be called a 'third' strain of PEDV in the U.S. The PEDV PC177 and Minnesota188 are probably the mutants of the U.S. PEDV prototype strains. Therefore, there are at least two genetically different PEDV strains currently circulating in U.S. swine: U.S. PEDV prototype strain and S-INDEL-variant strain.

The U.S. PEDV prototype strains have been successfully isolated and propagated in cell culture by several groups [7, 10, 12, 13]. A number of serological assays, including an indirect fluorescent antibody (IFA) assay, a virus neutralization (VN) test, a whole virus-based enzyme-linked immunosorbent assay (ELISA), a recombinant S1 protein-based ELISA, and recombinant nucleocapsid protein-based ELISAs, have been developed for the detection of PEDV-specific antibodies [14–18]. All of these serological assays are based on the U.S. PEDV prototype strains.

In this study, we isolated a U.S. PEDV S-INDEL-variant strain in cell culture. Pigs were experimentally inoculated with a U.S. PEDV prototype strain and the newly isolated U.S. PEDV S-INDEL-variant strain, respectively, to generate strain-specific antisera. Subsequently, the generated swine antisera were subjected to an in vitro evaluation for serological cross-reactivity and cross-neutralization between the two strains. Specifically, 1) PEDV IFA antibody assays (using the prototype and S-INDEL-variant strains as indicator viruses, respectively) and ELISAs (PEDV prototype strain whole virus-based ELISA, PEDV prototype strain S1-based ELISA, and PEDV S-INDEL-variant strain S1-based ELISA) were conducted to evaluate the antibody cross-reactivity of the two U.S. strains; and 2) VN tests using the prototype and S-INDEL-variant strains as indicator viruses were conducted to evaluate the in vitro cross-neutralization of two U.S. strains.

Methods

Isolation of U.S. PEDV S-INDEL-variant strain in cell culture

Sixty-eight clinical samples (27 fecal swabs, 24 feces, 13 small intestines and 4 oral fluids), which were tested positive by a PEDV N gene-based real-time RT-PCR [17, 19] at the Iowa State University Veterinary Diagnostic Laboratory (ISU VDL) and confirmed positive for the U.S. PEDV S-INDEL-variant strain but negative for the U.S. prototype strain by a PEDV S gene-based differential real-time RT-PCR (Chen et al., unpublished), were selected to attempt virus isolation in Vero cells (ATCC CCL-81) following previously described procedures [7].

Among the aforementioned 68 clinical samples positive for the U.S. PEDV S-INDEL-variant strain, one small intestine homogenate (with PEDV N gene-based real-time RT-PCR cycle threshold (Ct) value of 16.1) [17, 19] from a pig located in Illinois was inoculated orogastrically into three PEDV-naïve weaned pigs at 3 weeks of age (10 ml per pig). The homogenate used for inoculation was confirmed negative for transmissible gastrointestinal virus (TGEV), porcine rotavirus groups A, B, C and porcine deltacoronavirus (PDCoV) by virus-specific RT-PCRs at the ISU VDL. Rectal swabs and feces were collected from each inoculated pig twice a day and tested by the PEDV real-time RT-PCR on the same day. Once the RT-PCR Ct values of the rectal swabs were <15, the pig was euthanized and necropsied within 24 h. Small intestine tissues and cecum contents were collected for attempting virus isolation in cell culture as previously described [7]. This animal study was performed according to the procedures approved by the Iowa State University Institutional Animal Care and Use Committee (IACUC, approval number 3-14-7766-S).

The whole genome sequence of the U.S. PEDV S-INDEL-variant strain cell culture isolate USA/IL20697/2014 obtained in this study was determined by next-generation sequencing (NGS) technology using an Illumina MiSeq platform as described previously [7]. The PEDV S1 portion sequences of the isolate USA/IL20697/2014 and the clinical sample from which the virus isolate was derived were determined by Sanger sequencing following the previously described procedures [7].

Generation of antisera against the U.S. prototype and S-INDEL-variant PEDVs

Fifteen 3-week-old pigs, negative for PEDV as confirmed by a real-time RT-PCR on rectal swabs and by IFA antibody assay on sera, were first segregated by weight and then assigned randomly into 3 groups with 5 pigs per group and with similar average weight per group, one group per room. Five pigs within each group were housed together in one room on a solid floor. After acclimation for 3 days, three groups of pigs were orogastrically inoculated with a U.S. PEDV prototype cell culture isolate USA/IN19338/2013 (Pro group) [7], a U.S. PEDV S-INDEL-variant cell culture isolate USA/IL20697/2014 (Var group), and virus-negative culture medium (Neg group), respectively, with virus titers of 10^4 $TCID_{50}$/ml, 10 ml per pig. Rectal swabs were collected from all pigs daily between 0 and 7 DPI, and then at 10, 14, 21 and 28 DPI, and tested by a PEDV N gene-based quantitative real-time RT-PCR [20] to confirm infection. Serum samples were collected from all pigs at 0, 7, 14, 21 and 28 days post inoculation (DPI) for cross-reactivity and cross-neutralization evaluations. This animal study was performed according to the procedures approved by the Iowa State University IACUC committee (approval number 6-14-7809-S).

Twenty-five serum samples collected at 0, 7, 14, 21, and 28 DPI from the Pro group (Pro antisera), 25 serum samples collected from the Var group (Var antisera), and 25 serum samples collected from the Neg group (Neg antisera), were tested by various serological assays in this study. In addition, one pig antiserum against the European PEDV CV777 strain, one pig antiserum against the TGEV Purdue strain, one pig antiserum against the porcine heamagglutinating encephalomyelitis virus (PHEV), one pig antiserum against the porcine respiratory coronavirus (PRCV), and one pig antiserum against PDCoV were included in this study for evaluations. Antisera against PEDV CV777, TGEV Purdue, and PHEV strains were purchased from National Veterinary Service Laboratory, Ames, IA. Antisera against PRCV and PDCoV were positive control sera obtained from the ISU VDL.

Indirect fluorescent antibody (IFA) assay

Eighty serum samples were tested by the PEDV prototype strain-based IFA (Pro IFA) and S-INDEL-variant strain-based IFA (Var IFA) following the previously described procedures [20]. The PEDV prototype isolate USA/IN19338/2013 was used as the indicator virus in the Pro IFA assay and the S-INDEL-variant isolate USA/IL20697/2014 was used as the indicator virus in the Var IFA assay. A positive signal at a serum dilution of 1:40 or higher was considered to be IFA antibody positive.

PEDV ELISAs for antibody detection

The U.S. PEDV prototype strain whole virus-based indirect ELISA (ProWV ELISA) was developed and validated at the ISU VDL for detection of PEDV-specific IgG antibody [15, 16]. All serum samples were tested by this ProWV ELISA following the procedures that had been previously described in detail [20]. The sample-to-positive (S/P) ratio of >0.8 was considered antibody positive, an S/P ratio between 0.6 and 0.8 was considered suspect, and an S/P ratio <0.6 was considered negative.

A previously published U.S. PEDV prototype strain S1-based indirect ELISA (ProS1 ELISA) was used to test all the serum samples in this study for the IgG antibody following the previously described procedures [14]. The S/P ratio of >0.2 was considered antibody positive, 0.14–0.2 was considered suspect, and an S/P ratio <0.14 was considered negative.

A U.S. PEDV S-INDEL-variant strain S1-based indirect ELISA (VarS1 ELISA) was developed in this study to detect the IgG antibody. The region encoding the S1 portion (aa 1–735) of the U.S. PEDV S-INDEL-variant strain was codon optimized and synthesized with the addition of a 5′ Kozac sequence, a 5′ eukaryotic signal sequence, and a 3′ 6×-His tag by GeneArt® Gene Synthesis (Thermo Fisher Scientific, Waltham, MA, USA). The resultant 2,358 base pair DNA fragment was cloned into a Zoetis proprietary eukaryotic expression vector (pZOE15). The authenticity and orientation of the insert in the recombinant plasmid was confirmed by sequencing. The recombinant plasmid was transiently transfected into human embryonic kidney (HEK) 293 cells using a Zoetis proprietary PEI transfection method. At 7 days post-transfection, culture supernatants were harvested and filter sterilized. The recombinant protein was purified via Ni-NTA Purification System (Thermo Fisher Scientific). The optimum antigen concentration and the optimum serum dilutions for the VarS1 ELISA were determined using a checkerboard titration. Polystyrene 96-well microtitration plates (Nunc®, Thermo Fisher Scientific) were coated (100 µl per well) with PEDV variant S1 protein and incubated overnight at 4 °C. After 5 washes with phosphate buffered saline (PBS), the plates were blocked (300 μl/well) with PBS containing 1 % bovine serum albumin (Jackson ImmunoResearch Inc., West Grove, PA, USA) for 2 h at 25 °C. Plates were dried at 37 °C for 4 h and stored at 4 °C in a sealed bag with desiccant packs until use. Serum samples were diluted 1:50 and added to the coated plates (100 μl/well). Plates were incubated at 25 °C for 1 h and then washed 5 times with PBS. Subsequently 100 μl of peroxidase-conjugated goat anti-porcine IgG (H + L) (Jackson ImmunoResearch Inc., West Grove, PA, USA) at 1:25,000 dilution was added and plates were incubated at 25 °C for 1 h. After a washing step, 100 μl tetramethylbenzidine-hydrogen peroxide substrate (TMB, Dako North America Inc., Carpinteria, CA, USA) was added. Plates were incubated at room temperature for 5 min and the reaction was stopped by adding 50 μl stop solution (1 M sulfuric acid). Reactions were measured as optical density (OD) at 450 nm using an ELISA plate reader operated with commercial software (Biotek® Instruments Inc., Winooski, VT, USA). The serum antibody response was presented as sample-to-positive (S/P) ratios calculated as: S/P ratio = (sample OD – negative control mean OD)/(positive control mean OD – negative control mean OD). The PEDV VarS1 ELISA was validated using 29 field serum samples collected from a farm with documented exposure to the U.S. PEDV S-INDEL-variant strain (serum samples were collected from 29 weaned pigs one month after they were found positive for S-INDEL-variant strain by PCR) and 20 PEDV-negative field serum samples. The S/P ratio of >0.3 was considered antibody positive, 0.2–0.3 was suspect, and <0.2 was negative.

Virus neutralization (VN) test

Serum samples were tested by a U.S. PEDV prototype strain-based VN (Pro VN) and a U.S. PEDV S-INDEL-variant strain-based VN (Var VN) following the previously described procedures [20]. The PEDV prototype isolate USA/IN19338/2013 was used as the indicator virus in the Pro VN assay and the S-INDEL-variant isolate USA/IL20697/2014 was used as the indicator virus in the Var VN assay. The reciprocal of the highest serum dilution resulting in >90 % reduction of staining as compared to the negative serum control was defined as the VN titer of the serum sample. A VN titer of ≥8 was considered positive.

Statistical analysis

The Log_2 (IFA titer/10) of the Pro antisera and the Var antisera tested by Pro IFA and Var IFA were analyzed in a generalized linear mixed model (GLIMMIX). Days post inoculation and antigen were used as independent variables, and pig ID and the interaction of pig ID and antigen were set as random effects. The Log_2 (VN titer) of the Pro antisera and the Var antisera tested by Pro VN and Var VN were analyzed in a similar way. For ELISA analysis, ELISA antigen, pig ID and DPI were used as independent variables. All statistical analyses were performed with Statistical Analysis System (SAS) version 9.3 (SAS institute, Cary, NC, USA), with p value <0.05 considered significantly different.

Results

Isolation of the U.S. PEDV S-INDEL-variant strain in cell culture

Virus isolation was first attempted on 68 clinical samples received at the ISU VDL that tested positive for the U.S. PEDV S-INDEL-variant strain but virus isolation attempts in cell culture were unsuccessful. Subsequently a PEDV S-INDEL-variant strain-positive intestine homogenate was used to inoculate three 3-week-old pigs. The rectal swab of one pig had a PEDV RT-PCR Ct < 15 at 2 DPI and the pig was euthanized and necropsied at 3 DPI. The rectal swabs of the other two pigs had PEDV RT-PCR Ct < 15 at 3 DPI and both pigs were euthanized and necropsied at 4 DPI. The small intestine tissues and cecum contents collected at necropsy were used to attempt virus isolation in Vero cells. The U.S. PEDV S-INDEL-variant strain was successfully isolated from small intestine homogenates and cecum contents collected from all 3 pigs. Typical PEDV cytopathic effects including syncytial body formation and cell detachment were observed and the virus growth was confirmed by immunofluorescence staining using PEDV-specific monoclonal antibody.

One U.S. PEDV S-INDEL-variant isolate designated as USA/IL20697/2014 was selected for further propagation and characterization. This isolate was serially passed in Vero cells and the infectious titers ranged from 10^3–10^5 $TCID_{50}$/ml for the first ten passages. The whole genome sequences of the isolate USA/IL20697/2014 at passage 5 (P5) had 99.3–99.9 % nucleotide identity to other U.S. PEDV S-INDEL-variant sequences available in GenBank. The S1 sequences of the USA/IL20697/2014 cell culture isolate P5 had 99.8 % nucleotide identity (only 4 nucleotide differences) to the original intestine homogenate from which the virus isolate was derived. The USA/IL20697/2014 isolate was tested at the ISU VDL and confirmed negative for TGEV, PRCV, PDCoV, porcine rotavirus A, B, C, influenza A virus, porcine reproductive and respiratory syndrome virus, and porcine circovirus 2 by virus-specific PCRs.

Generation of antisera against the U.S. prototype and S-INDEL-variant PEDVs

The U.S. PEDV prototype isolate USA/IN19338/2013 and S-INDEL-variant isolate USA/IL20697/2014 successfully established infections in all inoculated pigs as evidenced by PCR testing of the rectal swabs. In prototype group, 4/5, 5/5, 5/5, 5/5, 5/5, 5/5, and 3/5 pigs shed the virus in rectal swabs at 2, 4, 7, 10, 14, 21, and 28 DPI, respectively, as tested by PEDV real-time RT-PCR. In S-INDEL-variant group, 3/5, 5/5, 5/5, 5/5, 4/5, 3/5 and 1/5 pigs shed the virus in rectal swabs at 2, 4, 7, 10, 14, 21 and 28 DPI, respectively. The rectal swabs of the negative control pigs remained PEDV PCR negative throughout the study period. In total, 25 antisera were collected from the prototype strain-inoculated pigs (Pro antisera), 25 antisera collected from the variant strain-inoculated pigs (Var antisera), and 25 antisera collected from negative control group (Neg antisera), at 0, 7, 14, 21, and 28 DPI.

Evaluation of cross-reactivity of antibodies against the U.S. PEDV prototype strain and S-INDEL-variant strain by PEDV IFA antibody assays

As shown in Fig. 1, the Pro antisera tested antibody negative (0/5) at 0 and 7 DPI and 100 % positive (5/5) at 14, 21, and 28 DPI by the prototype strain-based IFA antibody assay (Pro IFA). The variant strain-based IFA (Var IFA) gave similar results on the Pro antisera except that one serum collected at 14 DPI was negative by the Var IFA assay. When the antibody titers were compared, the positive Pro antisera overall reacted better to the Pro IFA assay than to the Var IFA assay, with 1.4 log2 higher titer on average (Fig. 1).

The Var antisera tested negative (0/5) at 0 and 7 DPI and 100 % positive (5/5) at 14, 21, and 28 DPI by both the Pro IFA and Var IFA antibody assays. When the antibody titers were compared, the positive Var antisera reacted similarly to both Pro IFA and Var IFA assays, with less than 0.1 log2 titer differences on average (Fig. 1).

The antisera collected from the negative control group (Neg antisera) were antibody negative by both PEDV Pro IFA and Var IFA assays throughout the study. The pig antiserum against the European PEDV CV777 strain had similar antibody titers by the Pro IFA assay (titer 320) and by the Var IFA assay (titer 160). The antisera against TGEV Purdue, PHEV, PDCoV, and PRCV viruses were all negative by both PEDV Pro IFA and Var IFA assays.

Evaluation of cross-reactivity of antibodies against the U.S. PEDV prototype strain and S-INDEL-variant strain by various PEDV ELISAs

As shown in Fig. 2, the Pro antisera collected at 0 and 7 DPI were all antibody negative by ProWV ELISA, ProS1 ELISA, and VarS1 ELISA. For the Pro antisera collected at 14 DPI, 2 sera were positive and 3 were in the suspect

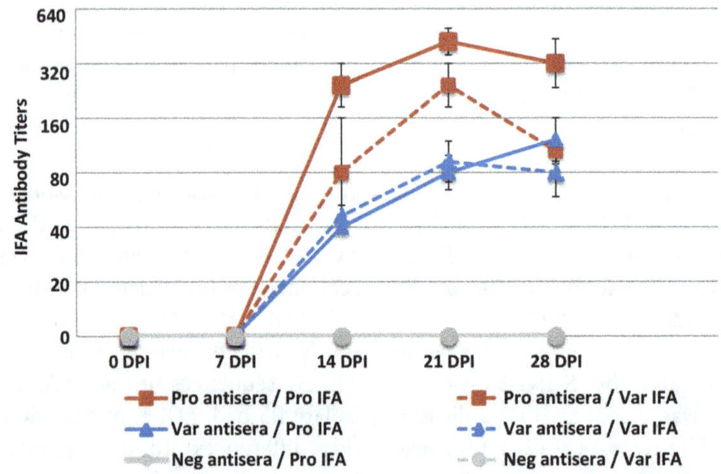

	Pro antisera		Var antisera		Neg antisera	
	Pro IFA +	Var IFA +	Pro IFA +	Var IFA +	Pro IFA +	Var IFA +
0 DPI	0	0	0	0	0	0
7 DPI	0	0	0	0	0	0
14 DPI	5	4	5	5	0	0
21 DPI	5	5	5	5	0	0
28 DPI	5	5	5	5	0	0

Fig. 1 IFA antibody testing of antisera against the U.S. PEDV prototype and S-INDEL-variant strains. The average IFA antibody titers are shown at the top and the number of IFA antibody positive samples is shown at the bottom. Pro antisera: antisera collected from the U.S. PEDV prototype strain-inoculated pigs; Var antisera: antisera collected from the U.S. PEDV S-INDEL-variant strain-inoculated pigs; Neg antisera: antisera collected from negative control pigs; Pro IFA: the U.S. PEDV prototype strain-based IFA; Var IFA: the U.S. PEDV S-INDEL-variant strain-based IFA

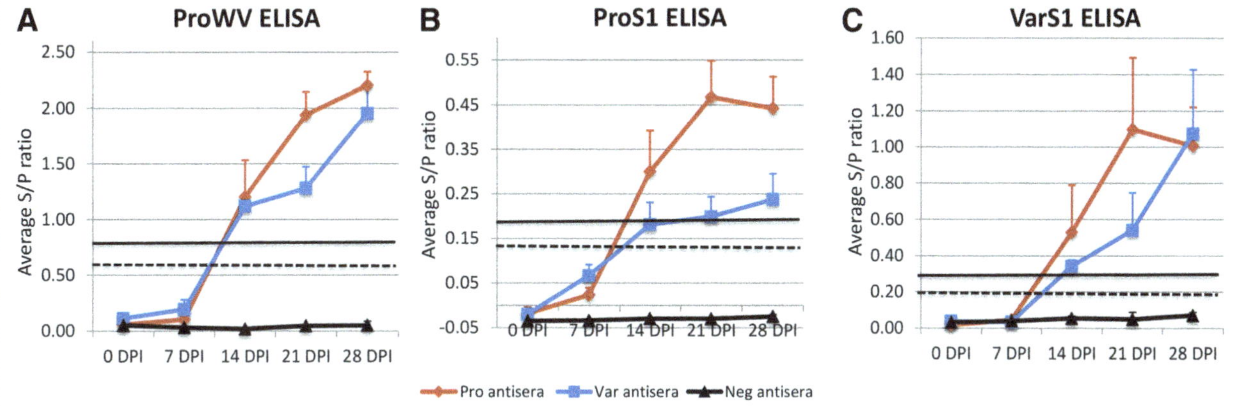

	Pro antisera			Var antisera			Neg antisera		
	ProWV ELISA Pos (Suspect)	ProS1 ELISA Pos (Suspect)	VarS1 ELISA Pos (Suspect)	ProWV ELISA Pos (Suspect)	ProS1 ELISA Pos (Suspect)	VarS1 ELISA Pos (Suspect)	ProWV ELISA Pos (Suspect)	ProS1 ELISA Pos (Suspect)	VarS1 ELISA Pos (Suspect)
0 DPI	0	0	0	0	0	0	0	0	0
7 DPI	0	0	0	0	0 (1)	0	0	0	0
14 DPI	2 (3)	3 (1)	2 (1)	5	3 (1)	4 (1)	0	0	0
21 DPI	5	5	5	4 (1)	2 (2)	3 (2)	0	0	0
28 DPI	5	5	5	5	3 (1)	5	0	0	0

Fig. 2 Testing of antisera against the U.S. PEDV prototype and S-INDEL-variant strains by ProWV ELISA (**a**), ProS1 ELISA (**b**) and VarS1 ELISA (**c**). For each assay, the solid black line indicates the S/P ratio above which the sample was positive; the dot black line indicates the S/P ratio below which the sample was negative; samples with S/P ratios between the solid and dot black line were suspect. ProWV ELISA: the U.S. PEDV prototype strain whole virus-based ELISA; ProS1 ELISA: the U.S. PEDV prototype strain S1-based ELISA; VarS1 ELISA: the U.S. PEDV S-INDEL-variant strain S1-based ELISA

range by the ProWV ELISA; 3 positives and 1 suspect by the ProS1 ELISA; 2 positives and 1 suspect by the VarS1 ELISA. The Pro antisera collected at 21 and 28 DPI were all positive by three ELISAs. When comparing the total number of positive Pro antisera at 14, 21 and 28 DPI by each ELISA, there were no significant differences among three ELISAs to detect antibody against the U.S. PEDV prototype strain.

The Var antisera collected at 0 and 7 DPI were antibody negative by all three ELISAs, with the exception of one serum at 7 DPI that was in the suspect range by the ProS1 ELISA (Fig. 2). The Var antisera collected at 14, 21 and 28 DPI had variable numbers of positive, suspect and negative results by three ELISAs (Fig. 2). Overall for the Var antisera, the ProWV ELISA detected 14 sera as antibody positive, 1 as suspect, and 10 as negative; the ProS1 ELISA detected 8 sera as positive, 5 as suspect, and 12 as negative; the VarS1 ELISA detected 12 sera as positive, 3 as suspect, and 10 as negative. When comparing the total number of positive Var antisera at 14, 21 and 28 DPI by each ELISA, the ProWV ELISA was significantly better than the ProS1 ELISA to detect antibody against the U.S. PEDV S-INDEL-variant strain ($p = 0.0079$). However, there were no significant differences between the ProWV ELISA and VarS1 ELISA ($p = 0.3643$), or between the ProS1 ELISA and VarS1 ELISA ($p = 0.0723$), to detect antibody against the U.S. PEDV S-INDEL-variant strain.

The antisera collected from the negative control group (Neg antisera) were antibody negative by all three PEDV ELISAs throughout the study period 0–28 DPI. The pig antiserum against the European PEDV CV777 strain was antibody positive by all three PEDV ELISAs. The antisera against TGEV Purdue, PHEV, PDCoV, and PRCV viruses were all negative by three PEDV ELISAs.

Evaluation of cross-neutralization of antibodies against the U.S. PEDV prototype strain and S-INDEL-variant strain by virus neutralization tests

As shown in Fig. 3, VN antibodies were detected as early as 7 DPI in sera of most of the pigs inoculated with either a prototype strain or an S-INDEL-variant strain, regardless of testing by Pro VN or Var VN assays. Serum samples collected at 14, 21 and 28 DPI from all pigs inoculated with PEDV prototype strain or S-INDEL-variant strain were VN antibody positive by both Pro VN and Var VN assays.

The positive Pro antisera had similar VN antibody titers by the Pro VN and Var VN assays and there was no significant difference between the two assays. The positive Var antisera had similar VN antibody titers by the Pro VN and Var VN assays and overall there was no significant difference between the two assays ($p = 0.42$)

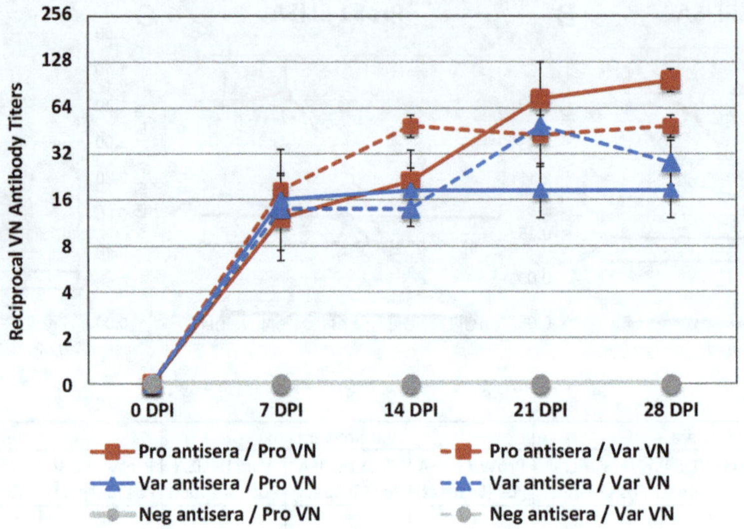

	Pro antisera		Var antisera		Neg antisera	
	Pro VN +	Var VN +	Pro VN +	Var VN +	Pro VN +	Var VN +
0 DPI	0	0	0	0	0	0
7 DPI	4	5	4	5	0	0
14 DPI	5	5	5	5	0	0
21 DPI	5	5	5	5	0	0
28 DPI	5	5	5	5	0	0

Fig. 3 Virus neutralization antibody testing of antisera against the U.S. PEDV prototype and S-INDEL-variant strains. The average VN antibody titers are shown at the top and the number of VN antibody positive samples is shown at the bottom. Pro VN: the U.S. PEDV prototype strain-based VN; Var VN: the U.S. PEDV S-INDEL-variant strain-based VN

although the average VN antibody titers of Var antisera at 21 and 28 DPI were slightly higher by the Var VN assay than by the Pro VN assay (Fig. 3).

The VN antibody titers of the positive Pro antisera tested by the homologous Pro VN assay were, on average, 0.8 log2 higher than the VN antibody titers of the positive Var antisera tested by the homologous Var VN assay (Fig. 3).

The antisera collected from the negative control group (Neg antisera) were antibody negative by both Pro VN and Var VN assays throughout the study period 0–28 DPI. The pig antiserum against the European PEDV CV777 strain was antibody positive by the Pro VN assay (titer 64) and by the Var VN assay (titer 16). The antisera against TGEV Purdue, PHEV, PDCoV, and PRCV viruses were all negative by both PEDV Pro VN and Var VN assays.

Discussion

Our lab has previously isolated the U.S. PEDV prototype strains in Vero cells [7]. In order to obtain a cell culture isolate of U.S. PEDV S-INDEL-variant strains to generate strain-specific antisera for evaluation, virus isolation was first attempted in Vero cells using 68 PEDV S-INDEL-variant strain-positive clinical samples submitted to the ISU VDL. However, attempts to isolate S-INDEL-variant virus in cell culture from these samples were unsuccessful. This could be due to multiple factors such as low concentration of virus in samples, cytotoxicity of some samples, and variable storage conditions of the clinical samples after collection. Next, among the 68 clinical samples, one intestine homogenate containing the S-INDEL-variant PEDV was inoculated into pigs to generate more fresh materials with abundant virus load for virus isolation attempts in cell culture. Using this approach, U.S. S-INDEL-variant PEDV was successfully isolated in Vero cells. It is speculated that high concentration of virus in the samples and immediate virus isolation attempts on the fresh samples are the key to success of virus isolation in cell culture. For other viruses under occasions that there is difficulty to isolate those viruses in cell cultures directly from the clinical samples of naturally infected animals, the approach described in this study can be considered, namely amplifying the virus in host animals to obtain fresh samples with high concentration of virus for virus isolation attempts in cell cultures.

Some field serum samples collected from swine farms were submitted to the ISU VDL for PEDV antibody detection. However, due to the lack of clear exposure history of these cases as well as the possibility of infection with multiple pathogens or with more than one PEDV strain, these field serum samples were not ideal for evaluating serological cross-reactivity of different PEDV strains. Therefore, in the present study, antisera against the U.S. PEDV prototype and S-INDEL-variant strains were generated in weaned pigs under strict experimental conditions, for evaluation of cross-reactivity by various serological assays.

The positive antisera against the prototype strain reacted with both prototype and S-INDEL-variant viruses, and the positive antisera against the S-INDEL-variant strain also reacted with both prototype and S-INDEL-variant viruses, as examined by IFA antibody assays. When taking the antibody titers into consideration, antibodies against the prototype strain reacted better to the Pro IFA assay than to the Var IFA assay whereas antibodies against the S-INDEL-variant strain reacted similarly to the Var IFA and Pro IFA assays. Thus, the current U.S. PEDV prototype strain-based IFA antibody assay offered at veterinary diagnostic laboratories can be used to detect antibodies against both U.S. PEDV strains.

The ProWV ELISA and ProS1 ELISA have been previously developed and validated to detect PEDV-specific antibodies [14–16]. A PEDV VarS1 ELISA was developed in this study. However, this VarS1 ELISA was only validated using a limited number of field antisera against the U.S. PEDV S-INDEL-variant strain before testing the experimentally generated antisera in this study. Further validation of this VarS1 ELISA using large number of serum samples would be needed to determine the performance of this assay. All three PEDV ELISAs reacted with the Pro antisera and Var antisera. The three ELISAs detected Pro antisera similarly. However, it appeared that the ProS1 ELISA used in this study was not as efficient as the ProWV ELISA and the VarS1 ELISA to detect the antibodies against the U.S. PEDV S-INDEL-variant strain under the conditions of this study.

The antibodies against the U.S. prototype strain and the antibodies against the U.S. S-INDEL-variant strain neutralized both virus strains to similar titers. The U.S. PEDV prototype strain-based VN tests currently run in the laboratories can be used to detect antibodies against both U.S. PEDV strains.

Both the prototype and S-INDEL-variant PEDV-inoculated pigs developed detectable IFA and ELISA antibodies in sera starting from 14 DPI in this study. In contrast, both groups of pigs developed low levels of serum neutralizing antibodies starting from 7 DPI. The IFA and ELISA assays in this study detected IgG antibodies; the VN tests could potentially detect any antibody isotype with neutralizing activity. It is unclear whether this contributes to the observed early detection of low-level VN antibody. In a previous study, it has also been reported that PEDV VN antibody could be detected as early as 7 DPI [20].

The distinct genetic differences between the U.S. prototype and S-INDEL-variant PEDVs are located in the S1 region (nucleotides 1–2214 corresponding to aa 1–738, according to positions in the prototype strain USA/IN19338/2013, GenBank accession number KF650371), especially the N-terminal region of the S gene (nucleotides 1–1170 corresponding to aa 1–390) whereas the remaining portions of the genomes are relatively conserved between the two U.S. strains [4, 8, 10]. The PEDV prototype strain S1 protein used for the ProS1 ELISA and the PEDV S-INDEL-variant strain S1 protein used for the VarS1 ELISA had 92 % amino acid identity. The reported PEDV neutralizing epitopes are located in the S protein amino acid residues 499–638, 744–759, 756–771, and 1368–1374 [1, 21]. The protein sequences in these locations harboring the neutralizing epitopes are conserved between the U.S. prototype and S-INDEL-variant PEDVs. This can explain why the antibodies against the two PEDV strains were able to cross-neutralize two virus strains. The ProS1 and VarS1 ELISAs were developed using the recombinant PEDV S1 proteins (aa 1–738). Although the U.S. prototype and S-INDEL-variant PEDVs have considerable differences in aa 1–390, the two strains still have some common epitopes in this region. In addition, the recombinant S1 proteins of two PEDV strains have relatively conserved sequences from aa 390–738 including the neutralizing epitopes in this region. These may be the reasons why the ProS1 and VarS1 ELISAs can detect antibodies against both U.S. PEDV strains despite of possible differences on the sensitivity between assays. The IFA antibody assay and ProWV ELISA are supposed to detect antibodies against multiple antigenic proteins of PEDV and thus they are expected to detect antibodies against both U.S. prototype and S-INDEL-variant PEDVs. Other laboratories have developed nucleocapsid protein-based ELISAs [18] that were not evaluated in this study. Considering that the nucleocapsid protein is rather conserved among PEDVs, it is expected that the nucleocapsid protein-based ELISAs should detect antibodies against both U.S. PEDV strains. We also included one pig antiserum against the classical European PEDV CV777 strain for evaluation and the PEDV CV777 antibody was detected by all serological assays evaluated in this study. However, antisera against TGEV Purdue, PHEV, PDCoV and PRCV had no cross-reactivity with PEDV serological assays evaluated in this study.

In a previous study by Lin et al [22], hyperimmune pig antisera against U.S. PEDV prototype strain, U.S. PEDV S-INDEL-variant strain, TGEV Purdue strain, and TGEV Miller strain were generated and tested by cell culture immunofluorescence (CCIF) assay (similar to our IFA antibody assay) and fluorescent focus reduction virus neutralization (FFRVN) assay (similar to our VN test). They found that antisera against the U.S. PEDV prototype strain, S-INDEL-variant strain, and European CV777 strain all had cross-reactivity by CCIF and FFRVN assays. Our findings are consistent with their results. In addition to similar serological assays used by Lin et al, we also evaluated PEDV serological reactivity via three PEDV ELISAs. Also, we tested sequential serum samples (0–28 DPI) from pigs experimentally infected with two U.S. PEDV strains, providing useful information about the kinetics of PEDV antibody production in weaned pigs. An interesting finding in the Lin et al study was that hyperimmune antisera against TGEV Miller strain rather than TGEV Purdue strain cross-reacted with all PEDV strains by CCIF assay but not by FFRVN assay. They further demonstrated that one epitope on the N-terminal region of PEDV/TGEV N protein may contribute to this cross-reactivity. We did not include an antiserum against TGEV Miller strain in our study and could not evaluate its cross-reactivity in our PEDV assays.

Conclusions

The data in the present study indicate that the antibodies against U.S. PEDV prototype and S-INDEL-variant strains cross-reacted and cross-neutralized both strains in vitro. The current serological assays based on U.S. PEDV prototype strain can detect antibodies against both U.S. PEDV strains. However, the cross-protection efficacy of these two PEDV strains needs to be determined by in vivo pig studies. Goede et al [23] showed that sows exposed to S-INDEL-variant PEDV infection 7 months ago could provide partial protection to newborn piglets challenged with a U.S. PEDV prototype strain. But more in vivo studies in this respect are needed to reveal whether a U.S. PEDV prototype strain or the S-INDEL-variant strain or both should be used to develop a vaccine for providing protection against both PEDV strains circulating in U.S. swine.

Consent for publication

Not applicable.

Abbreviations

ELISA: enzyme-linked immunosorbent assay; IFA: indirect fluorescent antibody; Neg antisera: antisera collected from negative control pigs; PED: porcine epidemic diarrhea; PEDV: porcine epidemic diarrhea virus; Pro antisera: antisera collected from the U.S. PEDV prototype strain-inoculated pigs; Pro IFA: the U.S. PEDV prototype strain-based IFA; Pro VN: the U.S. PEDV prototype strain-based VN; ProS1 ELISA: the U.S. PEDV prototype strain S1-based ELISA; ProWV ELISA: the U.S. PEDV prototype strain whole virus-based ELISA; S INDEL: spike gene insertions and deletions; Var antisera: antisera collected from the U.S. PEDV S-INDEL-variant strain-inoculated pigs; Var IFA: the U.S. PEDV S-INDEL-variant strain-based IFA; Var VN: the U.S. PEDV S-INDEL-variant strain-based VN.; VarS1 ELISA: the U.S. PEDV S-INDEL-variant strain S1-based ELISA; VN: virus neutralization.

Competing interests

The authors declare that they have no competing interests.

Authors' contributions

Conceived and designed the experiments: JZ. Isolated and characterized U.S. PEDV S-INDEL-variant strain: QC, JTT, PCG, DMM, YZ, GL and JZ. Performed animal studies to generate PEDV antisera: QC, JTT, PCG, DMM, DRM, and JZ. Performed IFA and VN antibody tests: QC. Cloned, expressed and purified PEDV S-INDEL-variant S1 protein: JMH and QG. Performed PEDV whole virus-based ELISA and PEDV variant S1-based ELISA: LGG. Performed PEDV prototype S1-based ELISA: PFG and TO. Conducted data analysis: QC and JZ. Prepared and revised the manuscript: QC, JZ, JTT, LGG, JMH, QG, PFG, TO, YZ, GL, PCG, DMM, and DRM. All authors read and approved the final manuscript.

Acknowledgements

This study was supported by Zoetis and the Iowa State University College of Veterinary Medicine Start-up fund awarded to Dr. Jianqiang Zhang. We are grateful to the Iowa State University Veterinary Diagnostic Laboratory faculty and staff for assistance with some testing. We also thank the Iowa State University Laboratory Animal Resources staff for animal care. Q.C. was partially supported by a fellowship sponsored by Zoetis.

Author details

[1]Department of Veterinary Diagnostic and Production Animal Medicine, College of Veterinary Medicine, Iowa State University, 1800 Christensen Drive, Ames, IA 50011, USA. [2]Zoetis, Kalamazoo, MI, USA. [3]The Roslin Institute and The Royal (Dick) School of Veterinary Studies, University of Edinburgh, Roslin, Midlothian, Edinburgh EH25 9RG, UK.

References

1. Song D, Park B. Porcine epidemic diarrhoea virus: a comprehensive review of molecular epidemiology, diagnosis, and vaccines. Virus Genes. 2012;44(2):167–75.
2. Stevenson GW, Hoang H, Schwartz KJ, Burrough ER, Sun D, Madson D, Cooper VL, Pillatzki A, Gauger P, Schmitt BJ et al. Emergence of Porcine epidemic diarrhea virus in the United States: clinical signs, lesions, and viral genomic sequences. J Vet Diagn Invest. 2013;25(5):649–54.
3. Pasick J, Berhane Y, Ojkic D, Maxie G, Embury-Hyatt C, Swekla K, Handel K, Fairles J, Alexandersen S. Investigation into the role of potentially contaminated feed as a source of the first-detected outbreaks of porcine epidemic diarrhea in Canada. Transbound Emerg Dis. 2014;61(5):397–410.
4. Vlasova AN, Marthaler D, Wang Q, Culhane MR, Rossow KD, Rovira A, Collins J, Saif LJ. Distinct Characteristics and Complex Evolution of PEDV Strains, North America, May 2013-February 2014. Emerg Infect Dis. 2014;20(10):1620–1628.
5. ICTV. International Committee on Taxonomy of Viruses. 2012. Virus Taxonomy: 2012 Release. 2012. http://ictvonline.org/virusTaxonomy.asp?version=2012. Accessed 2 Jan 2015.
6. Huang YW, Dickerman AW, Pineyro P, Li L, Fang L, Kiehne R, Opriessnig T, Meng XJ. Origin, evolution, and genotyping of emergent porcine epidemic diarrhea virus strains in the United States. MBio. 2013;4(5):e00737–00713.
7. Chen Q, Li G, Stasko J, Thomas JT, Stensland WR, Pillatzki AE, Gauger PC, Schwartz KJ, Madson D, Yoon KJ, et al. Isolation and characterization of porcine epidemic diarrhea viruses associated with

the 2013 disease outbreak among swine in the United States. J Clin Microbiol. 2014;52(1):234–43.
8. Wang L, Byrum B, Zhang Y. New variant of porcine epidemic diarrhea virus, United States, 2014. Emerg Infect Dis. 2014;20(5):917–9.
9. Zhang J, Chen Q, Gauger PC, Harmon KM, Yoon KJ. Reply to "classification of emergent U.S. strains of porcine epidemic diarrhea virus by phylogenetic analysis of nucleocapsid and ORF3 genes". J Clin Microbiol. 2014;52(9):3511–4.
10. Oka T, Saif LJ, Marthaler D, Esseili MA, Meulia T, Lin CM, Vlasova AN, Jung K, Zhang Y, Wang Q. Cell culture isolation and sequence analysis of genetically diverse US porcine epidemic diarrhea virus strains including a novel strain with a large deletion in the spike gene. Vet Microbiol. 2014;173(3-4):258–69.
11. Marthaler D, Bruner L, Collins J, Rossow K. Third strain of porcine epidemic diarrhea virus, United States. Emerg Infect Dis. 2014;20(12):2162–3.
12. Hoang H, Killian ML, Madson DM, Arruda PH, Sun D, Schwartz KJ, Yoon KJ. Full-Length Genome Sequence of a Plaque-Cloned Virulent Porcine Epidemic Diarrhea Virus Isolate (USA/Iowa/18984/2013) from a Midwestern U.S. Swine Herd. Genome Announc. 2013;1(6):e01049–13.
13. Lawrence PK, Bumgardner E, Bey RF, Stine D, Bumgarner RE. Genome sequences of porcine epidemic diarrhea virus: in vivo and in vitro phenotypes. Genome Announc. 2014;2(3):e00503–14.
14. Gerber PF, Gong Q, Huang YW, Wang C, Holtkamp D, Opriessnig T. Detection of antibodies against porcine epidemic diarrhea virus in serum and colostrum by indirect ELISA. Vet J. 2014;202(1):33–6.
15. Gimenez-Lirola LG. Porcine epidemic diarrhea virus antibody tests available at ISU VDL. In: Swine Health Monitoring Projecct. 9/26/2014th ed. 2014.
16. Gimenez-Lirola LG, Baum D, Bower L, Chen Q, Sun D, Johnson J, Kalkwarf E, Madson D, Magtoto R, Yoon KJ et al et al. Porcine epidemic diarrhea virus: antibody-based test development. In: The 22nd Annual Swine Disease Conference for Swine Practitioners. 2014. Ames, Iowa 2014: 34-37.
17. Madson DM, Magstadt DR, Arruda PH, Hoang H, Sun D, Bower LP, Bhandari M, Burrough ER, Gauger PC, Pillatzki AE, et al. Pathogenesis of porcine epidemic diarrhea virus isolate (US/Iowa/18984/2013) in 3-week-old weaned pigs. Vet Microbiol. 2014;174(1-2):60–8.
18. Okda F, Liu X, Singrey A, Clement T, Nelson J, Christopher-Hennings J, Nelson EA, Lawson S. Development of an indirect ELISA, blocking ELISA, fluorescent microsphere immunoassay and fluorescent focus neutralization assay for serologic evaluation of exposure to North American strains of Porcine Epidemic Diarrhea Virus. BMC Vet Res. 2015;11:180.
19. Lowe J, Gauger P, Harmon K, Zhang J, Connor J, Yeske P, Loula T, Levis I, Dufresne L, Main R. Role of transportation in spread of porcine epidemic diarrhea virus infection, United States. Emerg Infect Dis. 2014;20(5):872–4.
20. Thomas JT, Chen Q, Gauger PC, Gimenez-Lirola LG, Sinha A, Harmon KM, Madson DM, Burrough ER, Magstadt DR, Salzbrenner HM et al. Effect of Porcine Epidemic Diarrhea Virus Infectious Doses on Infection Outcomes in Naive Conventional Neonatal and Weaned Pigs. PLoS One. 2015;10(10): e0139266.
21. Sun D, Feng L, Shi H, Chen J, Cui X, Chen H, Liu S, Tong Y, Wang Y, Tong G. Identification of two novel B cell epitopes on porcine epidemic diarrhea virus spike protein. Vet Microbiol. 2008;131(1-2):73–81.
22. Lin CM, Gao X, Oka T, Vlasova AN, Esseili MA, Wang Q, Saif LJ. Antigenic relationships among porcine epidemic diarrhea virus and transmissible gastroenteritis virus strains. J Virol. 2015;89(6):3332–42.
23. Goede D, Murtaugh MP, Nerem J, Yeske P, Rossow K, Morrison R. Previous infection of sows with a "mild" strain of porcine epidemic diarrhea virus confers protection against infection with a "severe" strain. Vet Microbiol. 2015;176(1-2):161–4.

7

Molecular identification and investigations of contagious ecthyma (Orf virus) in small ruminants

Mebrahtu Tedla[1*], Nega Berhan[2], Wassie Molla[3], Wudu Temesgen[4] and Sefinew Alemu[3]

Abstract

Background: Orf virus, the prototype of parapoxvirus, is the main causative agent of contagious ecthyma. Little is known about the status of the disease in Ethiopia and this study was aimed at determining its status using PCR as a confirmatory tool.

Methods: a total of 400 randomly selected sheep and goat was screened for the identification of the virus using amplification of B2L gene and transfection of mammalian cells (VERO cells).

Results: Out of 400 animals screened for infection of the virus, 48 animals were found positive to PCR and revealed an overall incidence of 12%. Different epidemiological parameters were considered to look at the association with incidence of the disease and of which, only species of the animal(sheep), non-vaccinated and non-treated animals, nursing animals, poor body condition animals, extensively managed animals, animals having mouth lesion, and study areas having outbreak history showed higher prevalence. A univariate logistic regression analysis showed statistically significant difference in all variables ($P < 0.05$). Whereas, age and sex of animals showed no significant difference ($P < 0.05$).

Conclusion: The result of the present finding showed high incidence of Orf virus in the region as confirmed through PCR.

Keywords: Orf virus, Incidence, Cytopathic effect, PCR, Sheep and goat, Risk factors

Background

Small ruminants have a tremendous importance in terms of generating income in the form of meat, wool, hide and occasionally milk in small scale farming. However, infectious diseases are still the health challenges by hindering the production and productivity and this causes huge economic loss [1, 2]. Contagious ecthyma or alternatively called contagious pustular dermatitis is a viral disease of sheep and goat caused by Orf virus which belongs to the family of poxviridae and based on the classification of international committee on taxonomy of viruses(ICTV), it is one of the notifiable viral disease known to have a zoonotic importance [1, 3, 4]. It is characterized to have a benign nature, and it can cause a large tumor like vascularized lesions which can be treated using antiviral drugs or removed surgically. It is transmitted through direct contact with infected animals and environmental contamination [5, 6].

Although the rate of morbidity is generally higher than the mortality rate, younger animals such as lambs are more susceptible for the disease and the mortality is significantly higher [7]. Currently, there are live Orf vaccines which can control the disease, but it has a spreading potential to the environment and increasing the risk of another animals [7]. Infected animals can show a common clinical picture such as infectious pustules around the lip area, mouth, tongue, and very rarely on udder and teats and unsurprisingly, the disease in various outbreaks is named as Orf, contagious ecthyma, pustular dermatitis, infectious labial dermatitis, scabby mouth, or sore mouth [8].

The pathogenesis starts with the development of skin erythema and progresses in to vesicle and pustules formation and finally scab formation. One of the typical

* Correspondence: mebvet2002@gmail.com
[1]Department of Biomedical Sciences, University of Gondar, College of Veterinary Medicine and Animal Sciences, P.O. Box: 196, Gondar, Ethiopia
Full list of author information is available at the end of the article

characteristics of the disease is proliferative and sometimes self-limited lesions on the infected regions of the skin, mucosa of oral cavity and nostrils [9]. The morphology of the virus under electron microscope looks like an ovoid with diagonally woven structures or bands [10, 11].

The virus genome consists of linear double-stranded DNA ranging from 134 up to 139 kb [6]. The envelope gene (B2L) of the virus encodes for a highly immunogenic envelope protein [12]. And amplification of this gene has been used for the detection of ORFV by PCR [13–15]. A gene called vascular endothelial growth factor is identified as a potential cause of Orf virus pathology due to its ability of stimulating endothelial cells to promote vascular permeability [16–18]. A sequencing analysis of the virus has been studied and Peralta et al. 2015 [19] identified five genes namely, B2L, ORFO20, ORF109, ORF127, ORF117 genes from virus outbreaks in Argentina. Furthermore, Delhon G.et al. 2004 [20] sequenced the whole genome of the virus and phylogenic analysis has been carried out from various isolates from around the world such as Korea [21], Brazil [22], china [23, 24] and India [25].

The disease has a global distribution [25–27] and it affects not only sheep and goat but also a wide range of animals such as dog, cattle, camel and wild animals and it is endemic in countries where these animals are common [6]. Outbreaks of contagious ecthyma has been frequently occurred in Ethiopia. However, there is no detail report on the molecular identification of the disease so far and this study was aimed for the first time to identify the status of the disease in the study area.

Methods

Identification of study area

The present study was conducted in three districts. Namely, Ambagiorgis from highland, Gondar Zuria from midland, and Addis Zemen from lowland areas. The study areas are depicted in the map showed in Fig. 1, modified from (https://no.wikipedia.org/wiki/Amhara_(region)(region)). The study areas were represented considering presence of adequate study animals and diversity in agroecology.

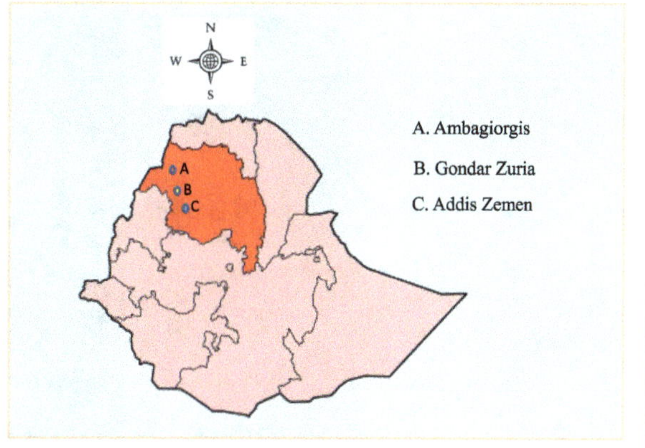

Fig. 1 Geographic location of the study areas

Screening and sampling procedure

This study involved a total of 400 randomly selected animals (200 sheep and 200 goat). The sampling procedure involves first step of screening infected animals having a characteristic Orf lesions as shown in Fig. 2 followed by taking tissue samples from the lesion. Fresh lesion scraping was taken immediately from the animal aseptically using diethyl ether. Dried scabs, papular fluids, crusts, and nodules collected were stored in ice box using 1% PBS supplied with pen strep and transported to national veterinary institute for confirmation. Data related to different risk factors or variables were collected through direct observation or by direct interviewing of animal owners. Ethical approval for animal studies was approved by the animal ethics and welfare committee of the University of Gondar. Informed consent was obtained from animal owners who participated in the study.

Viral isolation, culture and PCR amplification

Tissue samples were first washed using 1% PBS supplied with antibiotics three times and from the third wash, tissues were centrifuged at 14,000 rpm for 10 min. Then 500 µl of viral supernatant was taken for the infection of VERO cells. Cells were cultured on 25cm^2 culture flask using sterilized GMEM (Sigma Aldrich) and with the addition of 10% FCS. Then cells were incubated for 5 days at 37 °C, 5% CO_2. The confluency of the cells and the cytopathic effects was regularly checked [28]. DNA was extracted following Commercial Purlink ™ genomic DNA kit(Invitrogen) and purified DNA was stored at -20 °C until the next use.

Polymerase chain reaction

After isolating genomic DNA from the virus, B2L gene was amplified using forward primers (5′-TGA GCT GGT TGG CGC TGT CCT-3′) and reverse primers (5'-CGC AGA CGT GGC TCA GTA CGT-3′). The reaction set up was prepared as follows: 5X standard reaction buffer (5 µl), 2 mM dNTPs (0.5 µl), 500 nM forward primer (1.25 µl), 500 nM reverse primer (1.25 µl), template DNA (5 µl), 2.5 U Taq DNA Polymerase (0.25 µl), nuclease-free water (to 25 µl). The thermal profile was set as follows: Initial denaturation (94 °C, 5 min, 1X cycle), Denaturation (94 °C, 1 min), Annealing (55 °C, 60 s, 35X), Extension (68 °C, 70 s), Final extension (68 °C, 5 min, 1X).

The size of DNA fragments was estimated using agarose gel electrophoresis. The DNA samples was mixed thoroughly with a loading dye at a ratio of 1:6. The mixed DNA samples were carefully loaded in to the gel and 1 kb plus DNA marker was used to gauge the size of the DNA. The

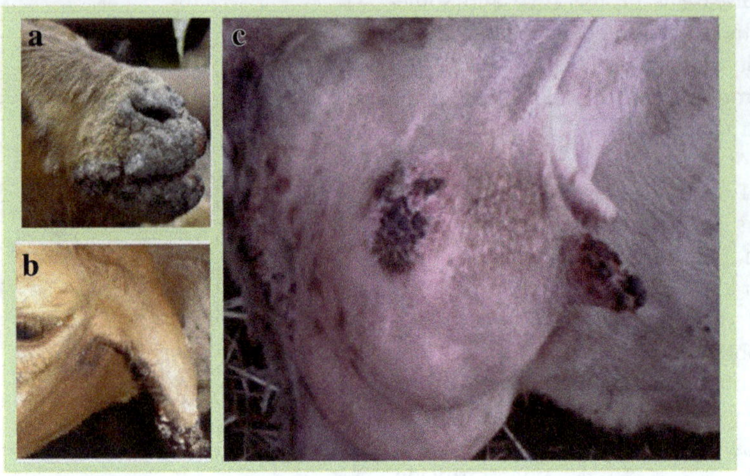

Fig. 2 Typical clinical lesions of contagious ecthyma in different body parts. **a**) nostrils and mouth region, **b**) ear, **c**) teat and udder

fragments were separated at a voltage of 100 V for a run time of 60 min. DNA bands were analyzed using UV transilluminator.

Data management and analysis

All date collected from the study were recorded in a microsoft excel spreadsheet and the statistical analysis was performed using STATA version 13. prevalence was calculated by dividing the number of positive animals to total animals examined multiplied by 100. Univariate logistic regression analysis was used to indicate the association of different risk factors with the occurrence of Orf virus infection.

Results

Cytopathic effect (CPE), characterized by the degenerative changes in VERO cells due to multiplication of the viruses in the cells was used as a first step screening of the samples by examining the morphology of cells after virus transfection of cells and a peculiar feature of evident syncytia formation was observed. Hence, different passages of cells were examined to identify the cytopathic effect of the virus and a total of 48 samples were processed for viral isolation and observation of CPE and the result revealed all the viral suspensions were toxic to the cells which was pre- confirmatory test for the virus. The morphology of VERO cells before and after transfection by the virus is illustrated in Fig. 3. Furthermore, genomic DNA from all clinical samples was extracted to amplify the B2L gene of the virus using a specific primer and revealed a PCR product of 140 bp size as confirmed by agarose gel electrophoresis. A representative sample assigned from S1 to S10 showed samples which were positive for the virus as indicated in Fig. 4.

For investigating the association of the disease with different putative risk factors, a total of 400 animals were screened for the identification of any signs of Orf such as contagious pustular dermatitis in different body parts of the animal including the mouse, nostrils, udder, teat, reproductive organs, interdigital space and the result showed an overall incidence of 12%. In addition, the questionnaire survey administered to the animal owners also indicated that animals having a Orf lesion showed a mortality rate of 4.8%. Orf identification based on the location of the lesion on the animal body revealed a prevalence of 19.8, 10.5, 8.97 and 2% on mouth, nostrils, teat and udder, and lower legs respectively. The univariate logistic regression analysis showed a strong association ($P < 0.05$) between the prevalence of Orf and the lesion development in various organs of the animal body with higher prevalence in mouth and lower prevalence in lower legs of the animal (Table 1).

Analysis on the prevalence of Orf virus based on the species of the animal showed a higher prevalence (15.5%) on sheep than goat (8.5%). The statistical association showed species has an impact on the prevalence of the disease (Table 1). Out of 190 male animals examined, 21 (11.05%) were positive for Orf virus and out of 210 female animals examined, 27 (12.85) were positive for the virus (Table 1). Although there was a difference in the prevalence of the virus among both sex groups, no statistically significant association was observed ($P < 0.05$). A higher prevalence (17.4%) of Orf virus was recorded in poor body conditioned animals than medium (9.2%) and good (7.8%) body conditioned animals (Table 1). The statistical analysis of these variables related to the prevalence of the disease showed a significant difference ($P < 0.05$). The prevalence based on age of the animal was recorded, and highest prevalence rate was recorded in the age group of 1–2 years (16.5%) than < 1 years (6.4%), 2-3 years (9.2%), and > 4 years (13.2%). Though there was a slight difference in the prevalence of each age groups, the statistical association showed no

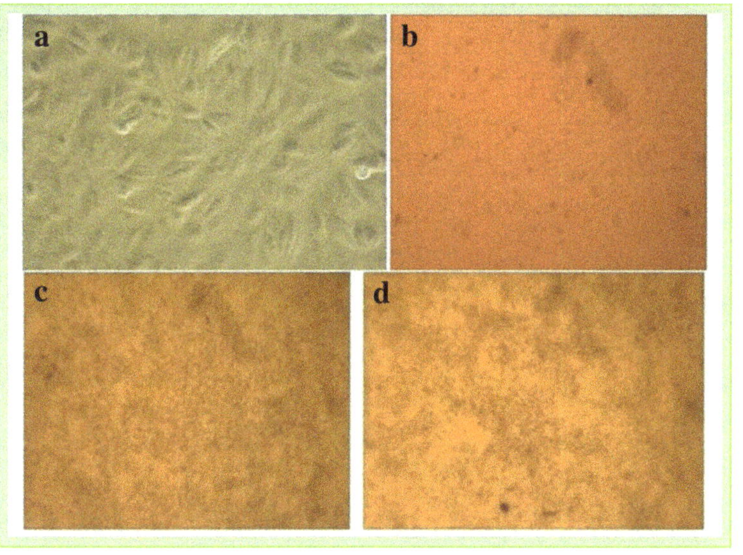

Fig. 3 a) Normal cells before viral transfection; **b**) Cells are trypsinized and appeared as a single cell; **c** & **d**) showing the peculiar feature of the cytopathic effects after 2 days of incubation

significant ($P > 0.05$). The result of the present study showed a prevalence of 17.04% in animals which are nursing. Whereas, a prevalence of 10.57% was recorded in non-nursing animals. The statistical analysis revealed a strong association between the nursing status and prevalence of Orf in the study area ($P < 0.05$). The prevalence of Orf virus in animals having either treatment and vaccination history was studied and showed a prevalence of 9.1% (anthelmintic treated animals), 14. %(no anthelmintic treated animals), 8% (antibiotic treated animals), 17.14%(no antibiotic treated animals), 15.21% (vaccinated animals), 21.62% (non-vaccinated animals). The statistical analysis revealed a significance difference among each group in relation to prevalence of the disease ($P < 0.05$).

By considering the management system of the study animals, we investigated whether there is an effect on the prevalence of the disease or not and the result showed a high prevalence of Orf virus in free housing animals and extensively managed animals with a prevalence of 18.18 and 14.15% respectively. The result of statistical analysis also showed that there was a strong association between management system and prevalence of the disease (Table 1. The prevalence on different study areas also showed a variation in the status of the disease in which higher prevalence was recorded in Addis Zemen (12.38%), Amba Giorgis (10.37%), and Gondar Zuria (13. 12%).However, we statistically found no significant difference in the prevalence of the disease in all the study areas ($P > 0.05$).

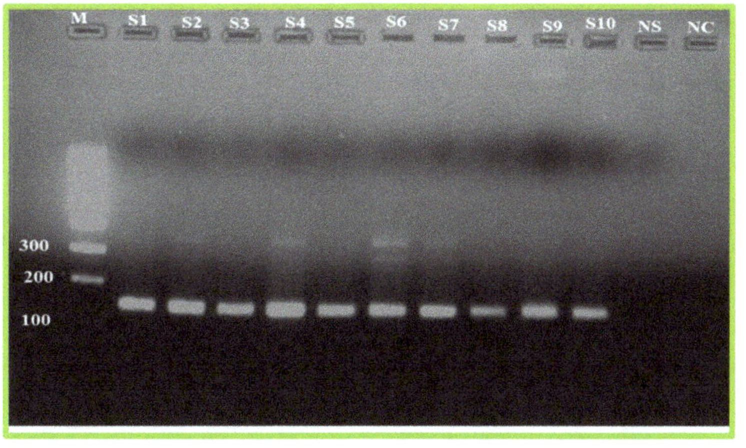

Fig. 4 The band size of 140 bp is the amplified product of B2L gene which is a confirmatory for the presence of the Orf virus on the clinical samples. M represents a 10,000 bp molecular weight marker and S1-S10 represents the unknown samples tested and NS is the negative sample. Whereas, NC is the negative control

Table 1 Univariate logistic regression analysis of the prevalence of Orf Virus infection with different putative risk factors

Body part lesion	N	No. Positive	Prevalence, % (95% CI)	*P*- value
Mouth	121	24	19.80 (14.71–23.22)	
Nostrils	153	16	10.50 (8.03–12.45)	0.041
Teat and udder	78	7	8.97 (5.98–11.32)	
Lower leg	50	1	2.00 (0.98–3.45)	
Total	400	48	12.00 (11.21–14.87)	
Species				
Goat	200	17	8.5 (7.23–10.11)	0.054
Sheep	200	31	15.5 (13.43–17.26)	
Total	400	48	12.00 (11.21–14.87)	
Sex				
Male	190	21	11.05 (9.86–14.36)	0.32
Female	210	27	12.85 (10.03–15.88)	
Total	400	48	12.00 (11.21–14.87)	
Body condition				
Poor	155	27	17.4 (14.01–19.23)	0.043
Medium	130	12	9.20 (7.01–12.87)	
Good	115	9	7.80 (5.44–9.06)	
Total	400	48	12.00 (11.21–14.87)	
Age				
< 1 year	47	3	6.4 (4.49–9.67)	
1–2 year	133	22	16.5 (12.54–19.98)	0.65
2–3 year	152	14	9.2 (6.31–12.03)	
> 4 years	68	9	13.2 (12.79–15.02)	
Total	400	48	12.00 (11.21–14.87)	
Nursing				
Yes	88	15	17.04 (14.01–21.39)	0.047
No	312	33	10.57 (7.75–11.64)	
Total	400	48	12.00 (11.21–14.87)	
Treatment and Vaccination				
Treated with anthelmentics	121	11	9.1 (7.01–12.20)	0.021
Not treated with anthelmentics	49	7	14.3 (11.10–17.09)	
Treated with antibiotics	112	9	8.0 (6.93–10.05)	
Not treated with antibiotics	35	6	17.14 (13.67–21.39)	
Any vaccination history	46	7	15.21 (12.32–17.66)	
No any vaccination history	37	8	21.62 (17.31–24.89)	
Total	400	48	12.00 (11.21–14.87)	
Management System				
Extensive	106	15	14.15 (11.05–17.08)	0.042
Semi extensive	94	11	11.70 (7.88–13.09)	
Mixed	81	9	11.11 (7.64–13.04)	
Free housing	56	10	18.18 (15.03–21.80)	
Protected housing	63	3	4.76 (2.44–7.42)	
Total	400	48	12.00 (11.21–14.87)	

Table 1 Univariate logistic regression analysis of the prevalence of Orf Virus infection with different putative risk factors *(Continued)*

Body part lesion	N	No. Positive	Prevalence, % (95% CI)	*P*- value
Study Area				
Gondar Zuria	160	21	13.12 (10.19–15.32)	0.65
Ambagiorgis	135	14	10.37 (7.83–13.09)	
Addis Zemen	105	13	12.38 (8.21–14.39)	
Total	400	48	12.00 (11.21–14.87)	
Type of Treatment		No. Responding		
Moist dressing		32	15.2 (12.1–19.64)	0.032
Surgical removal		57	27.1 (21.3–31.24)	
Culling		26	12.4 (9.02–15.62)	
Antibiotics		95	45.2 (39.56–45.42)	
Total		210		
Outbreak history				
Yes		280	70 (64.10–74.50)	0.012
No		120	30 (27.21–34.52)	
Total		400		

Furthermore, a total of 210 animal owners were interviewed on the treatment practices of their animals after they got infected and most (45.2%) use antibiotics followed by surgical removal (27.1%), moist dressing (15.2%) and culling (12.4%) as treatment options. In addition, the response of the owners and animal health workers on the outbreak history of the disease in the area showed a higher prevalence of Orf virus (70%) in areas having an outbreak history and lower (30%) in areas having no outbreak history (Table 1).

Discussion

In this study, we presented the first clinical report of Orf virus in small ruminants based on molecular identification in north western regions of Ethiopia. The disease has a high morbidity rate but low mortality rate and as a result, less attention has been given by the owners. However, the loss of production and productivity of the animals due to the disease significantly jeopardize the market value. Over the study period, we have recognized lack of adequate diagnosis and effective treatment of clinical cases which is the main contributing factor for the occurrence of disease outbreaks at any time points. The traditional methods of diagnosis which depends on the characteristic clinical signs is inaccurate, but virus isolation and culturing is thought to be a gold standard method of confirmation though it is time-consuming [29]. With the development of molecular biology, PCR technique has become widely used to amplify the desired genomic fragments from tissue specimens, and it has become a powerful tool in molecular diagnosis. This method is recommended for proper identification of the pathogen through gene amplification using specific forward and reverse primers [30]. Various researchers in different parts of the world have reported contagious ecthyma as common outbreak of sheep and goats [31] and indicated that PCR is a quick confirmatory test for Orf virus [32].

In the present study, we showed the distribution of the disease using tests such as the cytopathic effect(CPE) of the virus in mammalian cells followed PCR amplifications of B2L gene. In addition, this study showed the association of different variables that we classified them as risk factors with the incidence and prevalence of the disease. In this study, we found that the infection of Orf virus is common in mouth and nostrils of the animal. This is due to the close confinement and grazing habit of the animals which causes the formation of minor abrasions on the mouth and lips of the animal during feeding. A very low incidence of the virus was also observed on the teat and udder of the animal particularly in nursing animals in which the infected lambs could possibly be the source of infection during suckling. Furthermore, species of the animal showed a significant impact on the prevalence of the disease in which sheep were more sensitive than goat with a prevalence of 15.5% in sheep and 8.5% in goat. Though the prevalence is higher in sheep than goat, the severity of infection is vice versa and this finding is consistent with the work of Nandi et al. 2011 [33] who described as goat were more sensitive to the infection than sheep which was characterized with a proliferative lesions in the first 1–2 months. Sex of the animal showed no association with prevalence of the disease and this might be due to the reason that both sex groups in the area were kept under the same management system.

Body condition of the animal was strongly correlated with prevalence of the virus in which poor body conditioned animals showed a higher prevalence comparing to good and medium body conditioned animals. This is associated with the development of strong immunity in well-nourished animals comparing to less nourished animals. The immune system protects animal health and contributes to animal well-being. Nutrition is an important modulator of immune function and can often balance between health and disease [34, 35]. The diet provides substrates such as energy and amino acids, that contribute to the development, maintenance and use of the immune system. In young animals, a severe deficiency of virtually any nutrient impairs many indices of immunocompetence [36]. Age of the study animals was also considered as a risk factor of infection but there was no significant difference among young and old animals although there was a slight difference in the prevalence of the disease and this might be because all animals in the study area were kept under similar husbandry and management systems. Regardless of disease prevalence, the severity of infection was higher in the young age group (< 1 year) due to the exposure to primary infections and poor immunity against infections. Nursing animals showed higher prevalence than non-nursing animals due to the difference in the chance of contact with the infected neonates during suckling period and in addition, nursing animals had more likely to develop stress and compromised immunity due to suckling which makes them more vulnerable for infection.

Management system of the animals were also another risk factor and animals kept under extensive management system and free housing developed more chance of infection due to high chance of contact and transmission of the virus. The effect of vaccination on developing infection was also explored and revealed that vaccinated animals were less likely to develop infection than non-vaccinated animals. The host immune response of Orf virus after vaccination has widely studied and many live attenuated vaccines can induce a strong immune response in vaccinated animals by stimulating lymph node originated lymphocytes to combat infections [37]. In addition, animals with treatment history of anthelmintic and antibiotics has also shown a less prevalence of viral infections and this is justified from the perspective of indirect effect on the inhibition of bacterial and parasitic infections which might help improving host immunity. Finally, study area also showed no difference in the incidence of the disease and epidemiologically, this finding might be interpreted from the point of having a similar agroecology for the survival of the virus and the management system of the animals and equal chance of exposure to infection in general.

Conclusion

In conclusion, diagnosis of Orf based on traditional method is not accurate to identify the level of infection and as a result, we established a molecular diagnostic approach using PCR for confirmation of the virus and discriminating from other bacterial and viral pathogens. Future works will be focused on the detail phylogenetic analysis of the viral strains in all regions of the country.

Acknowledgements

We are highly grateful to the University of Gondar for funding this project and the National Veterinary Institute for the provision of laboratory supplies and technical supports.

Funding

This work was funded by the University of Gondar.

Authors' contributions

MT proposed the idea and performed the experimental works, analyzed data and drafted the paper, NB, WM, WT, SA reviewed and commented the draft paper. All authors read and approved the final version of the draft paper.

Consent for publication

Not applicable

Competing interests

The authors declare that they have no competing interests.

Author details

[1]Department of Biomedical Sciences, University of Gondar, College of Veterinary Medicine and Animal Sciences, P.O. Box: 196, Gondar, Ethiopia. [2]Department of Biotechnology, University of Gondar, College of Natural and Computational Sciences, P.O. Box: 196, Gondar, Ethiopia. [3]Department of Clinical Studies, University of Gondar, College of Veterinary Medicine and Animal Sciences, P.O. Box: 196, Gondar, Ethiopia. [4]Department of Veterinary Epidemiology and Public Health, University of Gondar, College of Veterinary Medicine and Animal Sciences, P.O. Box: 196, Gondar, Ethiopia.

References

1. Nadeem M, Curran P, Cooke R, Ryan CA, Connolly K. Orf: contagious pustular dermatitis. Ir Med J. 2010;03(5):152–3.
2. Koufakis T, Katsaitis P, Gabranis I. Orf disease: a report of a case. Braz J Infect Dis. 2014;18(5):568–9. https://doi.org/10.1016/j.bjid.2014.04.001
3. Damon I. Poxviridae and their replication. In: Fields Virology. New York: Raven Press Ltd; 2007. p. 2079–81.
4. Pal M, Tesfaye S, Dave P. Zoonoses occupationally acquired by abattoir workers. J Environ Occu Sci. 2013;2(3):155–62.
5. Almagro M, Maestre JR, Martinez P, Malagon I, Perez E, Herrera I. Milker's nodes: transmission by fomites and virological identification. Enferm Infecc Microbiol Clin. 1991;9:286–8.
6. Haig DM, Mercer AA. Ovine diseases. Orf Vet Res. 1998;29:311–26.
7. Kumar R, et al. Contagious Pustular dermatitis (Orf disease) – epidemiology, diagnosis, control and public health concerns. Adv Anim Vet Sci. 2015;3(4):560–9.
8. Wet C, Murie J. Lamb pays lip service: two cases of ecthyma contagiosum (Orf). Scott Med J. 2011;56(1):59. https://doi.org/10.1258/smj.2011.011092

9. Vikoren T, Lillehaug A, Akerstedt J, Bretten T, Haugum M, Tryland M. A severe outbreak of contagious ecthyma (Orf) in a free-ranging musk ox (Ovibos Moschatus) population in Norway. Vet Microbiol. 2008;127:10–20.
10. Mercer AA, Ueda N, Friederichs SM, Hofmann K, Fraser KM, Bateman T, Fleming SB. Comparative analysis of genome sequences of three isolates of Orf virus reveals unexpected sequence variation. Virus Res. 2006;116:146–58.
11. Zhao K, Song D, He W, Lu H, Zhang B, Li C, Chen K, Gao F. Identification and phylogenetic analysis of an Orf virus isolated from an outbreak in sheep in the Jilin province of China. Vet Microbiol. 2010;142:408–15. https://doi.org/10.1016/j.vetmic.2009.10.006
12. Sullivan JT, Mercer AA, Fleming SB, Robinson AJ. Identification and characterization of an orf virus homologue of the vaccinia virus gene encoding the major envelope antigen p37K. Virology. 1994;202:968–73.
13. Hosamani, M., Bhanuprakash, V., Scagliarini, A., 2006. Singh, R.K., comparative sequence analysis of major envelope protein gene (B2L) of Indian orf viruses isolated from sheep and goats. Vet Microbiol; 116:317-324.
14. Guo, J, Zhang, Z., Edwards, J. F, Ermel, R.W., Taylor, C. Jr., de la, Concha-Bermejillo A. Characterization of a north American orf virus isolated from a goat with persistent, proliferative dermatitis. Virus Res; 2003 93:169-179.
15. Guo, J., Rasmussen, J., Wunschmann, A., de La, Concha-Bermejillo A. Genetic characterization of orf viruses isolated from various ruminant species of a zoo. Vet Microbiol; 2004 99:81-92.
16. Scagliarini A, Pozzo FD, Gallina L, Guercio A, Vaccari F, Battilani M, Ciulli S, Prosperi S. In vitro activity of VEGF-E produced by orf virus strains isolated from classical and severe persistent contagious ecthyma. Vet Microbiol. 2006;114(1–2):142–7.
17. Wise LM, Savory LJ, Dryden NH, Whelan EM, Fleming SB, Mercer AA. Major amino acid sequence variants of viral vascular endothelial growth factor are functionally equivalent during Orf virus infection of sheep skin. Virus Res. 2007;128(1–2):115–25. http://dx.doi.org/10.1016/j
18. Harvey R, McCaughan C, Wise LM, Mercer AA, Fleming SB. Orf virus inhibits interferon stimulated gene expression and modulates the JAK/STAT signaling pathway. Virus Res. 2015;208:180–8. http://dx.doi.org/10.1016/j
19. Peralta A, Robles C, Martínez A, Alvarez L, Valera A, Calamante G, Konig GA. Identification and molecular characterization of Orf virus in Argentina. Virus Genes. 2015;50(3):381–8. https://doi.org/10.1007/s11262-015-1189-6
20. Delhon G, Tulman ER, Afonso CL, Lu Z, de la Concha-Bermejillo A, Lehmkuhl HD, Piccone ME, Kutish GF, Rock DL. Genomes of the parapoxviruses Orf virus and bovine papular stomatitis virus. J. Virol. 2004;78(1):166–7.
21. Oem JK, Chung JY, Kim YJ, Lee KK, Kim SH, Jung BY, Hyun BH. Isolation and characterization of orf viruses from Korean black goats. J Vet Sci. 2013;14(2): 227–30. https://doi.org/10.4142/jvs.2013.14.2.227
22. Martins M, Cargnelutti JF, Weiblen R, Flores EF. Pathogenesis in lambs and sequence analysis of putative virulence genes of Brazilian orf virus isolates. Vet Microbiol. 2014;174(1–2):69–77. https://doi.org/10.1016/j.vetmic.2014.09.005
23. Yang H, Meng Q, Qiao J, Peng Y, Xie K, Liu Y, Zhao H, Cai X, Chen C. Detection of genetic variations in Orf virus isolates epidemic in Xinjiang China. J Basic Microbiol. 2014;54(11):1273–8. https://doi.org/10.1002/jobm.201300911
24. Zhang K, Liu Y, Kong H, Shang Y, Liu X. Comparison and phylogenetic analysis based on the B2L gene of orf virus from goats and sheep in China during 2009-2011. Arch Virol. 2014;159(6):1475–9. https://doi.org/10.1007/s00705-013-1946-6
25. Kuhl JT, Huerter CJ, Hashish H. A case of human orf contracted from a deer. Cutis. 2003;71:288–90.
26. Georgiades G, Katsarou A, Dimitroglou K. Human ORF (ecthyma contagiosum). J Hand Surg. 2005;30(4):409–11.
27. Uzel M, Sasmaz S, Bakaris S, Cetinus E, Bilgic E, Karaoguz A, Ozkul A, Arican O. A viral infection of the hand commonly seen after the feast of sacrifice: human orf (orf of the hand). Epidemiol. Infection. 2005;133:653–7. https://doi.org/10.1017/S0950268805003778
28. Office for International Epizootics, 2012. Manual of diagnostic tests and vaccines for terrestrial animals.
29. Chan KW, Lin JW, Lee SH, Liao CJ, Tsai MC, Hsu WL, Wong ML, Shih HC. Identification and phylogenetic analysis of orf virus from goats in Taiwan. Virus Genes. 2007;35:705–12.
30. McKeever DJ, Jenkinson DM, Hutchison G, Reid HW. Studies of the pathogenesis of orf virus infection in sheep. J Comp Pathol. 1998;99:317–28.
31. Joern K, Morten T. Characterization of parapoxviruses isolated from Norwegian semi-domesticated reindeer (*Rangifer tarandus tarandus*). Virol J. 2005; 2–79
32. Murphy FA, Gibbs EP, Horzinek MC, Studdert MJ. Veterinary virology. 3rd ed. New York: Elsevier; 2001.
33. Nandi S, De UK, Chowdhury S. Current status of contagious ecthyma or orf disease in goat and sheep-a global perspective. Small Rumin Res. 2011; 96(2–3):73–82.
34. Athanasiadou S, Huntley JF. Emerging technologies and their applications in interactions between nutrition and immunity to gastrointestinal parasites in sheep. Parasite Immunol. 2008;30(2):101–11.
35. Sordillo LM. Nutritional strategies to optimize dairy cattle immunity. J Dairy Sci. 2016;99(6):4967–82.
36. Cook ME. Nutrition and the immune response of the domestic fowl. Cr Rev Poult Biol. 1991;3:167–90.
37. Zhao K, He W, Gao W, Lu H, Han T, Li J, Zhang X, et al. Orf virus DNA vaccines expressing ORFV 011 and ORFV 059 chimeric protein enhances immunogenicity. Virol J. 2011;8(1):562.

8

Serological testing of Schmallenberg virus in Swedish wild cervids from 2012 to 2016

A. Malmsten[1*], J. Malmsten[2,3], G. Blomqvist[4], K. Näslund[4], C. Vernersson[4], S. Hägglund[5], A.-M. Dalin[1], E. O. Ågren[2] and J.-F. Valarcher[5,6]

Abstract

Background: Schmallenberg virus (SBV) first emerged in Europe in 2011, and in Sweden in late 2012. The virus was still circulating in parts of Europe in 2015. In recent testing, the virus has not been detected in Swedish domestic animals, indicating that it is no longer circulating in Sweden. It is not known if the virus has circulated and is still circulating in Swedish wild cervid populations and whether wildlife can act as virus reservoirs. The aim of this study was to investigate whether SBV has circulated, and is still circulating among wild cervids in Sweden.

Results: Ninety-two sera from moose (*Alces alces*, $n = 22$), red deer (*Cervus elaphus*, $n = 15$), fallow deer (*Dama dama*, $n = 44$), and roe deer (*Capreolus capreolus*, $n = 11$) were collected and analyzed for antibodies against SBV. The sampling occurred in the southern and middle part of Sweden during three time periods: 1) before the vector season in 2012, 2) after the vector season in 2012, and 3) after the vector season in 2015. Animals from periods 1 and 2 were of varying ages, whereas animals collected in period 3 were born after the vector season 2013. Animals from period 1 ($n = 15$) and 3 ($n = 47$) were seronegative, but, 53% (16 of 30) of animals from period 2 were seropositive, determined by SBV competitive ELISA. Samples from period 2 were additionally analyzed for SBV-neutralizing antibodies. Such antibodies were detected in 16/16 SBV-N-antibody-positive, 3/12 negative and 2/2 doubtful sera. The two tests were in accordance at SBV-neutralizing antibody titers of 1:32 or higher.

Conclusion: Our results show that SBV circulated among wild cervids during the vector season of 2012. Three years later, no SBV-antibodies were detected in animals born after the vector season 2013. The likely absence of SBV circulation in Sweden, in contrast to other parts of Europe, might be explained by the annual occurrence of a vector-free season due to climate conditions. Interpretations are limited by the small sample-size, but the results suggest that the SBV competitive ELISA has high specificity but might have slightly lower sensitivity compared to a seroneutralization assay, when using samples from wild cervids.

Keywords: SBV, Moose, Roe deer, Red deer, Fallow deer, Serology, Orthobunyavirus, Scandinavia, Wildlife

Background

When an emerging disease affects an animal or human population, there are often social, economic and welfare consequences. This was the case in 2011 and 2012, when Schmallenberg virus (SBV) was detected in Europe [1]. Initially, clinical signs were observed mainly in cattle, and included diarrhea, pyrexia, and a drop in milk yield. Infection during the first part of gestation was followed by stillbirths and birth defects in the offspring. No relation to any current and known circulating pathogen was identified [2]. Shortly thereafter, the causative agent was shown to be a novel *Orthobunyavirus* of the family *Bunyaviridae* [3] that is transmitted by biting midges (*Culicoides* spp.) [4]. The virus has the ability to cross the placental barrier and cause lesions in fetuses and neonates [5]. It infects a number of domestic and wild animal species including cattle, sheep, goats [6], alpaca [7] red deer, roe deer [8], fallow deer, moose, bison [9], wild boar [10], dogs [11], and a number of zoo animals [12]. In 2014 and 2015 the virus was still circulating in continental Europe [13, 14]. In Sweden, SBV was first detected in 2012 in domestic animals in the south. The virus spread rapidly north beyond the Arctic Circle, and occurred in high prevalence in tested animals [15]. However, it was not known if the virus

* Correspondence: anna.malmsten@slu.se
[1]Department of Clinical Sciences, Division of Reproduction, Swedish University of Agricultural Sciences, Box 7054750 07 Uppsala, Sweden
Full list of author information is available at the end of the article

did circulate (in 2012) or still is circulating in wildlife ruminant populations, and if they could act as reservoirs for the virus [16].

The aim of this study was to investigate if SBV is circulating among wild cervids in Sweden. Two hypotheses were tested: a) SBV-specific serum antibodies can be detected in Swedish wild cervids to the same extent and during the same time periods as SBV was diagnosed in domestic ruminants. b) SBV is still widely circulating in wild ruminant populations, despite likely being absent in the domestic ruminant population.

Methods

Sampling collection

Sera from moose (*Alces alces*, $n = 22$), red deer (*Cervus elaphus*, $n = 15$), fallow deer (*Dama dama*, $n = 44$), and roe deer (*Capreolus capreolus*, $n = 11$) were collected during three time periods: 1) before the vector season in 2012 (February, samples collected for biobanking), 2) after the vector season in 2012 (October 2012 - February 2013) and, 3) after the vector season in 2015 (November 2015 - January 2016, see Table 1 for species and sample distribution).

In time period 1, captured live adult moose aged >2 years were sampled. In time periods 2 and 3, hunter-killed moose, red deer, fallow deer, and roe deer were sampled. The animals from time period 2 were of varying age. In time period 3 samples were collected from animals that were born after the vector season 2013 and aged between 0.5 to 1.5 years to avoid testing animals that could have been exposed to SBV in earlier time periods.

Age in all sampled species was determined by investigating tooth eruption patterns, and antler development status. All sampling occurred in the southern and middle parts of Sweden (Fig. 1) where domestic ruminants previously had been tested positive for antibodies against SBV [15], whereas recent testing had shown negative results. Blood samples were collected in sterile dry tubes (BD Vacutainer®, Franklin Lakes, USA) kept at room temperature 24 h before centrifugation at 3000×g for ten minutes. The sera were stored in −20 °C prior to analysis.

Serology

All sera were analyzed by competitive ELISA (cELISA, ID Screen® Schmallenberg virus Competition Multi-species) according to the manufacturer's instructions [17]. This ELISA detects antibodies by competition with conjugated antibodies specific to the SBV nucleoprotein (N). The sera were tested undiluted in duplicate and results were expressed as competition percentage (S/N%), based on the mean optical density $(OD)_{Sample}/OD_{Negative\ Control}$ X100. As indicated in the instructions, sera with S/N% greater than 50% were considered as negative, >40-50% were classified as doubtful, and ≤40% as positive. A positive control provided with the kit was included in each run.

Sera collected during the initial SBV outbreak in Sweden [15] (time period 2) were additionally analyzed for SBV-neutralizing antibodies. The sera were heat-inactivated, 2-fold diluted from 1:8 to 1:512 and analyzed in duplicate. Fifty microliters of each dilution was mixed with an equal volume of EMEM containing 150 tissue culture infectious dose 50% ($TCID_{50}$) SBV (BH80/11-4, kindly provided by the Friedrich-Loeffler Institute, Germany) and was incubated for one hour at 37 °C. Thereafter, approximately 20,000 BHK-21 cells in a volume of 50 µl in EMEM supplemented with 20% fetal calf serum were added to each well. The plates were then incubated for 3-4 days at 37 °C under 5% CO_2. The cells were examined daily in a light microscope for the presence of SBV-specific cytopathogenic effects (cpe). The neutralizing titer of a serum was determined as the highest dilution in which the cell monolayer was intact. A serum sample was considered negative if cpe was observed at and from a dilution of 1:8 [18, 19].

Results

All analyzed samples collected from wild cervids before the vector season 2012 ($n = 15$) as well as those collected after the vector season 2015 animals ($n = 47$, born after the vector season 2013) were seronegative for SBV by cELISA (Table 1). In sera collected during time period 2 after the vector season 2012, SBV-N-specific antibodies were detected by cELISA in 16 sera out of 30

Table 1 Results of serological testing by cELISA of Swedish wild cervids for the detection of specific antibodies directed against Schmallenberg virus in different time periods

Species	Time period 1 (Feb 2012) No. positive/ no. tested (%)	Time period 2 (Nov 2012 - Feb 2013) No. positive/ no. tested (%)	Time period 3 (Nov 2015 - Jan 2016) No. positive/ no. tested (%)
Moose	0/15 (0)	3/4 (75.0)	0/3 (0)
Roe deer		2/6 (33.3)	0/5 (0)
Red deer		0/4 (25.0)	0/11 (0)
Fallow deer		11/16 (75.0)	0/28 (0)
Total	0/15 (0)	16/30 (60.0)	0/47 (0)

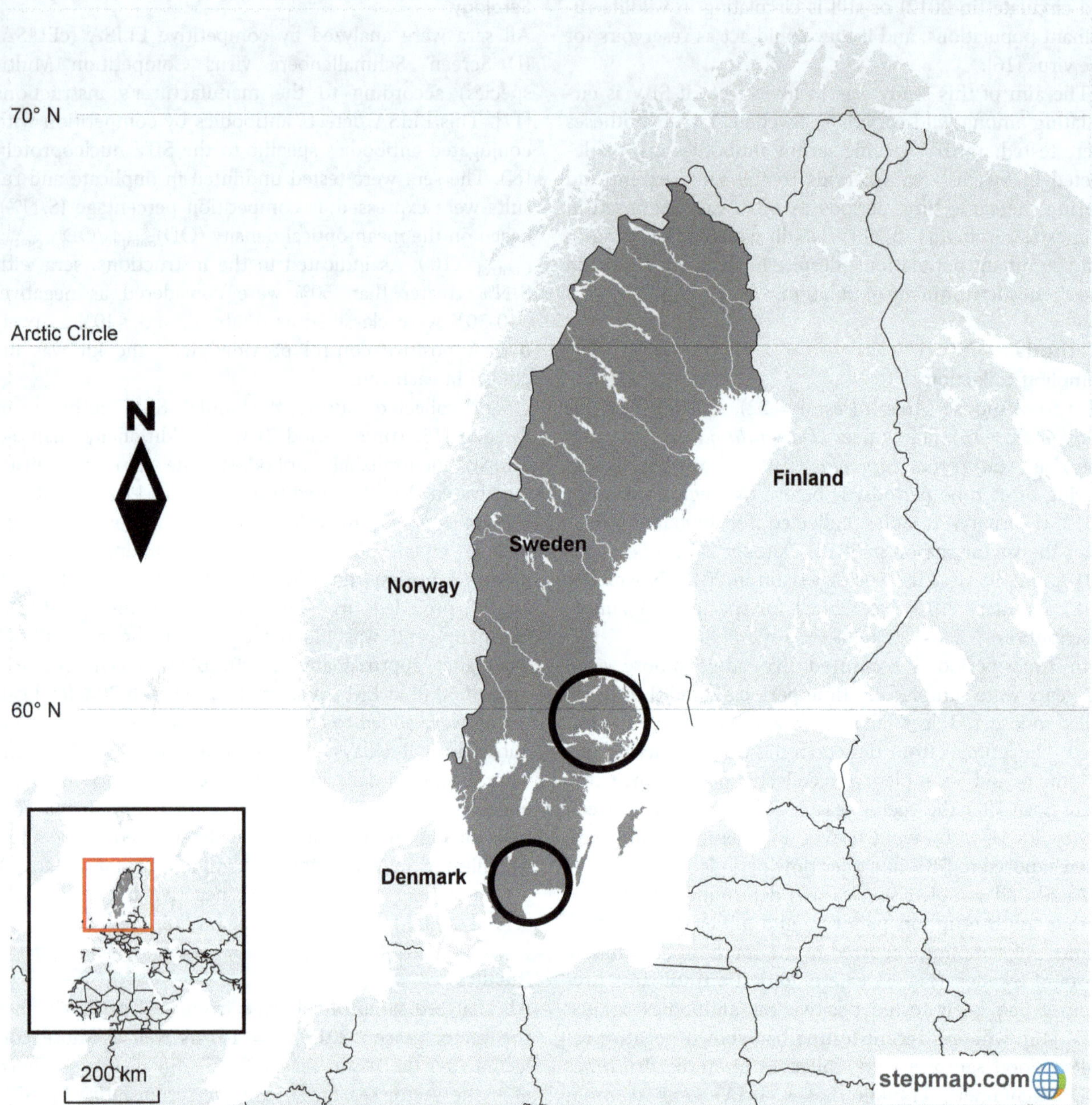

Fig. 1 Map of Sweden with circles indicating sampling regions where Swedish wild cervids were sampled and tested for antibodies against Schmallenberg virus

(53%) (Table 1). One red deer and one fallow deer showed doubtful reaction in cELISA (Table 2).

Sera from time period 2 were additionally analyzed for SBV-neutralizing antibodies. Such antibodies were detected in 16/16 SBV-N-antibody-positive sera, in 3/12 SBV-N-antibody negative and 2/2 doubtful sera. No SBV-specific antibodies were detected by any of the techniques in nine animals (Table 2). Seropositive animals were found in all sampling areas and in all tested cervid species (moose, roe deer, red deer, and fallow deer). The SBV-neutralizing antibody titers varied between species (Table 2), but low sample sizes precluded statistical analyzes with regards to inter- and intraspecies titer variation. These data show a very good agreement between both tests for negative samples or when the SBV-neutralizing antibody titers were >1/16. Five samples with an SBV-neutralizing antibody titer of 1/8 (n = 3) or 1/16 (n = 2) were found doubtful (n = 2) or negative (n = 3) by cELISA.

Discussion

This is the first report of findings of SBV-specific antibodies in Scandinavian wildlife, showing that wild

Table 2 Sera from wild cervids sampled in Sweden between November 2012 and February 2013, and tested for SBV antibodies by serum neutralization test (SNT), and competitive ELISA (cELISA)

SNT		cELISA		
Titer	No	No positive (≤40%)	No doubtful (>40-50%)	No negative (>50%)
<8	9 (3 red deer, 3 fallow deer, 3 roe deer)	-	-	9 (3 red deer, 3 fallow deer, 3 roe deer)[a]
8	7 (1 red deer, 4 fallow deer, 2 roe deer)	4 (3 fallow deer, 1 roe deer)[a]	1 (1 red deer)	2 (1 fallow deer, 1 roe deer)
16	6 (1 moose, 4 fallow deer, 1 roe deer)	4 (3 fallow deer, 1 roe deer)[a]	1 (1 fallow deer)	1 (1 moose)
32	3 (1 moose, 2 fallow deer)	3 (1 moose, 2 fallow deer)[a]	-	-
64	5 (2 moose, 3 fallow deer)	5 (2 moose, 3 fallow deer)[a]	-	-

[a]Indicates agreement of the results of the two tests

cervids in Sweden were exposed to the virus in the summer of 2012 and probably not after the vector season 2014. Moreover, this study indicates that SBV infection in wildlife and domesticated animals follows the same pattern in the same area in which cattle were seropositive in 2012 and 2013 but seronegative in a recent serological survey when born after the vector season 2013 (S. Zohari, personal communication). Schmallenberg virus does not seem to circulate in Sweden anymore, in contrast to other European countries such as Germany [13]. The difference between Sweden and countries in central and southern Europe is that Sweden has a long vector-free season. Virus transmission and spread is possible at temperatures around 15 °C with a temperature optimum between 18 °C and 19 °C due to vector limitations [20]. In Sweden, such daily mean temperatures are usually limited to May-August [21], but may occur in September as well. Virus persistence depends on the winter survival of adult midges which must have access to a naïve ruminant population. The absence of SBV antibodies in the tested animals suggests that the virus does not persist in ruminants (wild or domestic) or in the environment during the vector-free season. However, to completely verify that the infection is not present in Swedish cervid populations, a larger and predetermined number of animals need to be tested.

A seroneutralization test (SNT) was used at first to test wildlife following the emergence of SBV in Europe, since no cELISA was available to measure specific antibodies against SBV. Since then, a cELISA has been developed with high sensitivity and specificity for domestic ruminant samples [17], and in addition, is easier to perform. Our results indicate that the two methods are in agreement for most samples tested and the level of agreement increases with increasing titer. It is possible that none of the techniques perform well for samples with low titers. Our data suggest that the cELISA lacks sensitivity for sera with low antibody titers. The SNT, on the other hand, might lack specificity for sera at low dilution, as previously observed for sheep [22]. Nevertheless, in contrast to in the sera collected between November 2012 and February 2013, no specific antibodies were detected by cELISA in sera collected in 2015 from animals aged between 0.5 and 1.5 years of age, which suggest that the SBV has not recently circulated among wild cervids in the investigated area.

The effect of SBV in wildlife is still unknown. No clinical signs of SBV were reported in Swedish wildlife during the summer and early autumn of 2012 when the outbreak was detected. Possible signs of SBV infection in Swedish wild or fenced cervids, in the form of abortions and congenital malformations, were not reported during 2013 [23]. However, it is unlikely to make such observations in wild animals for a number of reasons such as scavenging birds and mammals. Furthermore, it requires a primary maternal infection and viremia during a particular period of pregnancy, i.e. after the first placentoma has developed and before the fetuses are immunocompetent [24]. The circulation of SBV most likely did not coincide with the placentoma formation in wild cervids in Sweden. Hence, delayed consequences of SBV infection in Swedish cervids are presumed to be minimal.

Conclusion

Schmallenberg virus was circulating among Swedish wild cervids during the vector season 2012, but no serological evidence of SBV was found during subsequent testing in 2015 and 2016. Based on Swedish climate conditions and the results of this study, we can assume that Sweden has an unfavorable climate for SBV-overwintering vectors. This might have contributed to the fact that the virus infection has seemingly not become endemic or possibly not reoccurred in Sweden. Midge activity and the reproductive season of Swedish wild cervids, is a seasonal and biological mismatch for the virus, which may explain that SBV has little impact on Swedish wild ruminant health. These animals are thus highly unlikely to be reservoirs of this virus.

Abbreviations

cELISA: Competitive enzyme-linked immunosorbent assay; CPE: Cytopathogenic effects; N: Nucleoprotein; OD: Optical density; SBV: Schmallenberg virus; SNT: Seroneutralization test; TCID: Tissue culture infectious dose

Acknowledgements
The authors are thankful to members of the Swedish Association for Hunting and Wildlife Management and its "wildlife sampling organization" (Viltprovtagarna), Eriksberg Wildlife Park, and the Department of Wildlife, Fish, and Environmental Studies at the Swedish University of Agricultural Sciences in Umeå for supplying the samples for this study. We are also most grateful to the gamekeepers of the two estates that have contributed with additional samples. We also thank Anna Johansson Gordon for language review and editing.

Funding
This work was supported by the Swedish National Veterinary Institute in Uppsala, Sweden, and by the Department of Clinical Sciences at the Swedish University of Agricultural Sciences in Uppsala, Sweden. Both institutions jointly supported equal amounts of internal funding for time allocated and costs for the design of the study, sample collection, analyzes, interpreting the data, and writing the manuscript.

Authors' contributions
AM, JM, and JFV were involved in the design and coordination of the study, AM, JM and EÅ collected/coordinated the sampling. GB, KN, CV, SH were responsible for the seroneutralization test and ELISA. AM, JM, JFV GB, KN, CV, SH, AMD, and EÅ contributed analyzing data and in drafting the manuscript. All authors have read and approved the final manuscript.

Competing interests
The authors declare that they have no competing interests.

Consent for publication
Not applicable.

Author details
[1]Department of Clinical Sciences, Division of Reproduction, Swedish University of Agricultural Sciences, Box 7054750 07 Uppsala, Sweden. [2]Department of Pathology and Wildlife Diseases, National Veterinary Institute, 751 89 Uppsala, Sweden. [3]Department of Wildlife, Fish, and Environmental studies, Swedish University of Agricultural Sciences, 901 83 Umeå, Sweden. [4]Department of Microbiology, National Veterinary Institute, 751 89 Uppsala, Sweden. [5]Department of Clinical Sciences, Host Pathogen Interaction Group, DOS, Swedish University of Agricultural Sciences, Box 7054750 07 Uppsala, Sweden. [6]Department of Clinical Sciences, Host Pathogen Interaction Group, Ruminant medicine, Swedish University of Agricultural Sciences, Box 7054750 07 Uppsala, Sweden.

References

1. Spiegel Online 'Schmallenberg-Virus. Neue Tierseuche breitet sich rasant aus. http://www.spiegel.de/wissenschaft/natur/schmallenberg-virus-neue-tierseuche-breitet-sich-rasant-aus-a-817671.html. Accessed 1 May 2016 (in German).
2. ProMED-mail: Schmallenberg virus – Europe (26): Vector morphology. March 10: 20120311.1066949. 2012. http://www.promedmail.org. Accessed Mar 8 2013.
3. Hoffmann B, Scheuch M, Höper D, Jungblut R, Holsteg M, Schirrmeier H, Eschbaumer M, Goller KV, Wernike K, Fischer M, Breithaupt A, Mettenleiter TC, Beer M. Novel orthobunyavirus in cattle, Europe, 2011. Emerg Infect Dis. 2012;18:469–72. doi:10.3201/eid1803.111905.
4. De Regge N, Deblauwe I, De Deken R, Vantiegheim P, Madder M, Geysen D, Smeets F, Losson B, van den Berg T, Cay AB. Detection of Schmallenberg virus in different Culicoides spp. by real-time RT-PCR. Transbound Emerg Dis. 2012;59:471–5. doi:10.1111/tbed.12000.
5. Garigliany MM, Bayrou C, Kleijnen D, Cassart D, Jolly S, Linden A, Desmecht D. Schmallenberg virus: a new Shamonda/Sathuperi-like virus on the rise in Europe. Antivir Res. 2012;95:82–7. doi:10.1016/j.antiviral.2012.05.014.
6. van den Brom R, Luttikholt SJ, Lievaart-Peterson K, Peperkamp NH, Mars MH, van der Poel WH, Vellema P. Epizootic of ovine congenital malformations associated with Schmallenberg virus infection. Tijdschr Diergeneeskd. 2012;137:106–11.
7. Jack C, Anstaett O, Adams J, Noad R, Brownlie J, Mertens P. Evidence of seroconversion to SBV in camelids. Vet Rec. 2012;170:603. doi:10.1136/vr.e3939.
8. Linden A, Desmecht D, Volpe R, Wirtgen M, Gregoire F, Pirson J, Paternostre J, Kleijnen D, Schirrmejer H, Beer M, Garigliany MM. Epizootic spread of Schmallenberg virus among wild cervids, Belgium, fall 2011. Emerg Infect Dis. 2012;18:2006–8. doi:10.3201/eid1812.121067.
9. Larska M, Krzysiak M, Smreczak M, Polak MP. Zmudsinski. First detection of Schmallenberg virus in elk (*Alces alces*) indicating infection of wildlife in Bialowieza National Park in Poland. Vet J. 2013;198:279–81. doi:10.1016/j.tvjl.2013.08.013.
10. Mouchantat S, Wernike K, Lutz W, Hoffmann B, Ulrich RG, Börner K, Wittstatt U, Beer M. A broad spectrum screening of Schmallenberg virus antibodies in wildlife animals in Germany. Vet Res. 2015;46. doi: 10.1186/s13567-015-0232-x.
11. Sailleau C, Boogaerts C, Meyrueix A, Laloy E, Bréard E, Viarouge C, Desprat A, Vitour D, Doceul V, Boucher C, Zientara S, Nicolier A, Grandjean D. Schmallenberg virus infection in dogs, France, 2012. Emerg Infect Dis. 2013; 19:1896–8. doi:10.3201/eid1911.130464.
12. Molenaar FM, La Rocca SA, Khatri M, Lopez J, Steinbach F, Dastjerdi A. Exposure of Asian elephants and other exotic ungulates to Schmallenberg virus. PLoS One. 2015;10:e0135532. doi:10.1371/journal.pone.0135532.
13. Wernike K, Hoffmann B, Conraths FJ, Beer M. Schmallenberg virus recurrence, Germany, 2014. Emerg Infect Dis. 2015;21:1202–4. doi:10.3201/eid2107.150180.
14. Poskin A, Théron A, Hanon JB, Saegerman C, Vervaeke M, Van der Stede Y, Cay B, De Regge N. Reconstruction of the Schmallenberg virus epidemic in Belgium: Complementary use of disease surveillance approaches. Vet Microbiol. 2016;183:50–61. doi:10.1016/j.vetmic.2015.11.036. Epub 2015 Nov 30
15. Chenais E, Ståhl K, Frössling J, Blomqvist G, Näslund K, Svensson L, Renström L, Mieziewska K, Elvander M, Valarcher JF. Schmallenberg virus beyond latitude 60°N. Transbound Emerg Dis. 2013;62:11–8.
16. Talavera S, Muñoz-Muñoz F, Durám M, Verdún M, Soler-Membrives A, Oleaga Á, Arenas A, Ruiz-Fons F, Estrada R, Pagès N. Culicoides species communities associated with wild ruminant ecosystems in Spain: tracking the way to determine potential bridge vectors for arboviruses. PLoS One. 2015;28: e0141667. doi:10.1371/journal.pone.0141667. eCollection 2015
17. Comtet L, Pourquier, P. (IDvet, France). ID Screen® Schmallenberg virus Competition Multi-species: validation of a competitive ELISA for the detection of antibodies directed against the Schmallenberg virus nucleoprotein. Brussels, Belgium: Poster presented at the Epizone 7th Annual Meeting; 2013. doi: 10.1038/nplants.2017.32.
18. Näslund K, Blomqvist G, Vernersson C, Zientara S, Bréard E, Valarcher JF. Development and evaluation of an indirect enzyme-linked immunosorbent assay for serological detection of Schmallenberg virus antibodies in ruminants using whole virus antigen. Acta Vet Scand. 2014;56:71. doi:10.1186/s13028-014-0071-1.
19. van der Poel WH, Cay B, Zientara S, Steinbach F, Valarcher JF, Bøtner A, Mars MH, Hakze-van der Honing R, Schirrmeier H, Beer M. Limited interlaboratory comparison of Schmallenberg virus antibody detection in serum samples. Vet Rec. 2014;174:380. doi:10.1136/vr.102180. Epub 2014 Mar 3
20. EFSA (European Food Safety Authority). "Schmallenberg" virus: Analysis of the epidemiological data and Impact assessment. http://www.efsa.europa.eu/en/efsajournal/doc/2768.pdf. Accessed 10 Mar 2013.
21. Climatemps.com, 2013: Sweden climate graph. http://www.sweden.climatemps.com/#brief. Accessed 10 Mar 2013.
22. Loeffen W, Quak S, de Boer-Luijtze E, Hulst M, van der Poel W, Bouwstra R, Maas R. Development of a virus neutralisation test to detect antibodies against Schmallenberg virus and serological results in suspect and infected herds. Acta Vet Scand. 2012;54:44. doi:10.1186/1751-0147-54-44.
23. Statens veterinärmedicinska anstalt. Sjukdomsövervakning av vilda djur i Sverige 2014. SVA:s Rapportserie 31 ISSN 1654-7098 (in Swedish).
24. Garigliany MM, Bayrou C, Kleijnen D, Cassart D, Desmecht D. Schmallenberg virus in domestic cattle, Belgium, 2012. Emerg Infect Dis. 2012;18:1512–4. doi:10.3201/eid1809.120716.

9

Genetic variation analysis of PCV1 strains isolated from Guangxi Province

Liang Cao[1,2], Wenchao Sun[2], Huijun Lu[2], Mingyao Tian[2], Changzhan Xie[1,2], Guanyu Zhao[2,4], Jicheng Han[2], Wei Wang[2], Min Zheng[3], Rui Du[1*], Ningyi Jin[1,2*] and Aidong Qian[1*]

Abstract

Background: Porcine circovirus type 1 (PCV1) was discovered in 1974 as a contaminant of a porcine kidney (PK-15) cell line and was generally accepted to be nonpathogenic. But recently it was shown to cause lesions in experimentally infected pig fetuses. Serological evidence and genetic studies suggested that PCV1 was widespread in domestic pigs. Thus, the molecular epidemiology and genetic variation of PCV1 are still necessary to understand.

Results: Here 247 tissue samples were collected from piglets in Guangxi Province, China and performed whole-genome sequencing of the PCV1 genome. Thirteen PCV1 strains were sequenced from the samples. Similarity analysis showed that there were 97.8% to 99.6% nucleotide similarity to each other and 97.1% to 99.8% nucleotide similarity to the 40 reference strains. Besides, based on sequence analysis, we found one putative recombinant virus named GXdx84 strain contained the open-reading frame 1 (ORF1) of PCV1 and the ORF2 of PCV2d-2, which was consistent with the results of phylogenetic analysis that compared PCV1 and PCV2 strains. Variation analysis of the amino acids of the capsid protein revealed that the GXyl224 strain, which encoded 235 amino acids, had two amino acids more than other strains. This is the first study to report that a *cap* gene mutation resulted in lengthening of in the gene sequence.

Conclusions: These data contribute to the understanding of PCV1 evolution and molecular epidemiology that will facilitate programs for its control and prevention.

Keywords: Porcine circovirus 1, Genetic variation, Phylogenetic study, Putative recombinant virus

Background

Porcine circovirus 1 (PCV1) is a small, non-enveloped, circular single-stranded DNA virus with a genome length of 1.7kb. It is a member of the family *Circoviridae* and genus *Circovirus* [1, 2]. PCV has two genotypes: PCV1 and PCV2. PCV1 was first identified as a contaminant in a pig kidney cell culture (PK-15) [3, 4]. PCV2 is the causative agent of porcine circovirus-associated disease (PCVAD) in swine, and result in substantial economic losses for the pig industry in the world [5].

The genome organization of PCV1 and PCV2 are highly similar. The cis-acting and trans-acting replication factors of both viruses are interchangeable for DNA replication [6–8]. The overall DNA sequence similarity within the PCV1 or PCV2 isolations is greater than 90%, while the similarity between PCV1 and PCV2 isolations is 68% to 76%. There are two major open-reading frames, ORF1 and ORF2, which diverge from the Ori expressing four proteins [9]. ORF1 (*rep* gene) is transcribed in a clockwise direction and encodes two viral replication-associated proteins Rep and Rep'. These two proteins are the main factors for initiation of viral DNA replication. ORF2 (*cap* gene) is transcribed in an anti-clockwise direction, and encodes the immunogenic capsid protein which builds the capsid of the virus [10, 11]. In addition to the replication ORF1 and the capsid protein ORF2, another fragment recognized to be involved in modulation of virulence was encoded by ORF3. PCV1 and PCV2 utilize similar

* Correspondence: durui71@126.com; ningyik@126.com; qianaidong0115@163.com
[1]College of Animal Science and Technology, Jilin Agricultural University, Changchun 130118, People's Republic of China
Full list of author information is available at the end of the article

initiation and termination signals at comparable locations within the viral genome. However, they differ from each other with respect to specific RNA expression level as well as splice-junction selection is unique to each virus. Previous research shows that thirteen RNAs reported as PCV1, while ten RNAs to be PCV2 during virus replication in PK-15 cells [12, 13]. Besides, the *cap* of PCV2 encodes the viral capsid protein (Cap) and ORF3-RNA which encodes the apoptosis-associated protein. While the functions of the respective protein are the same, ORF3 of PCV1 is 612nt in length, twice the size of PCV2 [13].

Although PCV1 DNA has been isolated from lymph nodes of a piglet with a wasting condition, it is generally accepted that PCV1 is nonpathogenic but widespread in pigs and porcine cell line PK-15 [14, 15]. However, PCV1 can produce pathology in the lungs of porcine fetuses in foetal life [16]. Clinical data shows that PCV1 infection is common in pigs and that pigs can produce antibodies against PCV1 [6, 17, 18].

The main objective of this study is to analyze the prevalence of PCV1 and the evolutionary patterns as well as the relationships among PCV1 genomes isolated from Guangxi Province of China and compare them with data on PCV1 and recombination of PCV1 and PCV2 published worldwide.

Methods

Clinical samples

A total of 247 spleen and lymph node samples were collected from piglets (All piglets were euthanized by an anesthetic overdose with the pentobarbital before collected the samples) in Guangxi Province, China, in 2015. All the pigs displayed signs of progressive weight loss, inguinal lymph node edema and hemorrhage, pulmonary edema, and other lesions. Clinical tissues were homogenized for DNA extraction and stored at -80 °C.

DNA isolation and polymerase chain reaction (PCR)

Viral DNA was extracted using a TIANamp Genomic DNA kit (TIANGEN, Beijing, China). Two pair of specific PCR primers named PCV1-F and PCV1-R, PCV2-F and PCV2-R were designed according to published PCV1 and PCV2 sequences to amplify the complete genome (Table 1). The PCR assays were performed in a 25μL reaction mixture consisting of 3ng tissue-isolated DNA templates, containing final concentrations of 1.25mM $MgCl_2$, 2.5μL 10 × PCR buffer, 1mM of each dNTP, 0.5μM of each primer and 2.5U of *Taq* DNA polymerase (TAKARA, Dalian, China). The DNA was amplified with an initial denaturation of 95 °C for 5 min, followed by 35 cycles of amplification (95°C for 30s, 57°C for 30s, and 72°C for 2min) and a final extension of 72°C for 10min.

Genome cloning and sequencing

The amplified PCR products were separated by electrophoresis on a 1% agarose. The bands were extracted and purified using the AxyPrep DNA Gel Extraction Kit (AxyGene, USA). Then, the PCR products were ligated into the pMD-18T Vector System (Takara Co. Dalian, China), and the recombinant plasmids were sequenced by Takara Co. (Dalian, China).

Phylogenetic analysis

To understand the genetic relationship between the PCV1 isolates from Guangxi, 40 published genomic sequences were downloaded from GenBank (Table 1). All sequences were aligned with Clustal W [19] and were analyzed. The phylogenetic tree was calculated using the Maximum Likelihood (ML) method with 1000 bootstrap replicates and the genetic distance of *rep* genes, *cap* genes and complete genomes were calculated using the Kimura 2-parameter, Hasegawa-kishino-Yano and Tamura-Nei model respectively by MEGA6 program [20].

Recombination analysis

Recombination event analysis was carried out by analyzing the complete genome of potential recombinant of GXdx84 since the strain clustered as a separate branch located between PCV1 and PCV2 in the phylogenetic tree based on complete genome as well as *cap* gene and *rep* gene. In the recombination events, possible breakpoint were identified using two programs based on different approaches: the RDP4 (http://web.cbio.uct.ac.za/~darren/rdp.html) [21] and SimPlot(http://sray.med.som.jhmi.edu/RaySoft) [22]. The RDP tests the recombination events by six methods (GENECONV, BootScan, MaxChi, Chimaera, SiScan and RDP) and the setting for each method was adjusted account for the dataset features according to the RDP manual recommendations. Recombination events detected by more than 4 methods, where a significance value$<10^{-5}$ (P-value$<10^{-5}$) and Bonferroni

Table 1 Primers used to amplify the whole genomes of PCV

Name	Sequence (5′-3′)	Tm(°C)	Genome position	Size of amplicons	PCV type
PCV1-F	GGTACCCGAAGGCCGATTTG	56.5	920-939	1759bp	PCV 1
PCV1-R	GGGTACCTCCGTGGATTGTTCT	58.5	905-926		PCV 1
PCV2-F	GCCAGAATTCAACCTTAACCTTTCT	63	1430-1454	1769bp	PCV 2
PCV2-R	GAATTCTGGCCCTGCTCCC	61	1421-1439		PCV 2

correction were accepted. The recombination signal and sequences of recombination parental lineages were analyzed by SimPlot. SimPlot analysis was performed with three groups of complete genome: a group of major parent (PCV1G, JN398656), a group of minor parent (PCV2b, AF112862) and a group of potent recombinant (GXdx84, KY437725).

Selection pressure analysis

The selective pressure analysis of genome was assessed by calculating the difference between the dN and dS rates for the aligned *rep* and *cap* genes by using MEGA version 6.0 software [23]. The entropy was used to measure the genetic complexity which was calculated by BioEdit [24]. The difference in entropy was plotted between dN and dS [25]. If the dN rate was higher than the dS rate, i.e., dN–dS>0, the genes would be considered to be under positive selection; otherwise, the genes would be considered to be under purified selection (dN–dS<0). If the dN rate was approximately equal to the dS rate, i.e., dN–dS=0, the genes would be considered to be under neutral evolution [26].

Results

Screening for PCV1 prevalence in clinical samples

Clinical samples (n=247) were collected from the lungs, spleen and lymph nodes of apparently healthy pigs (n=172) and sick pigs (n=75) from different regions of Guangxi Province in 2015. Among collected samples, 32 positive samples are PCV1 (positive rate, 12.95%); among these ones, 21 were from the 75 sick pigs (21/75, 28%) and 11 were from the 172 apparently healthy pigs (11/172, 6.39%). Besides of the 247 samples, 214 were PCV2 positive (positive rate 86.6%). 65 samples were from sick pigs (65/75, 86.67%), 149 were from apparently healthy pig (149/172, 86.62%). Both PCV1 and PCV2 were detected in samples from both diseased and apparently healthy pigs.

Phylogenetic analysis of the PCV1 isolates

Fourteen complete genome sequences were randomly selected from the 32 positive samples of PCV1 by PCR (Table 2). Of these samples, 13 strains had a whole-genome length of 1759 nucleotides, and only the GXdx84 strain had a genome length of 1757 nucleotides. Regarding the length of the *cap* gene, 12 strains had a length of 702 nucleotides, similar to other strains. But the GXyl224 strains had a length of 708 nucleotides (Fig. 1a). As the stop codon TAA mutated to TAT and added Y and K amino acids were added to the end of the Cap protein. This is the first case of PCV1 wherein a structural gene mutation resulted in gene extension. Considering the complete genome, the similarity among the 13 strains (except GXdx84) in this study ranged from 97.8% to 99.6%. In addition, the nucleotide similarity to the other 40 comparison strains of PCV1 ranged from 97.1% to 99.8%. The percentage of mutations were 13.47% (237 mutations) in the whole genome, 16.24% (114 mutations) in *cap*, and 11.40% (107 mutations) in *rep*. The nucleotide sequence similarity for the complete gene of GXdx84 strains ranged from 86.8% to 89.0% comparing to PCV2 strains used in this study and 86.8% to 89.0% comparing to the other 40 PCV1 strains. The similarity of *rep* gene ranged from 92.2% to 94% in PCV1 and 87.6% to 88.3% in PCV2. While the similarity of *cap* gene ranged from 65.3% to 66.5% in PCV1, and 88.1% to 99.5% in PCV2, especially the similarity to PCV2d-2 was as high as 99.5%. These results indicated that strain of GXdx84 might contain a *rep* came from PCV1 and a *cap* came from PCV2.

We also identified several novel amino acid substitutions in the ORF2 genes from PCV1 isolated in this study. The PCV1 isolates showed 6 amino acid substitutions differed from the PCV1 reference strains: 60 (K to E), 63 (Y to H), 72 (H to Q), 74 (K to R), 176 (H to Q) and 233 (K to E) (Fig. 1b).

To understand the genetic relationship among the PCV1 isolates in this study, a maximum likelihood (ML) phylogenetic tree was constructed with the 14 strains collected from Guangxi Province, 40 other comparison PCV1 strains, and 4 PCV2 strains with complete genomic nucleotide sequences available in GenBank. Except for the GXdx84 strain, all isolated strains belonged to the PCV1 and showed geographical differences, but these differences were not evident. In particular, the ML phylogenetic tree analysis showed that the GXdx84 strain was different from the other strains (Fig. 2). The GXdx84 strain was located in the branch of neither PCV1 nor PCV2 strains as shown by the whole nucleotide analysis. With regard to the *cap* and *rep* gene of the samples, *cap* of the strain was located in the branch of PCV2, and *rep* of the strain was located in the branch of PCV1 but was distantly related to other strains of PCV1. These results indicated that the GXdx84 strain might have underwent recombination.

Recombination analysis

The putative recombination events were identified using the Recombination Detection Program (RDP). For 14 PCV1 isolation strains, one recombination event was detected, in which the GXdx84 strain (P-value=1.54×10^{-13}) with the potential parental of PCV1 subtype strain PCV1G and PCV2 subtype strain PCV2b. The number and location of the breakpoints were also determined using similarity plots. When the PCV1G and PCV2b strains were used as potential parental strains, they shared one breakpoint location at 694nt (Fig. 3). It indicated that PCV2b and PCV1G strains might be the minor and major parents of GXdx84 strain.

Table 2 Summary of the complete PCV genomes sequenced used in this study

Strain name	Accesion Number	Country	Collection Date	Genotype	Length(nt)	Source	Linical condition/tissue origin of isolation
BJ-1	FJ475129	Beijing, China	07/5/2009	PCV1	1759bp	GenBank	Lymph nodes, spleen, lung and other tissue materials
PCV1	AY193712	Zhijiang, China	17/2/2003	PCV1	1759bp	GenBank	Lymph nodes, spleen, lung and other tissue materials
PCV1-Hun	KJ408799	Hungary	16/4/2014	PCV1	1759bp	GenBank	lymph nodes, spleen, lung and other tissue materials
PCV1-Eng-1970	KJ408798	United Kingdom	16/4/2014	PCV1	1759bp	GenBank	lymph nodes, spleen, lung and other tissue materials
PCV1-XFD-Beijing	KC447455	Beijing, China	16/4/2013	PCV1	1759bp	GenBank	lymph nodes, spleen, lung and other tissue materials
PCV1/G	JN398656	Harbin, China	31/8/2011	PCV1	1759bp	GenBank	Contaminated PK-15 cell
HZ2006	EF533941	Hangzhou, China	01/5/2007	PCV1	1759bp	GenBank	Lymph nodes, spleen, lung and other tissue materials
NMB	GU799575	USA	28/2/2011	PCV1	1759bp	GenBank	Lymph nodes, spleen, lung and other tissue materials
Jiangsu	GU722334	Jiangsu, China	03/3/2010	PCV1	1759bp	GenBank	Lymph nodes, spleen, lung and other tissue materials
Tian Jin	GU371908	Tianjin, China	06/2/2010	PCV1	1759bp	GenBank	Lymph nodes, spleen, lung and other tissue materials
ZY	KF732857	Guiyang, China	08/1/2014	PCV1	1759bp	GenBank	Lymph nodes, spleen, lung and other tissue materials
DY	KC924758	Guiyang, China	13/8/2013	PCV1	1759bp	GenBank	Lymph nodes, spleen, lung and other tissue materials
GY	KC894933	Guiyang, China	06/8/2013	PCV1	1759bp	GenBank	Lymph nodes, spleen, lung and other tissue materials
Guiyang	KC878437	Guiyang, China	30/7/2013	PCV1	1759bp	GenBank	Lymph nodes, spleen, lung and other tissue materials
ZZ-3	KC733436	Zhengzhou, China	18/6/2013	PCV1	1759bp	GenBank	Lymph node
NJ03	JX566507	Nanjing, China	06/5/2013	PCV1	1759bp	GenBank	Congenital tremors/lymph nodes, spleen, lung and other tissue materials
CT-PCV-P7	AY099501	USA	19/5/2009	PCV1	1759bp	GenBank	Lymph nodes, spleen, lung and other tissue materials
CCL33-UGent	JN133303	Belgium	12/11/ 2011	PCV1	1759bp	GenBank	Lymph nodes, spleen, lung and other tissue materials
3384	JN133302	United Kingdom	12/11/ 2011	PCV1	1759bp	GenBank	Lymph nodes, spleen, lung and other tissue materials
HRB-09	GQ449671	Beijing, China	24/10/ 2011	PCV1	1758bp	GenBank	PK-15 cell culture
PCV3_Rotarix_con1	HM143844	USA	20/6/2010	PCV1	1759bp	GenBank	Lymph nodes, spleen, lung and other tissue materials
SC-10	DQ659154	Guangdong, China	19/6/2006	PCV1	1759bp	GenBank	Pig serum
SC-9	DQ659153	Guangdong, China	19/6/2006	PCV1	1759bp	GenBank	Pig serum
SC-8	DQ494788	Guangdong, China	06/5/2006	PCV1	1759bp	GenBank	Pig serum
SC-7	DQ494787	Guangdong, China	06/5/2006	PCV1	1759bp	GenBank	Pig serum
SC-5	DQ472016	Guangdong, China	24/4/2006	PCV1	1759bp	GenBank	Pig serum
SC-6	DQ472015		24/4/2006	PCV1	1759bp	GenBank	Pig serum

Table 2 Summary of the complete PCV genomes sequenced used in this study *(Continued)*

Strain name	Accesion Number	Country	Collection Date	Genotype	Length(nt)	Source	Linical condition/tissue origin of isolation
		Guangdong, China					
SC-4	DQ472014	Guangdong, China	24/4/2006	PCV1	1759bp	GenBank	Pig serum
SC-3	DQ472013	Guangdong, China	24/4/2006	PCV1	1759bp	GenBank	Pig serum
SC-2	DQ472012	Guangdong, China	24/4/2006	PCV1	1759bp	GenBank	Pig serum
NT70719	FJ159693	Jiangsu, China	23/9/2008	PCV1	1759bp	GenBank	Lymph nodes, spleen, lung and other tissue materials
TZ70717	FJ159692	Jiangsu, China	23/9/2008	PCV1	1759bp	GenBank	Lymph nodes, spleen, lung and other tissue materials
SD-73-3	KJ746930	Shandong, China	15/7/2014	PCV1	1759bp	GenBank	Lymph nodes, spleen, lung and other tissue materials
TJ1307	KJ808815	Beijing, China	18/8/2014	PCV1	1759bp	GenBank	Lymph nodes, spleen, lung and other tissue materials
SD-73-1	KJ746929	Shandong, China	15/7/2014	PCV1	1759bp	GenBank	Lymph nodes, spleen, lung and other tissue materials
PK	DQ650650	Jiangsu, China	08/7/2006	PCV1	1759bp	GenBank	Lymph nodes, spleen, lung and other tissue materials
Aust4	AY754015	Australia	21/3/2014	PCV1	1759bp	GenBank	PK-15 cell culture
Aust3	AY754014	Australia	21/3/2014	PCV1	1759bp	GenBank	PK-15 cell culture
SC-1	DQ358813	Guangdong, China	01/3/2006	PCV1	1759bp	GenBank	Pig serum
WB-H-8	DQ648032	Hungary	02/7/2006	PCV1	1759bp	GenBank	Lymph nodes, spleen, lung and other tissue materials
YZ70719	FJ159691	Jiangsu, China	23/9/2008	PCV1	1759bp	GenBank	Lymph nodes, spleen, lung and other tissue materials
YZ70722	FJ159689	Jiangsu, China	23/9/2008	PCV1	1759bp	GenBank	Lymph nodes, spleen, lung and other tissue materials
PCV2a	AF027217	Canada	19/3/2009	PCV2a	1768bp	GenBank	Suspected PMWS/ lymph nodes, spleen, lung and other tissue materials
PCV2b	AF112862	Canada	12/10/ 2005	PCV2b	1768bp	GenBank	Suspected PMWS/ lymph nodes, spleen, lung and other tissue materials
PCV2c	AF109398	Canada	23/7/2001	PCV2c	1768bp	GenBank	Suspected PMWS/ lymph nodes, spleen, lung and other tissue materials
PCV2d-1(P2425NT)	JX099786	Viet Nam	01/5/2014	PCV2d-1	1767bp	GenBank	Suspected PMWS/ lymph nodes, spleen, lung and other tissue materials
PCV2d-2(CS5)	KX161667	Hunan, China	05/6/2016	PCV2d-2	1767bp	GenBank	Suspected PMWS/ lymph nodes, spleen, lung and other tissue materials
GXdx115	KX827778	Guangxi, China	00/7/2015	PCV1	1759bp	This study	Lungs, spleen, and lymph nodes
GXdx105	KX827779	Guangxi, China	00/7/2015	PCV1	1759bp	This study	Lungs, spleen, and lymph nodes
GXdx64	KX827780	Guangxi, China	00/7/2015	PCV1	1759bp	This study	Lungs, spleen, and lymph nodes
GXdx51	KX827781	Guangxi, China	00/7/2015	PCV1	1759bp	This study	Lungs, spleen, and lymph nodes
GXbb158	KX827782	Guangxi, China	00/7/2015	PCV1	1759bp	This study	Lungs, spleen, and lymph nodes
GXyl225	KX827783	Guangxi, China	00/7/2015	PCV1	1759bp	This study	Lungs, spleen, and lymph nodes

Table 2 Summary of the complete PCV genomes sequenced used in this study *(Continued)*

Strain name	Accesion Number	Country	Collection Date	Genotype	Length(nt)	Source	Linical condition/tissue origin of isolation
GXyl224	KX827784	Guangxi, China	00/7/2015	PCV1	1759bp	This study	Lungs, spleen, and lymph nodes
GXlsh19	KX827785	Guangxi, China	00/7/2015	PCV1	1759bp	This study	Lungs, spleen, and lymph nodes
GXlsh12	KX827786	Guangxi, China	00/7/2015	PCV1	1759bp	This study	Lungs, spleen, and lymph nodes
GXlsh11	KX827787	Guangxi, China	00/7/2015	PCV1	1759bp	This study	Lungs, spleen, and lymph nodes
GXlsh10	KX827788	Guangxi, China	00/7/2015	PCV1	1759bp	This study	Lungs, spleen, and lymph nodes
GXlsh7	KX827789	Guangxi, China	00/7/2015	PCV1	1759bp	This study	Lungs, spleen, and lymph nodes
GXlsh2	KX827790	Guangxi, China	00/7/2015	PCV1	1759bp	This study	Lungs, spleen, and lymph nodes
GXdx84	KY437725	Guangxi, China	00/7/2015	PCV1/2d	1757bp	This study	Lungs, spleen, and lymph nodes

Selection-pressure analysis of PCV1

The selection-pressure of PCV1 strains was analyzed by calculating the difference in non-synonymous substitution (dN) and synonymous substitution (dS) rates for *rep* and *cap*. The differences of dN–dS were -0.09127±0.0251 for the *rep* gene and -0.2111±0.0541 for the *cap* gene. These results suggested that the *rep* gene and the *cap* gene of PCV1 are under purified selection. Moreover, entropy was coupled with dN–dS to indicate diversity and complexity. The vast majority of Rep and Cap protein amino acid residues exhibited low level or zero entropy (Fig. 4). It indicated that the Rep and Cap protein had low complexity. Only the Cap protein amino acid sequences which were at 50-80, 161-180 and 230-233 had high complexity.

Discussion

PCV1 is considered to be non-pathogenic and economically unimportant and therefore, little is known about its epidemiology and worldwide distribution. More research on PCV1 has focused on the chemic vaccine of PCV1-2 to prevent PCV2 infected in pigs [27, 28]. Recent research found that PCV1 can replicate efficiently and produce pathology in the lungs of porcine fetuses and have a certain impact on porcine alveolar macrophages [16]. It is difficult to rule out the potential damage of PCV1 to the immune system of piglets.

Recombinant events of PCV among different genotypes or different virus isolates have been reported, including recombinant event between PCV2a and PCV2b, and between PCV1 and PCV2a. In this study, we found a recombination GXdx84 strain which was recombinant by PCV1 and PCV2d-2 had a breakpoint at 694nt. Previous research found that the *rep* gene of the PCV2 can be divided into three regions, and the third region has the highest level of selective pressure which makes the fragment more changeable than the other two [1, 29]. The PCV1 and PCV2 are highly similarity of *rep* gene and this might be the reason why recombinant event occurred at 694nt.

Most studies on the genetic characterization of PCV2 were based on the *cap* gene, which is the ideal marker for phylogenetic analysis because this region is considered to be the most variable region in the PCV2 genome and the same phylogenetic tree constructed on the basis of the full genome can be reconstructed with ORF2. However, analysis based on the complete genome is necessary, as it may help identify genetic variability, particularly in terms of recombination events. In this study, genotypic analysis based on the *cap* gene and complete genome resulted in different phylogenetic trees. The GXdx84 strain was divided into different branches of the phylogenetic tree. Analysis of the *cap* and *rep* genes showed that the new strain was clustered in *cap* in PCV2 and in *rep* in PCV1. Besides, *cap* of the GXdx84 strain was highly similar to the genotype of PCV2d-2. In a recent report from China, the positive rate of PCV2d out of PCV2 positive samples ranged from 55% (22/40) [30] to 68.2% (45/66) [31]. It had become the predominant PCV2 subtype [32]. PCV2d can be classified into PCV2d-1 and PCV2d-2, with substantial genetic divergence between the two subtypes. PCV2d-1 strains were first identified in China in 2002 [33], whereas PCV2d-2 strains were first identified in China in 2008 and had been linked with increased virulence [34, 35].

As for the isolated PCV1 strains, the *cap* gene in the GXyl224 strain spanned 708 nucleotides (codes 235aa), while the other PCV1 strains spanned 702 nucleotides (codes 233aa). This was the first case to report that the capsid protein contains 235 amino acids. Previous studies

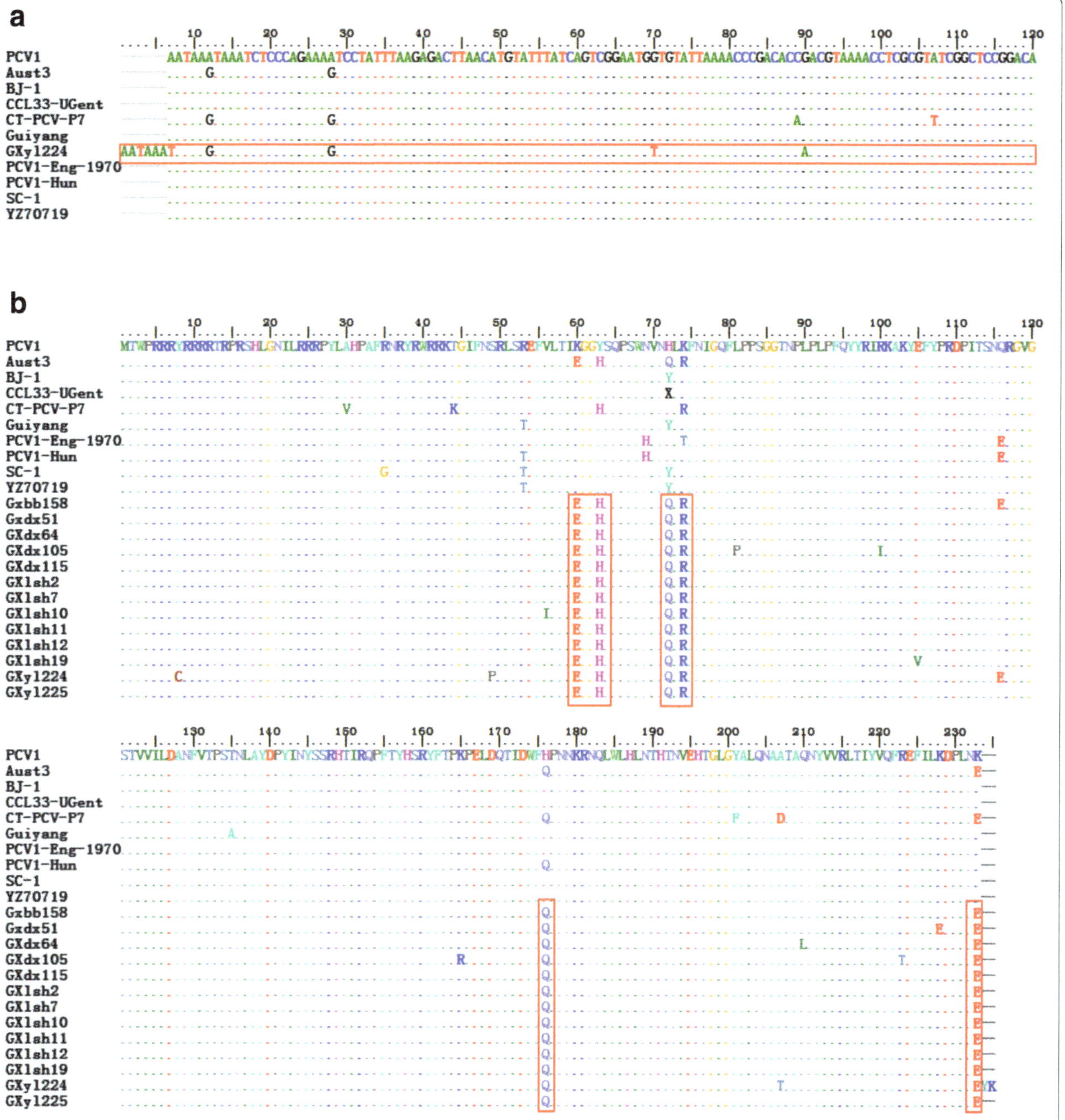

Fig. 1 Alignment of the nucleotide sequence and deduced amino acid for the *cap* gene, and Cap protein of partial strains analyzed in this study. Conserver residues are indicated by dashed lines. PCV1 is used as the majority sequence for this alignment (AY193712). **a** The *cap* gene of GXyl224 inside the red box is one wherein the stop codon mutation led to an increase in the number of nucleotides. **b** The major nucleotide mutation sites of Cap protein are presented within the red box

suggested that the immunoreactive regions of the capsid protein were potential candidate regions involved in the emergence of PCV2 variants [36, 37]. Although PCV1 has no obvious pathogenicity, clinical trials have shown that PCV1 and PCV2 mixed infection generally exhibits the presence of a recombinant strain [38]. Unfortunately, we have not isolated the virus. In the future, we will aim to separate the virus and study its pathogenicity.

In the present study, we also analyzed the selective pressure by calculating the dN and dS rates and the entropy. Very low levels of variability were detected at the nucleotide and amino acid level. Further, the dN–dS values showed that most codons are under neutral or negative selection [39, 40]. Another previous study showed that the average genomic substitution rate for PCV1 was two-fold lower than that for PCV2 [41],

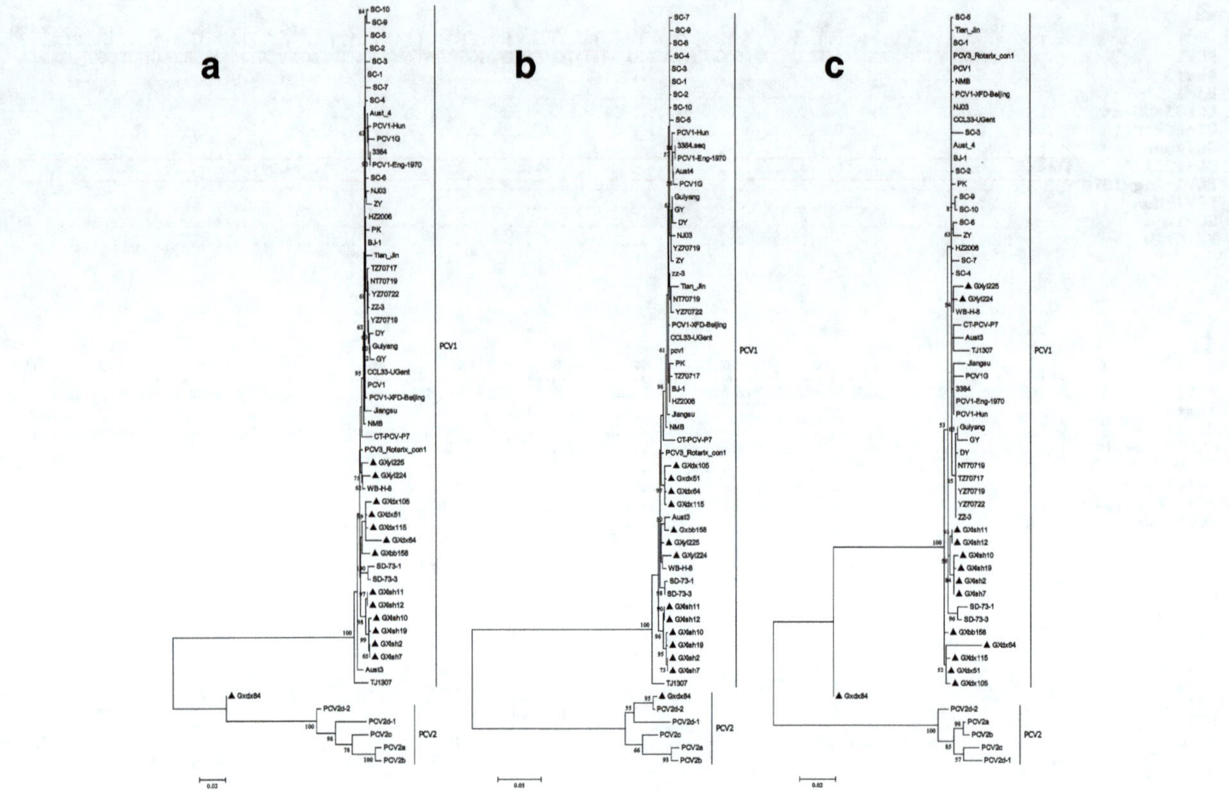

Fig. 2 Phylogenetic tree analysis based on the nucleotide sequences of the complete genome (**a**), *cap* gene (**b**), and *rep* gene (**c**), performed using the ML method. Numbers along the branches indicate the percentage of confidence in the ML analysis. Only bootstrap support values of >50% are indicated. PCV1 strains isolated in this study are denoted by triangle (▲)

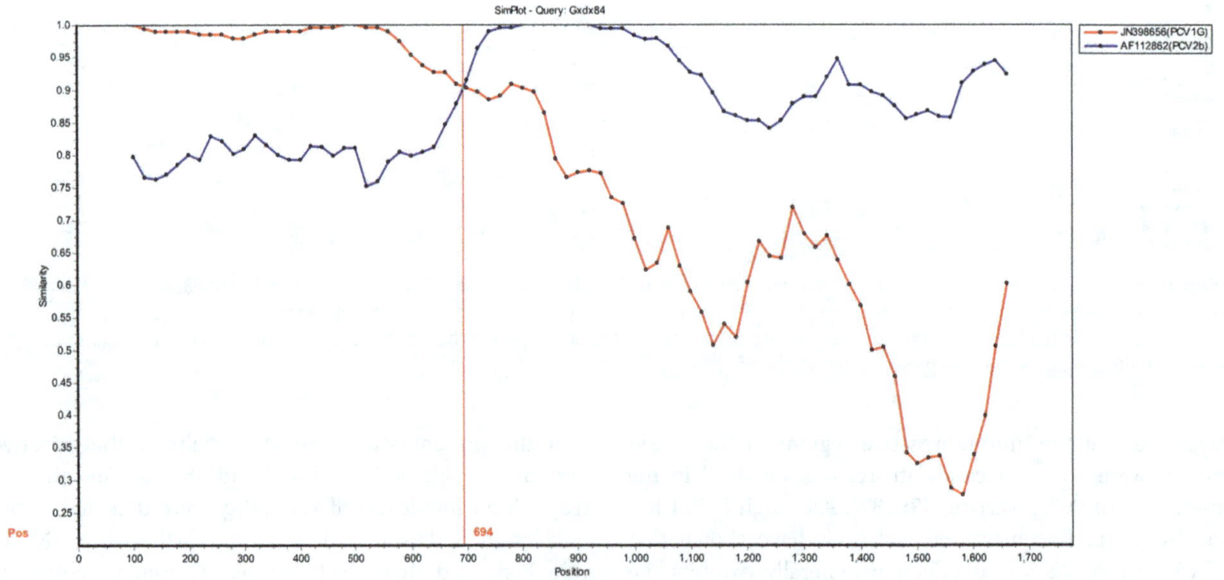

Fig. 3 Simplot analysis the recombination events. One recombination event might be occurred in GXdx84 strain with the PCV1G strain (JN398656) and PCV2b strain (AF112862) as two parent groups. The Y-axis refers to the percentage of similarity. The X-axis refers to the nucleotide position in alignment. The crossed point might be the potential location of recombination event

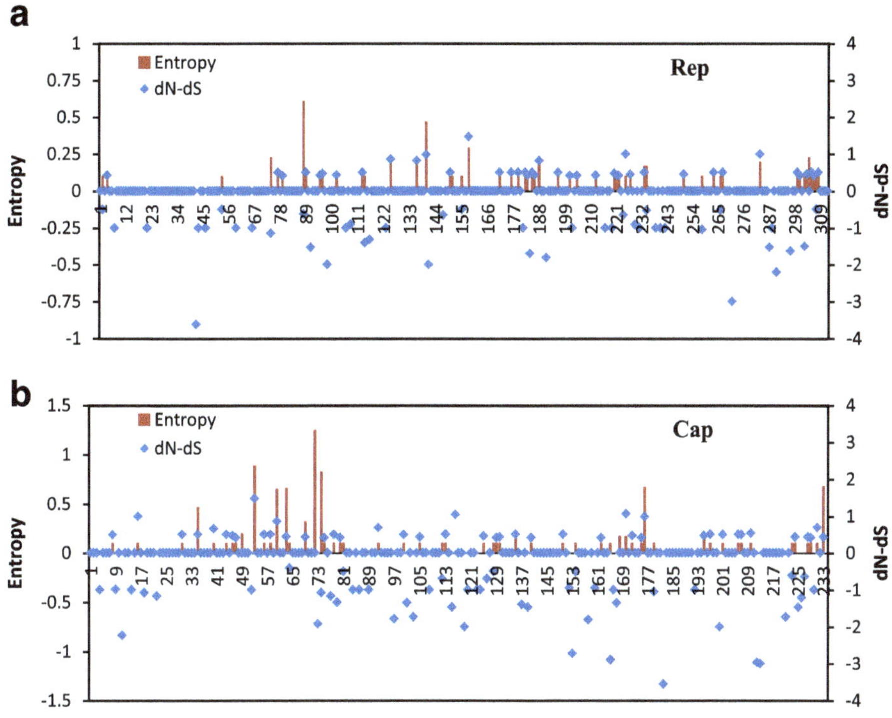

Fig. 4 Plot for the difference between non-synonymous and synonymous rates (dN–dS) and amino acid entropy rate for the *rep* (**a**) and *cap* (**b**) genes

which indicated that the PCV1 genome lacked variation. Entropy of Cap and Rep protein coupled with a low complexity, but the Cap protein amino acid sequence which were at 60-80, 161-180 and 230-233 had high complexity (Fig. 4). It was reported that Cap protein was the main antigenic determinant of the PCV2, and contained different epitopes within residues 47-85, 165-200 and the last of the four C-terminal amino acid of the PCV2 capsid protein [42]. Three high complexity regions of PCV1 researched in this study might be the epitopes regions of PCV1. Besides, the Cap protein of GXyl224 coded 235 amino acids, which is two amino acids more than other strains. By analysising the antigenic of GXyl224 by IEDB (http://tools.iedb.org/bcell/), we found that the last six amino acids (230-235aa) were the potential epitope region, other strains of PCV1 were the last four amino acid (230-233aa). Two additional amino acids may result in increased antigenicity of Cap protein, which still need further verification.

Conclusion

In summary, we have sequenced 14 strains suspected to be PCV1 from Guangxi Province, China. ML phylogenetic tree analysis showed that 13 of these strains belonged to PCV1 and 1 strain named GXdx84 belonged neither to PCV1 nor PCV2: it was a chimeric PCV1 and PCV2 strain. In addition, another stain named GXyl224 with ORF2 spans 708 nucleotides by gene sequencing. This is the first study to report that a *cap* gene mutation resulted in lengthening of in the gene sequence. The correlation between epitope mutations and pathogenicity as well as immunogenicity of GXyl224 and GXdx84 needs further investigation.

Abbreviations

dN: Non-synonymous substitution; dS: Synonymous substitution; ORF: Open-reading frame; PCV: Porcine circovirus; PMWS: Post-weaning multi-systemic wasting syndrome; RDP: Recombination detection program

Acknowledgements

We would like to thank the native English staff of Elixigen Company (Huntington Beach, California) for editing the manuscript. And we would like to thank Ningning Hu for her assistance with reagent preparation.

Funding

This study was funded by the National Program on Key Research Project of China [grant number 2017YFD0500101 and 2016YFD0500401] and the National Natural Science Foundation of China [grant number 31272573].

Authors' contributions

LC performed the research, data analysis and wrote the manuscript. WCS, HJL and MYT helped in the writing of the manuscript. CZX, GYZ, JCH, WW and MZ participated in sample collection and research testing. RD, NYJ and ADQ designed the research. All authors read and approved the final manuscript.

Ethics approval and consent to participate
Experimental protocols for obtaining pigs clinical samples used in this study were obtained from Guangxi Center for Animal Disease Control and Prevention and carried out in strict accordance with the Animal Ethics Procedures and Guidelines of the People's Republic of China. All pigs were euthanized by an anesthetic overdose with the pentobarbital before collected the samples and all pig owners agree the samples' usage before participation in the study.

Consent for publication
Not applicable.

Competing interests
The authors declare that they have no competing interests.

Author details
[1]College of Animal Science and Technology, Jilin Agricultural University, Changchun 130118, People's Republic of China. [2]Institute of Military Veterinary, Key Laboratory of Jilin Province for Zoonosis Prevention and Control, Academy of Military Sciences, Changchun 130122, People's Republic of China. [3]Guangxi Center for Animal Disease Control and Prevention, Nanning 530001, People's Republic of China. [4]College of Veterinary Medicine, Jilin University, Changchun 130062, People's Republic of China.

References
1. Olvera A, Cortey M, Segales J: Molecular evolution of porcine circovirus type 2 genomes: phylogeny and clonality. Virology 2007, 357(2):175-185.
2. Cortey M, Segales J. Low levels of diversity among genomes of Porcine circovirus type 1 (PCV1) points to differential adaptive selection between Porcine circoviruses. Virology. 2012;422(2):161–4.
3. Tischer I, Gelderblom H, Vettermann W, Koch MA. A very small porcine virus with circular single-stranded DNA. Nature. 1982;295(5844):64–6.
4. Tischer I, Rasch R, Tochtermann G. Characterization of papovavirus-and picornavirus-like particles in permanent pig kidney cell lines. Zentralblatt fur Bakteriologie, Parasitenkunde, Infektionskrankheiten und Hygiene Erste Abteilung Originale Reihe A: Medizinische Mikrobiologie und Parasitologie. 1974;226(2):153–67.
5. Allan G, Meehan B, Todd D, Kennedy S, McNeilly F, Ellis J, Clark EG, Harding J, Espuna E, Botner A, et al. Novel porcine circoviruses from pigs with wasting disease syndromes. Vet Rec. 1998;142(17):467–8.
6. Beach NM, Juhan NM, Cordoba L, Meng XJ. Replacement of the replication factors of porcine circovirus (PCV) type 2 with those of PCV type 1 greatly enhances viral replication in vitro. J Virol. 2010;84(17):8986–9.
7. Cheung AK. Comparative analysis of the transcriptional patterns of pathogenic and nonpathogenic porcine circoviruses. Virology. 2003; 310(1):41–9.
8. Mankertz A, Mueller B, Steinfeldt T, Schmitt C, Finsterbusch T. New reporter gene-based replication assay reveals exchangeability of replication factors of porcine circovirus types 1 and 2. J Virol. 2003;77(18):9885–93.
9. Cheung AK. Porcine circovirus: transcription and DNA replication. Virus Res. 2012;164(1-2):46–53.
10. Mankertz A, Caliskan R, Hattermann K, Hillenbrand B, Kurzendoerfer P, Mueller B, Schmitt C, Steinfeldt T, Finsterbusch T. Molecular biology of Porcine circovirus: analyses of gene expression and viral replication. Veterinary microbiology. 2004;98(2):81–8.
11. Nawagitgul P, Morozov I, Bolin SR, Harms PA, Sorden SD, Paul PS. Open reading frame 2 of porcine circovirus type 2 encodes a major capsid protein. J Gen Virol. 2000;81(Pt 9):2281–7.
12. Bratanich AC, Blanchetot A. PCV2 replicase transcripts in infected porcine kidney (PK15) cells. Virus Genes. 2002;25(3):323–8.
13. Chaiyakul M, Hsu K, Dardari R, Marshall F, Czub M. Cytotoxicity of ORF3 proteins from a nonpathogenic and a pathogenic porcine circovirus. J Virol. 2010;84(21):11440–7.
14. Tischer I, Bode L, Peters D, Pociuli S, Germann B. Distribution of antibodies to porcine circovirus in swine populations of different breeding farms. Arch Virol. 1995;140(4):737–43.
15. Rodriguez-Arrioja GM, Segales J, Balasch M, Rosell C, Quintant J, Folch JM, Plana-Duran J, Mankertz A, Domingo M. Serum antibodies to porcine circovirus type 1 and type 2 in pigs with and without PMWS. *Vet Rec.* 2000; 146(26):762–4.
16. Saha D, Lefebvre DJ, Ducatelle R, Doorsselaere JV, Nauwynck HJ. Outcome of experimental porcine circovirus type 1 infections in mid-gestational porcine foetuses. BMC Vet Res. 2011;7:64.
17. Calsamiglia M, Segales J, Quintana J, Rosell C, Domingo M. Detection of porcine circovirus types 1 and 2 in serum and tissue samples of pigs with and without postweaning multisystemic wasting syndrome. Journal of clinical microbiology. 2002;40(5):1848–50.
18. Fenaux M, Opriessnig T, Halbur PG, Xu Y, Potts B, Meng XJ. Detection and in vitro and in vivo characterization of porcine circovirus DNA from a porcine-derived commercial pepsin product. The Journal of general virology. 2004; 85(Pt 11):3377–82.
19. Thompson JD, Higgins DG, Gibson TJ. CLUSTAL W: improving the sensitivity of progressive multiple sequence alignment through sequence weighting, position-specific gap penalties and weight matrix choice. Nucleic acids research. 1994;22(22):4673–80.
20. Tamura K, Peterson D, Peterson N, Stecher G, Nei M, Kumar S. MEGA5: molecular evolutionary genetics analysis using maximum likelihood, evolutionary distance, and maximum parsimony methods. Molecular biology and evolution. 2011;28(10):2731–9.
21. Martin DP, Lemey P, Lott M, Moulton V, Posada D, Lefeuvre P. RDP3: a flexible and fast computer program for analyzing recombination. Bioinformatics. 2010;26(19):2462–3.
22. Lole KS, Bollinger RC, Paranjape RS, Gadkari D, Kulkarni SS, Novak NG, Ingersoll R, Sheppard HW, Ray SC. Full-length human immunodeficiency virus type 1 genomes from subtype C-infected seroconverters in India, with evidence of intersubtype recombination. Journal of virology. 1999; 73(1):152–60.
23. Pond SL, Frost SD, Muse SV. HyPhy: hypothesis testing using phylogenies. Bioinformatics. 2005;21(5):676–9.
24. Wolinsky SM, Korber BT, Neumann AU, Daniels M, Kunstman KJ, Whetsell AJ, Furtado MR, Cao Y, Ho DD, Safrit JT. Adaptive evolution of human immunodeficiency virus-type 1 during the natural course of infection. Science. 1996;272(5261):537–42.
25. Zhang Z, Jia R, Lu Y, Wang M, Zhu D, Chen S, Yin Z, Chen X, Cheng A. Identification, genotyping, and molecular evolution analysis of duck circovirus. Gene. 2013;529(2):288–95.
26. Hughes AL, Nei M: Nucleotide substitution at major histocompatibility complex class II loci: evidence for overdominant selection. Proceedings of the National Academy of Sciences of the United States of America 1989, 86(3):958-962.
27. Seo HW, Oh Y, Han K, Park C, Chae C. Reduction of porcine circovirus type 2 (PCV2) viremia by a reformulated inactivated chimeric PCV1-2 vaccine-induced humoral and cellular immunity after experimental PCV2 challenge. BMC Vet Res. 2012;8:194.
28. Han S, Xiao Y, Zheng D, Gu Y, Xuan Y, Jin Y, Pang W, Huang Y, Li X, Deng J, et al. Establishment and application of a competitive enzyme-linked immunosorbent assay differentiating PCV2 antibodies from mixture of PCV1/PCV2 antibodies in pig sera. *BMC Vet Res.* 2016;12(1):175.
29. Cheung AK. Identification of an octanucleotide motif sequence essential for viral protein, DNA, and progeny virus biosynthesis at the origin of DNA replication of porcine circovirus type 2. Virology. 2004;324(1):28–36.
30. Cai L, Ni J, Xia Y, Zi Z, Ning K, Qiu P, Li X, Wang B, Liu Q, Hu D, et al. Identification of an emerging recombinant cluster in porcine circovirus type 2. *Virus Res.* 2012;165(1):95–102.
31. Wei C, Zhang M, Chen Y, Xie J, Huang Z, Zhu W, Xu T, Cao Z, Zhou P, Su S, et al. Genetic evolution and phylogenetic analysis of porcine circovirus type 2 infections in southern China from 2011 to 2012. *Infect Genet Evol.* 2013;17:87–92.
32. Perez LJ, Diaz de Arce H, Frias MT. Genetic characterization and phylogenetic analysis of porcine circovirus type 2 strains present in Cuban swine herds. Res Vet Sci. 2010;89(2):301–5.
33. Cortey M, Olvera A, Grau-Roma L, Segales J. Further comments on porcine circovirus type 2 (PCV2) genotype definition and nomenclature. Veterinary microbiology. 2011;149(3-4):522–3.

34. Guo LJ, Lu YH, Wei YW, Huang LP, Liu CM. Porcine circovirus type 2 (PCV2): genetic variation and newly emerging genotypes in China. Virology journal. 2010;**7**:273.
35. Xiao CT, Halbur PG, Opriessnig T. Global molecular genetic analysis of porcine circovirus type 2 (PCV2) sequences confirms the presence of four main PCV2 genotypes and reveals a rapid increase of PCV2d. J Gen Virol. 2015;96(Pt 7):1830–41.
36. Lv QZ, Guo KK, Zhang YM. Current understanding of genomic DNA of porcine circovirus type 2. Virus genes. 2014;49(1):1–10.
37. Larochelle R, Magar R, D'Allaire S. Genetic characterization and phylogenetic analysis of porcine circovirus type 2 (PCV2) strains from cases presenting various clinical conditions. Virus Res. 2002;90(1-2):101–12.
38. Gagnon CA, Music N, Fontaine G, Tremblay D, Harel J. Emergence of a new type of porcine circovirus in swine (PCV): a type 1 and type 2 PCV recombinant. Vet Microbiol. 2010;144(1-2):18–23.
39. Csagola A, Kiss I, Tuboly T. Detection and analysis of porcine circovirus type 1 in Hungarian wild boars: short communication. Acta veterinaria Hungarica. 2008;56(1):139–44.
40. Muhling J, Raye WS, Buddle JR, Wilcox GE. Genetic characterisation of Australian strains of porcine circovirus types 1 and 2. Australian veterinary journal. 2006;84(12):421–5. discussion 416
41. Firth C, Charleston MA, Duffy S, Shapiro B, Holmes EC. Insights into the evolutionary history of an emerging livestock pathogen: porcine circovirus 2. Journal of virology. 2009;83(24):12813–21.
42. Lekcharoensuk P, Morozov I, Paul PS, Thangthumniyom N, Wajjawalku W, Meng XJ. Epitope mapping of the major capsid protein of type 2 porcine circovirus (PCV2) by using chimeric PCV1 and PCV2. J Virol. 2004;78(15): 8135–45.

Post-epidemic Schmallenberg virus circulation: parallel bovine serological and *Culicoides* virological surveillance studies in Ireland

Á. B. Collins[1,2], D. Barrett[3], M. L. Doherty[2], M. Larska[4] and J. F. Mee[1*]

Abstract

Background: Schmallenberg virus (SBV) emerged in northern-Europe in 2011 resulting in an epidemic of ruminant abortions and congenital malformations throughout the continent. In the years following the epidemic there have been reports of SBV overwintering and continued circulation in several European countries. When the population-level of immunity declines in exposed regions, re-introduction of SBV could result in further outbreaks of Schmallenberg disease. The aims of this study were to determine the SBV seroprevalence in previously exposed Irish dairy herds in 2014 and to investigate if SBV continued to circulate in these herds in the three years (2013–2015) following the Irish Schmallenberg epidemic.

Whole-herd SBV serosurveillance was conducted in 26 herds before (spring) and following the 2014 vector-season (winter), and following the 2015 vector-season (winter). In spring 2014, 5,531 blood samples were collected from 4,070 cows and 1,461 heifers. In winter 2014, 2,483 blood samples were collected from 1,550 youngstock (8–10 months old) and a subsample (n = 933; 288 cows, 645 heifers) of the seronegative animals identified in the spring. Youngstock were resampled in winter 2015. *Culicoides* spp. were collected in 10 herds during the 2014 vector-season and analysed for SBV; a total of 138 pools (3,048 *Culicoides*) from 6 SBV vector species were tested for SBV RNA using real-time PCR.

Results: In spring 2014, animal-level seroprevalence was 62.5 % (cows = 84.7 %; heifers = 0.6 %). Within-herd seroprevalence ranged widely from 8.5 %–84.1 % in the 26 herds. In winter 2014, 22 animals (0.9 %; 10 cows, 5 heifers, 7 youngstock) originating in 17 herds (range 1–4 animals/herd) tested seropositive. In winter 2015 all youngstock, including the 7 seropositive animals in winter 2014, tested seronegative suggesting their initial positive result was due to persistence of maternal antibodies. All of the *Culicoides* pools examined tested negative for SBV-RNA.

Conclusions: SBV appears to have recirculated at a very low level in these herds during 2013 and 2014, while there was no evidence of SBV infection in naïve youngstock during 2015. A large population of naïve animals was identified and may be at risk of infection in future years should SBV re-emerge and recirculate as it has done in continental Europe.

Keywords: Schmallenberg virus, Cattle, Surveillance, Serology, *Culicoides* spp, Ireland

* Correspondence: john.mee@teagasc.ie
[1]Animal and Bioscience Research Department, AGRIC, Teagasc, Moorepark, Fermoy, Co. Cork, Ireland
Full list of author information is available at the end of the article

Background

Schmallenberg virus (SBV) is a novel Orthobunyavirus (family *Bunyavirudae*) which was first identified at the Friedrich Loeffler Institute in Germany in October 2011 by metagenomic analyses of blood samples collected from dairy cattle presenting non-specific clinical signs [1]. Cattle, sheep and goats are the main species affected by the virus; however SBV has also been detected in other ruminants including camelids and deer [2]. The virus is transmitted by a range of *Culicoides* spp. biting midges [3, 4]. Infection in adult cattle is typically mild; clinical signs include short-duration fever, diarrhoea and a drop in milk yield in dairy cows [1]. If susceptible ruminants become infected with SBV during the gestation-susceptible period (estimated to be between day 62–173 in cattle and day 28–56 in sheep) [2], transplacental foetal infection can occur resulting in abortions, stillbirths and congenital malformations of the musculoskeletal and central nervous system (arthrogryposis-hydranencephaly syndrome) in neonates [4].

Following the initial emergence of SBV in Germany in 2011, the virus rapidly disseminated throughout the continent reaching an almost pan-European distribution by the end of the 2011–2012 vector-season [5] with herd seroprevalence rates nearing 100 % in many regions [2, 4]. The first Irish SBV case confirmed by RT-PCR was in a bovine foetus with pathognomonic SBV lesions in October 2012 [6]. National cattle SBV sero-surveys conducted in Ireland at the end of 2012 and in 2013 demonstrated that much of the south and south east of the country had been exposed to SBV during 2012, while the north and north-west remained predominantly uninfected [7]. There was little evidence of further spread of SBV (expansion of the area exposed to SBV) in Ireland over the course of the second vector season (2013) [7]; this is in contrast with other European countries such as Germany [8] and Belgium [9], where SBV appeared to re-emerge in cattle herds and sheep flocks in 2012. In the three years (2012, 2013 and 2014) following the European Schmallenberg epidemic there have been a number of reports of SBV overwintering and continued virus circulation in several countries [10–15]. Currently (2016), it is unknown whether SBV continues to be present and active in previously exposed regions in Ireland.

Cattle are the preferred host for the most common *Culicoides* arbovirus vector species [16, 17] and are often used as sentinel animals in surveillance programs for vector-borne diseases [18, 19]. Hence, simultaneous monitoring of *Culicoides* and their preferred bovine host species for evidence of infection is an established method to investigate arbovirus circulation in a region. The aims of the present study were (i) to determine the seroprevalence of SBV infection in 26 previously exposed Irish dairy herds in 2014 (two years after SBV first emerged in Ireland in 2012) and (ii) to investigate whether there was evidence of SBV circulation in these herds in the three years (2013–2015) following the Irish Schmallenberg epidemic, and if so to what extent.

Methods

Sampling design

For the purpose of this study the timespan before, during and after the Irish Schmallenberg epidemic was divided into five time periods; Year −1 to Year +4. Year −1 is the year prior to SBV emergence in Ireland (and the year of the European Schmallenberg epidemic, 2011/2012), Year 0 is the year of the Irish epidemic (2012/2013) and Year +1, Year +2 and Year +3 are one, two and three years after the Irish epidemic, respectively. Each year-long period ranges from May until April of the following year (Fig. 1). This period corresponds with the start of the vector-active season (May), [20], and the end of the peak period of congenital Schmallenberg malformations (end of peak spring calving period in April) associated with that particular vector-active season (1 May- 1 November) [20].

In order to investigate the prevalence of SBV infection and virus re-circulation, we monitored cattle herds and SBV *Culicoides* vector species for evidence of infection in the three years (2013, 2014 and 2015) following the Irish Schmallenberg epidemic. In 2014, a total of 36 Irish dairy farmers located in a region where SBV circulated

Year	2011	2012	2013	2014	2015
Year relative to Irish SBV epidemic	-1 (European epidemic)	0 (Irish epidemic)	1	2	3
Vector seasons	V -1	V 0	V +1	V +2	V +3
Sampling periods			S1	*Culicoides* S2	S3

Fig. 1 Sampling design. This SBV surveillance study was conducted in the three years following the 2012/2013 Irish Schmallenberg epidemic; Year +1, Year +2, Year +3 correspond to years one, two and three after the Irish epidemic, respectively. Surveillance years correspond with the beginning of the vector-season (V-1 to V + 3) and end with the drop in the peak of congenital malformations (end of spring calving period) associated with that particular vector-season. Blood samples were collected during three sampling periods (S1, S2, and S3); before (S1) and after (S2) the 2014 vector-season and after the 2015 vector-season. *Culicoides* spp. were collected on farms during the 2014 vector-season, (V +2)

extensively during the Irish Schmallenberg epidemic [7] were invited to participate in an epidemiological study on SBV surveillance. These herds were selected from a sampling frame of 111 farmers for a separate calf mortality study [21]. These herds were screened for spring-calving (January–May), more than 50 calvings/year, calf mortality rate, farmers with a history of good record keeping and farm located within a 1.30 h driving time radius of Moorepark. Twenty-six of the 36 dairy herds distributed at random in an SBV exposed region (Fig. 2) were successfully enrolled in the two year study which commenced in spring 2014.

A total of 7,081 animals (n = 9,454 blood samples) were evaluated for evidence of SBV infection during the study period (Table 1). Blood samples were collected during three sampling periods; S1 (spring 2014: 18th March – 5th April), S2 (winter 2014: 1st November–11th December) and S3 (winter 2015: 18th November–10th December). *Culicoides* were collected during the 2014 vector-active season (V +2).

During the first sampling period (S1) whole-herd SBV serology was conducted in order to determine animal-level and herd-level SBV seroprevalence. A total of 5,531 individual animal blood samples were collected from 4,070 cows (born in 2012 and earlier) and 1,461 replacement heifers (born in spring 2013) in 26 study herds (range 73–561 animals/herd) and evaluated for SBV-specific antibodies. This sample size was sufficient to estimate animal-level SBV true seroprevalence in this population of animals with 99 % confidence and 1 % precision using *a priori* herd prevalence estimate of 60 % in cattle herds in this region after the 2013 vector-season [7, 22] and ELISA test sensitivity and specificity of 97.6 and 100 %, respectively (ID Screen® internal validation report) [22, 23].

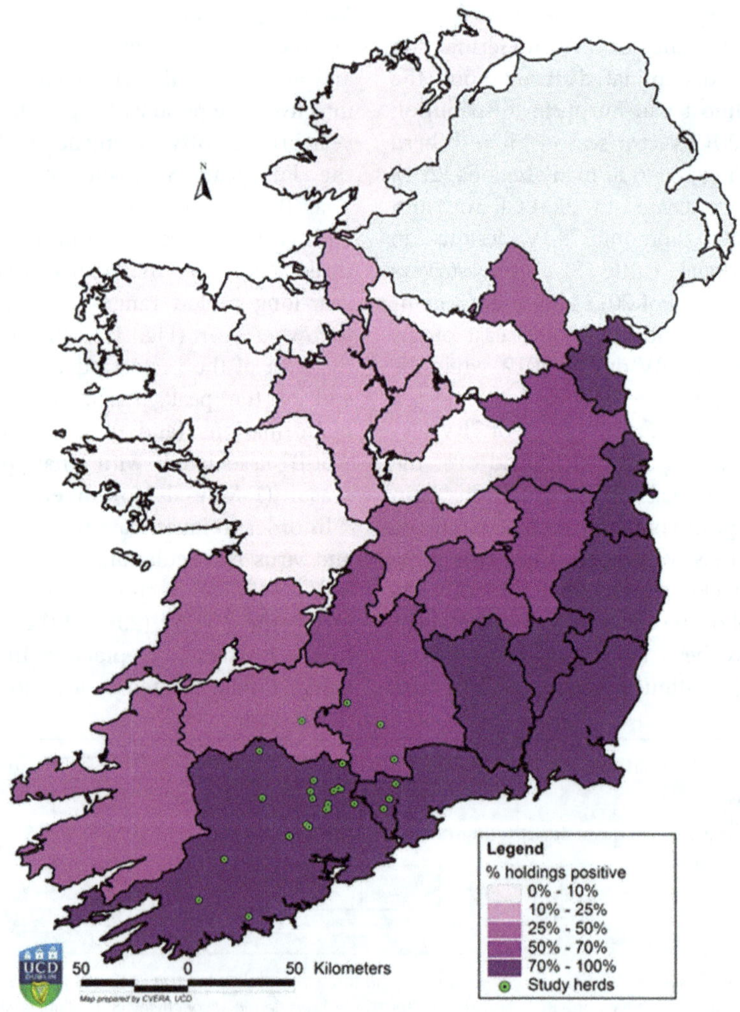

Fig. 2 Herd locations. Spatial distribution of study surveillance herds in a region exposed to SBV during the 2012/2013 Irish Schmallenberg epidemic, including county-level percentage of SBV antibody positive herds in Ireland in December 2013 [7]. The original published map has been modified to include the present study herd locations and county-level percentage of SBV antibody-positive herds only

Table 1 Number of animals blood sampled in each animal group

Animal type	Sampling period 1	Sampling period 2	Sampling period 3
	Spring 2014	Winter 2014	Winter 2015
Lactating cows	4070	288	n/s
Heifers	1461	645	n/s
Youngstock	n/s	1550	1440
Total	5531	2483	1440

(*n/s* not sampled)

During the second sampling period (S2), a subsample of the seronegative animals identified in spring 2014 (n = 933; range 6–87 animals/herd) were resampled in each herd after the 2014 vector-season (V +2) and evaluated for evidence of SBV infection during 2014. This sample size was sufficient to demonstrate freedom of SBV circulation in these animals in 2014 with 99 % confidence using the present study spring 2014 heifer estimated true prevalence results of 0.6 % (99 % CI: 0.2–1.4 %).

Blood samples were collected from 1,550 youngstock (range 25–118 animals/herd) from 25 of the present study herds (one herd opted out of the study) in winter 2014 (S2) and monitored prospectively for one year. Youngstock were resampled in winter 2015 (S3) and evaluated for SBV exposure during 2015. For this evaluation it was assumed that the duration of persistence of maternal antibodies was between 6–8 months [24]; hence, only animals between 8–10 months of age were included in the study. This sample size was sufficient to demonstrate freedom of SBV circulation in these herds in 2015 with 99 % confidence using our winter 2014 youngstock estimated true prevalence results of 0.5 % (99 % CI: 0–0.9 %).

Serum samples were analysed for SBV-specific antibodies using a competitive ELISA (ID Screen Schmallenberg virus Competition Multi-species, IDVet, Montpellier, France) in accordance with manufacturer's guidelines. The assay specificity and sensitivity were reported by the manufacturer at 100 % (95 % CI: 99.64–100 %) and 97.6 %, respectively (manufacturer internal validation report). Optical density (OD) values measured by the ELISA reader were transformed to sample-to-negative percentage ratios (S/N %) using the manufacturer's set of positive and negative controls using the formula: S/N% ratio = $(OD_{Sample} / OD_{Negative\ control}) \times 100$. Serum samples with an S/N% value less than or equal to 40 %, greater than 40 % and less than or equal to 50 %, and greater than 50 %, were considered as positive, inconclusive and negative, respectively.

Culicoides collection

Ultraviolet light trapping for *Culicoides* spp. was carried out on 10 of the study farms during the 2014 vector-active season (V2) as part of a separate entomological study investigating the species, abundance and ecological habitats of biting midges in Irish cattle herds, and their potential role as arbovirus vectors [25]. Each site was sampled fortnightly over a period of 16 weeks from 21st July to 5th November 2014; one Onderstepoort Veterinary Institute UV light trap (OVI trap) was run overnight in the vicinity of livestock. Catches were transferred immediately into 80 % ethanol. A total of 24,094 *Culicoides* were caught during the sampling period which included 6,621 pigmented (or so called *parous*; ovoposited and blood-fed at least once) *Culicoides* from six known SBV vector species *(C. obsoletus/scoticus, C. pulicaris, C. punctatus, C. dewulfi, C. chiopterus*). The midges were morphologically identified to species level and parity status using the keys of Campbell and Pelham-Clinton (1960) [26] and pooled accordingly.

Pools comprising approximately 23 pigmented midges from the six known SBV vector species were prepared for PCR analysis; each pool contained specimens from each catch collection for one specific site. Sample size calculation for the demonstration of freedom (detection of disease) in *Culicoides* using pooled testing was calculated using a design prevalence of 0.15 %; this figure was estimated from a review of published reports of SBV detection in field-caught *Culicoides* between 2011 and 2012 in Belgium, Denmark, Netherlands, Italy, Poland and France [4] and in field-caught *Culicoides* in Poland between 2013 and 2015 (Larska et al., unpublished observations) as the prevalence of SBV in Irish *Culicoides* spp. is unknown. Real time rt-PCR test sensitivity was assumed to be 100 % for the purpose of this sample size calculation as no data are available defining the rt-RT-PCR test sensitivity for the detection of SBV RNA in *Culicoides* insect specimens.

Hence, a sample size of 138 pools (n = 3,043 pigmented *Culicoides*) was used to detect SBV infection on these farms during the sampling period with 95 % confidence. The number of pools for each species tested was determined from the *Culicoides* spp. prevalence on these farms; the most abundant species identified were *C. obsoletus/scoticus* complex (37.6 %; n = 46 pools) and *C. dewulfi* (35.9 %; n = 46 pools), followed by *C. pulicaris* (9.0 %; n = 20 pools), *C. punctatus* (5.6 % n = 12 pools) and *C. chiopterus* (4.5 % n = 14 pools). The species *C. nubeculosis* were underrepresented, while the other 14 *Culicoides* spp. identified are not considered SBV vectors; these species were therefore omitted from the virological testing. *Culicoides* spp. pools were tested for SBV RNA using real-time RT-PCR, adapted from the method described previously [3]. Insects were homogenised in RLT buffer using Lysing Matrix D tubes containing ceramic beads in a ribolyzer (Thermo

Electron Corp., Milford, USA) for 90 s at 6.5 m/s speed. Total RNA was purified using RNeasy Mini Kit (Qiagen®) in the Qiacube automatic station (Qiagen®). Duplex real-time RT-PCR pairs of primers designed to detect SBV S segment and the 18S midge gene fragment in *C. obsoletus/scoticus* complex, *C. chiopterus, C. pulicaris, C. punctatus* as internal control were used. For the specific detection of *C. dewulfi* RNA, an additional set of primers flanking a fragment of mitochondrial cytochrome oxidase 1 gene was used [27]. Samples were analysed in the in-house optimised rt-RT-PCR using AgPath-ID OneStep RT-PCR Reagents kit (Ambion, Applied Biosystem) in a StepOne Real-Time PCR system (Life Technologies) as previously described [3]. A threshold cycle (C_t) value of ≤40 was considered the cut off value to detect SBV positive pools.

Statistical methods

Epidemiological analyses, including apparent prevalence (AP) and estimated true prevalence (TP) rates, and sample size calculations were completed using an online epidemiological calculator (EpiTools) [22].

Results

Spring 2014 (S1)

Seroprevalence results are shown in Table 2. In total, 3,375 animals tested positive for SBV-specific antibodies, which gave an animal-level AP of 61.0 % (CI 99 %: 59.3–62.6 %)

Table 2 Animal-level and within herd SBV seroprevalence in previously exposed Irish dairy herds in 2014 and 2015, with number of positives animals and respective TP (true prevalence) rates in each herd/animal group

	Sampling period 1					Sampling period 2						Sampling period 3	
	Spring 2014					Winter 2014						Winter 2015	
	Whole herd					Seronegative animals				Youngstock		Youngstock	
Herd ID	Herd size	No. of positives	Herd TP (%)	Cows TP (%)	Heifers TP (%)	Sample size	No. of positives	Cows positive	Heifers positive	Herd size	No. of positives	Sample size	No. of positives
1	148	101	69.9	99.5	2.3	Farmer opted out of study							
2	390	198	52	72.2	0	86	1	0	1	99	0	94	0
3	180	15	8.5	10.7	2.2	75	0	0	0	30	0	29	0
4	196	138	72.1	96.2	0	30	1	0	1	44	1	43	0
5	117	85	74.4	94.7	0	16	1	1	0	20	0	20	0
6	106	79	76.4	92	0	9	1	0	1	75	0	66	0
7	284	166	59.9	71.2	0	55	3	2	1	28	0	28	0
8	169	119	72.1	91.7	0	14	0	0	0	33	0	32	0
9	73	58	81.4	100	0	8	0	0	0	20	0	20	0
10	241	27	11.5	16.2	0	87	0	0	0	79	0	77	0
11	142	59	42.6	63	0	36	0	0	0	39	0	23	0
12	379	261	70.6	95.8	1	52	2	2	0	106	0	105	0
13	338	232	70.3	99.9	1	53	1	0	1	106	1	106	0
14	123	88	73.3	100	0	18	1	1	0	36	0	35	0
15	283	180	77.5	99.2	0	43	0	0	0	84	1	81	0
16	561	435	79.4	100	0	55	2	2	0	118	1	115	0
17	338	209	63.4	96.5	0	50	1	1	0	77	1	76	0
18	217	143	67.5	90.4	0	34	0	0	0	81	1	62	0
19	206	169	84.1	98.9	0	17	0	0	0	50	0	49	0
20	163	94	59.1	89.1	1.8	32	0	0	0	81	0	76	0
21	89	65	74.8	95	5.1	6	0	0	0	34	0	9	0
22	212	117	56.5	77.5	3.4	50	1	1	0	66	1	65	0
23	106	66	63.8	96.6	0	19	0	0	0	44	0	41	0
24	218	154	72.4	99.9	0	27	0	0	0	115	0	114	0
25	113	26	23.6	30.6	0	37	0	0	0	35	0	30	0
26	139	91	67.1	100	2.1	24	0	0	0	50	0	44	0
Total	5531	3375	62.5	84.7	0.6	933	15	10	5	1550	7	1440	0

and TP of 62.5 % (99 % CI: 60.8–64.2 %) when correcting for imperfect test characteristics. Seropositive animals were present in all 26 herds. Within-herd TP ranged widely from 8.5 to 84.1 % (median 70.1 %) across the 26 herds. In cows, animal-level AP was 82.7 % (99 % CI: 81.1–84.2 %), TP was 84.7 % (99 % CI: 83.1–86.3 %) and ranged between 10.7 % and 100 % across the 26 herds. In heifers, animal-level AP was 0.6 % (99 % CI: 0.3–1.4 %) and TP was 0.6 % (99 % CI: 0.2–1.4 %). Seropositive heifers (n = 9) originated in 8 herds and ranged from 1–2 animals per herd (Table 3). Of all the seronegative animals identified in spring 2014, 68.5 % were spring 2013-born heifers; of which 98.8 % were seronegative. Inconclusive blood results were re-tested and confirmed using the same ELISA testing kit.

Winter 2014 (S2)

Of the 933 seronegative animals re-sampled in winter 2014, 891 [95.5 %] animals (268 [28.7 %] cows and 623

Table 3 SBV ELISA-positive animals detected in surveillance Year +1, Year +2 and Year +3 in cows (C), heifers (H), youngstock (Y) in each herd, with the number of positive animals detected per herd in each surveillance year, blood sampling dates, ELISA S/N% results, Positive (P), Negative (N), S/N% value from the ELISA threshold cut-off and date of birth and age (months) of animals at first blood sampling

Surveillance year	Herd ID	Animal type	Number of positives	Blood sample 1						Blood sample 2			
				Date	ELISA S/N %	Result	S/N% from cut off	Date of birth	Age (months)	Date	ELISA S/N %	Result	S/N % from cut off
Year +1 (2013)[a]	1	H	1	29-Mar-14	6.9	P	33.1	15-Mar-13	31.2	–	–	–	–
	3	H	1	28-Mar-14	4.9	P	35.1	13-Mar-13	31.3	–	–	–	–
	12	H	1	21-Mar-14	25.0	P	15.0	07-Mar-13	31.2	–	–	–	–
	13	H	1	21-Mar-14	32.8	P	7.2	14-Feb-13	33.1	–	–	–	–
	20	H	1	14-Mar-14	37.6	P	2.4	15-Feb-13	32.4	–	–	–	–
	21	H	1	28-Mar-14	33.1	P	6.9	16-Mar-13	31.0	–	–	–	–
	22	H	2	22-Mar-14	31.4	P	8.6	26-Mar-13	29.7	–	–	–	–
	22	H	2	22-Mar-14	7.6	P	32.4	26-Mar-13	29.7	–	–	–	–
	26	H	1	26-Mar-14	6.6	P	33.4	18-Feb-13	33.2	–	–	–	–
Year +2 (2014)	4	C	2	19-Mar-14	57.8	N	7.8	–	–	25-Nov-14	37.3	P	2.7
	7	C	3	21-Mar-14	64.1	N	14.1	–	–	28-Nov-14	33.9	P	6.1
	7	C	3	24-Mar-14	76.9	N	26.9	–	–	17-Nov-14	11.5	P	28.5
	12	C	2	19-Mar-14	50.7	N	0.7	–	–	27-Nov-14	23.2	P	16.8
	12	C	2	18-Mar-14	55.0	N	5.0	–	–	27-Nov-14	9.5	P	30.5
	14	C	1	21-Mar-14	50.7	N	0.7	–	–	01-Dec-14	30.4	P	9.6
	16	C	2	28-Mar-14	68.9	N	18.9	–	–	14-Nov-14	19.6	P	20.4
	16	C	2	27-Mar-14	51.0	N	1.0	–	–	20-Nov-14	30.5	P	9.5
	17	C	1	21-Mar-14	54.2	N	4.2	–	–	28-Nov-14	34.0	P	6.0
	22	C	1	18-Mar-14	77.4	N	27.4	–	–	27-Nov-14	7.2	P	32.8
	2	H	1	27-Mar-14	69.2	N	19.2	–	–	20-Nov-14	13.3	P	26.7
	4	H	1	27-Mar-14	81.1	N	31.1	–	–	20-Nov-14	23.1	P	16.9
	6	H	1	21-Mar-14	71.6	N	21.6	–	–	28-Nov-14	39.5	P	0.5
	7	H	3	14-Mar-14	72.4	N	22.4	–	–	24-Nov-14	34.6	P	5.4
	13	H	1	19-Mar-14	78.1	N	28.1	–	–	27-Nov-14	15.0	P	25.0
Year +3 (2015)	4	Y	1	24-Nov-14	38.8	P	1.2	19-Jan-14	10.17	17-Nov-15	74.4	N	24.4
	13	Y	1	28-Nov-14	34.0	P	6.0	17- Feb-14	9.37	02-Dec-15	86.0	N	36.0
	15	Y	1	19-Nov-14	34.7	P	5.3	14-Mar-14	8.17	08-Dec-15	105.4	N	55.4
	16	Y	2	27-Nov-14	32.5	P	7.5	13-Feb-14	9.47	25-Nov-15	71.7	N	21.7
	16	Y	1	27-Nov-14	37.6	P	2.4	19-Feb-14	9.27	25-Nov-15	79.7	N	29.7
	18	Y	1	12-Dec-14	36.0	P	4.0	30-Mar-14	8.40	20-Nov-15	85.7	N	35.7
	22	Y	1	01-Dec-14	34.2	P	5.8	05-Mar-14	8.87	09-Dec-15	95.8	N	45.8

[a]Surveillance year +1 = positive heifers only; positive cows are excluded as they are likely to have been exposed to SBV during the 2012 Irish SBV epidemic

[66.8 %] heifers) remained seronegative after the 2014 vector-season. Fifteen animals (10 cows and 5 heifers) originating in 11 herds (1–3 animals per herd) tested positive for SBV-specific antibodies resulting in animal-level AP of 1.6 % (99 % CI: 0.8–3.1 %) and TP of 1.6 % (99 % CI: 0.08–3.0 %) in this group of animals. Six out of these 15 seropositive animals had an S/N% result near the ELISA S/N% cut-off threshold (Table 3). Of the 1,550 youngstock blood sampled, a total of seven animals originating in seven herds tested positive for SBV-specific antibodies (Table 3) resulting in an animal-level AP of 0.5 % (99 % CI: 0.2–1.1 %) and TP of 0.05 % (99 % CI: 0.01–1.1 %) in youngstock. Nineteen (1.23 %) animals had inconclusive results. Positive and inconclusive blood results were re-tested and confirmed using the same ELISA testing kit.

Winter 2015 (S3)

In winter 2015, 1,440 youngstock were resampled; 110 animals originating in 25 herds (range 1–25 animals per herd) had been culled/sold prior to the sampling date. All youngstock blood sampled, including the 7 animals with a positive ELISA test result in winter 2014, had a negative ELISA result when retested in winter 2015 (Table 3).

SBV analysis of Culicoides spp

A total of 3,043 pigmented *Culicoides* (138 pools) were analysed for the presence of SBV RNA. Seven pools (two *C. obsoletus/scoticus*, three *C. chiopterus*, two *C. punctatus*) containing a total of 84 specimens (range 3–24 specimens per pool) had a negative internal control (IC) reading and were excluded from the analysis. Of the 131 pools successfully analysed all tested negative for SBV RNA; one *C. dewulfi* pool was weakly positive on initial first test (SBV $C_t = 38.11$, IC $C_t = 19.15$) but was negative when retested using rt-RT-PCR and was negative on gel electrophoresis. Internal control C_t values for the 131 pools evaluated ranged from 19.4 to 29.28.

Discussion

The first incursion of SBV into Ireland occurred in August 2012 [28] which resulted in an epidemic of SBV-associated congenital malformations and abortions in cattle and sheep in autumn 2012 and spring 2013. In spring 2014, one year after the Schmallenberg epidemic in Ireland, animal-level seroprevalence in the present study herds was high [62.5 %; 99 % CI: 60.8–64.2 %]. Interestingly, almost all (99.7 %) of the seropositive animals detected in these herds in spring 2014 were cows; animal-level seroprevalence was significantly higher in cows [84.7 % (CI: 99 %: 83.1–86.3 %)] when compared to heifers [0.6 % (99 % CI: 0.2–1.4 %)] suggesting that cows were most likely exposed to SBV during the 2012 vector-season. Seropositive heifers identified in spring 2014 were most likely exposed to SBV during the 2013 vector-season. However, the possibility of in-utero infection of these heifers during the 2012 vector-season should also be considered; one study in Germany found that high SBV-specific antibody titres can be found in clinically healthy calves before colostrum intake [29]. The large population of seronegative heifers (born in spring 2013) identified in these herds in spring 2014 also demonstrates that there was a substantial decrease in SBV circulation in these herds during 2013 when compared to the year of the epidemic. These findings are consistent with similar surveillance studies in continental Europe in the first year following the epidemic; where seroprevalence remained high in adult cattle [2, 4] while a lower level of virus circulation was evident in youngstock in a number of regions [10, 13, 15].

Both between-herd (BH) and within-herd (WH) seroprevalence in the 26 herds ranged widely in spring 2014; BH range 8.5 to 84.1 %, and WH range 10.7 to 100 % in cows and 0 and 5.1 % in heifers. This highlights that despite high levels of virus circulation during the Schmallenberg epidemic in this region, individual herds and within-herd animal groupings in these herds, displayed widely different levels of immunity, and as a consequence, susceptibility to new infection during the 2014 vector season. The herds in the present study are all spring-calving, pasture-managed dairy herds; the habitats where cows grazed and where *Culicoides* spp. were collected in 2014 were predominantly improved grassland, which included a mix of semi-natural woodland and hedges [25]. Hence, the variation observed in BH and WH seroprevalence in these herds is unlikely to be due to differences in herd management practices (housing conditions, pasture management etc.). Rather it is likely a consequence of the distribution and extent of spread of SBV during the 2012/2013 Irish epidemic where there was a lower percentage of positive herds in the north and west of Ireland when compared to the south and the east [7]. In the present study, the herds with low WH seroprevalence were located further west in the country when compared to herds with high WH seroprevalence, which were located in the east.

In winter 2014, only 15 animals (10 cows and 5 heifers; originating in 11 herds) which were identified as seronegative in spring 2014, showed evidence of seroconversion during the 2014 vector-season. This low prevalence of SBV infection [AP = 1.6 % (99 % CI: 0.8–3.1 %) and TP = 1.6 % (99 % CI: 0.8–3.0 %)] in naïve animals in these herds after the 2014 vector-season suggests that SBV continued to circulate in these herds during 2014, albeit at a very low level. A similar pattern of continued virus circulation has been observed in several European countries in the years following the European

Schmallenberg Epidemic [10–15]. It is important to note however, that these 15 seropositive animals were distributed at random across 11 herds and that the individual animal ELISA S/N% results varied widely between 0.5 and 32.8 % from the cut-off; some animals (n = 6) were near the cut-off a suggesting a 'weak' positive result, while the remaining animals had 'highly' positive serology results. The positive and inconclusive blood results in these animals were repeated and confirmed using the same ELISA test. Given the high specificity of the ELISA test used, the probability of a repeated false-positive result is close to zero, while the high sensitivity of this test demonstrates improved sensitivity for sera with low antibody titres (IDVet internal validation report).

Interestingly, when 46.0 % of the six known SBV *Culicoides* vector spp. specimens trapped in these herds during the 2014 vector-active season (which was sufficient to detect an individual SBV positive pool with 95 % confidence using an estimated prevalence of 0.15 %) were analysed for evidence of SBV infection, one *C. dewulfi* pool was weakly positive (SBV $C_t = 38.11$, IC = C_t 19.15) indicating that SBV may have also been present and circulating in *Culicoides* in these herds during 2014. However, this pool was negative when retested using rt-RT-PCR and was also negative on gel electrophoresis. These findings are consistent with the bovine serosurveillance work conducted on the same farms in the same year, supporting the lack of evidence of notable SBV circulation in these herds in 2014.

When all youngstock (born in spring 2014) in these herds were blood sampled in winter 2014 only 7 animals [AP of 0.5 % (99 % CI: 0.02–1.2 %) and TP of 0.5 % (99 % CI: 0.1–1.1 %)] originating in 6 herds had a seropositive result. The ELISA results in these 7 youngstock were all weakly positive; their S/N% results ranged between 1.2 and 7.5 % from the ELISA cut-off threshold suggesting that youngstock in these herds were exposed to SBV in 2014 at a low level. When the serology results collected from heifers and youngstock during the three study sampling periods were evaluated simultaneously, it revealed that in animals (n = 3011) born after the Irish Schmallenberg epidemic (born in spring 2013 or spring 2014), only 21 animals (14 heifers and 7 youngstock) originating in 17 herds (1–4 animals per herd) tested positive for SBV antibodies. This equates to an animal-level AP of 0.7 % (CI 99 %: 0.4–1.2 %) and TP of 0.7 % (CI 99 %: 0.4–1.2 %) in animals born after the Schmallenberg epidemic suggesting that SBV continued to circulate at low levels in these herds in 2013 and 2014.

When youngstock were retested in winter 2015, all animals, including the 7 seropositive animals identified in winter 2014, tested negative for SBV-specific antibodies demonstrating that SBV did not circulate in these herds in 2015. These 7 youngstock were aged between 8–10 months at first sampling; when they were retested 12 months later all 7 animals had a negative result suggesting that the initial 'weak' positive ELISA result was due to persistent maternally-derived SBV antibodies. Similar results were found in an SBV sero-survey of youngstock in the Netherlands where animals between the ages of 9–15 months tested positive at first sampling but subsequently had a negative result when retested a few months later [15]. There are limited data on the duration of SBV maternally-derived antibodies in calves and the half-life of SBV maternally-derived antibodies is unknown. However, a study in the Netherlands reported an average duration of 180 days (range 120–140) in 13 calves in one herd [24]. Furthermore, there are scant reports describing the course of decay of maternally-derived antibodies against other Orthobunyaviruses in ruminants [30]. These findings highlight the need for further research in this area; this information would be particularly useful when designing SBV vaccination protocols and for identifying the most appropriate age to vaccinate animals. Moreover, these results highlight that a large population of naïve animals may be at risk of infection should SBV re-circulate in Ireland in the future at it appears to have done in continental Europe [10–15]. This population of susceptible animals is likely to increase each year SBV does not circulate as older animals are replaced by naïve younger animals. A similar naïve population of animals is also likely to be increasing in the UK and in continental Europe [10, 15].

It is surprising that so few animals showed evidence of SBV infection in these herds during the study period despite the presence of a large population of susceptible animals in each herd during this time. It is possible that the high rate of herd-immunity at the beginning of the study (animal-level seroprevalence was 62.5 % in spring 2014) may have reduced the virus's ability to circulate in this population of animals in the subsequent vector-seasons. The lack of clustering of seroconverted naïve animals within a herd is somewhat inconsistent with the transmission characteristics of SBV; SBV is typically highly efficient in spreading in herds in the presence of transmitting vector species [31]. This is due to the rapid rate of virus replication and the high probability of transmission from host to vector [32]. This is supported by high within-herd seroprevalence rates in cattle and sheep after the 2011/2012 epidemic [4]. These epidemiological characteristics of SBV result in a high basic reproductive number (R_0), estimated to be as high as 6.2 in cattle herds [32], which reduces the probability of finding low numbers of seropositive animals once the virus has circulated in a naïve ruminant population [15]. Using this R_0 value, it is interesting to note that the effective reproductive number ($R_e = R_0 \times$ fraction of the population of susceptible animals) in animals in these herds in spring 2014 (one year after the Irish Schmallenberg epidemic) would have been greater than one (R_e = 2.33; $R_e = 6.2 \times 0.375$) highlighting the potential for SBV to re-circulate in these herds during 2014, despite a high rate of herd immunity. In addition, variations in the genome of SBV have occurred in the time since the virus first emerged in 2011 [11, 33, 34]. It remains to be determined if these genetic variations have caused important enough mutations in the SBV genome to alter the immunogenicity or the transmissibility of the virus.

The mechanism by which SBV infection persists from season to season (overwinter) remains unclear [4]. Limited data suggest SBV may overwinter in vectors, possibly via vertical/trans-ovarial transmission [3]. This is supported by reports of SBV infections during the winter months despite very low vector activity [35]. Furthermore, it has been suggested in Germany, that atypical warm weather conditions during winter months may have facilitated low levels of vector activity and in turn enabled SBV transmission during the winter months [35]. SBV did not appear to circulate at the borders of the area affected in Ireland in 2012/2013 [7]. It has been suggested that the adverse weather conditions experienced in spring and early summer of 2013 [7, 36] were likely to have delayed resumption of midge activity at the start of the 2013 vector-season; this may have impeded SBV overwintering and continued circulation of the virus subsequently. A model which estimated the spread of SBV in Europe in 2011 demonstrated that the majority of SBV infections in the UK occurred as a result of infected midges being transported through downwind movement facilitated by prevailing winds from Europe [37]. The emergence of SBV in Ireland is likely to have occurred in a similar way. Moreover, during the present study, SBV was circulating at considerably lower levels in neighbouring European countries; in France in 2013/2014 and in the UK SBV circulated at a low intensity [12, 38]. This low level of virus circulation in neighbouring European countries coupled with unfavourable weather conditions in Ireland early in the 2013 vector-season [36] are likely to have reduced the risk of further incursions of SBV infected midges into Ireland during this time.

Arbovirus surveillance programs which solely monitor vectors (*Culicoides* spp. and/or mosquitos) for evidence of infection are not considered the most effective programs to detect virus circulation or emergence. This may be due to lower virus detection rates (sensitivity) in insect specimens comparing to mammalian samples. The detection of SBV in midges can be ambiguous as it does not always mean the virus is present at transmissible levels; bimodal distributions of C_t values for SBV in *Culicoides* spp. are reported suggesting that the virus can be present in the vector at transmissible and subtransmissible levels [3, 39]. Hence, arbovirus surveillance programs which combine serological, virological and entomological studies, such as the National Arbovirus Monitoring Program (NAMP) in Australia [18] are considered the most effective for arbovirus surveillance work.

Akabane virus (AKAV) is a Simbu serogroup Orthobunyavirus present in Africa, Asia, Oceania and the Middle East which is similar to SBV; AKAV is also transmitted by *Culicoides* spp. and can cause similar fatal congenital defects as SBV in infected foetuses (arthrogryposis-hydrancephaly syndrome) [40]. In Australia, *Culicoides* are distributed in well-defined geographical regions [41]. In these areas AKAV is endemic and virus transmission occurs frequently and usually each year resulting in most animals developing long-lasting protective antibodies prior to breeding age [40]. As a result, outbreaks of Akabane disease are rare and typically only occur when there is a disruption or alternation to the endemic cycle [40]. Changes in climatic conditions, expansion of the distribution of virus vectors [42] or the introduction of susceptible animals into an endemic region can influence disease outbreaks [43]. SBV appears to have followed a similar cyclical pattern of virus recirculation and re-emergence as AKAV, in Europe.

The present study suggests that SBV circulated at very low levels in previously exposed Irish cattle herds in 2013 and 2014. There was no evidence of virus circulation in youngstock in the same herds in 2015 and it is unlikely that SBV is circulating currently (2016). However, if SBV becomes endemic in continental Europe, which is possible considering the continued low levels of virus circulation in many European countries [8–15], SBV could re-emerge in Ireland in a similar fashion to AKAV re-emergence at the border zones of AKAV endemic regions. Periods of favourable weather conditions which could facilitate the mechanical transport of SBV-infected vectors, or the export of SBV-infected animals from endemic regions to susceptible regions, could result in SBV re-circulation and re-emergence in susceptible populations in the future. Furthermore, other arbovirus diseases, notably bluetongue virus which re-emerged in France in 2015 [44] and was recently identified as a potential risk to the UK in 2016 [45], could also emerge in Ireland in a similar way. This is likely to be driven and made possible by climate change [46].

Implications

The results of the present study demonstrate that it would be prudent to continue monitoring immunologically naïve animals in previously exposed and unexposed regions for evidence of SBV infection. Furthermore, animal surveillance work for arboviruses such as SBV and bluetongue virus should be complemented with

Culicoides spp. entomological surveillance work. In Australia, NAMP has proven effective in monitoring arboviruses such as Akabane, bluetongue and bovine ephemeral fever viruses [18]. This program monitors sentinel farms throughout the country (endemic areas, border regions and disease/vector free areas) on a permanent basis using serology, virus isolation and vector surveillance (*Culicoides*/mosquitos). Future arbovirus surveillance work in Ireland could be based on such a program.

Conclusions

This SBV surveillance study indicated that SBV circulated at a very low level in previously exposed cattle herds in Ireland in 2013 and 2014. However there was no evidence of SBV circulation in youngstock in these herds in 2015. Moreover, a large population of seronegative animals was identified in these herds which may be at risk of SBV infection should SBV re-emerge or recirculate in the future.

Abbreviations

AKAV: Akabane virus; Ap/Tp: Apparent/True prevalence; CI: Confidence interval; Ct: Cycle threshold; ELISA: Enzyme-Linked Immunosorbent Assay; IC: Internal control; OD: Optical density; OVI: Onderstepoort Veterinary Institute; RNA: Ribonucleic acid; RT-PCR: Real-time polymerase chain reaction; S/N: Sample-to-negative ratio; S1/S2/S3: Sampling period 1/ Sampling period 2/ Sampling period 3; SBV: Schmallenberg virus; Spp: Species; UV: Ultraviolet; V −1 V 0, V + 1, V + 2, V +3: 2011, 2012, 2013, 2014, 2015 vector-season

Acknowledgements

We acknowledge the significant contribution of Dr. Marion England (The Pirbright Institute, UK) in assisting with *Culicoides* identification and Julia Kęsik (National Veterinary Research Institute Poland) for assisting with *Culicoides* PCR analysis. We are grateful for the contributions of Jonathon Kenneally and John Heffernan (Teagasc), Isabella Prunner (University of Veterinary Medicine, Vienna) and numerous veterinary students (University College Dublin) in assisting with sample collection. We thank the farmers for access to their herds and their data.

Funding

This research was funded in the Teagasc project MKAB-6520 and the Teagasc Walsh Fellowship Scheme. The rt-RT-PCR testing of *Culicoides* was financed from the National Centre for Research and Development (NCBiR) in Poland project No PBS2/A8/24/2013.

Authors' contributions

All authors participated in the design of the study. ÁC and JFM were involved in sample collection and analysis. ML oversaw the *Culicoides* rt-RT-PCR. AC and JFM wrote the first draft of the manuscript, with all authors involved in reviewing. All authors read and approved the final manuscript.

Competing interests

The authors declare that they have no competing interests.

Consent for publication

Not applicable.

Ethics approval and consent to participate

This study was ethically approved locally by the Teagasc Animal Ethics Committee (TAEC) and nationally by the Health Products Regulatory Authority (HPRA). All institutional and national guidelines for the care and use of animals were followed. This study complies with all relevant permissions and licensing outlined by the aforementioned regulatory bodies. Informed consent was obtained from all animal owners for the use of animals enrolled in the study and all animals received best practice of veterinary care.

Author details

[1]Animal and Bioscience Research Department, AGRIC, Teagasc, Moorepark, Fermoy, Co. Cork, Ireland. [2]School of Veterinary Medicine, University College Dublin, Dublin 4, Ireland. [3]Sligo RVL, Department of Agriculture, Food and the Marine, Doonally, Co. Sligo, Ireland. [4]Department of Virology, National Veterinary Research Institute, Puławy, Poland.

References

1. Hoffmann B, Scheuch M, Höper D, Jungblut R, Holsteg M, Schirrmeier H, et al. Novel orthobunyavirus in cattle, Europe, 2011. Emerg Infect Dis. 2012;18(3):469–72.
2. European Food Safety Authority (EFSA). "Schmallenberg" virus: analysis of the epidemiological data (May 2013), Supporting Publications 2013; EN-429 [22pp.] http://www.efsa.europe.eu/publications. Accessed 1 Mar 2016.
3. Larska M, Lechowski L, Grochowska M, Żmudziński J. Detection of the Schmallenberg virus in nulliparous *Culicoides* obsoletus/scoticus complex and *C.* punctatus- the possibility of transovarial virus transmission in the midge population and of a new vector. Vet Micro. 2013;166(3–4):467.
4. European Food Safety Authority (EFSA). Schmallenberg virus: state of art. EFSA Journal. 2014;12(5):3681. doi:10.2903/j.efsa.2014.3681. 54 pp.
5. Afonso A, Abrahantes JC, Conraths F, Veldhuis A, Elbers A, Roberts H, et al. The Schmallenberg virus epidemic in Europe 2011–2013. Prev Vet Med. 2014;116(4):391–403.
6. Bradshaw B, Mooney J, Ross P, Murphy C, O'Donovan J, Sanchez C, Gomez-Parada M, Toolan D. Schmallenberg virus cases identified in Ireland. Vet Rec. 2012;171:540–1.
7. Barrett D, More S, O'Neill R, Bradshaw B, Casey M, Keane M, McGrath G, Sammin D. Prevalence and distribution of exposure to Schmallenberg virus in Irish cattle during October 2012 to November 2013. BMC Vet Res. 2015;11(1):1.
8. Conraths FJ, Kamer D, Teske K, Hoffmann B, Mettenleiter TC, Beer M. Reemerging Schmallenberg virus infections, Germany. Emerg Infect Dis 2013. 2012;19(3):513–5.
9. Claine F, Coupeau D, Wiggers L, Muylkens B, Kirschvink N. Schmallenberg virus among female lambs, Belgium, 2012. Emerg Infect Dis. 2013;19(7):1115–7.
10. Méroc E, Poskin A, Van Loo H, Van Driessche E, Czaplicki G, Quinet C, et al. Follow-up of the Schmallenberg Virus Seroprevalence in Belgian cattle. Transbound Emerg Dis. 2015;62(5):e80–4.
11. Wernike K, Hoffmann B, Conraths FJ, Beer M. Schmallenberg virus recurrence, Germany, 2014. Emerg Infect Dis. 2015;21(7):1202.
12. Gache K, Hosteing S, Perrin J-B, Zientara S, Bournez L, Touratier A. Surveillance du virus Schmallenberg en France: une circulation peu intense en. 2014. http://bulletinepidemiologique.mag.anses.fr/sites/default/files/BEP-mg-BE72-art6.pdf. Accessed 20 March 2016.
13. Balmer S, Gobet H, Nenniger C, Hadorn D, Schwermer H, Vögtlin A. Schmallenberg virus activity in cattle in Switzerland in 2013. Vet Rec. 2015;177(11):289.
14. Elbers ARW, Meiswinkel R, van Weezep E, Kooi EA, van der Poel WHM. Schmallenberg virus in *Culicoides* biting midges in the Netherlands in 2012. Transbound Emerg Dis. 2015;62(3):339–42.
15. Veldhuis AMB, Mars MH, Roos CAJ, van Wuyckhuise L, van Schaik G. Two years after the Schmallenberg virus epidemic in the Netherlands: does the virus still circulate? Transbound Emerg Dis. 2015. doi:10.1111/tbed.12349.
16. Ayllon T, Nijhof A, Weiher W, Bauer B, Allene X, Clausen P-H. Feeding behaviour of *Culicoides* spp. (Diptera: Ceratopogonidae) on cattle and sheep in northeast Germany. Parasites & Vectors. 2014;7(1):34. doi:10.1186/1756-3305-7-34.

17. Bartsch S, Bauer B, Wiemann A, Clausen P-H, Steuber S. Feeding patterns of biting midges of the *Culicoides* obsoletus and *Culicoides* pulicaris groups on selected farms in Brandenburg. Germany Parasitol Res. 2009;105(2):373–80.
18. Kirkland P, Ellis T, Melville L, Johnson S. Australian national arbovirus monitoring program-a model for studying bluetongue epidemiology in China, Proceedings of the Australian Centre for International Agricultural Research (ACIAR). 1996. p. 95–9.
19. Racloz V, Griot C, Stärk KDC. Sentinel surveillance systems with special focus on vector-borne diseases. Anim Health Res Rev. 2006;7(1–2):71–9.
20. McCarthy TK, Bateman A, Nowak D, Lawless A. National BTV Vector Surveillance Programme 2007–2009. https://www.agriculture.gov.ie/media/migration/animalhealthwelfare/diseasecontrols/bluetonguedisease/2008%20vector%20monitoring%20report%20final.pdf. Accessed 15Apr 2016.
21. Mee JF, Grant J, Sánchez-Miguel C, Doherty M. Pre-calving and calving management practices in dairy herds with a history of high and low bovine perinatal mortality. Animals. 2013;3(3):866–81.
22. Sergeant ESG. Epitools epidemiological calculators. Aus Vet Animal Health Services and Australian Biosecurity Cooperative Research Centre for Emerging Infectious Disease. 2016. http://epitools.ausvet.com.au. Accessed 10 March 2016.
23. Humphry RW, Cameron A, Gunn GJ. A practical approach to calculate sample size for herd prevalence surveys. Prev Vet Med. 2004;65(3–4):173–88.
24. Elbers A, Stockhofe-Zurwieden N, van der Poel W. Schmallenberg virus antibody persistence in adult cattle after natural infection and decay of maternal antibodies in calves. BMC Vet Res. 2014;10(1):103.
25. Collins ÁB, Mee JF, Barrett D, Doherty M, England ME. Species composition, abundance and new geographical species identification of *Culicoides* biting midges on dairy farms, Proceedings of the 29th World Buiatrics Congress. 2016. p. 358.
26. Campbell JA, Pelham-Clinton EC. Taxonomic review of the British species of Culicoides Latreille (Diptera, Ceratopogonidae). Proceedings of the Royal Entomological Society of London (B). 1960;67:181–302.
27. Wenk CE, Kaufmann C, Schaffner F, Mathis A. Molecular characterization of Swiss Ceratopogonidae (Diptera) and evaluation of real-time PCR assays for the identification of *Culicoides* biting midges. Vet Parasitology. 2012;184(2–4):258–66.
28. O'Neill R, Boland C, Ross P. Retrospective profiling of the 2012 Schmallenberg virus incursion into Ireland, Proceedings of the BSAS and AVTRW annual conference. 2014. p. 28–30.
29. Wernike K, Holsteg M, Schirrmeier H, Hoffmann B, Beer M. Natural infection of pregnant cows with Schmallenberg virus–a follow-up study. PloS ONE. 2014;9(5):e98223.
30. Tsutsui T, Yamamoto T, Hayama Y, Akiba Y, Nishiguchi A, Kobayashi S, Yamakawa M. Duration of maternally derived antibodies against Akabane virus in calves: survival analysis. J Vet Med Sci. 2009;71(7):913–9.
31. Wernike K, Silaghi C, Nieder M, Pfeffer M, Beer M. Dynamics of Schmallenberg virus infection within a cattle herd in Germany, 2011. Epidemiol Infect. 2014;142(07):1501–4.
32. Gubbins S, Turner J, Baylis M, van der Stede Y, van Schaik G, Abrahantes JC, Wilson AJ. Inferences about the transmission of Schmallenberg virus within and between farms. Prev Vet Med. 2014;116(4):380–90.
33. Rosseel T, Scheuch M, Höper D, De Regge N, Caij AB, Vandenbussche F, Van Borm S. DNase SISPA-next generation sequencing confirms Schmallenberg virus in Belgian field samples and identifies genetic variation in Europe. PLoS One. 2012;7(7):e41967.
34. Fischer M, Hoffmann B, Goller KV, Hoeper D, Wernike K, Beer M. A mutation 'hot spot'in the Schmallenberg virus M segment. J Gen Virol. 2013;94(6):1161–7.
35. Wernike K, Kohn M, Conraths FJ, Werner D, Kameke D, Hechinger S, Kampen H, Beer M. Transmission of Schmallenberg virus during winter, Germany. Emerg Infect Dis. 2013;19(10):1701.
36. Anon. Met Eireann, summary weather reports. 2014. http://www.met.ie/climate/monthly-weather-reports.asp Accessed 12 Mar 2016.
37. Sedda L, Rogers DJ. The influence of the wind in the Schmallenberg virus outbreak in Europe. Sci Rep. 2013;3:3361.
38. King B, O'Shea Brown T, Tarlinton R, Daly JM. Seroprevalence of Schmallenberg virus in the United Kingdom and the Republic of Ireland: 2011–2013. Vet Micro. 2015;180(1):36–40.
39. De Regge N, Madder M, Deblauwe I, Losson B, Fassotte C, Demeulemeester J, Smeets F, Tomme M, Cay AB. Schmallenberg virus circulation in *Culicoides* in Belgium in 2012: field validation of a real time RT-PCR approach to assess virus replication and dissemination in midges. PLoS One. 2014;9(1):e87005.
40. Kirkland PD. Akabane and bovine ephemeral fever virus infections. Veterinary Clinics of North America: Food Ani Pract. 2002;18(3):501–14.
41. Cybinski DH, St George TD, Paull NI. Antibodies to Akabane virus in Australia. Aust Vet J. 1978;54(1):1–3.
42. Shepherd NC, Gee CD, Jessep T, Timmins G, Carroll SN, Bonner RB. Congenital bovine epizootic arthrogyyposis and hydranencephaly. Aust Vet J. 1978;54(4):171–7.
43. Jagoe S, Kirland PD, Harper PA. An outbreak of Akabane virus—induced abnormalities in calves after agistment in an endemic region. Aust Vet J. 1993;70(2):56–8.
44. Sailleau C, Bréard E, Viarouge C, Vitour D, Romey A, Garnier A, Fablet A, Lowenski S, et al. Re-Emergence of Bluetongue Virus Serotype 8 in France, 2015. Transbound Emerg Dis. 2015. doi:10.1111/tbed. 12453.
45. Anon. Department for Environment, Food and Rural Affairs (DEFRA), 2016 Qualitative risk assessment for entry into the UK by bluetongue virus (BTV-8) in 2016 www.gov.uk/government/publications. Accessed 12 Mar 2016.
46. Purse BV, Mellor PS, Rogers DJ, Samuel AR, Mertens PPC, Baylis M. Climate change and the recent emergence of bluetongue in Europe. Nat Rev Micro. 2005;3(2):171–81.

IRES-mediated translation of foot-and-mouth disease virus (FMDV) in cultured cells derived from FMDV-susceptible and -insusceptible animals

Takehiro Kanda[1], Makoto Ozawa[1,2] and Kyoko Tsukiyama-Kohara[1,2*]

Abstract

Background: Foot-and-mouth disease virus (FMDV) possess a positive sense, single stranded RNA genome. Internal ribosomal entry site (IRES) element exists within its 5′ untranslated region (5′UTR) of the viral RNA. Translation of the viral RNA is initiated by internal entry of the 40S ribosome within the IRES element. This process is facilitated by cellular factors known as IRES trans-acting factors (ITAFs).
Foot-and-mouth disease (FMD) is host-restricted disease for cloven-hoofed animals such as cattle and pigs, but the factors determining the host range have not been identified yet. Although, ITAFs are known to promote IRES-mediated translation, these findings were confirmed only in cells derived from FMDV-insusceptible animals so far.
We evaluated and compared the IRES-mediated translation activities among cell lines derived from four different animal species using bicistronic luciferase reporter plasmid, which possesses an FMDV-IRES element between *Renilla* and *Firefly* luciferase genes. Furthermore, we analyzed the effect of the cellular factors on IRES-mediated translation by silencing the cellular factors using siRNA in both FMDV-susceptible and -insusceptible animal cells.

Results: Our data indicated that IRES-mediated translational activity was not linked to FMDV host range. $ITAF_{45}$ promoted IRES-mediated translation in all cell lines, and the effects of poly-pyrimidine tract binding protein (PTB) and eukaryotic initiation factor 4E-binding protein 1 (4E-BP1) were observed only in FMDV-susceptible cells. Thus, PTB and 4E-BP1 may influence the host range of FMDV.

Conclusions: IRES-mediated translation activity of FMDV was not predictive of its host range. $ITAF_{45}$ promoted IRES-mediated translation in all cells, and the effects of PTB and 4E-BP1 were observed only in FMDV-susceptible cells.

Keywords: FMDV, IRES, ITAF, $ITAF_{45}$, 4E-BP1, PTB, Translation

Background

Foot-and-mouth disease (FMD) is a highly contagious infectious disease in cloven-hoofed animals such as cattle, pigs, and other related species [1]. It is considered an endemic in several countries in Asia, Africa, and South America. Typical clinical signs of FMD include vesicle formation, and erosion of cutaneous mucosae and hairless parts of the skin proximal to the mouth and the hoofs. While FMD is rarely lethal in adult animals, it can induce myocarditis in newborn animals, which leads to high mortality [2]. In countries with endemic FMD, FMD-related mortality of young animals and decreased productivity (reduced milk production and animal weight loss) in adult animals can lead to major economic losses. In industrialized countries that are normally free of FMD, the costs associated with the control and eradication of an outbreak can reach several billion US dollars, which also include indirect losses due to trade restrictions on animal products [3].

* Correspondence: kkohara@vet.kagoshima-u.ac.jp
[1]Department of Animal Hygiene, Joint Facility of Veterinary Medicine, Kagoshima University, Kagoshima, Kagoshima, Japan
[2]Transboundary Animal Disease Center, Joint Facility of Veterinary Medicine, Kagoshima University, Kagoshima, Kagoshima, Japan

FMDV possesses a positive sense, single stranded RNA as its viral genome and belongs to the *Aphtovirus* genus of the *Picornaviridae* family. FMDV possesses an internal ribosomal entry site (IRES) element within the 5′ untranslated region (5′UTR), and virus proteins are synthesized by IRES-mediated translation [1, 4]. It is known that, like FMDV, poliovirus (PV) and encephalomyocarditis virus (EMCV) belonging to the *Picornaviridae* family, and hepatitis C virus (HCV) belonging to the *Flaviviridae* family, possesses a virus-specific IRES element within the 5′UTR, and virus proteins are synthesized by IRES-mediated translation [5, 6]. According to the RNA secondary structure, picornavirus IRESs can be classified into five types designated I (PV), II (FMDV), III (hepatitis A virus), IV (HCV-like), and V (aichivirus-like) [7]. Although FMD primarily affects cloven-hoofed animals such as cattle and pigs [1], the factors that determine the host range of FMDV have not yet been identified. Usually, eukaryotic mRNA is translated by cap-dependent translation, which is initiated by recognition of the cap structure at the 5′ end of the mRNA by the 43S ribosome [8]. Virus mRNA with a short 5′UTR (<100 nucleotides) containing no AUG can facilitate protein synthesis in a cap-dependent manner, similar to most types of eukaryotic mRNAs [5, 6]. Cap-independent translation is mediated by the IRES [5, 6] and involves 3′-UTR cap-independent translation enhancer (3′-CITE)-mediated initiation [9, 10]. Vpg interacts with the cap-binding protein eIF4E to modulate translation [11, 12]. The translation of eukaryotic mRNA is halted or significantly suppressed by cleavage of eIF4G with picornavirus protease (e.g., PV $2A^{pro}$ and FMDV L^{pro}), whereas protein synthesis directed by PV or EMCV-IRES is stimulated [13, 14]. FMDV L^{pro} can enhance translation driven by all picornavirus IRESs, even after inactivation of eIF2 by phosphorylation [15].

The FMDV-IRES element contains five domains, and each of these domains forms a specific three-dimensional conformation to directly bind to the 40S ribosome and initiate IRES-mediated translation [16, 17]. In addition to canonical eukaryotic initiation factors (eIFs), which are essential to initiate cap-dependent translation, IRES trans-acting factors (ITAFs), which specifically bind to the individual domains of the IRES element and stabilize its three-dimensional structure, are required to facilitate IRES-mediated translation [18, 19]. In previous reports, it was revealed that $ITAF_{45}$ and polypyrimidin tract binding protein (PTB) plays an important role in facilitating IRES-mediated translation of FMDV [20–22].

On the other hand, eukaryotic initiation factor 4E (eIF4E), a cap-binding protein, is an essential cellular factor that initiates cap-dependent translation; however, some viral mRNAs with IRESs can escape the eIF4E regulatory pathway [23]. The translation inhibitor, eIF4E-binding protein 1 (4E-BP1), binds eIF4E in its dephosphorylated form and is phosphorylated by stimulation with insulin or epidermal growth factors to dissociate from eIF4E [24, 25] after phosphorylation by mammalian target of rapamycin complex 1 (mTORC1) [26]. The free-eIF4E can promote cap-dependent translation by forming eIF4F with other eIFs [27]. However, once 4E-BP1 is dephosphorylated due to stress, it binds to eIF4E tightly, and cap-dependent translation is suppressed because eIF4F cannot be formed [28, 29]. EMCV and PV have been reported to dephosphorylate 4E-BP1, which may block host protein synthesis [29]. Because eIF4E is not essential for some types of virus IRES-mediated translation, it is possible that dephosphorylation of 4E-BP1 could facilitate IRES-mediated translation of FMDV [29–31].

However, these results were obtained in an experiment using cell lines derived from mice or hamsters, which are not the host animals of FMDV. Hence, whether these findings are also observed in cells derived from the FMDV host animals have not yet been analyzed.

Clove-hoofed animals are the main FMDV hosts, but the virus or cellular factors that determine the host range have not yet been identified. In this study, to analyze whether the host range of FMDV is determined by its IRES-mediated translation or not, we evaluated and compared IRES-mediated translation activities among the cell lines derived from different animal species, including both host and non-host animals (host animals: bovine and swine, non-host animals: human and canine). Furthermore, to confirm whether previous findings about ITAFs and 4E-BP1 were also observed in the host animal cells of FMDV, we analyzed the effect of the ITAFs and 4E-BP1 for IRES-mediated translation of FMDV in both host and non-host animal cells.

Results

Evaluation and comparison of IRES-mediated translation activity of FMVD in various animal cell lines

To evaluate IRES-mediated translational activity, we constructed a bicistronic reporter plasmid [30]. *Eco*RV and *Hpa*I were used to excise the reporter gene from pRF/FMDV-IRES, which has an FMDV-IRES element between *Renilla* luciferase and firefly luciferase genes. The extracted reporter gene was then inserted into the pCAGGS/MCS(F) vector, as the CAG promoter is functional in most cell types [32]. This plasmid construct was named pCAGGS/FMDV-IRES (Fig. 1).

This plasmid was then transfected into cell lines derived from the kidney epithelium of different animal species (HEK293 cells: human, MDCK cells: canine, MDBK cells: bovine, and CPK cells: swine). Amongst the assessed animal species, bovine and swine cell lines were derived from animals that are the natural hosts for FMDV. The bicistronic mRNA that contains the FMDV-IRES element

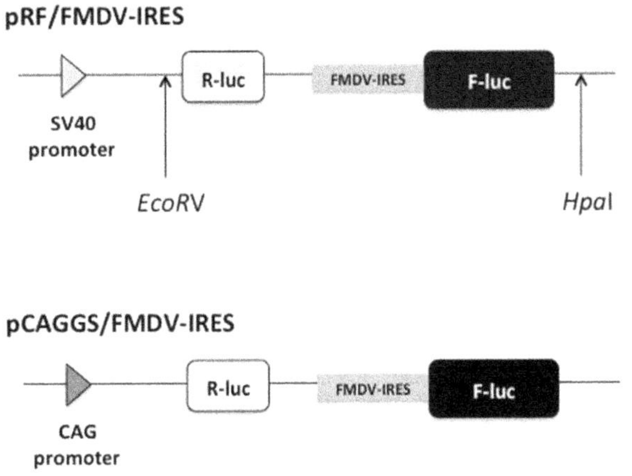

Fig. 1 pRF/FMDV-IRES and pCAGGS/FMDV-IRES plasmid construction. Structure of the bicistronic luciferase reporter construct containing the FMDV-IRES element located between *Renilla* luciferase and firefly luciferase (pRF-FMDV-IRS). Reporter gene was excised from this plasmid construct using the restriction enzymes *EcoRV* and *HpaI*, and was o the pCAGGS/MCS(F) vector treated with *SmaI* and rAPid Alkaline Phosphatase using Mighty Mix

between *Renilla* luciferase and firefly luciferase genes was produced in the transfected cells. 24 h following transfection, both *Renilla* luciferase and firefly luciferase activities in the cells were serially measured. *Renilla* luciferase activity represented cap-dependent translation, and firefly luciferase activity represented IRES-mediated translation. To evaluate IRES-mediated translational activity, the ratio of IRES-mediated translation to cap-dependent translation was calculated (Fig. 2). It was assumed that IRES-mediated translational activity of FMDV would be much higher in the cell lines derived from host animals of FMDV compared with cells derived from animals that are not natural hosts of FMDV. Previous studies have shown that IRES-mediated translational activity in CPK cells was higher than in MDBK cells, which may be due to efficient FMDV replication in swine cells [33]. In this study, although differences in IRES-mediated translational activity were observed among the cell lines, the translation activity of FMDV in FMDV-susceptible-host-derived cells was comparable to that of FMDV-insusceptible-host-derived cells. Furthermore, IRES-mediated translational activity in CPK cells was lower than that in MDCK cells, which were derived from canines (non-host animal of FMDV). Therefore, IRES-mediated translation activity cannot be used to accurately determine the host range of FMDV.

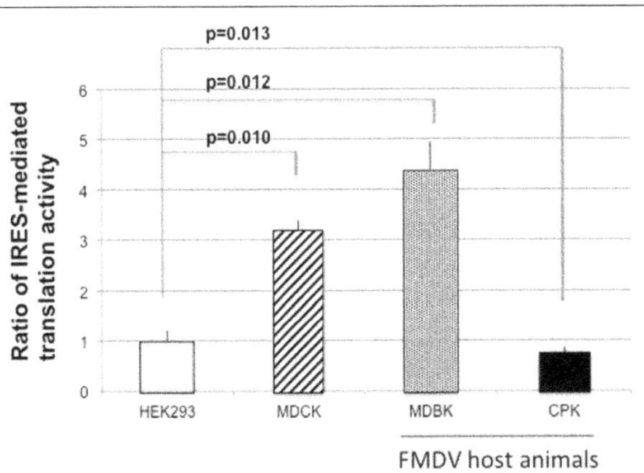

Fig. 2 Evaluation of IRES-mediated translation activity. HEK293, MDCK, MDBK, and CPK cells were transfected with pCAGGS/FMDV-IRES. 24 h following transfection, *Renilla* luciferase and firefly luciferase units were measured using the Dual-Luciferase Reporter Assay System, and the ratio of IRES-mediated translation activity to that in HEK293 cells was evaluated. Experiments were performed in triplicates and error bars indicate S.D. Student's *t*-tests were performed to calculate *p* values

The effects of cellular factors on IRES-mediated translation of FMDV

The cellular factors ITAF and eIF play important roles in facilitating IRES-mediated translation [20–22]. However, these findings were obtained by using cell lines derived from FMDV-insusceptible animals.

Therefore, to analyze the effect of ITAFs and 4E-BP1, the expression of $ITAF_{45}$, PTB, and 4E-BP1 was inhibited using siRNAs. The effect of siRNA was assessed by western blot analysis (Fig. 3). Following siRNA treatment, cells were further transfected with the reporter plasmid and evaluated for IRES-mediated translational activity (Figs. 4, 5 and 6). We found that inhibition of $ITAF_{45}$ expression suppressed IRES-mediated translational activity in cell lines derived from both FMDV-susceptible and FMDV-insusceptible animals. Inhibition of PTB and 4E-BP1 reduced IRES-mediated translational activity only in the FMDV-susceptible host cell lines (MDBK $p < 0.05$, and CPK $p < 0.01$). Our results show silencing of $ITAF_{45}$, PTB and 4E-BP1 in CPK cells can significantly suppress IRES-mediated translational activity.

Discussion

In this study, we evaluated IRES-mediated translational activity in HEK293, MDCK, MDBK, and CPK cells to determine whether this process differs between cells derived from FMDV-susceptible and FMDV-insusceptible animals. Although difference in IRES-mediated translational activity was observed among these cell lines, it was not predictive of FMDV host range. Thus, other cellular processes/interactions that are distinct from IRES-mediated translation are needed when determining the host range of FMDV. For example, it was recently reported that the amino acid sequence of integrin protein, which is a candidate FMDV receptor, is different between host and non-host animals [34]. In the host animals, there is also a difference in the expression of integrin proteins between FMDV-susceptible organs and FMDV-insusceptible organs [35]. Furthermore, diverse innate

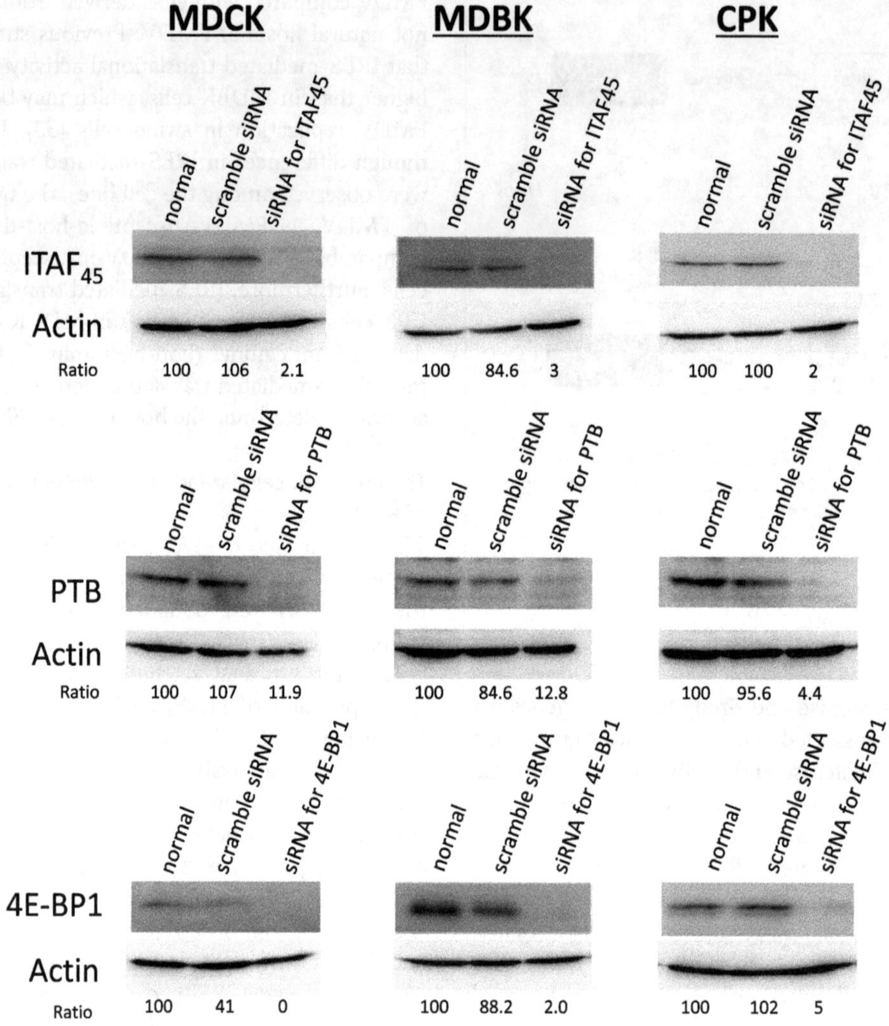

Fig. 3 The effect of siRNAs on the cellular factors. The siRNAs targeting ITAF45, PTB, and 4E-BP1 were reverse transfected into MDCK, MDBK, and CPK cells using Lipofectamine RNAiMAX, and incubated for 48 h. After 48-h treatment, western blot analysis was performed on cell lysates to confirm the effect of siRNAs. Protein bands were quantified using an LAS1000UVmini. The protein intensity was divided by that of actin, and the normalized ratio (100 %) was indicated

immune reactions have been shown to be initiated against FMDV infection in different animal species, including the host animals of FMDV [33]. The data obtained in this study indicate that IRES-mediated translation cannot be used to accurately define FMDV host range.

Next, we analyzed the effect of $ITAF_{45}$, PTB, and 4E-BP1 on IRES-mediated translation of FMDV in cell lines derived from FMDV-susceptible and FMDV-insusceptible animals. Inhibition of $ITAF_{45}$ expression suppressed IRES-mediated translation activity in all cell lines. However, silencing of PTB and 4E-BP1 suppressed IRES-mediated translation activity only in the cell lines derived from FMDV host animals. The active subunits of some cellular factors, including PTB, are generated by proteolysis, which has been correlated to FMDV-induced cytopathic effects [36]. Our findings from this study indicate that PTB, along with some other unidentified factors may be involved in facilitating IRES-mediated translation in FMDV-susceptible animals. The role of ITAFs in IRES-mediated translation has not yet been thoroughly characterized. Additional studies are required to determine the role of ITAFs in regulating FMDV-susceptibility of cells through IRES-mediated translation.

The inhibition of 4E-BP1 expression suppressed IRES-mediated translation activity in MDCK, MDBK, and CPK cells. These unexpected results suggest that IRES-mediated translation is dependent on 4E-BP1 (indicated by decrease in firefly luciferase activity, data not shown). Overexpression of 4E-BP1 has been previously shown to promote IRES-mediated translation of EMCV, and eIF4E availability has been shown to regulate IRES-mediated translation efficiency [37]. Although the translation of

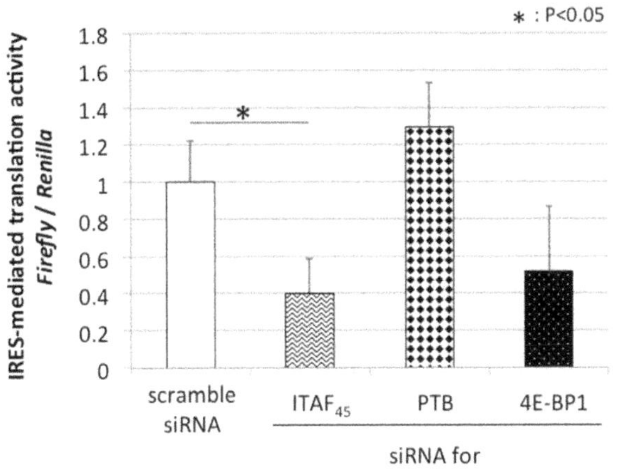

Fig. 4 The effect of siRNAs on IRES-mediated translation in MDCK cells. After 48 h of siRNA treatment, cells were further transfected with plasmid construct. 24 h following transfection, *Renilla* luciferase and firefly luciferase units were measured using the Dual-Luciferase Reporter Assay System and IRES-mediated translation activity in MDCK cells. Experiments were performed in triplicates and error bars indicate S.D

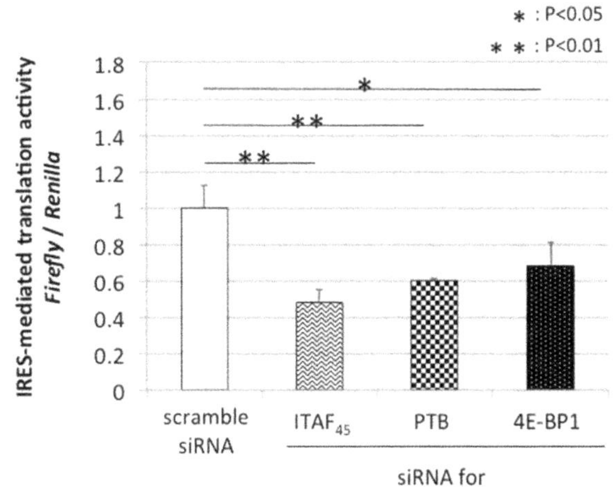

Fig. 6 The effect of siRNAs on IRES-mediated translation in CPK cells. After 48 h of siRNA treatment, cells were further transfected with plasmid construct. 24 h following transfection, *Renilla* luciferase and firefly luciferase units were measured using the Dual-Luciferase Reporter Assay System and IRES-mediated translation activity in CPK cells. Experiments were performed in triplicates and error bars indicate S.D

some viruses, such as poliovirus and vesicular stomatitis virus, has been shown to be promoted by phosphorylation of 4E-BP1, the translation of other viruses, such as adenovirus, has been shown to be promoted by dephosphorylation of 4E-BP1 [33, 38]. Furthermore, 4E-BP1 was previously shown to be involved in other cell activities such as regulation of cell growth and oncogenesis [39, 40]. Together with previous findings, our study indicates that 4E-BP1 regulates IRES-mediated translation of FMDV through complex mechanisms, and may play differential roles among various animal species. Further studies are required to characterize these potential novel functions of 4E-BP1.

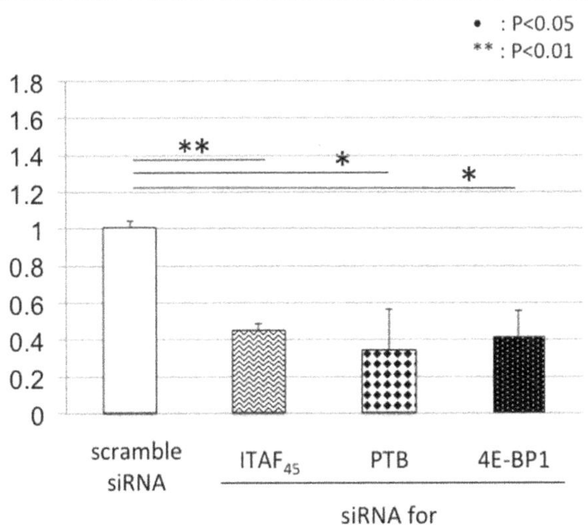

Fig. 5 The effect of siRNAs on IRES-mediated translation in MDBK cells. After 48 h of siRNA treatment, cells were further transfected with plasmid construct. 24 h following transfection, *Renilla* luciferase and firefly luciferase units were measured using the Dual-Luciferase Reporter Assay System and IRES-mediated translation activity in MDBK cells. Experiments were performed in triplicates and error bars indicate S.D

Conclusions

IRES-mediated translation activity of FMDV was not predictive of its host range. $ITAF_{45}$ promoted IRES-mediated translation in all cells, and the effects of PTB and 4E-BP1 were observed only in FMDV-susceptible cells. Eukaryotic initiation factor 4E-BP1 unexpectedly interacted with IRES-mediated translation in cells.

Methods

Cell lines and culture

The human kidney cell line (HEK293) and bovine kidney cell line (MDBK) used in this study were obtained from the American Type Culture Collection (ATCC), and were maintained in Dulbecco's modified Eagle's medium (DMEM; Nissui) supplemented with 10 % fetal calf serum (FCS; Bovogen). The canine kidney cell line (MDCK) was originally from ATCC and was maintained in Eagle's minimum essential medium (MEM; Life Technologies) supplemented with 5 % newborn calf serum (NCS; Hazleton). The porcine kidney cell line (CPK) [41] was maintained in MEM supplemented with 10 % FCS. All cell lines were cultured at 37 °C in 5 % CO_2.

Plasmids

The pRF/FMDV-IRES plasmids were kindly provided to us by Dr. Hirasawa (Memorial University of Newfoundland). Reporter genes were excised from pRF/FMDV-IRES using the restriction endonucleases *Eco*RV (Toyobo) and *Hpa*I (NEB). pCAGGS/FMDV-IRES was generated by inserting a reporter gene into pCAGGS/MSC(F), which was then treated with SmaI (Takara) and rAPid Alkaline Phosphatase (Roche) using Mighty Mix (Takara). DNA fragments were purified with the Big Dye XTerminator Purification kit, followed by sequencing via capillary electrophoresis on the ABI PRISM310 genetic analyzer.

Short interfering RNA assay

Short interfering RNAs (siRNAs) targeting human-$ITAF_{45}$ were used for MDCK, and MDBK cells. The siRNAs targeting mouse-$ITAF_{45}$ were used for CPK cells. Both types of $ITAF_{45}$-targeting siRNAs were composed of a mixture containing 3 siRNAs with 19–25 nucleotides (Santa Cruz Biotechnology). The siRNAs targeting human-PTB and human-4E-BP1 were as follows: 5′-GGCAGGAAATTC TGTATTG-3′, and 5′-GAGTCACAGTTTGAGATGGA CATTTAA-3′, respectively (Life Technologies).

Transfection

Cells (10^5/well) were grown in 24-well plates with culture medium for 24 h to achieve 50–70 % confluency for transfection. Plasmid transfection was performed using Lipofectamine 2000 reagent (Invitrogen) according to manufacturer's specification. The siRNA reverse transfection was performed using Lipofectamine RNAiMIX reagent (Invitrogen) according to manufacturer's specification.

Luciferase assay

Cells were washed once with PBS (–), and lysed with passive lysis buffer (Promega). *Renilla* luciferase and firefly luciferase activities were measured using the Dual-Luciferase Reporter Assay System (Promega). Cell lysates (10 μL) were mixed with a 10-fold diluted reagent (100 μL), and luminescence was measured with the GloMax 96 Microplate for 10 s. Luciferase activity was quantified as the relative fluorescent intensity in the 10-s interval.

Western blot analysis

Cells were washed twice with PBS, and lysed with RIPA buffer containing 0.1 % SDS, 10 μg aprotinin/mL, 100 μg PMSF/mL and 1 % phosphatase inhibitor cocktail (Sigma). Cell lysates were subjected to SDS-PAGE, and the resolved proteins were transferred to a PVDF membrane (Millipore). The membrane was blocked with 5 % Block Ace (Yukijirushi) in Tris buffered saline (TBS) containing 0.1 % Tween-20, and was probed with the following primary antibodies: anti-ITAF45 (Santa Cruz Biotechnology), anti-PTB (Cell Signaling), anti-4E-BP1 (Cell Signaling), and anti-βactin (SIGMA)]. The membranes were then washed 3 times with 0.05 % Tween- 20-TBS for 10 min. Secondary antibodies (peroxidase-conjugated anti-rabbit or anti-mouse IgG; DAKO) were subsequently added, and specific protein bands were visualized with enhanced chemical luminescence (GE Healthcare).

Statistical analysis

All data are presented as means ± SEM from three independent experiments. Statistical analysis was performed using Student's *t*-test to evaluate significant differences ($*P < 0.05$, $**P < 0.01$).

Consent for publication

Not applicable.

Abbreviations

FMDV: Foot-and-mouth disease virus; IRES: Internal ribosomal entry site; 5′ UTR: 5′ untranslated region; ITAFs: IRES trans-acting factors; PTB: Poly-pyrimidine tract binding protein; 4E-BP1: 4E-binding protein1.

Competing interests

The authors do not have any financial or personal relationship with organizations or people that could influence the content or conclusions of the study.

Authors' contributions

TK performed experiment, KTK made experimental design, and MO and KTK wrote manuscript. All authors read and approved the final manuscript.

Acknowledgement

We would like to thank Dr. Hirasawa for providing the pRF/FMDV-IRES plasmid.

Funding

This study was supported by the grant from the ministry of education, science and culture, Japan (15 K14781).

References

1. Grubman MJ, Baxt B. Foot-and-mouth disease. Clin Microbiol Rev. 2004;17: 465–93.
2. Ryan E, Horsington J, Durand S, Brooks H, Alexandersen S, Brownlie J, Zhang Z. Foot-and-mouth disease virus infection in young lambs: pathogenesis and tissue tropism. Vet Microbiol. 2008;127:258–74.
3. Jamal SM, Belsham GJ. Foot-and-mouth disease: past, present and future. Vet Res. 2013;44:116.
4. Belsham GJ, Brangwyn JK. A region of the 5′ noncoding region of foot-and-mouth disease virus RNA directs efficient internal initiation of protein synthesis within cells: involvement with the role of L protease in translational control. J Virol. 1990;64:5389–95.
5. Jackson RJ, Kaminski A. Internal initiation of translation in eukaryotes: the picornavirus paradigm and beyond. RNA. 1995;1:985–1000.
6. Tsukiyama-Kohara K, Iizuka N, Kohara M, Nomoto A. Internal ribosome entry site within hepatitis C virus RNA. J Virol. 1992;66:1476–83.

7. Lozano G, Martinez-Salas E. Structural insights into viral IRES-dependent translation mechanisms. Curr Opin Virol. 2015;12:113–20.
8. Shatkin AJ. mRNA cap binding proteins: essential factors for initiating translation. Cell. 1985;40:223–4.
9. Truniger V, Nieto C, Gonzalez-Ibeas D, Aranda M. Mechanism of plant eIF4E-mediated resistance against a Carmovirus (Tombusviridae): cap-independent translation of a viral RNA controlled in cis by an (a)virulence determinant. Plant J. 2008;56:716–27.
10. Miras M, Sempere RN, Kraft JJ, Miller WA, Aranda MA, Truniger V. Interfamilial recombination between viruses led to acquisition of a novel translation-enhancing RNA element that allows resistance breaking. New Phytol. 2014;202:233–46.
11. Michon T, Estevez Y, Walter J, German-Retana S, Le Gall O. The potyviral virus genome-linked protein VPg forms a ternary complex with the eukaryotic initiation factors eIF4E and eIF4G and reduces eIF4E affinity for a mRNA cap analogue. FEBS J. 2006;273:1312–22.
12. Eskelin K, Hafren A, Rantalainen KI, Makinen K. Potyviral VPg enhances viral RNA Translation and inhibits reporter mRNA translation in planta. J Virol. 2011;85:9210–21.
13. Ziegler E, Borman AM, Deliat FG, Liebig HD, Jugovic D, Kean KM, Skern T, Kuechler E. Picornavirus 2A proteinase-mediated stimulation of internal initiation of translation is dependent on enzymatic activity and the cleavage products
of cellular proteins. Virology. 1995;213:549–57.
14. Borman AM, Kirchweger R, Ziegler E, Rhoads RE, Skern T, Kean KM. eIF4G and its proteolytic cleavage products: effect on initiation of protein synthesis from capped, uncapped, and IRES-containing mRNAs. RNA. 1997;3:186–96.
15. Moral-Lopez P, Alvarez E, Redondo N, Skern T, Carrasco L. L protease from foot and mouth disease virus confers eIF2-independent translation for mRNAs bearing picornavirus IRES. FEBS Lett. 2014;588:4053–9.
16. Kieft JS. Viral IRES RNA structures and ribosome interactions. Trends Biochem Sci. 2008;33:274–83.
17. Filbin ME, Kieft JS. Toward a structural understanding of IRES RNA function. Curr Opin Struct Biol. 2009;19:267–76.
18. Martinez-Salas E. The impact of RNA structure on picornavirus IRES activity. Trends Microbiol. 2008;16:230–7.
19. Yu Y, Abaeva IS, Marintchev A, Pestova TV, Hellen CU. Common conformational changes induced in type 2 picornavirus IRESs by cognate trans-acting factors. Nucleic Acids Res. 2011;39:4851–65.
20. Pilipenko EV, Pestova TV, Kolupaeva VG, Khitrina EV, Poperechnaya AN, Agol VI, Hellen CU. A cell cycle-dependent protein serves as a template-specific translation initiation factor. Genes Dev. 2000;14:2028–45.
21. Andreev DE, Fernandez-Miragall O, Ramajo J, Dmitriev SE, Terenin IM, Martinez-Salas E, Shatsky IN. Differential factor requirement to assemble translation initiation complexes at the alternative start codons of foot-and-mouth disease virus RNA. RNA. 2007;13:1366–74.
22. Monie TP, Perrin AJ, Birtley JR, Sweeney TR, Karakasiliotis I, Chaudhry Y, Roberts LO, Matthews S, Goodfellow IG, Curry S. Structural insights into the transcriptional and translational roles of Ebp1. EMBO J. 2007;26:3936–44.
23. Deforges J, Locker N, Sargueil B. mRNAs that specifically interact with eukaryotic ribosomal subunits. Biochimie. 2015;114:48–57.
24. Pause A, Belsham GJ, Gingras AC, Donze O, Lin TA, Lawrence Jr JC, Jr., Sonenberg N. Insulin-dependent stimulation of protein synthesis by phosphorylation of
a regulator of 5′-cap function. Nature. 1994;371:762–7.
25. Tsukiyama-Kohara K, Poulin F, Kohara M, DeMaria CT, Cheng A, Wu Z, Gingras AC, Katsume A, Elchebly M, Spiegelman BM, et al. Adipose tissue reduction in mice lacking the translational inhibitor 4E-BP1. Nat Med. 2001; 7:1128–32.
26. Sekiyama N, Arthanari H, Papadopoulos E, Rodriguez-Mias RA, Wagner G, Leger-Abraham M. Molecular mechanism of the dual activity of 4EGI-1: Dissociating eIF4G from eIF4E but stabilizing the binding of unphosphorylated 4E-BP1. Proc Natl Acad Sci U S A. 2015;112:E4036–45.
27. Pyronnet S, Imataka H, Gingras AC, Fukunaga R, Hunter T, Sonenberg N. Human eukaryotic translation initiation factor 4G (eIF4G) recruits mnk1 to phosphorylate eIF4E. EMBO J. 1999;18:270–9.
28. Fernandez J, Yaman I, Mishra R, Merrick WC, Snider MD, Lamers WH, Hatzoglou M. Internal ribosome entry site-mediated translation of a mammalian mRNA is regulated by amino acid availability. J Biol Chem. 2001;276:12285–91.
29. Gingras AC, Svitkin Y, Belsham GJ, Pause A, Sonenberg N. Activation of the translational suppressor 4E-BP1 following infection with encephalomyocarditis virus and poliovirus. Proc Natl Acad Sci U S A. 1996;93:5578–83.
30. Licursi M, Komatsu Y, Pongnopparat T, Hirasawa K. Promotion of viral internal ribosomal entry site-mediated translation under amino acid starvation. J Gen Virol. 2012;93:951–62.
31. Connor JH, Lyles DS. Vesicular stomatitis virus infection alters the eIF4F translation initiation complex and causes dephosphorylation of the eIF4E binding protein 4E-BP1. J Virol. 2002;76:10177–87.
32. Czudai-Matwich V, Schnare M, Pinkenburg O. A simple and fast system for cloning influenza A virus gene segments into pHW2000- and pCAGGS-based vectors. Arch Virol. 2013;158:2049–58.
33. Toka FN, Golde WT. Cell mediated innate responses of cattle and swine are diverse during foot-and-mouth disease virus (FMDV) infection: a unique landscape of innate immunity. Immunol Lett. 2013;152:135–43.
34. Du J, Gao S, Chang H, Cong G, Lin T, Shao J, Liu Z, Liu X, Cai X. Bactrian camel (Camelus bactrianus) integrins alphavbeta3 and alphavbeta6 as FMDV receptors: molecular cloning, sequence analysis and comparison with other species. Vet Immunol Immunopathol. 2009;131:190–9.
35. Zhu JJ, Arzt J, Puckette MC, Smoliga GR, Pacheco JM, Rodriguez LL. Mechanisms of foot-and-mouth disease virus tropism inferred from differential tissue gene expression. PLoS One. 2013;8:e64119.
36. Rodriguez Pulido M, Serrano P, Saiz M, Martinez-Salas E. Foot-and-mouth disease virus infection induces proteolytic cleavage of PTB, eIF3a, b, and PABP RNA-binding proteins. Virology. 2007;364:466–74.
37. Svitkin YV, Herdy B, Costa-Mattioli M, Gingras AC, Raught B, Sonenberg N. Eukaryotic translation initiation factor 4E availability controls the switch between cap-dependent and internal ribosomal entry site-mediated translation. Mol Cell Biol. 2005;25:10556–65.
38. Gingras AC, Sonenberg N. Adenovirus infection inactivates the translational inhibitors 4E-BP1 and 4E-BP2. Virology. 1997;237:182–6.
39. Petroulakis E, Parsyan A, Dowling RJ, LeBacquer O, Martineau Y, Bidinosti M, Larsson O, Alain T, Rong L, Mamane Y, et al. p53-dependent translational control of senescence and transformation via 4E-BPs. Cancer Cell. 2009;16: 439–46.
40. She QB, Halilovic E, Ye Q, Zhen W, Shirasawa S, Sasazuki T, Solit DB, Rosen N. 4E-BP1 is a key effector of the oncogenic activation of the AKT and ERK signaling pathways that integrates their function in tumors. Cancer Cell. 2010; 18:39–51.
41. Komaniwa H, Fukusho A, Shimizu Y. Micro method for performing titration and neutralization test of hog cholera virus using established porcine kidney cell strain. Natl Inst Anim Health Q (Tokyo). 1981;21:153–8.

12

Seroprevalence and risk factors associated with *Pseudorabies virus* infection in Tibetan pigs in Tibet

Qingxia Wu[1*†], Hui Zhang[2†], Hailong Dong[1], Khalid Mehmood[2,3], Zhenyu Chang[1], Kun Li[2], Suozhu Liu[1], Mujeeb Ur Rehman[2], Fazul Nabi[2], Muhammad Tariq Javed[4], Hongyun Zhu[1*] and Jiakui Li[1,2*]

Abstract

Background: Pseudorabies (PR) is an important emerging infectious disease that is characterized by fever, extreme itching and encephalomyelitis. However, it is still unclear whether Tibetan pigs are exposed to Pseudorabies virus (PRV) or not.
The present study was conducted to investigate the seroprevalence of PRV infection in Tibetan pigs in Nyingchi area of Tibet through enzyme-linked immunosorbent assay (ELISA). A total of 368 serum samples from Tibetan pigs were collected during 2015.

Results: Results showed that 58 (15.76%) samples were found positive for PRV antibodies with further distribution of 18.23%, 13.42% and 6.25% from Nyingchi, Mainling and Gongbo'gyamda areas on the Tibetan plateau, respectively; along with 12.10%, 17.71% and 17.57% prevalence of PRV in juveniles, sub-adults and adults, respectively. The prevalence of PRV infection between male (14.61%) and female (16.84%) showed non-significant difference ($P > 0.05$). The risk factors of infection were found to be associated with feed type, age and altitude.

Conclusions: The present study depicts a serious concern with a new emerging infectious disease in Tibetan pigs in Tibet, China.

Keywords: Pseudorabies (PR), Seroprevalence, Risk factors, Tibetan pigs, Tibet

Background

Pseudorabies (PR) or Aujeszky's disease is one of the highly contagious diseases, which is responsible for devastating outbreaks and considerable economic losses to the swine industry in China. It is caused by Pseudorabies virus (PRV), which is the member of genus Varicellovirus, belonging to subfamily Alphaherpesvirinae, and family Herpesviridae [1–3]. The domestic and feral pigs are the main natural hosts of this disease [4]. The PR is usually characterized by reproductive disorders such as miscarriage, fetal death and mummified fetus. The mortality rate of newborn piglets and abortion are up to 100% in some cases [5]. The infection in growing pigs usually leads to decrease in semen quality, and even death in some cases. Pseudorabies is highly hazardous and widely distributed contagious disease, and world health organization (OIE) has listed PR as class B animal disease, and listed as the secondary kind of animal disease in China [6].

The PR is an endemic and widespread swine disease in China from the last 5 years, and it is planned as one of the priority swine diseases for control [7, 8]. Recently, with the use of PRV vaccines, this situation has been controlled on large-scale pig farms [2]; however, the prevention and control of PR on small pig farms and free-ranging pigs is still a big challenge [9]. The regional elimination and eradication program of PRV is required in China as no region is declared free from PRV yet [6].

In China, PRV was first reported in cats in 1947, and subsequently found in swine [7]. Tibetan pig is relatively ancient in origin, indigenous and rare plateau type pig breed in the world and is the only high-altitude pasture pig breed in China [10, 11]. It is distributed in the

* Correspondence: wuqx2014@sina.com; zh0561@sina.com; lijk210@sina.com
†Equal contributors
[1]Key laboratory of clinical veterinary medicine in Tibet, Tibet Agriculture and Animal Husbandry College, Linzhi 860000, Tibet, People's Republic of China
Full list of author information is available at the end of the article

Qinghai-Tibetan Plateau in China (Qinghai, Sichuan, Yunnan and eastern Tibet region). The seroprevalence of PRV infection in pigs in Qinghai, Sichuan and Yunnan areas is reported in local Chinese journals but hardly accessible to international readers, and that is summarized in Table 1.

To date, no survey has been conducted to elucidate PRV infection and risk factors on PR in Tibetan pigs. The current study is conducted for the first time on seroprevalence of PRV infection in Tibetan pigs and it provides a reference basis for the PRV research in the future.

Methods

The study sites

The present study was carried out in Nyingchi Prefecture in southeastern Tibet, China. This area is geographically isolated from Tibet and Sichuan Provinces by Himalayan Mountains, and shares its borders with Yunnan and Qinghai Provinces [10–12]. Nepal is located on the southwest, while India and Myanmar in the south of the Nyingchi. The average elevation of the surveyed area is more than 3100 m above the sea level (Fig. 1).

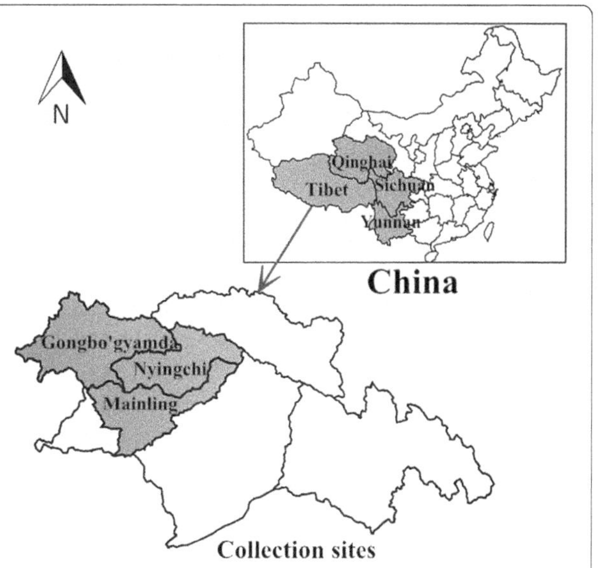

Fig. 1 Geographic location of Aujeszky's disease virus in four provinces, China. Map was created by using Mapinfo software; data are from the National Fundamental Geographic System website (www.dituhui.com)

Samples

A total of 368 blood samples were collected from different slaughterhouses of three counties (Nyingchi, Mainling and Gongbo'gyamda) in Tibet during 2015 (Fig. 1). All samples were collected from non-vaccinated pigs. The blood samples were collected by anterior vena cava of pigs. After collection of blood samples, each sample was centrifuged at 3000×g for 20 min to separate the serum which was subsequently stored at − 20 °C. These samples were transported in ice bag to Huazhong Agricultural University for further analysis.

The serum samples were used for detection of IgG antibodies for PRV by a commercially available ELISA kit (Wuhan Keqian Biology Co., Ltd). All the protocols were followed according to the manufacturer's instructions and the results were interpreted accordingly.

The results were based on the critical value (cut off) according to the formula: Critical Value = the average of Negative control OD_{630} + 0.15. The validity was ensured as: the average of Negative control OD_{630} - Positive control OD_{630} was ≥0.4. The samples were interpreted as negative: if sample OD_{630}/ Negative controlOD_{630} was > 0.7 (cut off). The samples were interpreted as positive if sample OD_{630}/ Negative control OD_{630} was ≤0.7 (cut off).

Statistical analysis

The data were analyzed by the chi-square test using the procedure of SAS (Statistical Analysis System, Version 8.0). Statistically significant levels within factors and interactions were recognized, when probability (*P*) value was found $P < 0.05$. Odds-ratios were determined for the risk factors associated PRV along with 95% confidence intervals.

Results

Seroprevalence of PRV

A total of 35 (16.36%) out of 214 serum samples were found positive for antibodies to PRV in large-scale Tibetan pig farms, with the further distribution of 23 (20.00%), 11 (12.64%) and 1 (8.33%) from Nyingchi, Mainling and Gongbo'gyamda areas, respectively. Antibodies against PRV were detected in 23 (14.94%) of 154 serum samples by ELISA in free-ranging Tibetan pigs, with the further distribution of 14 (15.91%), 9 (14.52%) and 0 from Nyingchi, Mainling and Gongbo'gyamda areas, respectively. The results were statistically

Table 1 Prevalence of Aujeszky's disease virus infection in pigs and in Tibetan pig distribution province, China

Province	No. tested	Test method	Positive (%)	Reference
Qinghai	456	ELISA	4.80%	Xiaoying Qi et al. 2015 (in Chinese)
Sichuan	1110	ELISA	17.61%	Kui Nie et al. 2013 (in Chinese)
Yunnan	1164	ELISA	35.40%	Xianghua Shu et al. 2010 (in Chinese)
Tibet	368	ELISA	15.76%	In present study

significant between large-scale and free-ranging Tibetan pigs ($P < 0.05$), as well as among different regions (Table 2).

The results of this study showed that a much higher proportion of seropositive were sub-adults (17.71%), followed by adults (17.57%) and juveniles (12.10%). There was non-significant difference between the sub-adults or adults and juveniles as shown in Table 3. The results revealed that the prevalence in female and male Tibetan pigs' was 14.61% and 16.84%, respectively. The seroprevalence was 21.43%, 15.70% and 11.11% at the altitude of 2800 m, 3200 m and 3700 m, respectively. Statistical analysis revealed that the prevalence of PRV was significantly different ($P < 0.05$) at different altitudes.

Table 3 Association between Tibetan pig characteristics and Aujeszky's disease virus serological status with corresponding chi square (χ^2), *p*-value, odds ratio (OR), and confidence interval (CI)

Characteristic	No. tested	Positive N	Positive %	95% CI	MH Chi-sq P value	OR/ reciprocal
Age						
Juveniles	124	15	12.10	6.9–19.2	$P = 0.229$	–
Sub-adults	96	17	17.71	10.7–26.8		–
Adults	148	26	17.57	11.8–24.7		–
Sex						
Male	178	26	14.61	9.8–20.7	–	0.84/ 1.18
Female	190	32	16.84	11.8–22.9	–	
Feed type						
Free-ranging	154	23	14.94	9.7–21.6	–	0.90 / 1.11
Large-scale	214	35	16.36	11.7–22.0	–	
Altitude						
3700 m	135	15	11.11	6.4–17.7	$P = 0.027$	–
3200 m	121	19	15.70	9.7–23.4		–
2800 m	112	24	21.43	14.2–30.2		–

Risk factors for seropositivity of PRV

We evaluated four pre-identified probable risk factors including age, sex, feed type and altitude. Our results showed that feed type, altitude and age were significantly associated with an increase risk of PRV seropositivity in Tibetan pigs (Table 3).

Discussion

Pseudorabies virus has been reported in many countries and it was first reported in the 19th century in the United States [7, 13, 14]. Infectious diseases have been serious threat for animal health and productivity in developing countries [15–19]. China is the world's largest producer of swine, and PRV has become a major infectious disease threat to pig industry and causes serious issue. The lack of awareness and control measures against common infectious disease is a major cause of PRV in population. Although, the vaccination program was applied on many pig farms, but there were often occurrence and epidemic of this disease. The previous reports showed that the prevalence of PRV infection in pigs in Qinghai (4.80%), Sichuan (17.61%) and Yunnan (35.40%) provinces were very serious [5, 20, 21]. Tibetan pigs are mainly distributed in Qinghai, Sichuan, Yunnan and the eastern Tibet region. There are no previous published data regarding the prevalence of PRV infection in pigs. To the best of our knowledge, the present study provides the first report of PRV infection in Tibetan pigs.

In our study, the overall PRV seroprevalence was 15.76% in Tibetan pigs in Tibet, which was lower than that reported in pigs in Shandong (56.7%), Henan (53.7%), Beijing (24.0%), Tianjing (17.1%), Hebei (16.9%) and Liaoning (16.8%) [1, 8, 22, 23]. The low seropositivity of PRV in Tibetan pigs may be due to the evolution difference and unique characteristics of the plateau environment. On the other hand, Tibet's unique mountains and rivers build a natural barrier to prevent or minimize the chances of spread of PRV.

Our results showed PRV infection among the different age groups of Tibetan pigs, a higher prevalence was detected in sub-adult (17.71%) or adult (17.57%) pigs, compared with the juveniles (12.10%). Some previous studies have also observed a higher seroprevalence of Aujeszky disease virus (ADV) between adults and juveniles [24]. However, non-significant difference ($P > 0.05$) was observed in *PR* seroprevalence between sex and feed type Tibetan pigs, which was different than the previous report [24]. Our results suggested that the incidence of PR was not related to the gender and feed type and there are several other possible reasons for this in Tibetan

Table 2 Descriptive characteristics and estimates of Aujeszky's disease virus seroprevalence at large-scale Tibetan pigs and free-range Tibetan pigs

Variable	Large-scale Tibetan pigs		Free-ranging Tibetan pigs		Total	
	Samples	NO. Positive (%)	Samples	NO. Positive (%)	Samples	NO. Positive (%)
Nyingchi	115	23(20.00%)	88	14(15.91%)	203	37(18.23%)
Mainling	87	11(12.64%)	62	9 (14.52%)	149	20(13.42%)
Gongbo'gyamda	12	1 (8.33%)	4	0	16	1(6.25%)

pigs. Firstly, it may be due to living in a similar environment and free-ranging system and secondly, each pig has the same chance to contact PRV [11, 25].

Hu et al. reported that the probability of reintroduction of PRV infection in large-scale Tibetan pig farms was positively different with free-ranging Tibetan pig farms [22]. However, our study has shown that feed type is associated with the infection of PRV. The subsequent univariate analysis indicated that the large-scale Tibetan pig farms were at higher risk for PRV seropositivity than free-ranging Tibetan pigs (OR: 1.11). Tibetan pigs are mainly fed by grazing in open environment [26]. Under such conditions, this animal gets more chance to expose to the external environment. Among these, sub-adults and adults have the longest time of outdoor activities which increases the risk of infection as compared with the juvenile Tibetan pigs.

Tibet is located in the Himalaya region and have high altitude with low temperature [10, 12, 26]. The local herdsmen have very less chance of interacting with the outside, which is not conducive to the survival of PRV. Tibet has unique mountains and rivers, forming a natural barrier structure, which is a different than reported earlier [27]. However, our study found that Tibetan pigs have been exposed to PRV and we discovered that the pigs living at low altitude (2800 m) were at higher risk for PRV seropositivity than those living at high altitude (3200 m and 3700 m). Current study reported PRV in Tibetan pig, and thus preventive and hygienic measures are suggested to minimize the serious economic losses. The vaccination, regular disinfection, and isolation of infected pigs are important to prevent the spread of PR from a particular area.

Conclusions

The present study demonstrated the seroprevalence of PRV infection in Tibetan pigs, and found that feed type, age and altitude are major risk factors associated with PRV herd seropositivity and possible source for the spread of PRV in Tibetan pigs.

Abbreviations

ELISA: Enzyme-linked immunosorbent assay; PR: Pseudorabies; PRV: Pseudorabies virus; SAS: Statistical Analysis System

Acknowledgments

The authors thanked Jiakui Li (Huazhong Agricultural University) for his positive advice on experimental design.

Funding

This study was supported Key Science Fund of Science and Technology Agency of Tibet Autonomous Region, Key laboratory of clinical veterinary medicine in Tibet in project designing and sample collection and projects in the National Science & Technology Pillar Program during the 12th Five-year Plan Period (2012BAD3B03) helped in data interpretation. Research and Application of Non-Grain Feed Development for Tibetan pigs in winter and spring helped in manuscript drafting.

Authors' contributions

JK L, HY Z, HZ, QX W, HL D, KL, KM, MU R, SZ L, ZY C, FN and MTJ contributed to study design, data analysis, and manuscript writing along with participated sufficiently in final approval of the paper. JK L, HY Z, HZ and QX W conceived and designed the experiments; HL D, KL and MU R performed the experiments; SZ L, ZY C, FN, and MTJ contributed reagents, materials, and analysis tools; SZ L, ZY C, and MTJ revised the manuscript. Furthermore, all the authors have read and approved the final manuscript.

Consent for publication

Not applicable

Competing interests

The authors declare that they have no competing interests.

Author details

[1]Key laboratory of clinical veterinary medicine in Tibet, Tibet Agriculture and Animal Husbandry College, Linzhi 860000, Tibet, People's Republic of China. [2]College of Veterinary Medicine, Huazhong Agricultural University, Wuhan 430070, People's Republic of China. [3]University College of Veterinary & Animal Sciences, the Islamia University of Bahawalpur, Bahawalpur 63100, Pakistan. [4]Departmet of Pathology, University of Agriculture, Faisalabad, Pakistan.

References

1. An TQ, Peng JM, Tian ZJ, Zhao HY, Li N, Liu YM, et al. Pseudorabies virus variant in Bartha-K61-vaccinated pigs, China, 2012. Emerg. Infect. Dis. 2015;19:1749–55.
2. Gu Z, Dong J, Wang J, Hou C, Sun H, Yang W, et al. A novel inactivated gE/gI deleted Pseudorabies virus (PRV) vaccine completely protects pigs from an emerged variant PRV challenge. Virus Res. 2015;195:57–63.
3. Klupp BG, Hengartner CJ, Mettenleiter TC, Enquist LW. Complete, annotated sequence of the pseudorabies virus genome. J Virol. 2004;78:424–40.
4. Kluge JP, Beran GW, Hill HT, Platt KB. Pseudorabies (Aujeszky's disease). Disease Swine. 1999;8:233–46.
5. Nie K, Li ZQ, Zeng Z, Yang ZL, Luo L. Seroepidemiological investigation and risk factor analysis of Pseudorabies in finishing pigs in some regions of Sichuan and Chongqing. J. Southwest Univ. 2013;35:7–12. (in Chinese)
6. The State Council of the People's Republic of China, National middle-to-long term plan for animal disease control (2012–2020), the bulletin of the state Council of the People's republic of China, 2012.
7. Sun Y, Luo Y, Wang CH, Jin Y, Na L, Song K. Control of swine pseudorabies in china: opportunities and limitations. Vet Microbiol. 2016;183:119–24.
8. Tong GZ, Chen HC. Pseudorabies epidemic status and control measures in China. China Journal Veterinary Science. 1999;19:1–2. (in Chinese)
9. Wang CH, Yuan J, Qin H, Luo Y, Cong X, Li Y, et al. A novel gE-deleted Pseudorabies virus (PRV) provides rapid and complete protection from lethal challenge with the PRV variant emerging in Bartha-K61-vaccinated swine population in China. Vaccine. 2014;32:3379–85.
10. Zhang H, Mujeeb UR, Li K, Luo HQ, Lan YF, Fazul N, et al. Epidemiologic survey of Japanese encephalitis virus infection, Tibet, China, 2015. Emerg Infect Dis. 2017;23(6):1023–4.
11. Zhang H, Mujeeb UR, Li K, Luo HQ, Lan YF, Fazul N, et al. Antimicrobial resistance of *Escherichia coli* isolated from Tibetan piglets suffering from white score diarrhea. Pak Vet J. 2016;37(1):43–6.
12. Zhang H, Luo HQ, Mujeeb UR, Fazul N, Li K, Lan YF, et al. Evidence of JEV in *Culex tritaeniorhynchus* and pigs from high altitude regions of Tibet, China. J. Vector Borne Dis. 2017;54(1):69–73.
13. Wu R, Bai CY, Sun JZ, Chang SK, Zhang X. Emergence of virulent pseudorabies virus infection in northern China. J. Vet. Sci. 2013;14:363–5.
14. Gortázar C, Vicente J, Fierro Y, León L, Cubero MJ, Gonzalez M. Natural Aujeszky's disease in a Spanish wild boar population. Ann N Y Acad Sci. 2012;969:210–2.

15. Ali F, Hussain R, Qayyum A, Gul ST, Iqbal Z, Hassan MF. Milk somatic cell counts and some hemato-biochemical changes in sub-clinical mastitic dromedary she-camels (*Camelus dromedarius*). Pak Vet J. 2016;36:405–8.
16. Elhaig MM, Selim A, Mahmoud MM, El-Gayar EK. Molecular confirmation of *Trypanosoma evansi* and *Babesia bigemina* in cattle from lower Egypt. Pak Vet J. 2016;36:409–14.
17. Qayyum A, Khan JA, Hussain R, Avais M, Ahmad N, Khan MS. Investigation of milk and blood serum biochemical profile as an indicator of subclinical mastitis in Cholistani cattle. Pak Vet J. 2016;36:275–9.
18. Wen XB, Jiang HT, Zhang YL, Lang XY, Liu J, Ni HB. Rapid and sensitive diagnosis of cattle anaplasmosis by loop-mediated isothermal amplification (LAMP). Pak Vet J. 2016;36:174–8.
19. Yilmaz R, Cangul IT, Onat K, Akkoc A, Ozyigit MO, Akkdesir E. Histopathological, immunohistochemical and bacteriological characterization of Mycoplasma bovis pneumonia in cattle. Pak Vet J. 2016;36:316–21.
20. Qi XY. Seroprevalence of Pseudorabies, infection in pigs in Qinghai of China. Chinese Qinghai Journal of Animal Veterinary Science. 2015;9:137–8. (in Chinese)
21. Shu XH, Yin GF, Li WG, Liu Y, Hou JF. Seroprevalence of respiratory disease, infection in pigs in some parts of Yunnan. China Animal Husbandry Veterinary. 2010;5:75–7. (in Chinese)
22. Hu D, Lv L, Zhang Z, Xiao Y, Liu S. Seroprevalence and associated risk factors of pseudorabies in Shandong province of China. J Vet Sci. 2016;17:361–8.
23. Yu X, Zhou Z, Hu D, Han T, Li X. Pathogenic pseudorabies virus, China, 2012. Emerge Infectious Disease. 2015;20:102–4.
24. Vicente J, Ruizfons F, Vidal D, Höfle U, Acevedo P, Villanúa D. Serosurvey of Aujeszky's disease virus infection in European wild boar in Spain. Vet Res. 2005;156:408–12.
25. Zhang XX, Lou ZZ, Huang SY, Zhou DD, Jia WZ, Su CL, et al. Genetic characterization of *Toxoplasma gondii* from Qinghai vole, plateau pika and Tibetan ground-tit on the Qinghai-Tibet plateau. China Parasite Vector. 2013;6:291.
26. Zhang NZ, Zhou DH, Huang SY, Wang M, Shi XC, Ciren DB. Seroprevalence and risk factors associated with *Haemophilus parasuis*, infection in Tibetan pigs in Tibet. Acta Tropical. 2014;132:94–7.
27. Solymosi N, Reiczigel J, Berke O, Harnos A, Szigeti S, Fodor L, et al. Spatial risk assessment of herd sero-status of Aujeszky's disease in a county in Hungary. Prev. Vet. Med. 2004;65:9–16.

13

H5N2 Highly Pathogenic Avian Influenza Viruses from the US 2014-2015 outbreak have an unusually long pre-clinical period in Turkey

Erica Spackman*, Mary J. Pantin-Jackwood, Darrell R. Kapczynski, David E. Swayne and David L. Suarez

Abstract

Background: From December 2014 through June 2015, the US experienced the most costly highly pathogenic avian influenza (HPAI) outbreak to date. Most cases in commercial poultry were caused by an H5N2 strain which was a reassortant with 5 Eurasian lineage genes, including a clade 2.3.4.4 goose/Guangdong/1996 lineage hemagglutinin, and 3 genes from North American wild waterfowl low pathogenicity avian influenza viruses. The outbreak primarily affected turkeys and table-egg layer type chickens. Three isolates were selected for characterization in turkeys: the US index isolate from December 2014 (A/northern pintail/WA/40964/2014), and two poultry isolates from April 2015 (A/chicken/IA/13388/2015 and A/turkey/MN/12528/2015).

Results: Four week old broad-breasted white turkeys were inoculated with one of three doses (10^2, 10^4 or 10^6 50% egg infectious doses [EID_{50}] per bird) of each of the isolates to evaluate infectious dose and pathogenesis. The mean bird infectious dose of A/northern pintail/WA/40964/2014 and A/turkey/MN/12528/2015 was 10^5 EID_{50} per bird, but was 10^3 EID_{50} per bird for A/chicken/IA/13388/2015, suggesting the latter had greater adaptation to gallinaceous birds. All three isolates had unusually long mean death time of 5.3–5.9 days post challenge, and the primary clinical signs were severe lethargy and neurological signs which started no more than 24 h before death (the average pre-clinical period was 4 days). Infected turkeys also shed high levels of virus by both the oropharyngeal and cloacal routes.

Conclusions: The unusually long mean death times, high levels of virus in feces, and increased adaptation of the later viruses may have contributed to the rapid spread of the virus during the peak of the outbreak.

Keywords: Highly pathogenic avian influenza virus, Clade 2.3.4.4 H5N2, Turkey disease, Avian influenza outbreak, Chicken disease

Background

An H5 HPAIV outbreak that began in December 2014 and lasted 6 months through June 2015 was the 5th highly pathogenic avian influenza virus (HPAIV) outbreak in the US since the 1920's and was the most geographically widespread. Direct and indirect costs to the US economy were estimated to be near $3.3 billion USD [1]. The hemagglutinin (HA) gene was determined to belong to clade 2.3.4.4 of the goose/Guangdong/1996 (GS/GD/96) H5 lineage of HPAIV and was subsequently named intercontinental group A (IcA) H5 [2, 3]. Wild waterfowl are thought to have carried viruses of this Eurasian lineage from Asia into North America during migration over the Bearing sea route [2, 4–6]. The GS/GD/96 lineage has circulated in wild and domestic birds throughout Asia since 1996 with occasional incursions into Europe and Africa. In December 2014, the IcA H5 HPAIVs were first discovered in poultry in Canada, and subsequently in the US a few weeks later [4, 7].

In North America four variants of the IcA H5 viruses were identified; an H5N8 with a genome that was

* Correspondence: Erica.spackman@ars.usda.gov
Southeast Poultry Research Laboratory, USDA-Agricultural Research Service, 934 College Station Rd, Athens, GA 30605, USA

completely Eurasian in lineage (≥98% identity among all gene segments with H5N8 virus isolates from South Korea); and three reassortants with a mixture of North American wild bird lineage genes, an H5N2, an H5N1 and an H5N8 [4, 8, 9]. The H5N2 was the variant that caused the most cases in commercial poultry in the US [10]. Turkey farms had the highest number of infected premises (153 of 211) during this outbreak, but table-egg layer chickens were the poultry type with the highest numbers of birds affected [10]. The goal of these studies was to characterize the pathobiology of the US index H5N2 HPAIV isolate collected from a wild Northern Pintail in December 2014 and to compare that with two poultry isolates from later in the outbreak (April 2015) in commercial broad breasted white turkeys.

Methods

Turkeys

Broad-breasted white turkeys were obtained from a commercial turkey producer and were reared in a commercial production environment from hatch until they were delivered to the Southeast Poultry Research Laboratory-USDA-ARS (SEPRL) at 4 weeks of age. Each bird was individually tagged for identification. The turkeys were housed and cared for in accordance with procedures approved by the SEPRL Institutional Animal Care and Use Committee. Serum was collected from turkeys immediately prior to challenge to confirm the absence of antibody to type A influenza by commercial ELISA (MultiS Screen, IDEXX Inc. Westbrook, ME).

Viruses

Three H5N2 HPAIV isolates were selected for evaluation: the US index H5N2 HPAIV isolate from December 2014, A/Northern Pintail/Washington/40964/2014 (NOPI/40964); and two isolates from commercial poultry operations collected in April 2015, A/turkey/MN/12582/2015 (TK/12582) and A/chicken/IA/13388/2015 (CK/13388). Viruses were provided by the National Veterinary Services Laboratories-USDA-APHIS (Courtesy of Dr. Mia Torchetti). Each isolate was passaged twice in embryonating chickens eggs (ECE) and titrated using standard procedures [11]. Inocula were diluted to the appropriate dose in brain heart infusion (BHI) broth.

Pathogenesis, infectious dose and transmission

To evaluate the infectious dose of each isolate and transmission to non-inoculated hatch-mates housed in the same isolator (contact exposed turkeys), three doses of virus: 10^2, 10^4 and 10^6 50% egg infectious doses (EID_{50}) per bird, were administered to groups of five turkeys as reported in Bertran et al. [12]. Virus was administered using a simulated respiratory route, the intrachoanal route, in 0.1 ml per bird. The contact exposed turkeys ($n = 3$) were added to each dose group 24 h post challenge (PC). Sixteen additional turkeys at the 10^6 EID_{50} per bird dose group were included to characterize the pathogenesis of the virus. Clinical signs and mortality were recorded a minimum of daily and birds that were euthanized due to severe illness were counted as dying the following day for mean death time (MDT) calculations. Turkeys were considered infected if virus was detected in oropharyngeal (OP) or cloacal (CL) swabs at any time point and/or if the bird seroconverted by the end of the experiment (14 days PC).

The later experiments with TK/12582 and CK/13388 had a modified swab collection schedule from what was done with NOPI/40964 because additional sample collection times were added to more precisely establish when the turkeys started to shed detectable levels of virus. For all three isolates, OP and CL swabs were collected from the directly inoculated turkeys at 2, 4, 7, 10 and 14 days PC, and OP and CL swabs were collected from contact exposure turkeys at 1, 3, 6, 9 and 13 days PC. Additional OP and CL samples collected from groups inoculated with TK/12582 and CK/13388 were at 12, 24 and 36 h PC. Virus titers in swabs were evaluated by quantitative real-time RT-PCR. Sera were collected from all surviving turkeys 14 days PC. Sera were tested for antibody by homologous hemagglutination inhibition (HI) assay.

Two to six birds at the 10^6 EID_{50} per bird dose group exposed to each virus were necropsied for tissue collection when clinical signs were apparent. A full set of tissue samples (lungs, bursa, kidneys, adrenal gland, thymus, bursa, brain, liver, heart, proventriculus, pancreas, intestine, spleen, trachea, Harderian gland, beak, and thigh muscle) were collected for microscopic evaluation and immunohistochemistry (IHC). Tissues were fixed in 10% neutral buffered formalin, sectioned, paraffin embedded, and stained with hematoxylin-and-eosin. Serial sections were stained by IHC methods [13] to visualize influenza antigen in individual tissues. An identical tissue set was collected from two non-inoculated hatch-mates to serve as negative controls.

Sera were collected from all surviving turkeys 14 days PC to evaluate infection status by antibody detection with homologous HI assay.

The infectious dose was calculated by the Reed-Muench method [14], using the criteria that turkeys were considered infected if they had clinical signs, died, shed virus or were positive for antibody 14 days PC.

Quantitative real-time RT-PCR

Quantitative real-time RT-PCR targeting the influenza M gene including the RNA extraction, was conducted as previously described [15]. The standard curve was run in duplicate using RNA from the same virus stock used to prepare the inocula. Virus quantity was reported as equivalents to infectious titer.

Hemagglutination inhibition assay

The HI assay was conducted using standard procedures [11]. Homologous isolates were used as antigens and were inactivated with 0.1% beta-propiolactone. A titer of 1:16 (2^4) or above was considered positive.

Statistics

Virus titers shed by time point for the same swab type (OP or CL) were tested among the viruses with Kruskal-Wallis H test (Prism 7, GraphPad Software, La Jolla, CA). A p value of ≤0.05 was considered significant.

Results

Infectious dose and transmission

Infection status was determined based on virus shed, clinical disease, mortality and seroconversion. Turkeys which survived to 14 days were not infected as indicated by lack of virus shed and seroconversion. At each dose and virus combination either 100% of the turkeys were infected or none were infected (Table 1). The 50% turkey infectious dose (TID_{50}) and 50% turkey lethal doses (TLD_{50}) were the same for each isolate and were approximately $10^5 EID_{50}$/bird for NOPI/40964 and TK/12582 but was two $\log_{10}$ lower for CK/13388 which was 10^3 EID_{50}/bird (Table 1).

Infection rates in the contact exposure groups were the same as the inoculated groups to which they were exposed; 100% of the contact exposure turkeys, with all three isolates, at $10^6 EID_{50}$/bird dose group were infected. The only lower dose group where the contact turkeys were infected was the $10^4 EID_{50}$/bird dose group exposed to CK/13388, where 100% (3 of 3) were infected. All the infected contact exposed birds presented with clinical signs similar to the inoculated turkeys and died.

Virus shed

No turkeys exposed to $10^2 EID_{50}$/bird shed detectable levels of virus at any time. Only one group exposed to $10^4 EID_{50}$/bird shed detectable levels of virus: the CK/13388 exposed group (Table 1). In this group, virus was only detected in OP swabs from 3 of 5 turkeys and in CL swabs from 2 of 5 turkeys, although the two turkeys from which virus was not detected both presented with clinical signs consistent with HPAIV and died (one at 24 h PC and the other at 5 days PC).

Oro-pharyngeal and CL shed titers for groups exposed to $10^6 EID_{50}$/bird are shown in Fig. 1. Oro-pharyngeal shedding was detectable at all times and peaked 3–4 days PC for all three isolates with titers exceeding $10^6 EID_{50}$/ml from birds exposed to TK/12528 and CK/13388. Although

Table 1 Mortality, mean death time, 50% infectious dose, 50% lethal dose and number of birds shedding for three H5N2 highly pathogenic avian influenza viruses in 4-week old directly inoculated and contact exposed broad-breasted white turkeys

Isolate	Dose (EID_{50}/bird)	Mortality		Mean death time (days)		Number of turkeys shedding		Seroconversion		50% Turkey infectious dose[e]
		Inoculated	Contact exposed	Inoculated	Contact exposed	Inoculated	Contact exposed	Inoculated	Contact exposed	
A/northern pintail/WA/40964/2014	10^2	0/5[a]	0/3[a]	NA[b]	NA	0/5[d]	0/3[d]	0/5[i]	0/3[i]	10^5 EID^f_{50}
	10^4	0/5	0/3	NA	NA	0/5	0/3	0/5	0/3	
	10^6	5/5	3/3	5.3 (4–7)[gh]	7.6 (7–8)[cg]	5/5	3/3	NA	NA	
	10^6	16/16	NA		NA	16/16	NA	NA	NA	
A/turkey/MN/12582/2015	10^2	0/5	0/3	NA	NA	0/5	0/3	0/5	0/3	10^5 EID_{50}
	10^4	0/5	0/3	NA	NA	0/5	0/3	0/5	0/3	
	10^6	5/5	3/3	5.9 (3–10)	8.0 (6–10)	5/5	3/3	NA	NA	
	10^6	16/16	NA		NA	16/16	NA	NA	NA	
A/chicken/IA/13388/2015	10^2	0/5	0/3	NA	NA	0/5	0/3	0/5	0/3	10^3 EID_{50}
	10^4	5/5	3/3	5.4 (1–7)	9.0 (6–10)	3/5	3/3	NA	NA	
	10^6	5/5	3/3	5.6 (3–13)	7.6 (2–13)	5/5	3/3	NA	NA	
	10^6	16/16	NA		NA	16/16	NA	NA	NA	

[a]Number dead/total
[b]*NA* not applicable. Either no mortality or no birds survived for antibody testing
[c]Calculated from the day of placement with the inoculated turkeys
[d]Number shedding/total
[e]50% infectious dose was equal to the 50% lethal dose for all isolates
[f]EID_{50} = 50% egg infectious dose
[g]Mean death time days (range of mortality in days). For inoculated birds includes data from all 21 turkeys exposed to 10^6 EID_{50}/bird
[h]Mean death times are combined for directly exposed turkeys in the same dose group for each isolate
[i]Number seroconverted/total

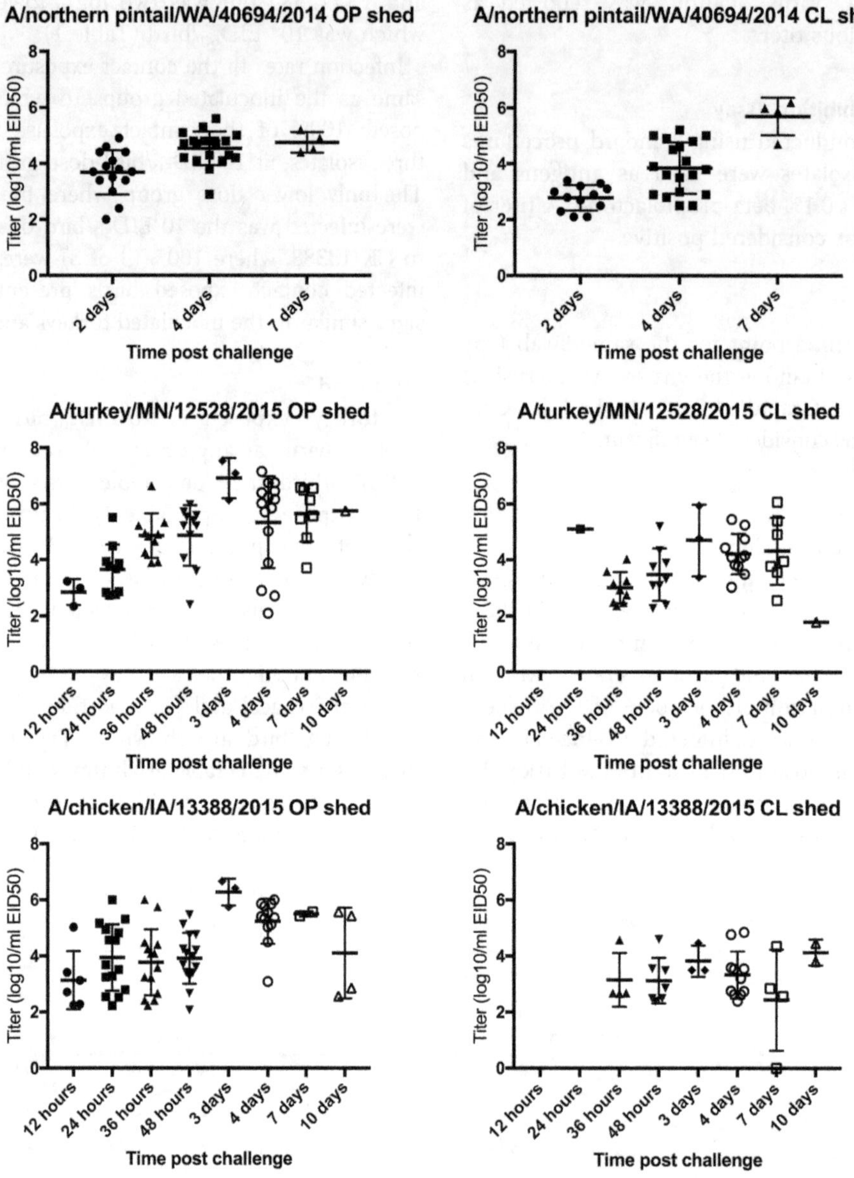

Fig. 1 Oropharyngeal (OP) and cloacal (CL) shed determined by real-time RT-PCR for each virus by time post challenge with 10^6 50% egg infectious doses (EID_{50}) per bird. Data are absent from the A/northen pintail/WA/40964/2014 isolates at 12, 24, 36 h and 3 days because the samples were not collected, at 10 and 14 days because no turkeys survived to these time points. *Thick bars* indicate the mean of the group and *error bars* represent one standard deviation

titers from birds exposed to NOPI/40964 were about one log_{10} lower the difference was not significant. Cloacal shedding also peaked at 3 days PC from birds exposed to TK/12528 and CK/133388, but was later for NOPI/40964 exposed birds where the highest titers were at 7 days PC. Turkeys in the 10^6EID_{50}/bird dose group that survived to 10 days PC were still shedding virus. There were no differences in the numbers of turkeys shedding among the isolates for the 10^6EID_{50}/bird dose group (all were 100%).

Shed titers were compared among all three isolates for all turkeys exposed to 10^6EID_{50}/bird by swab type at 2 and 4 days PC and between TK/12582 and CK/13388 at 12, 24, 36 h and 3DPC (at time points where five or fewer birds were shedding detectable levels of virus statistical analysis was not performed). At 36 h PC the OP titers from TK/12528 were significantly lower than CK/13388. Titers of shed among the viruses were only significantly different at two other times; CK/13388 OP shed titers were significantly lower than either NOPI/40964 or TK/12582 at 2 days PC, and CK/13388 titers were again significantly lower than either other virus with CL at 4 days PC.

Each group of contact exposed turkeys shed virus similarly to the inoculated groups with which they were housed. In the groups housed with the 10^6EID_{50}/bird dose group all (3 of 3) contact exposure turkeys shed virus. In the 10^4EID_{50}/bird dose group for CK/13388, which was the only middle or lower dose group to be infected; all three turkeys shed virus (data not shown).

Pathogenesis

The pathogenesis for all three isolates was similar. Mean death times for the inoculated turkeys were between 5.3 and 5.9 days and were between 7.6 and 9 days post placement for the contact exposed turkeys (Table 1). Clinical disease was not apparent until 24 h or less prior to death (turkeys that could not reach food or water were euthanized). With all three isolates, an average of 50% of the turkeys died without exhibiting any clinical signs within 12 h prior to death (i.e. they appeared normal at the late afternoon/evening observation period and were dead at the morning observation period).

The only clinical signs observed were neurological signs and lethargy. Lethargic birds tended to rest with ruffled body feathers. The severity of neurological signs and lethargy was similar among all three isolates. Neurological signs consisting of torticollis (Fig. 2), tremors or ataxia were observed in 28 and 23% of the turkeys infected with NOPI/40964 and TK/12582, and 50% of the turkeys infected with CK/13388.

Turkeys were selected for necropsy because they were presenting with clinical signs (neurological and/or lethargy). Tissues were collected from six turkeys exposed to NOPI/40964 (4 DPC) and from two turkeys exposed to TK/12582 and two turkeys exposed to CK/13388 (3DPC). Gross lesions were typically absent, however petechial hemorrhages were observed in the skeletal muscle of two turkeys: one infected with TK/12582 and CK/13388 each. The CK/13388 infected turkey with the muscle hemorrhage also had swollen kidneys. A third turkey, infected with TK/12582, also had swollen kidneys. Other lesions were non-specific and were consistent with anorexia and lethargy (i.e. approximately 10% of the turkeys had empty alimentary tracts). In addition, any turkeys dying or that were euthanized were necropsied, but no tissues were taken. Gross lesions were all similar to those observed in the turkeys from which tissues were collected.

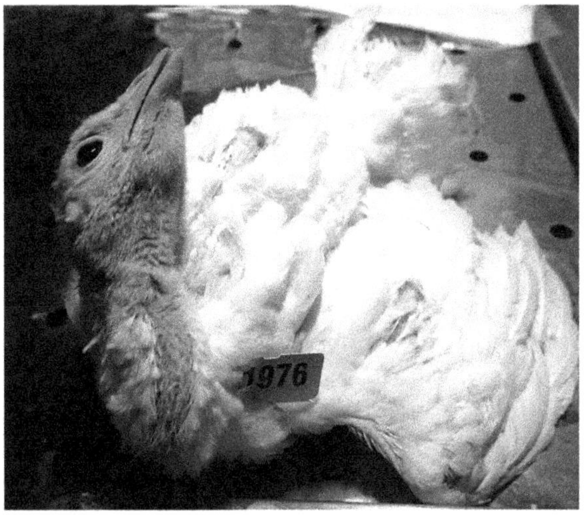

Fig. 2 Four week-old broad-breasted white turkey with torticollis after exposure to A/northern pintail/WA/40964/2014 H5N2 highly pathogenic avian influenza virus

Tissues were examined for microscopic lesions and viral antigen staining (Table 2 and Fig. 3). Microscopic lesions were similar among the eight birds examined, with only minor variations in severity. The most severe lesions were found in the nasal cavity, brain, heart, adrenal gland and pancreas. Moderate to severe rhinitis and sinusitis with multifocal necrosis of the nasal epithelium was common in all birds. Mild tracheitis and bronchitis, and mild to moderate interstitial pneumonia were also present. Mild to severe, randomly disseminated foci of neuronal and glial cell necrosis were observed in the cerebrum and cerebellum of all turkeys examined (Fig. 3a). Microgliosis, edema and mononuclear perivascular cuffs were also commonly observed in malacic areas of the brain. In the heart, mild to moderate multifocal myocyte necrosis was commonly observed (Fig. 3b). Moderate to severe multifocal necrosis of the pancreatic acinar epithelium was present in all birds (Fig. 2c). In the adrenal gland, mild to moderate multifocal to confluent areas of vacuolar degeneration to necrosis of corticotropic cells, and less commonly, chromaffin cells was observed in all but one turkey (Fig. 2d). Thymus, bursa and mucosa-associated lymphoid tissue had moderate to severe lymphoid depletion with apoptosis to necrosis in remaining lymphocytes (Fig. 2e). Mild to moderate depletion of the white pulp with multifocal lymphocytic necrosis was observed in the spleen. Mild to moderate necrosis of the epithelia of the Harderian glands and nasal glands was observed in most turkeys. Infrequently, the kidneys presented mild focal tubular necrosis, and the liver mild multifocal fibrinoid necrosis. Epithelial cell necrosis of the proventricular gland was observed in three turkeys. No lesions were observed in the intestine, eyelid, snood, or skeletal muscle.

Immunohistochemical staining was used to visualize virus distribution in tissues. All three viruses demonstrated similar tissue tropism where the highest levels of viral staining relative to other tissues were observed in the brain, heart, pancreas, and adrenal glands (Table 2). Staining for virus antigen was present in areas of necrosis in many tissues including brain, pancreas, adrenal gland lymphoid tissues, liver, and spleen. Virus antigen was found in parenchymal cells of organs including microglial

Table 2 Distribution of avian influenza virus antigen visualized by immunohistochemical staining in tissues by isolate

Bird ID	Detection of avian influenza virus antigen in tissues															
	Nasal epithelium	Nasal glands	Trachea	Lung	Heart	Brain	Liver	Kidney	Adrenal gland	Spleen	Intestine	Pancreas	Harderian gland	Thymus	Bursa	Proventric
A/Northern Pintail/WA/40964/2014																
1043	+	+	−	+	++	+++	+	+	+++	+	+	+++	−	−	+	−
1045	+	++	−	+	+	+++	−	−	+++	−	+	+++	++	++	+	−
1047	+	+	−	+	+	+++	+	+	+++	+	+	+++	+	+	++	+
1052	+	++	−	+	−	+++	+	++	++	−	−	+		+	+	−
1053	+	++	−	−	++	+++	+	+	++	−	++	+++	+	+	++	−
1056	++	++	+	++	++	+++	+	++	+++	−	+++	++	+	++	++	+
A/turkey/MN/12528/2015																
1093	++	+++	−	+	++	+++	−	+	−	−	−	++	+	+	+	−
1097	+	++	+	+	+++	+++	++	+	++	+	−	++	+++	+	+	+++
A/chicken/IA/13388/2015																
1040	+	+	−	+	+++	+++	+	+	+++	+	−	+++	+	−	+	−
1050	+	++	−	+	++	+++	−	+	++	−	−	+++	−	+	++	−

Turkeys were selected for examination because they were presenting with clinical illness at 4 days post challenge (DPC) (A/Northern Pintail/WA/40964/2014) or 3DPC (A/turkey/MN/12528/2015 and A/chicken/IA/13388/2015)

− = no positive cells; + = single positive cells; ++ = scattered groups of positive cells; +++ = widespread staining

Proventric. = proventriculus

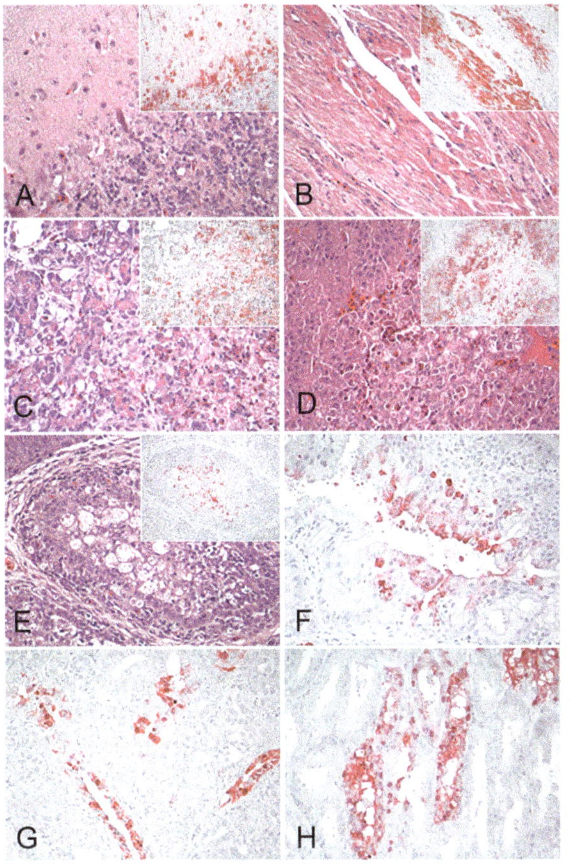

Fig. 3 Histological lesions and immunohistochemical detection of viral antigen in 4-week-old turkeys intranasally inoculated with H5N2 HPAI viruses. Tissues collected at 4 days post-inoculation. Virus antigen is stained in *red*. Magnifications 40×. **a** Cerebellum. Vacuolation of the molecular and granular layers of the cerebellum with necrosis of the Purkinge neurons. *Inset*: viral antigen in neurons and glial cells. **b** Heart. Focal hyalinization and fragmentation of cardiac myocytes. *Inset*: viral antigen in cardiac myocytes. **c** Pancreas. Diffuse pancreatic necrosis. *Inset*: viral staining in acinar epithelium. **d** Adrenal gland. Confluent necrosis of corticotrophic and chromaffin cells. *Inset*: viral antigen in adrenal corticotrophic and cromaffin cells. **e** Bursa de Fabricious. Lymphoid depletion with apoptosis to necrosis in remaining lymphocytes. *Inset*: viral antigen in phagocytic c and necrotic cells. **f** Harderian gland. Viral antigen present in epithelial cells and infiltrating phagocytes. **g** Nasal gland. Viral antigen present in glandular epithelial cells and infiltrating phagocytes. **h** Proventriculus. Viral antigen present in glandular epithelial cells

cells and neurons, cardiac myocytes, pancreatic acinar cells, adrenal corticotropic and chromaffin cells (Fig. 3a-d), hepatocytes, and kidney tubular epithelial cells. Viral staining was common in resident and infiltrating phagocytes of the thymus, bursa and spleen (Fig. 3e). Viral antigen was also present in epithelial cells and macrophage in the nasal turbinates, trachea, Harderian gland (Fig. 3f), nasal glands (Fig. 3g); and proventricular gland cells (Fig. 3h). No viral antigen was observed in vascular endothelial cells.

Discussion

The pathogenesis of three H5N2 HPAIV isolates from the US 2014–2015 outbreak were characterized in commercial broad breasted white turkeys. These H5N2 isolates, which were first isolated in North America in Canada, represent novel AIV reassortants with genes from Eurasian viruses: a GS/GD/96 derived HA, Eurasian PB2, PA, M and NS genes, and North American wild bid virus lineage PB1, NP, NA genes [7]. The US index isolate, NOPI/40964, was selected to represent the earliest introductions detected in the US and the H5N2 HPAIV variants which are mostly likely to be adapted to wild birds. Two later isolates from the Midwest, TK/12582 and CK/13388, were selected in real-time during the outbreak to represent isolates that had likely been passaged in gallinaceous poultry based on a relatively severe clinical presentation in the field and initial epidemiological information. Based on subsequent sequence analysis and field epidemiology, the TK/12582 isolate was probably an introduction either directly from waterfowl or soon thereafter and may not have been passaged extensively in gallinaceous poultry (unpublished data). In contrast, based on the same analysis, CK/13388 may have circulated in poultry longer. This would corroborate the infectious dose data where the TK/12582 and NOPI/40964 isolates each required a TID_{50} 2 log_{10} higher dose than the CK/13388.

In fact, the TID_{50} and TLD_{50} were the only differences observed among the three isolates. All three primarily presented with neurological signs and severe lethargy during the 24 h prior to death, and virus distribution among the tissues was similar. Microscopic lesions produced by all three isolates were typical for HPAIV in turkeys and other gallinaceous birds. Importantly, a high level of virus was observed in the brain by IHC, which could account for injury to the brain resulting in neurological signs.

Although the clinical presentations among all three isolates were similar, the pathogenesis of these isolates had some unusual characteristics for HPAIV. First, the MDT's, which were between 5.3 and 5.9 days, and the pre-clinical period were atypically long and mortality was distributed over a 10 day period with some turkeys dying as late as 13 days PC. By contrast, most HPAIV produce MDTs ranging between 2 and 4 days and death has been associated with replication of virus in blood vessel endothelial cells with vascular thrombosis or embolism and multi-organ failure [16, 17]. However, in this study, neural pathogenesis has been associated with direct replication of virus in neurons and neuropil support cells without vascular endothelial cells involvement, and accompanied by replication in other critical organ parenchymal cells leading to multi-organ failure, as has been shown with some previous HPAIV infections [17]. The even longer MDTs with the contact exposed turkeys are most likely because it took a day or two for the turkeys to become infected. Also, since the environment is artificial (e.g. grate floor isolators limiting coprophagy, high rate of airflow, etc.) the results with the contacts cannot be extrapolated directly to the field, and only provide a relative measure of transmissibility among isolates tested in similar ways.

Secondly, each of these viruses was shed at relatively high titers by the cloacal route. Highly pathogenic AIV is more often shed at the highest titers by the oral/respiratory route in gallinaceous birds [16]. It is possible that the late onset of morbidity and mortality, and high virus titers in manure contributed to the rapid spread of the virus in the Midwest, especially in light of the relatively high TID_{50}. Essentially the turkeys are infected and are shedding substantial amounts of virus in their manure and orally as early as 24–36 post infection for several days, but don't appear sick.

One aspect of the field situation that was not replicated in the laboratory was the age of the turkeys. During the outbreak 85% of the infected turkey flocks were at least 9 weeks of age (57% of affected turkeys were 12 or greater weeks of age) [10]. Unfortunately, facilities which can work with HPAIV often cannot accommodate broad-breasted white turkeys in isolation cabinets over about 7 weeks of age because of their size, so it was not possible to determine if turkey age affected susceptibility for biological reasons or whether older birds have a higher chance of exposure because they have been around for a longer period of time (or a combination of both) as animal facilities with the appropriate biosafety level for floor pen studies were not available.

Relatively little data has been reported regarding experimental infection of turkeys with HPAIV and none with isolates from this lineage (clade 2.3.4.4 H5 isolates). Experimental pathogenesis studies in birds have characterized H5N8 HPAIV isolates in chickens and ducks [18–23] and the pathogenesis of NOPI/40964 H5N2 HPAIV in chickens has been reported [12]. The 50% infectious dose in chickens was similar at $10^{5.7}$ EID_{50} (versus $10^{5.0}$ EID_{50} in turkeys). Notably there were differences between the pathogenesis of NOPI/40964 in chickens and turkeys: the MDT was 3 days in chickens versus 5.3 days in turkeys and the clinical presentation was also different. Neurological signs were more common in turkeys (only 1 of 10 chickens presented with neurological signs) and there were lesions unique to chickens: 1) petechial hemorrhages and cyanotic combs and wattles (turkey snoods appeared normal); and 2) infra-orbital swelling [12]. Differences in lesions between chickens and turkeys were also observed with H5N2 HPAI in the field in Canada [7] and with a 1997 H5N1 HPAIV GS/GD/96 lineage virus [24]. Similar clinical presentation (i.e. neurological signs) and gross lesions in turkeys in the field were observed in the UK with a GS/GD/96 lineage H5N1 HPAIV [25] and with the unrelated H5N8 HPAIV in Ireland in 1983 [26]. Based on limited information from field reports, lack of respiratory signs is not uncommon in turkeys with HPAIV [7, 25, 26], although respiratory signs were reported with an H5N2 HPAIV in Italy in 1997 [27]. However, in field cases the involvement of secondary bacterial infections cannot be ruled out.

Conclusions

High mortality is the most consistent sign of HPAIV infection in turkeys as there are some biological variations in the pathogenesis of the virus. In the case of these three isolates, the long pre-clinical period, late MDT and high titers of cloacal shed are unusual characteristics and may have contributed to spread despite the initially high exposure dose to produce infection; i.e. high TID_{50}. Also, neurological signs were the most common clinical sign after severe lethargy observed in the turkeys, which contrasts chickens, where hemorrhagic lesions are reported more frequently. This and a shorter reported MDT in chickens highlights the difference in pathogenesis of HPAIV between chickens and turkeys. Finally, there are many other factors involved in the spread of HPAIV in poultry; attention to biosecurity should be a priority regardless of the characteristics of the lineages involved.

Acknowledgements

The authors thank David Rives and Eric Gonder for providing turkeys; Carol Cardona for information on isolates in field; and Mia Torchetti for providing the viruses. We also thank: Scott Lee, Aniko Zsak, Diane Smith, Kira Moresco, Roger Brock, Gerald Damron for technical assistance with this work.

Funding

This research was supported by US Department of Agriculture, ARS CRIS Project 6612-32000-063-00D and with federal funds from the National Institute of Allergy and Infectious Diseases, National Institutes of Health, under IAA No. AAI12004-001-00001. Its contents are solely the responsibility of the authors and do not necessarily represent the official views of the NIH. Mention of trade names or commercial products in this manuscript is solely for the purpose of providing specific information and does not imply recommendation or endorsement by the U.S. Department of Agriculture. USDA is an equal opportunity provider and employer.

Authors' contributions

All authors contributed to the experimental design and editing the manuscript. ES: conducted the bird work and related lab work, and composed the manuscript. MPJ: evaluated the microscopic lesions and ran the immunohistochemistry. All authors read and approved the final manuscript.

Competing interests

The authors declare that they have no competing interests.

Consent for publication

Not applicable.

References

1. Testimony of Dr. Tom Elam. US Senate Committee on Agricultre, Nutrition and Forestry. Full Committee Hearing on Highly Pathogenic Avian Influenza: The Impact on the U.S. Poultry Sector and Protecting U.S. Poultry Flocks, July 7, 2015. http://www.agriculture.senate.gov/hearings/highly-pathogenic-avian-influenza-the-impact-on-the-us-poultry-sector-and-protecting-us-poultry-flocks
2. Lee DH, Torchetti MK, Winker K, Ip HS, Song CS, Swayne DE. Intercontinental spread of Asian-origin H5N8 to north America through Beringia by migratory birds. J Virol. 2015;89(12):6521–4.
3. Lee DH, Bahl J, Torchetti MK, Killian ML, Ip HS, DeLiberto TJ, Swayne DE. Highly pathogenic avian influenza viruses and generation of novel reassortants, United States, 2014–2015. Emerg Infect Dis. 2016;22(7):1283–5.
4. Ip HS, Torchetti MK, Crespo R, Kohrs P, DeBruyn P, Mansfield KG, Baszler T, Badcoe L, Bodenstein B, Shearn-Bochsler V, et al. Novel Eurasian highly pathogenic avian influenza A H5 viruses in wild birds, Washington, USA, 2014. Emerg Infect Dis. 2015;21(5):886–90.
5. Kwon JH, Lee DH, Swayne DE, Noh JY, Yuk SS, Erdene-Ochir TO, Hong WT, Jeong JH, Jeong S, Gwon GB, et al. Highly Pathogenic Avian Influenza A(H5N8) Viruses Reintroduced into South Korea by Migratory Waterfowl, 2014–2015. Emerg Infect Dis. 2016;22(3):507–10.
6. Verhagen JH, van der Jeugd HP, Nolet BA, Slaterus R, Kharitonov SP, de Vries PP, Vuong O, Majoor F, Kuiken T, Fouchier RA. Wild bird surveillance around outbreaks of highly pathogenic avian influenza A(H5N8) virus in the Netherlands, 2014, within the context of global flyways. Euro Surveill. 2015;20(12).
7. Pasick J, Berhane Y, Joseph T, Bowes V, Hisanaga T, Handel K, Alexandersen S. Reassortant highly pathogenic influenza A H5N2 virus containing gene segments related to Eurasian H5N8 in British Columbia, Canada, 2014. Sci Rep. 2015;5:9484.
8. Torchetti MK, Killian ML, Dusek RJ, Pedersen JC, Hines N, Bodenstein B, White CL, Ip HS. Novel H5 Clade 2.3.4.4 Reassortant (H5N1) Virus from a Green-Winged Teal in Washington, USA. Genome Announc. 2015;3(2): e00195–15.
9. Lee DH, Bahl J, Torchetti MK, Killian M, Ip HS, Deliberto T, Swayne DE. Asian H5N8 HPAI virus spread into North America in late 2014 and produced novel H5N1, H5N2, and H5N8 viruses by reassortment events. Emerg Infect Dis. 2016;22(7): in press
10. USDA-APHIS. Epidemiologic and Other Analyses of HPAI-Affected Poultry Flocks. September 9, 2015, Doc #300.0615 Version 5. https://www.aphis.usda.gov/aphis/ourfocus/animalhealth/animal-disease-information/avian-influenza-disease/ct_avian_influenza_disease. 2015
11. Pedersen JC. Hemagglutination-inhibition assay for influenza virus subtype identification and the detection and quantitation of serum antibodies to influenza virus. Methods Mol Biol. 2014;1161:11–25.
12. Bertran K, Swayne DE, Pantin-Jackwood MJ, Kapczynski DR, Spackman E, Suarez DL. Lack of chicken adaptation of newly emergent Eurasian H5N8 and reassortant H5N2 high pathogenicity avian influenza viruses in the U.S. is consistent with restricted poultry outbreaks in the Pacific flyway during 2014–2015. Virology. 2016;494:190–7.
13. Pantin-Jackwood MJ. Immunohistochemical staining of influenza virus in tissues. Methods Mol Biol. 2014;1161:51–8.
14. Reed LJ, Muench H. A simple method for estimating fifty percent endpoints. Am J Hyg. 1938;27:493–7.
15. Spackman E. Avian influenza virus detection and quantitation by real-time RT-PCR. Methods Mol Biol. 2014;1161:105–18.
16. Swayne DE, Suarez DL, Sims LD. Influenza. In: Swayne D, editor. Diseases of poultry. 13th ed. Ames: Blackwell; 2013. p. 181–218.
17. Swayne D, Pantin-Jackwood M. Pathobiology of avian influenza virus infections in birds and mammals. In: Swayne D, editor. Avian influenza. Ames: Blackwell; 2008. p. 87–122.
18. Kanehira K, Uchida Y, Takemae N, Hikono H, Tsunekuni R, Saito T. Characterization of an H5N8 influenza A virus isolated from chickens during an outbreak of severe avian influenza in Japan in April 2014. Arch Virol. 2015;160(7):1629–43.
19. Kang HM, Lee EK, Song BM, Jeong J, Choi JG, Jeong J, Moon OK, Yoon H, Cho Y, Kang YM, et al. Novel reassortant influenza A(H5N8) viruses among inoculated domestic and wild ducks, south Korea, 2014. Emerg Infect Dis. 2015;21(2):298–304.
20. Kim YI, Pascua PN, Kwon HI, Lim GJ, Kim EH, Yoon SW, Park SJ, Kim SM, Choi EJ, Si YJ, et al. Pathobiological features of a novel, highly pathogenic avian influenza A(H5N8) virus. Emerg Microbes Infect. 2014;3(10):e75.
21. Lee DH, Kwon JH, Noh JY, Park JK, Yuk SS, Erdene-Ochir TO, Lee JB, Park SY, Choi IS, Lee SW, et al. Pathogenicity of the Korean H5N8 highly pathogenic avian influenza virus in commercial domestic poultry species. Avian Pathol. 2016;45(2):208–11.
22. Lee EK, Song BM, Kang HM, Woo SH, Heo GB, Jung SC, Park YH, Lee YJ, Kim JH. Experimental infection of SPF and Korean native chickens with highly pathogenic avian influenza virus (H5N8). Poult Sci. 2016;95(5):1015–9.
23. Song BM, Kang HM, Lee EK, Jeong J, Kang Y, Lee HS, Lee YJ. Pathogenicity of H5N8 Highly Pathogenic Avian Influenza Virus in Chickens, South Korea. J Vet Sci. 2015;16(2):237-40.
24. Perkins LE, Swayne DE. Pathobiology of A/chicken/Hong Kong/220/97 (H5N1) avian influenza virus in seven gallinaceous species. Vet Pathol. 2001;38(2):149–64.
25. Irvine RM, Banks J, Londt BZ, Lister SA, Manvell RJ, Outtrim L, Russell C, Cox WJ, Ceeraz V, Shell W, et al. Outbreak of highly pathogenic avian influenza caused by Asian lineage H5N1 virus in turkeys in Great Britain in January 2007. Vet Rec. 2007;161(3):100–1.
26. McNulty MS, Allan GM, McCracken RM, McParland PJ. Isolation of a highly pathogenic influenza virus from turkeys. Avian Pathol. 1985;14(1):173–6.
27. Capua I, Marangon S, Selli L, Alexander DJ, Swayne DE, Pozza MD, Parenti E, Cancellotti FM. Outbreaks of highly pathogenic avian influenza (H5N2) in Italy during October 1997 to January 1998. Avian Pathol. 1999;28(5):455–60.

14

Canine influenza virus coinfection with *Staphylococcus pseudintermedius* enhances bacterial colonization, virus load and clinical presentation in mice

Dildar Hussain Kalhoro[†], Shanshan Gao[†], Xing Xie, Shan Liang, Su Luo, Yanbing Zhao and Yongjie Liu[*]

Abstract

Background: Canine influenza virus (CIV) and *Staphylococcus pseudintermedius* (Sp) are pathogens that cause respiratory disease in dogs. Considering bacterial infections following influenza are a leading cause of illness and death, it is of particular meaning to investigate the interaction between these two pathogens. In this study, BALB/c mice were used as a mouse model to assess whether inoculation with CIV H3N2 followed by *S. pseudintermedius* 72 h later resulted in exacerbation of disease. Disease was characterized by assessment of body weight loss, titration of virus and bacteria, histopathology, and cytokine production.

Results: There was a significantly greater decrease in body weight in the co-infected group compared with the CIV-only and SP-only groups. CIV inoculation increased bacterial colonization, whereas secondary infection with *S. pseudintermedius* elevated the viral RNA load of CIV in tissues. The histological lesions in the brain, spleen and lung were more severe in the CIV/Sp group than in the singly treated groups. Infection with CIV alone, Sp alone or coinfection stimulated a significantly higher release of cytokines, such as interferon-gamma (IFN)-γ, interleukin 6 (IL) -6, tumor necrosis factor (TNF-α) and lymphotactin (Lptn), than was observed in the mock-infected group (PBS). Moreover, the levels of IFN-γ in the spleen and lung were higher in the CIV/Sp group compared with the CIV-only and Sp-only groups.

Conclusion: Our findings provide the first demonstration that the secondary infection of mice with Sp leads to increased clinical signs and lesions during canine influenza.

Keywords: canine influenza virus, *Staphylococcus pseudintermedius*, coinfection, pathological lesions, mice

Background

Canine infectious respiratory disease (CIRD) is a common, worldwide disease syndrome, and involves a number of viral and bacterial pathogens. Canine influenza virus (CIV) is one of the viral causes of contagious respiratory disease [1]. In January 2004, CIV subtype H3N8 was first reported in racing greyhound dogs in Florida [2]. Subsequently, in 2007, a different influenza virus, subtype H3N2, caused an outbreak of canine respiratory disease in South Korea [3]. Recent reports suggest that H3N2 CIV has become endemic in the canine populations in China [4–6].

Bacterial pathogens associated with CIRD include *Bordetella bronchiseptica*, *Streptococcus equi* subspecies *zooepidemicus* and *Mycoplasma* [7]. In humans, Staphylococcal species are frequently identified as the cause of bacterial pneumonia [8, 9]. A study from our group showed that *Staphylococcus pseudintermedius* (Sp) was the most frequently isolated bacterial pathogen (24/40) from respiratory cases (unpublished data). This bacterium has been previously misidentified as *S. intermedius*. The name *S. pseudintermedius* is now given to the canine-specific strain of *S. intermedius* [10]. *S. pseudintermedius* is a common commensal of oral and nasal

* Correspondence: liuyongjie@njau.edu.cn
[†]Equal contributors
College of Veterinary Medicine, Nanjing Agricultural University, Nanjing 210095, China

vacities and the skin in healthy dogs, where it can also cause invasive disease [11, 12]. Sasaki et al. [13] isolated Sp from inpatient dogs (46.2 %) and outpatient dogs (19.4 %) in a Japanese veterinary teaching hospital. Some recent reports confirmed this bacterium can spread from pets to their owners [14, 15] and to the veterinary staff working in the veterinary clinics [16]. Furthermore, methicillin resistant *S. pseudintermedius* (MRSP) has emerged as an increasingly important cause of opportunistic infections in dogs [17]. It may emerge as a major and difficult-to-treat pathogen in the future.

In humans, co-infections of influenza virus and respiratory bacterial pathogens are common, and bacterial secondary infections have played an important role in influenza virus pandemics [18, 19]. Influenza pneumonia occurs mainly due to virus-bacteria interactions because of a synergistic effect that occurs during invasion of the respiratory tract [20]. Epithelial and mucosal degradation occurs due to viral replication, resulting in a reduced innate immune response to prevent secondary bacterial infections [21]. Thus, bacterial infections may be the main cause of death related to influenza virus infection in the absence of a pre-existing co-morbidity [22, 23].

Although CIV infection is typically self-limited with high-morbidity but low mortality, co-infections with respiratory bacterial pathogens may impact the pathogenicity and course of disease. It will be of particular importance considering the role of secondary bacterial infections as a major complication of influenza in pet clinics. To understand the treatment procedures for fighting viral and secondary bacterial infections, it is important to study the mechanisms involved in the interaction between influenza virus and bacterial organisms. In the present study, we investigated the interactions between CIV and Sp and evaluated pathological lesions in mice.

Methods

Infectious agents

The viral strain A/Canine/Jiangsu/06/2010 (H3N2) was used in this study. The viral strain was isolated from nasopharyngeal swabs of dogs with severe respiratory syndrome, which were collected from Animal Clinics of Nanjing Agricultural University in Jiangsu Province of China in 2010. The GenBank accession numbers are JN247615 to JN247623. Plaque assays were performed on monolayers of Madin-Darby canine kidney (MDCK) cells in 12-well tissue culture plates to determine the viral titres [24]. Viral aliquots were diluted in phosphate-buffered saline (PBS) supplemented with 0.1 % bovine serum albumin and adjusted to a final concentration of $1x10^5$ plaque forming units (PFU)/ml [25]. The Sp NJ-1 strain was isolated from a dog with respiratory syndrome. The bacterial species was identified based on its biochemical characteristics [26] and sequencing of the 16S rRNA gene. To prepare the inoculum, the bacterial strain was cultured in Luria–Bertani (LB) broth at 37 °C for 4 h. A suspension with approximately $1x10^9$ colony forming units (CFU)/ml was made in phosphate-buffered saline (PBS).

Mice

BALB/c mice (6 weeks of age, 18–20 g) were purchased from the Animal Experiment Centre, Yangzhou University, China. All of the mice were housed in individual compartments in stainless-steel wire cages. Before conducting the study, approval for conducting the experiments was obtained from the Animal Ethics Committee of Nanjing Agricultural University.

Animal experiments

One hundred mice were randomly divided into four groups with 25 mice per group. The mice in group 1 (Sp-only) were intranasally inoculated with Sp(1×10^9 CFU/ml, 50 μl/mouse) and 72 h later inoculated with non-infectious MDCK cell culture supernatant (50 μl/mouse); the mice in group 2 (CIV-only) were intranasally inoculated with PBS (50 μl/mouse) and 72 h later inoculated with CIV (1×10^5 PFU/ml, 50 μl/mouse); the mice in group 3 (CIV/Sp) were intranasally inoculated with CIV and 72 h later inoculated with Sp; and the mice in group 4 were inoculated with non-infectious MDCK cell culture supernatant and 72 h later inoculated with PBS. The groups were housed in individual isolation rooms.

The daily weight and clinical signs were recorded for up to five days. The observers were blinded as to the experimental treatments and they had veterinary medical qualifications to make assessments about clinical signs. Three mice from each group were killed humanely according to a pre-designated schedule at indicated time points. Blood samples from the experimental groups were collected using sodium heparin tubes from the eyeball capillary before collecting tissues, including spleen, lung and brain, at 1, 2, 3, 4 and 5 days post-infection (d.p.i.).

Pathological analysis

The lung, spleen and brain tissues from mice belonging to the various groups were harvested at 2 days post Sp challenge in the co-infected group and were fixed in 10 % formalin. After fixation, the tissues were embedded in paraffin wax. Tissue sections with a thickness of 4 μm were stained with haematoxylin and eosin (H&E) and assessed for the degree of inflammation and necrosis. The lungs were assigned a grade 0 to 3 based on the histological characteristics as described by Alymova et al. [27]. A score of 0 was given when no pathological changes could be detected. A score of 1 was given to findings representing mild pathologies, including minimal infiltrates of lymphocytes and plasma cells around airways and vessels, minimal epithelial hyperplasia, minimal leukocyte infiltration of alveolar spaces, and <10 % of the lung affected. A score of 2 was given for findings representing moderate pathologies, including moderate infiltrates of lymphocytes and plasma cells around airways and vessels, moderate epithelial hyperplasia with focal necrosis, focally extensive infiltration of the alveolar spaces by leukocytes with some consolidation, focal pleuritis, and >10 % but <30 % of the lung affected. A score of 3 was given for findings representing pathologies of greater severity, including extensive necrosis of airway epithelium and of interstitium, extensive leukocyte infiltration and consolidation, severe pleuritis, and lobar involvement. Grading and descriptions of pathology were performed by an experienced veterinary pathologist in a single-blinded manner.

Bacterial isolation

Samples of lung, spleen and brain from each mouse were weighed and homogenized individually in PBS to obtain a 10 % weight-to-volume suspension. The number of CFUs of Sp was determined by plating serial 10-fold dilutions of homogenates or blood on LB agar in duplicate. Therefore, the results are reported as CFU/ml for blood and as CFU/g for the lung, spleen and brain.

Determination of viral loads

The tissues were homogenized in lysates at a ratio of 1:1 (g/ml) and centrifuged at 10,000 *g* for 30 min, and the supernatants were collected for viral RNA extraction using a Virus Nucleic Acid Extraction Kit II (Geneaid, Taiwan). Quantitative RT-PCR (RT-qPCR) was performed to measure the viral loads in the above-mentioned organs and blood samples. The RNA from the samples was reverse-transcribed and run in an ABI 7300 Real-time PCR System using a SYBR1 Premix Ex Taq™ (Perfect Real Time) kit (TaKaRa, Dalian). The following primers were designed and used on the matrix gene region: 5′-TCTATCGTCCCATCAGGC/GGTCTTGT CTTTAGCCATTC-3′. Simple Vector pMD19-T (50 ng/μl; TaKaRa, Dalian) containing the target virus sequence was used as a reference standard. Series of eight 10-fold dilutions equivalent to 1×10^3-1×10^{10} copies per reaction were prepared to generate calibration curves and were run in parallel with the test samples [28].

Quantification of cytokine levels

The cytokine level was assessed to determine the correlation between severe disease and inflammatory cytokine production in the mice. The spleen and lung from the mice in all of the groups were homogenized in 1 ml of PBS/1 g of tissues. The homogenates were centrifuged, and the supernatants were frozen at −70 °C until testing. ELISAs for the levels of interferon-gamma (IFN-γ), interleukin 6 (IL-6), lymphotactin (Lptn) and tumor necrosis factor (TNF-α) on the lung and spleen from infected mice were performed using ELISA kits (Sigma-Aldrich, Beijing) according to the manufacturer's instructions.

Statistical analysis

The data were collected and analysed using MS Excel 2010 and SPSS Statistics v20.0 software. The weight loss/gain, bacterial load, viral load and cytokine levels were analysed by analysis of variance (ANOVA) followed by Turkey's multiple comparison test [29, 30]. Differences with $P<0.05$ were considered statistically significant, and differences with $P<0.01$ were considered highly significant.

Results

Clinical signs during experimental infection in the mice

The mice showed normal features after bacterial inoculation, but after 18 h post-infection (h.p.i), all the infected mice manifested with lethargy, anorexia, huddling and ruffled fur. It is notable that nervous signs appeared in the mice of SP (2/25) and CIV/Sp (4/25) groups at 20 h.p.i. On 2 d.p.i., this phenomenon was more pronounced. Distinct central nervous disturbances, including bending of their head towards one side and walking in circles, were observed in the Sp and CIV/Sp groups. More severe clinical signs were observed in the CIV/Sp group when the mice were lifted by the tail. Such neurological signs lasted until the end of experiment. But the number of affected mice did not increase. Mice with neurological signs lost more body weight compared with the other mice in the same group. In contrast, the mice in the CIV group did not show any neurological signs, but the signs, such as depression, decreased activity, huddling and ruffled fur, were witnessed in all the infected mice from 24 h.p.i., and lasted until the end of experiment

Body weight changes in mice

All of the infected groups exhibited a lowered body weight compared with the PBS group (Fig. 1, Additional file 1). Mice inoculated with virus alone showed mild to modest disease severity. There was a significant difference ($P<0.05$) between the sham and CIV groups only at 4 and 5 d.p.i. In contrast, Sp-alone-inoculated mice showed signs of more severe illness, and there was a significant difference between the sham and Sp groups ($P<0.001$) at each time point. Significant differences were also observed between the sham and CIV/Sp groups ($P<0.001$) at each time point. Mice coinfected with CIV and Sp lost more body weight compared with the mice in both the CIV-only ($P<0.001$) and Sp-only ($P<0.05$ or $P<0.01$) groups at 2, 3, 4 and 5 d.p.i., indicating that mice coinfected with

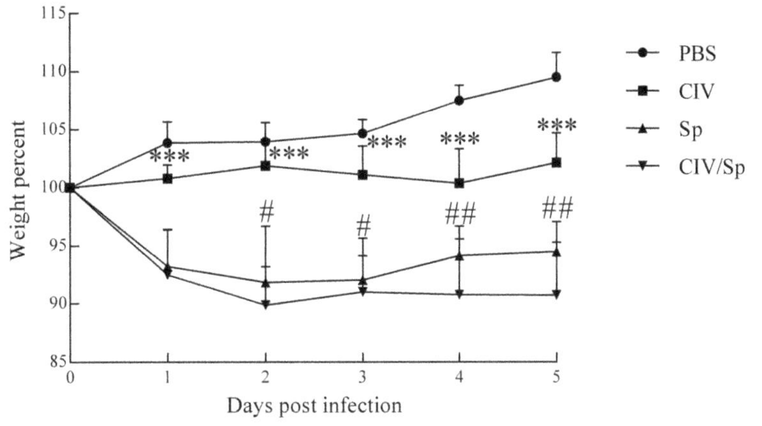

Fig. 1 Changes in the body weights of BALB/c mice that were infected with CIV or *S. pseudintermedius* alone, coinfected with both, or exposed to PBS as a control. The percentage of the body weight was calculated relative to the body weights recorded five days post-challenge. Analysis of variance (ANOVA) was performed for the statistical analysis. ***, $P < 0.001$, indicates a significantly different weight percent for CIV groups compared with CIV/Sp groups. #, $P < 0.05$, ##, $P < 0.01$, or ###, $P < 0.001$, indicates a significantly different weight percent for Sp groups compared with CIV/Sp groups

CIV followed by *S. pseudintermedius* developed more severe disease.

Determination of viable bacteria and viral RNA loads in the tissues of infected mice

The bacterial loads in the blood, brain, spleen and lungs of mice infected with bacteria alone and with both virus and bacteria were compared (Fig. 2, Additional file 1). At each time point, the bacterial load in all of the tissues of the coinfected group was relatively higher than that in the bacteria- alone group, but the statistically significant differences were not necessarily found in each tissue. At 1 d.p.i., the bacterial load in the blood, lung and brain was slightly higher in the CIV/SP group compared with that in the Sp-only group, but the difference was not significant (P>0.05). However, the bacterial loads in the spleen showed significantly higher level in the CIV/Sp group than in the Sp-only group (P<0.01). At 2 d.p.i., the bacterial loads in the blood, brain, spleen and lung had reached a peak level, and showed a significant higher level in the blood, spleen and lung of the coinfection group compared to the SP-lonely group (P<0.05 or P < 0.01). At 3 d.p.i., bacterial load was significantly higher in the spleen of CIV/Sp group than that in the SP-lonely group (P<0.01), and at 5 d.p.i., the bacterial loads in the blood, brain, spleen and lung were decreased to more than 10^2, 10^5, 10^4 and 10^4 CFU/g (CFU/ml) in both the two groups, respectively.

RT-qPCR was used to measure the viral loads in the above tissues of mice infected with virus alone and with both virus and bacteria (Fig. 3, Additional file 1). At all time-points that virus was detected at, the viral load in all the tissues of the coinfected group was higher than that in the virus-alone group. Statistically, compared to CIV-only group, the viral loads in the blood was significantly higher at 3, 4 and 5 d.p.i. in the CIV/Sp group. The brain showed more significant changes. At each time point, brain viral loads in the CIV/Sp group were higher. The viral loads in the CIV/Sp group showed significantly higher levels in the spleen at 4 d.p.i. and in the lung at 2 d.p.i than those in CIV-only group.

Histopathology

The extent of histological lesions in the brain, spleen and lungs of mice infected with CIV/Sp and with either Sp or CIV alone was compared at 2 d.p.i. All of the tissues tested in the Sp-only, CIV-only and CIV/Sp groups showed significant lesions, whereas the mice in the PBS group showed no lesions in the lungs, brain and spleen (Fig. 4).

The brain of the mice in the CIV-only group exhibited the dissolution of nerve fibres. In some areas, a diffused hyperplasia of microglial cells was noticed. In addition, the disintegration of neuronal cells was observed (Fig. 4a). The brain of the mice in the Sp-only group showed dissolution of a large area of nerve fibres. The microglial cells were severely diffused. The characterizing feature of the Sp group was the appearance of vascular cuff and neurophagia phenomena (Fig. 4b). Microscopic lesions in coinfected mice included changes seen in mice infected with single agents, but tended to be more severe than in mice infected with either agent alone. The nerve fibre dissolution observed in the CIV/Sp group was more obvious compared with that in the other two groups, and the disappearance of neurons was also observed (Fig. 4c). The spleen in the CIV-only group did not present any lesions (Fig. 4e). Histopathological lesions in spleens from Sp-infected mice were characterized by marked accumulations of macrophages, which expanded marginal zones, and there was hyperplasia of the lymphoid tissue in the spleen trabeculae (Fig. 4f). But the lesions in the spleens from the CIV/Sp group (Fig. 4g)

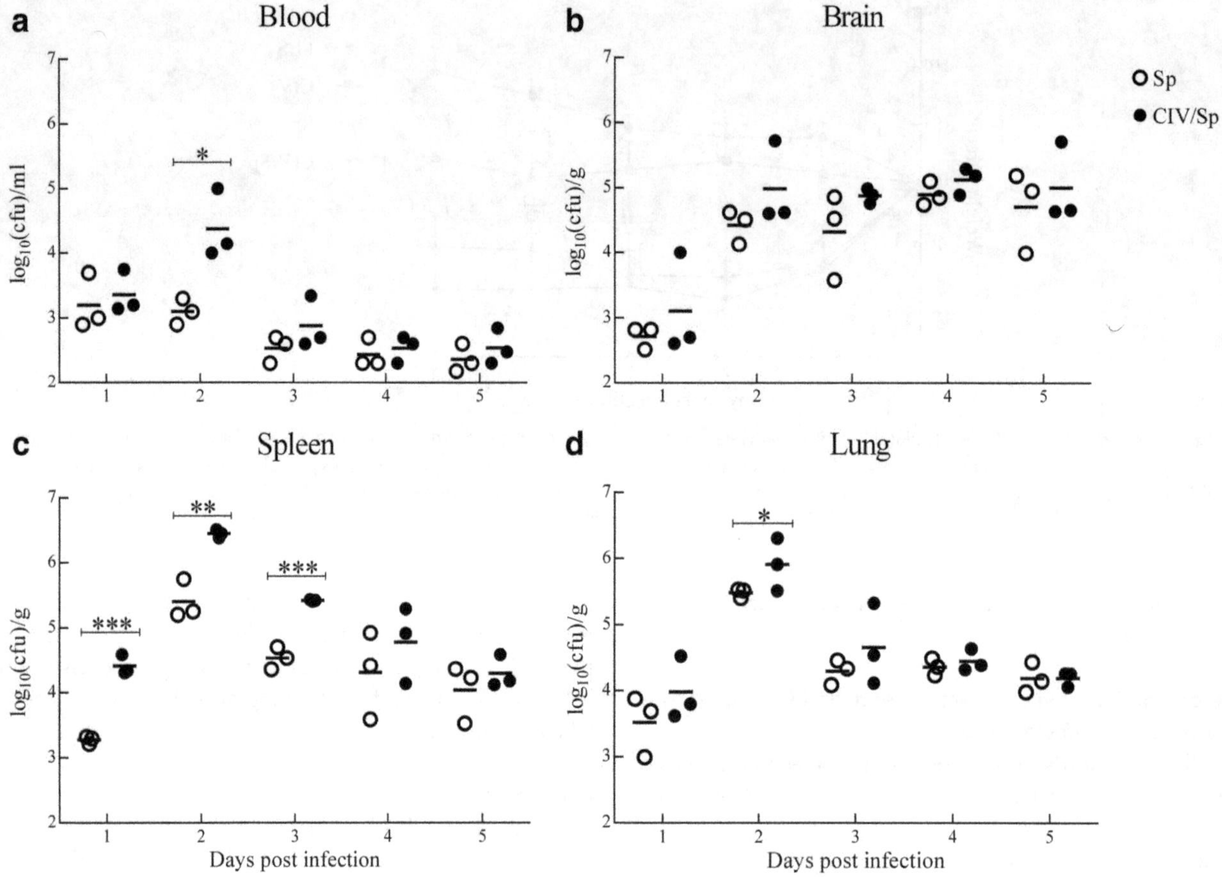

Fig. 2 Dynamic change in the bacteria loads in the blood, brain, spleen and lung (**a**, **b**, **c** and **d**) of mice infected with *S. pseudintermedius* alone or both *S. pseudintermedius* and CIV. The bacterial loads in the infected animals were measured on days 1, 2, 3, 4 and 5 post-challenge. The results are expressed as the mean log10 cfu/ml or log10 cfu/g. Each data point represents a single mouse, and the bar indicates the average for the group. Analysis of variance (ANOVA) was performed for the statistical analysis. *, $P < 0.05$, **, $P < 0.01$, or ***, $P < 0.001$

tended to be more pronounced than those in the Sp-only group. The lung of the mice in the CIV-only group revealed widening of the pulmonary interstitial and lung congestion (Fig. 4i). Microscopic lesions of the lung of mice infected with Sp alone typically consisted of multifocal areas of moderate to severe interstitial thickening of alveoli with mononuclear cells (Fig. 4j). The CIV/Sp group showed similar lung congestion but severe fibrin exudation along with accumulations of neutrophils in the bronchi and widened alveolar septa (Fig. 4k).

The histopathological scores for the H&E sections of the lungs from mice were determined (Fig. 5, Additional file 1). The histopathological score given to the lungs of the mice in the CIV/Sp group was significantly higher than those of the CIV group ($P<0.01$) and the Sp group ($P<0.05$).

Determination of cytokine concentrations

The levels of IFN-γ, TNF-α, IL-6 and Lptn in the spleen and lung of mice at 1, 3 and 5 d.p.i. were measured by ELISA (Fig. 6, Additional file 1). The levels of all four cytokines in the spleen and lung were elevated in the CIV-only, Sp-only and CIV/sp groups compared with the PBS group. The most pronounced difference was found at 3 d.p.i.. There were significant values ($P<0.01$ or $P<0.05$) between the three infection groups and the control group with the exception of the IFN-γ and IL-6 levels in the spleen between the Sp-only and PBS group and the TNF-α levels of the lung between the CIV-only or CIV/Sp group and the PBS group.

Compared with the CIV-only and Sp-only groups, at 1, 3 and 5 d.p.i., the levels of IFN-γ in the spleen and lung were higher in the CIV/Sp group, and IFN-γ level of the spleen reached the statistical significance at 1 d.p.i. ($P < 0.01$ or $P < 0.05$). At 1 d.p.i., the IL-6 levels of the spleen and lung showed a significant difference between the Sp and PBS groups. At 5 d.p.i., the IL-6 levels of the spleen in the Sp-only group were significantly higher compared with the levels in the CIV-only and CIV/Sp groups ($P<0.01$ or $P<0.05$), whereas there was no significant difference in the IL-6 levels in the lung between either the Sp-only or CIV-only

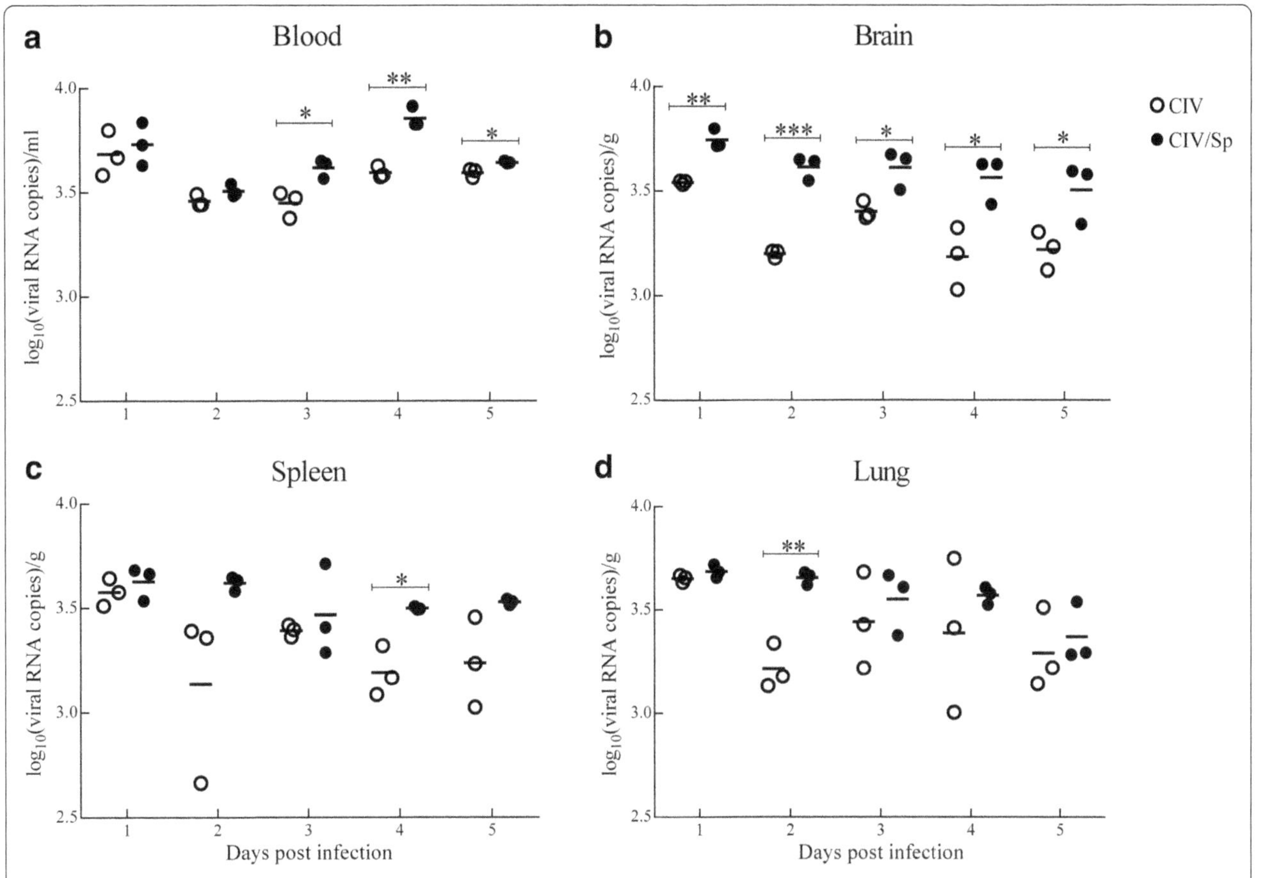

Fig. 3 Dynamic change in the viral loads in the blood, brain, spleen and lung (**a**, **b**, **c** and **d**) of mice infected with CIV alone, or both *S. pseudintermedius* and CIV. The viral loads in the infected animals were measured on days 1, 2, 3, 4 and 5 post-challenge. The results are expressed as the log10 RNA copy numbers per gram or per millilitre of sample. Each data point represents a single mouse, and the bar represents the average for the group. Analysis of variance (ANOVA) was performed for the statistical analysis. *, $P < 0.05$, **, $P < 0.01$, or ***, $P < 0.001$

group and the CIV/Sp group. In the case of TNF-α and Lptn, at 1 and 5 d.p.i., the highest levels in the spleen were observed in the Sp-only group, whereas the highest levels in the lung were found in the CIV-only group. There was no significant difference between the Sp-only or CIV-only group and the CIV/Sp group.

Discussion

Several studies have reported that influenza virus A is extremely contagious to humans and domestic animals, including avian, swine, equine, canine and feline species [31], and causes significant losses to animals and humans. Infection with influenza virus alone is rarely fatal but can encourage secondary bacterial infections that lead to death [32]. Sp is a common commensal in dogs and can cause opportunistic infections [33]. In this study, the coinfection of CIV and Sp resulted in more severe clinical signs and body weight loss in mice and an increased severity of microscopic lesions in the brain, spleen and lung compared with infection with either pathogen alone. The findings of this study showed that the interaction between the two pathogens appears to generate a more severe outcome than that observed with the individual pathogens by themselves.

Our study demonstrated increased bacterial loads in the blood, brain, spleen and lung of the mice in the CIV/Sp group compared with those in the Sp-only group. The finding is in agreement with observations from an earlier study conducted by Lee et al. [25] in which mice co-infected with virus and bacteria showed a higher bacterial load in the blood, spleen, kidneys and liver at 4 and 72 h after staphylococcal infection compared with the mice infected with bacteria alone. In another study, mice exposed to influenza virus followed by *S. pneumoniae* showed greater bacterial counts after 24 and 48 h of infection [34]. The nature of the interaction between CIV and Sp is unknown. However, studies have shown that influenza A virus infection leads to increased susceptibility of the host to secondary bacterial infection by damaging the respiratory epithelial barrier, upregulating host expression of receptors for bacteria, and impairing the innate immune response [35, 36]. Bacterial clearance can be prevented by viral-induced abnormalities in the immune response [37–39]. Previous data suggest that the increased bacterial titres in the lungs, blood and

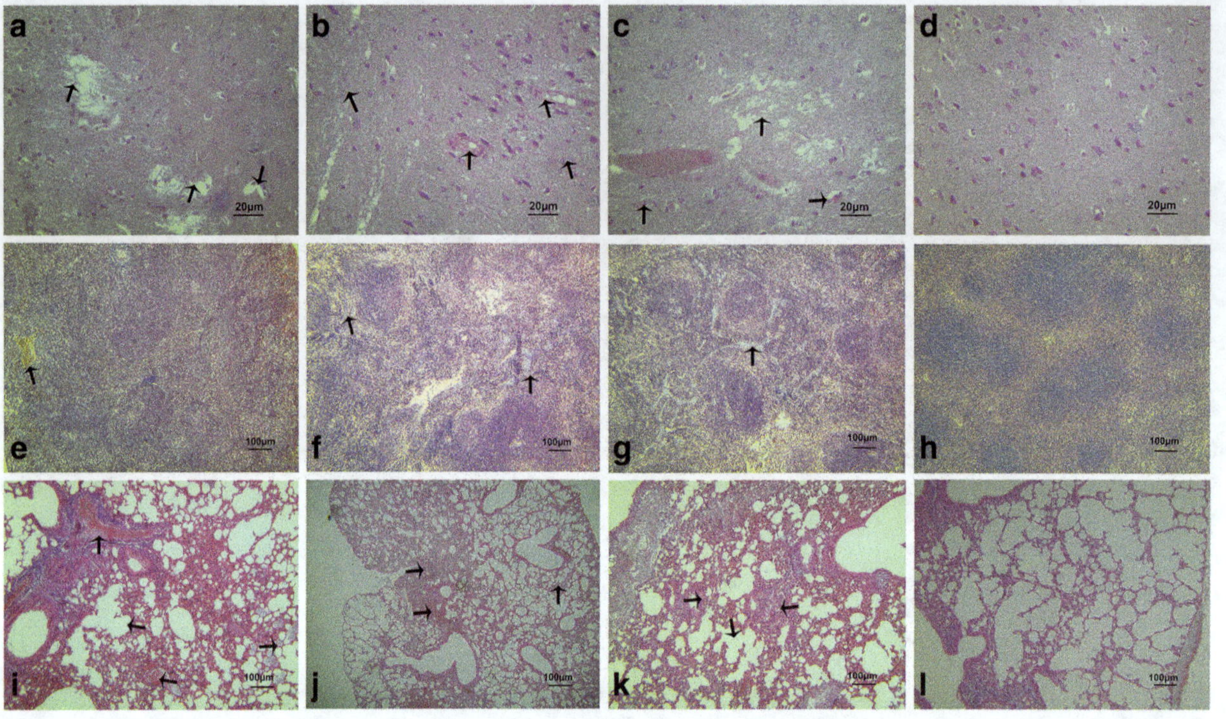

Fig. 4 Histopathological lesions at 2 days post Sp challenge in the co-infected group, shown by H&E staining in the brain, spleen and lung of mice infected with CIV alone, *S. pseudintermedius* alone, or both. **a** Representative brain image from the CIV-only group, showing diffused hyperplasia of microglial cells and disintegration of neuron cells (400×). **b** Representative brain image from the Sp-only group, showing dissolution of nerve fibres, vascular cuff phenomena and neurophagia phenomena (400×). **c** Representative brain image from the CIV/Sp group, showing nerve fibre dissolution and disappearance of neurons (400×). **e** Representative spleen image from the CIV-only group, showing no lesions (100×). **f** Representative spleen image from the Sp-only group, showing hyperplasia of the splenic trabeculae (100×). **g** Representative spleen image from the CIV/Sp group, showing hyperplasia and degeneration of the splenic trabeculae (100×). **i** Representative lung image from the CIV-only group, showing widening of the pulmonary interstitial (100×). **j** Representative lung image from the Sp-only group, showing widening of the alveolar septa (100×). **k** Representative lung image from the CIV/Sp group, showing severe fibrin exudation, appearance of neutrophils and widening of the alveolar septa (100×). **d**, **h**, **l** Representative brain, spleen and lung images of the control group, showing no histopathological lesions (400×, 400× and 100×)

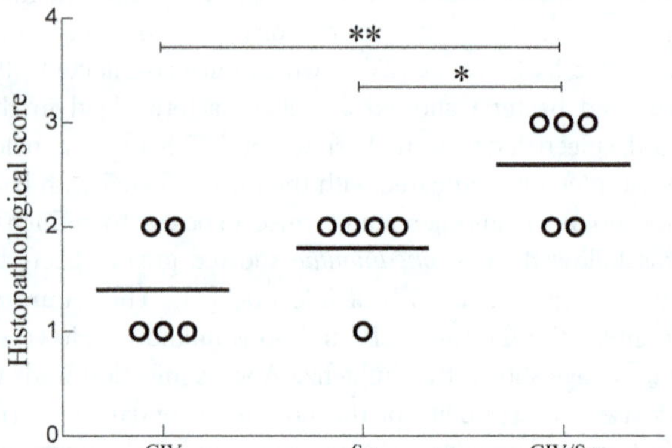

Fig. 5 Degree of lung injury present in mice after infection with CIV alone, *S. pseudintermedius* alone, or both. The lungs were assigned a grade from 0 to 3 based on the histological character of the lesions. Analysis of variance (ANOVA) was performed for the statistical analysis. *, $P < 0.05$, or **, $P < 0.01$

secondary organs cause high mortality and morbidity in groups of mice co-infected with *S. aureus* 3 and 7 d after influenza virus A infection [29]. However, in the present study, no mortality was noted; this finding may be because CIV H3N2 is not lethal to mice [5, 6].

The present study showed that the bacterial loads in the blood, brain, spleen and lungs peaked in Sp-only and CIV/sp groups on d.p.i. 2, indicating that the bacteria can enter the bloodstream, are transported to the other tissues and then pass through the blood–brain barrier into the brain, thus causing severe neurological signs. Distinct central nervous disturbances observed at this time, including bending of the head towards one side and walking in circles, support this hypothesis. More severe neurologic signs were observed in the coinfection group. Interestingly, in addition to an increased bacterial burden, we found that the viral loads in the blood, brain, spleen and lung were augmented following bacterial infection. Smith et al. [40] used a kinetic model to explore the coupled interactions of influenza A virus and *S. pneumoniae* and reported that the subsequent *S.*

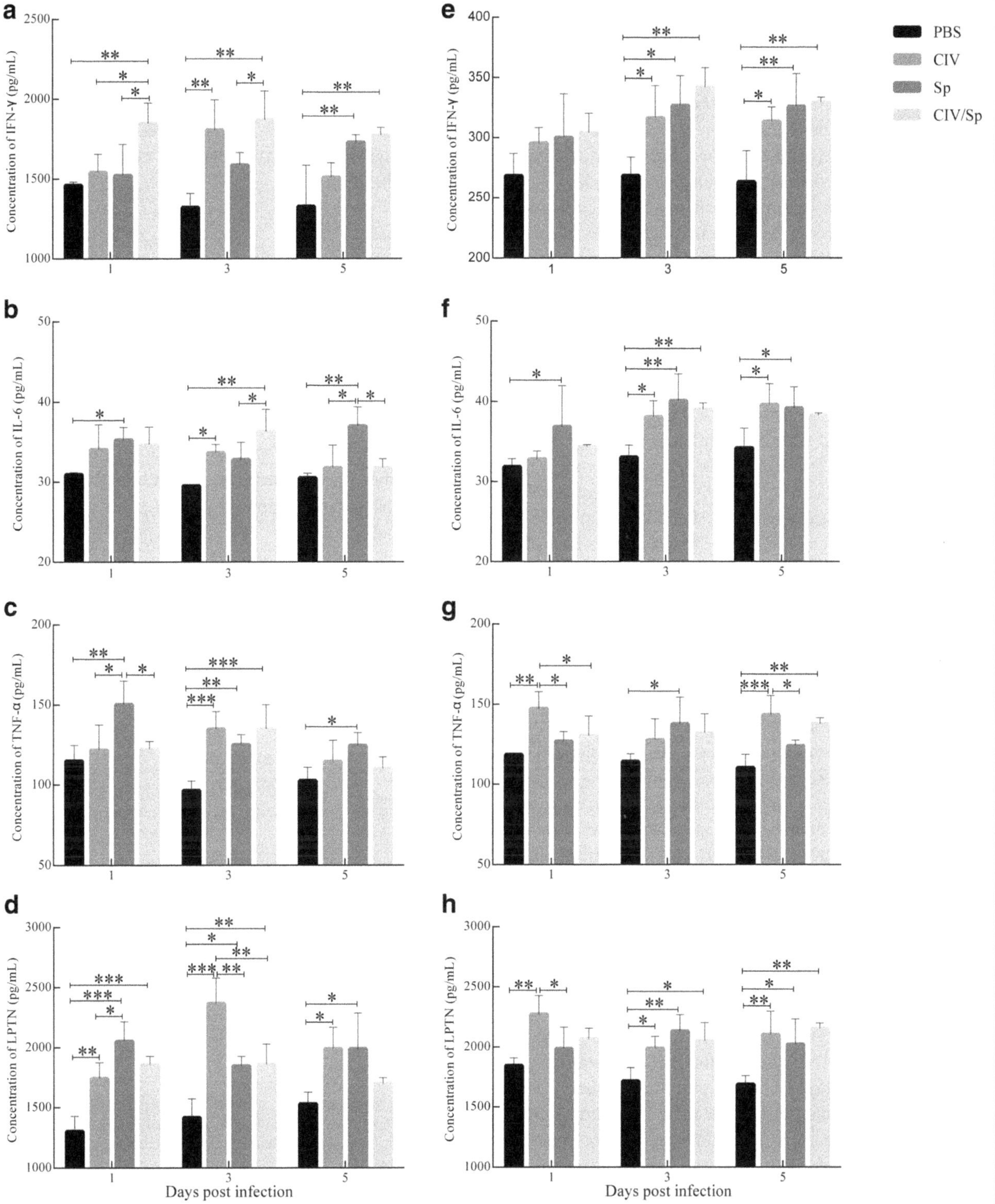

Fig. 6 Characterization of IFN-γ (**a**, **e**), IL-6 (**b**, **f**), TNF-α (**c**, **g**) and Lptn (**d**, **f**) secretion from the spleen (**a**, **b**, **c** and **d**) and lung (**a**, **b**, **c** and **d**) tissues of mice after CIV alone, *S. pseudintermedius* alone, or both. The concentrations in the supernatants of homogenates from the spleens and lungs on days 1, 3 and 5 post-challenge were measured by ELISA. The results are expressed in terms of pg/ml. Analysis of variance (ANOVA) was performed for the statistical analysis. *, $P < 0.05$, **, $P < 0.01$, or ***, $P < 0.001$

pneumoniae infection enhances viral release from infected cells. Therefore, we speculate that the observed increase in viral loads after bacterial infection may be due to increased virus release via bacterial proteases. Additionally, we cannot rule out the possible mechanism that elevated viral loads in the presence of bacteria are due to a reduction in viral clearance. Further work is necessary to study the precise mechanism involved.

The loads of both CIV and Sp in the coinfected mice were greater compared with those of singly infected mice. These results may help explain the increased severity of the lesions observed in the coinfected mice. Additionally, cytokine production after infection likely plays a role in the pathological changes observed during infection. A previous study reported that an excessive production of TNF-α leads to immunopathology [41]. The study conducted by Lee et al. [42] reported that the levels of IFN-γ and TNF-α in the lungs of dogs infected with H3N2 influenza virus increased rapidly, and the infected dogs developed severe bronchointerstitial pneumonia accompanied by a massive infiltration of immune cells. Lymphotactin is a chemokine that recruits T and NK cells, and can regulate or modulate T cell–mediated immune responses [43]. A previous report showed mycobacterial antigen could induce an increase of Lptn transcript, while Lptn has a regulation role in IFN-γ production [44]. A study from van Berke [45] reported that a gamma herpesvirus selective chemokine binding protein could inhibit Lptn action. In the present study, we determined the concentrations of IFN-γ, IL-6, TNF-α and Lptn in the lungs and spleen of mice infected with Sp alone, CIV alone or both CIV and Sp. In general, higher levels of cytokines were observed in all of the infection groups compared with the uninfected animals. We speculated that elevated levels of cytokines may be associated with the clinical manifestations observed in the infected mice. The comparison among the three infection groups revealed that IFN-γ showed the largest changes in the coinfected mice compared with the mice infected with either agent alone, particularly on day 1. These data are consistent with previous reports in which a higher level of IFN-γ expression was observed after coinfection with influenza virus and bacteria [25, 46]. IFN-γ is a Th1 cytokine that can activate macrophages to produce nitric oxide and other inflammatory mediators [47]. This finding may explain the increased severity of lesions observed early in the coinfected mice compared with the mice infected with bacteria or virus alone. With the exception of IFN-γ, the other cytokine or chemokine levels observed in coinfected mice showed no significant differences from those observed in mice infected with CIV or Sp alone. These data showed that coinfection did not influence the production levels of IL-6, TNF-α and Lptn.

Although mice are extensively used for influenza research, and they can be successfully infected with CIV [5, 6], the use of mouse model can be limited, however, due to the fact that mice are not natural hosts for CIV. The signs including lethargy, anorexia and body weight loss, huddling and ruffled fur, which are characteristic of influenza virus infection in mice [48], could be seen. However, some signs in dog disease such as coughing, nasal discharge and fever have not been observed. In the future study, we will further perform coinfection of CIV and Sp in beagles.

Conclusions

Taken together, the findings presented in this study showed that coinfection with CIV and Sp may worsen clinical signs and lesions in mice. This additive effect supports the need for improving the current strategies for the control of influenza and secondary bacterial infection. Because CIV is a relatively recently described canine pathogen, the available clinical data are relatively limited, and further epidemiological studies on the interactions between this virus and secondary bacterial infection are required.

Abbreviations

ANOVA, Analysis of variance; CFU, Colony forming unit; CIV, Canine influenza virus; ELISA, Enzyme Linked Immunosorbent Assay; IFN-γ, Interferon-gamma; IL-6, Interleukin 6; LPTN, Lymphotactin; MDCK, Madin-Darby canine kidney; PBS, phosphate-buffered saline; PCR, Polymerized chain reaction; PFU, Plague forming unit; RNA, Ribonucleic acid; SP, *Staphylococcus pseudintermedius*; TNF-α, Tumor necrosis factor.

Acknowledgements

The authors would like to acknowledge Prof. Shuxia Zhang for her critical advice on the project.

Funding

This work was supported by the International S&T Cooperation Program of China (2014DFG32770) and Priority Academic Program Development of Jiangsu Higher Education Institutions (PAPD).

Authors' contributions

Conceived and designed the experiments: DHK SSG XX SLiang SLuo YBZ YJL. Performed the experiments: DHK SSG XX SLiang. Analyzed the data: DHK SSG YJL. Contributed reagents/materials/analysis tools: YBZ YJL. Wrote the paper: DHK SSG XX SLiang SLuo YBZ YJL. All authors read and approved the final manuscript.

Competing interests

The authors declare that they have no competing interests.

Consent for publication

Not applicable.

References

1. Lee C, Jung K, Oh J, Oh T, Han S, Hwang J, et al. Protective efficacy and immunogenicity of an inactivated avian-origin H3N2 canine influenza vaccine in dogs challenged with the virulent virus. Vet Microbiol. 2010; 143(2):184–8.
2. Crawford P, Dubovi EJ, Castleman WL, Stephenson I, Gibbs E, Chen L, et al. Transmission of equine influenza virus to dogs. Science. 2005;310(5747):482–5.
3. Song D, Kang B, Lee C, Jung K, Ha G, Kang D, et al. Transmission of avian influenza virus (H3N2) to dogs. Emerg Infect Dis. 2008;14(5):741–6.
4. Zhao F, Li S, Zhou D, Chen N, Zhang Y, Qi W, et al. Seroprevalence of avian origin H3N2 canine influenza virus infection in pet dogs in Shenzhen, China. Afr J Microbiol Res. 2011;6:5960–3.
5. Lin Y, Zhao Y, Zeng X, Lu C, Liu Y. Genetic and pathobiologic characterization of H3N2 canine influenza viruses isolated in the Jiangsu Province of China in 2009–2010. Vet Microbiol. 2012;158(3):247–58.
6. Teng Q, Zhang X, Xu D, Zhou J, Dai X, Chen Z, et al. Characterization of an H3N2 canine influenza virus isolated from Tibetan mastiffs in China. Vet Microbiol. 2013;162(2):345–52.
7. Chalker VJ, Owen WM, Paterson C, Barker E, Brooks H, Rycroft AN, Brownlie J. Mycoplasmas associated with canine infectious respiratory disease. Microbiology. 2004;150:3491–7.
8. Finelli L, Fiore A, Dhara R, Brammer L, Shay DK, Kamimoto L, et al. Influenza-associated pediatric mortality in the United States: increase of *Staphylococcus aureus* coinfection. Pediatrics. 2008;122(4):805–11.
9. Centers for Disease Control and Prevention (CDC). Severe methicillin-resistant *Staphylococcus aureus* community-acquired pneumonia associated with influenza-Louisiana and Georgia, December 2006-January 2007. MMWR Morb Mortal Wkly Rep. 2007;56(14):325–9.
10. Blunt C, Van Vuuren M, Picard J. Antimicrobial susceptibility profiles of *Staphylococcus intermedius* isolates from clinical cases of canine pyoderma in South Africa. J S Afr Vet Assoc. 2013;84(1):E1–6.
11. Raus J, Love DN. Characterization of coagulase-positive *Staphylococcus intermedius* and *Staphylococcus aureus* isolated from veterinary clinical specimens. J Clin Microbiol. 1983;18(4):789–92.
12. Talan DA, Staatz D, Staatz A, Goldstein EJ, Singer K, Overturf GD. *Staphylococcus intermedius* in canine gingival and canine-inflicted human wound infections: laboratory characterization of a newly recognized zoonotic pathogen. J Clin Microbiol. 1989;27(1):78–81.
13. Sasaki T, Kikuchi K, Tanaka Y, Takahashi N, Kamata S, Hiramastu K. Methicillin-resistant *Staphylococcus pseudintermedius* in a veterinary teaching hospital. J Clin Microbiol. 2007;45(4):1118–25.
14. Soedarmanto I, Kanbar T, Ülbegi-Mohyla H, Hijazin M, Alber J, Lämmler C, et al. Genetic relatedness of methicillin-resistant *Staphylococcus pseudintermedius* (MRSP) isolated from a dog and the dog owner. Res Vet Sci. 2011;91(3):e25–7.
15. Frank LA, Kania SA, Kirzeder EM, Eberlein LC, Bemis DA. Risk of colonization or gene transfer to owners of dogs with meticillin-resistant *Staphylococcus pseudintermedius*. Vet Dermatol. 2009;20(5–6):496–501.
16. Paul NC, Moodley A, Ghibaudo G, Guardabassi L. Carriage of methicillin-resistant *Staphylococcus pseudintermedius* in small animal veterinarians: indirect evidence of zoonotic transmission. Zoonoses Public Health. 2011;58(8):533–9.
17. van Duijkeren E, Catry B, Greko C, Moreno MA, Pomba MC, Pyörälä S, et al. Review on methicillin-resistant *Staphylococcus pseudintermedius*. J Antimicrob Chemother. 2011;66(12):2705–14.
18. Morens DM, Taubenberger JK, Fauci AS. Predominant role of bacterial pneumonia as a cause of death in pandemic influenza: implications for pandemic influenza preparedness. J Infect Dis. 2008;198(7):962–70.
19. Hartshorn KL. New look at an old problem: bacterial superinfection after influenza. Am J Pathol. 2010;176(2):536–9.
20. Callan RJ, Hartmann FA, West SE, Hinshaw VS. Cleavage of influenza A virus H1 hemagglutinin by swine respiratory bacterial proteases. J Virol. 1997; 71(10):7579–85.
21. Mina MJ, McCullers JA, Klugman KP. Live attenuated influenza vaccine enhances colonization of *Streptococcus pneumoniae* and *Staphylococcus aureus* in mice. mBio. 2014;5(1):e01040–13.
22. Fowlkes AL, Arguin P, Biggerstaff MS, Gindler J, Blau D, Jain S, et al. Epidemiology of 2009 pandemic influenza A (H1N1) deaths in the United States, April–July 2009. Clin Infect Dis. 2011;52 Suppl 1:S60–8.
23. Louie J, Jean C, Chen T, Park S, Ueki R, Harper T, et al. Bacterial coinfections in lung tissue specimens from fatal cases of 2009 pandemic influenza A (H1N1)-United States, May-August 2009. MMWR Morb Mortal Wkly Rep. 2009;58(38):1071–4.
24. McCullers JA, Rehg JE. Lethal synergism between influenza virus and *Streptococcus pneumoniae*: characterization of a mouse model and the role of platelet-activating factor receptor. J Infect Dis. 2002;186(3):341–50.
25. Lee MH, Arrecubieta C, Martin FJ, Prince A, Borczuk AC, Lowy FD. A postinfluenza model of *Staphylococcus aureus* pneumonia. J Infect Dis. 2010;201(4):508–15.
26. Devriese LA, Vancanneyt M, Baele M, Vaneechoutte M, De Graef E, Snauwaert C, et al. *Staphylococcus pseudintermedius* sp. nov., a coagulase-positive species from animals. Int J Syst Evol Microbiol. 2005;55(4):1569–73.
27. Alymova IV, Green AM, van de Velde N, McAuley JL, Boyd KL, Ghoneim HE, McCullers JA. Immunopathogenic and antibacterial effects of H3N2 influenza A virus PB1-F2 map to amino acid residues 62, 75, 79, and 82. J Virol. 2011;85: 12324–33.
28. To KK, Chan KH, Li IW, Tsang TY, Tse H, Chan JF, et al. Viral load in patients infected with pandemic H1N1 2009 influenza A virus. J Med Virol. 2010;82(1):1–7.
29. Iverson AR, Boyd KL, McAuley JL, Plano LR, Hart ME, McCullers JA. Influenza virus primes mice for pneumonia from *Staphylococcus aureus*. J Infect Dis. 2011;203(6):880–8.
30. Xie X, Lin Y, Pang MD, Zhao YB, Kalhoro DH, Lu CP, Liu YJ. Monoclonal antibody specific to HA2 glycopeptide protects mice from H3N2 influenza virus infection. Vet Res. 2015;46:33.
31. Landolt GA, Olsen CW. Up to new tricks-a review of cross-species transmission of influenza A viruses. Anim Health Res Rev. 2007;8(1):1–21.
32. Layne SP, Beugelsdijk TJ, Patel C, Taubenberger JK, Cox NJ, Gust ID, et al. A global lab against influenza. Science. 2001;293(5536):1729.
33. Weese JS, van Duijkeren E. Methicillin-resistant *Staphylococcus aureus* and *Staphylococcus pseudintermedius* in veterinary medicine. Vet Microbiol. 2010; 140(3):418–29.
34. LeVine AM, Koeningsknecht V, Stark JM. Decreased pulmonary clearance of *S. Pneumoniae* following influenza A infection in mice. J Virol Methods. 2001;94(1–2):173–86.
35. Peltola VT, Mccullers JA. Respiratory viruses predisposing to bacterial infections: role of neuraminidase. Pediatr Infect Dis J. 2004;23(1):S87–97.
36. McCullers JA, McAuley JL, Browall S, Iverson AR, Boyd KL, Normark BH. Influenza enhances susceptibility to natural acquisition of and disease due to *Streptococcus pneumoniae* in ferrets. J Infect Dis. 2010;202(8):1287–95.
37. van der Sluijs KF, van Elden LJ, Nijhuis M, Schuurman R, Pater JM, Florquin S, et al. IL-10 is an important mediator of the enhanced susceptibility to pneumococcal pneumonia after influenza infection. J Immunol. 2004;172(12):7603–9.
38. Sun K, Metzger DW. Inhibition of pulmonary antibacterial defense by interferon-γ during recovery from influenza infection. Nat Med. 2008;14(5):558–64.
39. Didierlaurent A, Goulding J, Patel S, Snelgrove R, Low L, Bebien M, et al. Sustained desensitization to bacterial Toll-like receptor ligands after resolutionof respiratory influenza infection. J Exp Med. 2008;205(2):323–9.
40. Smith AM, Adler FR, Ribeiro RM, Gutenkunst RN, McAuley JL, McCullers JA, et al. Kinetics of coinfection with influenza A virus and *Streptococcus pneumoniae*. Plos Pathog. 2013;9(3), e1003238.
41. Zhang WJ, Sarawar S, Nguyen P, Daly K, Rehg JE, Doherty PC, et al. Lethal synergism between influenza infection and staphylococcal enterotoxin B in mice. J Immunol. 1996;157(11):5049–60.
42. Lee YN, Lee HJ, Lee DH, Kim JH, Park HM, Nahm SS, et al. Severe canine influenza in dogs correlates with hyperchemokinemia and high viral load. Virology. 2011;417(1):57–63.
43. Kelner GS, Kennedy J, Bacon KB, Kleyensteuber S, Largaespada D, et al. Lymphotactin: A cytokine that represents a new class of chemokine. Science. 1994;266(5189):1395–9.
44. Qiu B, Frait KA, Reich F, Komuniecki E, Chensue SW. Chemokine expression dynamics in mycobacterial (type-1) and schistosomal (type-2) antigen-elicited pulmonary granuloma formation. Am J Pathol. 2001;158(4):1503–15.
45. van Berkel V, Barrett J, Tiffany HL, Fremont DH, Murphy PM, et al. Identification of a gammaherpesvirus selective chemokine binding protein that inhibits chemokine action. J Virol. 2000;74(15):6741–7.

46. Damjanovic D, Lai R, Jeyanathan M, Hogaboam CM, Xing Z. Marked improvement of severe lung immunopathology by influenza-associated pneumococcal superinfection requires the control of both bacterial replication and host immune responses. Am J Pathol. 2013;183(3):868–80.
47. Ding AH, Nathan CF, Stuehr DJ. Release of reactive nitrogen intermediates and reactive oxygen intermediates from mouse peritoneal macrophages. Comparison of activating cytokines and evidence for independent production. J Immunol. 1988;141(7):2407–12.
48. Margine I, Krammer F. Animal models for influenza viruses: implications for universal vaccine development. Pathogens. 2014;3(4):845–74.

15

Seroprevalence of anti-hepatitis E virus antibodies in domestic pigs in Mexico

Montserrat Elemi García-Hernández[1], Mayra Cruz-Rivera[2], José Iván Sánchez-Betancourt[1], Oscar Rico-Chávez[1], Arely Vergara-Castañeda[3], María E. Trujillo[1] and Rosa Elena Sarmiento-Silva[1*]

Abstract

Background: Hepatitis E virus (HEV) infection is one of the most common causes of acute liver diseases in humans worldwide. In developing countries, HEV is commonly associated with waterborne outbreaks. Conversely, in industrialized countries, HEV infection is often associated with travel to endemic regions or ingestion of contaminated animal products. Limited information on both, human and animal HEV infection in Mexico is available. As a consequence, the distribution of the virus in the country is largely unknown. Here, we assessed the seroprevalence of HEV among swine in different geographical regions in Mexico.

Methods: Seroprevalence of anti-HEV antibodies in swine herds in Mexico was evaluated in a representative sample including 945 pig serum specimens from different regions of the country using a commercial enzyme-linked immunosorbent assay (ELISA).

Results: The overall prevalence of anti-HEV antibodies in swine was 59.4%. The northern region of Mexico exhibited the highest seroprevalence in the country (86.6%), while the central and southern regions in Mexico showed lower seroprevalence, 42.7% and 51.5%, respectively.

Conclusions: In Mexico, HEV seroprevalence in swine is high. Importantly, northern Mexico showed the highest seroprevalence in the country. Thus, further studies are required to identify the risk factors contributing to HEV transmission among pigs in the country. Assessment of HEV human infection in the context of viral transmission in swine is required to better understand the epidemiology of hepatitis E in Mexico.

Keywords: HEV, Mexico, Pigs, Seroprevalence

Background

Hepatitis E virus (HEV) infection is an emerging disease of increasing importance. HEV affects approximately ~20 million persons annually worldwide, causing ~70,000 deaths. In humans, HEV is transmitted primarily by the fecal-oral route [1, 2]. Clinically, hepatitis E is indistinguishable from other viral hepatitis. Hepatitis E is usually a self-limiting disease in immunocompetent individuals, commonly resulting in mild symptoms or asymptomatic disease [3–6]. Occasionally, and for reasons not completely understood, HEV infection can progress to fulminant hepatitis [7]. The overall mortality rate of HEV infection ranges from 0.5 to 4%; however, it is considerably higher among pregnant women (~20%) [2].

HEV is a non-enveloped virus with a single-stranded positive-sense RNA genome of ca. 7.2 (kb) in length. HEV is a member of the family *Hepeviridae* within the genus *Orthohepevirus*. This genus comprises four species: *Orthohepevirus A*, *Orthohepevirus B*, *Orthohepevirus C* and *Orthohepevirus D* –all grouping viruses that infect birds and different mammals. Based on its genetic variability, *Orthohepevirus A* is classified into seven main genotypes (HEV1–7). Genotypes 1 and 2 infect exclusively humans while all other are considered zoonotic. Genotypes 3 and 4 also affect pigs, wild boars, rabbits and mongoose. Genotype 5 and 6 have been identified from wild boar, while genotype 7 infects camels.

* Correspondence: rosass@unam.mx
[1]Facultad de Medicina Veterinaria y Zootecnia, Universidad Nacional Autónoma de México, Ciudad de México 04510, México
Full list of author information is available at the end of the article

HEV is endemic or epidemic to Africa and Asia. Epidemics of HEV in endemic regions are usually associated with water-borne outbreaks [1, 8]. Individuals from non-endemic regions who acquire HEV infection often have a history of traveling to endemic regions and/or consumption of contaminated animal products [9] evidence suggests that autochthonous HEV infections in developed countries also occur [7, 10]. HEV has been reported to circulate in different countries in Latin America, including Mexico [11]. After the first reported HEV outbreak in Mexico in 1987 [12], when HEV genotype 2 was originally described, several research groups have subsequently reported the circulation of HEV in the country in both, swine and humans [2, 13, 14]. In Mexico, HEV surveillance is not routinely performed; and as a result, diagnosis of HEV-related disease is underreported. Likewise, monitoring of HEV infection in pigs is rare [15]. Thus resulting in a profound lack of information about human and animal infection.

In pigs, reduced feed intake and mild diarrhea may be observed, but evident clinical disease signs such as elevation of liver enzymes or bilirubin levels are usually not detected. Upon infection, experimentally HEV-inoculated pigs seroconvert to anti-HEV immunoglobulin IgG, shedding of virus in feces is observed during approximately 23 days in contact infected pigs [16, 17]. Importantly, identification of HEV RNA in liver tissue and bile is not uncommon [18]. Higher anti-HEV antibody prevalence among individuals in close contact with pigs (handlers), in comparison to normal population has been previously reported [19]. In these settings, HEV-related disease has been related to consumption of contaminated meat products.

In this study we aimed to assess the seroprevalence of HEV in domesticated pigs in different geographical regions in Mexico.

Methods

Serum samples

Serum samples were obtained from different farms in 2014 and 2015 with informed consent from the owners. A total of 945 representative swine serum samples were selected for this study. Both, industrialized farms (95%) and backyard herds (5%) located in different counties from 27 states in Mexico were included. Samples were grouped according to their collection site and divided into three geographical regions (central, southern and northern Mexico) (Fig. 1). The sample size for statistical significant result for each region was calculated using the Daniel algorithm [20].

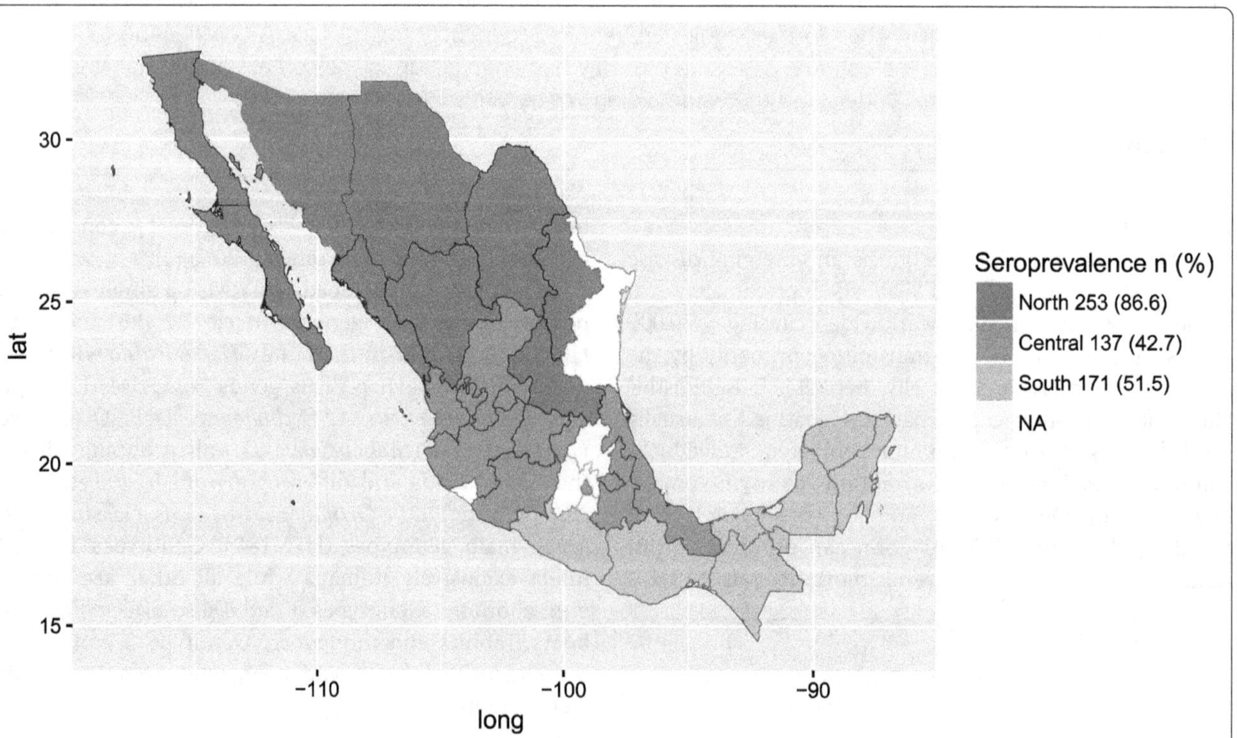

Fig. 1 Map showing the percentage of anti-HEV positive pigs and classification by region of the states included in the study. The central region included samples from Ciudad de Mexico, Guanajuato, Jalisco, Michoacán, Nayarit, Puebla, Queretaro, Aguascalientes, Tlaxcala, Veracruz and Zacatecas states, south from Quintana Roo, Campeche, Chiapas, Guerrero, Oaxaca, Tabasco and Yucatan; and northern states Baja California, Chihuahua, Coahuila, Durango, Nuevo Leon, Sinaloa, San Luis Potosi and Sonora. Latitude (Long). Latitude (lat). NA (Not available)

Detection of anti-HEV antibodies

Detection of anti-HEV antibodies was performed using a commercial enzyme-linked immunosorbent assay (ELISA) (Wantai Biopharmaceutical, Inc. Beijing, China), using horseradish peroxidase-labeled protein A (Bio-Rad, CA, USA) as reporting conjugate. Briefly, serum samples were diluted (1:10), and incubated for 30 min at 37 °C. After washing, the conjugate was added and incubated for 30 min at 37 °C. Plates were washed, and 100 μl of substrate solution (tetramethylbenzidine, Wantai Biopharmaceutical) were added. The reaction was stopped after 15 min with 50 μl of stop solution. The absorbance was measured at 450 nm using multi-scan EX spectrophotometer (Thermo Fisher, Waltham, MA). The cut off value was calculated after blanking as the mean absorbance of the negative controls +0.16 (mean absorbance value for negative controls +0.16) according to the manufacturer's instructions. Serum specimens exhibiting an absorbance value greater than the cut-off value were considered positive for anti-HEV antibodies.

Statistical analyses

Statistical analyses were performed using the Statistical Package for the Social Sciences (IBM SPSS Statistics v22.0, USA). All reported *p*-values were two-sided and a p-value of less than 0.05 was deemed statistically significant. Prevalence of positive serum among swine categories and regions were assessed by the chi- squared test and odds ratios were determined to evaluate the risk of positive/negative results for qualitative results, according to location and production stage.

In order to know the effect of each state in the corresponding region in the hepatitis seroprevalence we performed a general linear model (glm) with binomial distribution. The positive or negative result of hepatitis seroprevalence was used as dependent variable, while the region, state within region and production stage within region were used as independent variables. These analysis were performed selected the states with at least 10 observations, after the selection the sample size was equal to 878. A likelihood test was performed to determine the overall significance of the logistic model. The odd ratio of each state and region was calculated by exponentiating the model estimates. An analysis of variance was also calculated to know the statistically difference in hepatitis seroprevalence by state.

Results

A total of 945 samples were analyzed, 292 (30.8%) specimens were collected from the northern region of Mexico, and 332 sera from the southern (35.1%) and 321 central parts of Mexico (34%) and, when classified according to the production stage, a total of 299 samples corresponded to weaned production, 323 to fattening and 323 to reproducers animals (Table 1). No differences in distribution for this factor were found among the total of the samples.

The overall prevalence of anti-HEV IgG in the country was 59.4%. The highest seroprevalence was found in northern Mexico (86.6%), compared to 42.7 and 51.5% in the central and southern regions, respectively ($p < 0.001$) (Fig. 1). Based on the production stage, the chi- squared test showed no significant differences in positivity between the different production stages in the northern and central regions; however, in southern Mexico, a significant difference was observed in fattening swine compared to weaned and reproducer animals ($p = 0.012$) .

In the general linear model (glm) with binomial distribution, only the states with at least 10 observations were selected ($n = 878$), in this analysis, the production stage within region didn't show a statistical significance (LR chisq = 9.755, DF = 6, $p = 0.135$) (AIC = 948.84) while the state within region showed a statistical significance (LR chisq = 115.56, DF = 13 $p < 0.01$) (AIC = 946.6). The central region was used as intercept in the glm (Table 2). No significant difference was found in the analysis of variance in hepatitis seroprevalence by state (DF = 2, F = 2.59, $p = 0.118$).

Discussion

Here, we have shown a high prevalence of HEV-specific antibodies in domesticated pigs in different geographical regions of Mexico. The results suggested that animals in intensive pig farms are in contact with HEV at an early production stage. Few studies have reported the circulation of HEV in Mexico, particularly in pigs [15]. As a consequence, limited information about the seroprevalence of HEV in swine is available. A recent study, conducted in nine states located in central Mexico showed a seroprevalence of 30% [15]. The discrepancies between the seroprevalence found between the studies can be attributed to the difference in geographical areas tested and the methodology used by Merino-Ramos and cols which consisted of an ELISA test based on the use of recombinant HEV 3 ORF-2 expressed in *Trichoplusia ni* larvae as antigen. Performances of anti-HEV antibody detection methods vary significantly [21]. Here, we used a well-known commercial assay for the detection of antibodies in order to minimize

Table 1 Classification of analyzed samples by region and production stage

Category	Total	North	South	Central
Weaned	299 (31.6)	88 (29.4)	115 (38.4)	96 (32.1)
Fattening	323 (34.2)	94 (29.1)	116 (35.9)	113 (35)
Reproducers	323 (34.2)	110 (34)	101 (31.3)	112 (34.7)
		292 (30.8)	332 (35.1)	321 (34)

Data shown as n (%)

Table 2 Out put of general lineal model. The region and the state within region were used as independent variables. Only states with >10 observations were considered

Region	State	Estimate	Std. Error	z value	P	N	Prevalence (%)	OR	2.50%	97.50%
Center (intercept)		0.588	0.558	1.054	0.292	299	44.1	1		
	DF	−0.728	0.636	−1.144	0.253	43	46.5	0.483	0.13	1.637
	Guanajuato	−0.007	0.599	−0.011	0.991	92	64.1	0.993	0.285	3.127
	Jalisco	−1.314	0.6	−2.188	0.029*	92	32.6	0.269	0.077	0.847
	Michoacan	−2.821	0.825	−3.421	0.001*	31	9.7	0.06	0.01	0.271
	Queretaro	−0.588	0.843	−0.697	0.486	10	50.0	0.556	0.101	2.905
	Veracruz	−1.194	0.754	−1.583	0.113	17	35.3	0.303	0.064	1.282
North		2.105	0.627	3.356	0.001*	256	89.5	8.205	2.258	27.636
	Nuevo Leon	−1.083	0.618	−1.752	0.08	24	83.3	0.339	0.108	1.288
	Sinaloa	−2.162	0.491	−4.404	0.000*	27	63.0	0.115	0.044	0.305
South		1.284	0.774	1.658	0.097	323	52.0	3.611	0.794	17.653
	Chiapas	−3.163	0.636	−4.974	0.000*	51	21.6	0.042	0.011	0.134
	Guerrero	−1.664	0.654	−2.544	0.011*	29	55.2	0.189	0.047	0.638
	Oaxaca	−0.599	0.687	−0.872	0.383	32	78.1	0.549	0.13	2.051
	Tabasco	−4.27	1.174	−3.635	0.000*	12	8.3	0.014	0.001	0.098
	Yucatan	−1.765	0.559	−3.159	0.002*	169	52.7	0.171	0.049	0.463

Odds ratio (OR)
GLM
*$p < 0.05$

false antibody results [22–28]. Interestingly, HEV seroprevalence in pig herds in Mexico has been reported as high as 81% [2]. Both previous studies were focused in particular geographical regions in Mexico. Here, we undertook a nation-wide approach to assess the HEV seroprevalence in swine in the country, showing that northern Mexico is the most affected region by HEV infection in pigs. Nonetheless, high seroprevalence in all three geographical regions was observed. The reasons for these differences in seropositivity among different parts of Mexico could be associated with common practices in pig farms such as high population density, and shorter production cycles that significantly increased the risk for HEV infection [16].

Studies aimed to detect the virus in acutely infected animals are necessary to identify the routes of transmission exploited by the virus to warrant persistence in the pig population.

Conclusions

The relatively high seropositivity observed in all regions in Mexico suggests abundant circulation of HEV and high transmission rates among pigs. These findings highlight the importance of this zoonosis in Mexico. Further nation-wide studies on HEV prevalence in human population are required to better understand the epidemiology of HEV in Mexico. Assessing the prevalence of HEV infection in high-risk populations such as pig handlers and immunocompromised patients is critical to estimate HEV burden in the country. Implementation of adequate HEV surveillance in Mexico is important to implement proper control measures aimed to prevent virus spread.

Abbreviations

CI: Confidence interval; ELISA: Competitive enzyme-linked immunosorbent assay; HEV: Hepatitis E virus; OR: Odds ratio

Acknowledgements

MEGH and the founding for the project (CB221186) was supported by the Mexican National Council of Science and Technology (CONACYT). The authors would like to thank Jose Juan Martínez for critical reading of the manuscript.

Authors' contributions

Performed experiments and analyzed the data: MEGH, MCR, AVC, RESS. Wrote the manuscript: MEGH, MCR, AVC, RESS. Collected sample material and supported data analysis: MEGH, JISB, MET, RESS. Supervised and supported the study: RESS. All authors read and approved the final manuscript.

Competing interests

The authors declare that they have no competing interests.

Author details

[1]Facultad de Medicina Veterinaria y Zootecnia, Universidad Nacional Autónoma de México, Ciudad de México 04510, México. [2]Facultad de Medicina, Universidad Nacional Autónoma de México, 04510 Ciudad de México, México. [3]Facultad de Ciencias Químicas, Universidad La Salle, Benjamín Franklin 47, 06140 Ciudad de México, México.

References

1. Krawczynski K, Mast EE, Purdy MA. Hepatitis E: an overview. Minerva Gastroenterol Dietol. 1999;45(2):119–30. discussion 130-115
2. Cooper K, Huang FF, Batista L, Rayo CD, Bezanilla JC, Toth TE, Meng XJ. Identification of genotype 3 hepatitis E virus (HEV) in serum and fecal samples from pigs in Thailand and Mexico, where genotype 1 and 2 HEV strains are prevalent in the respective human populations. J Clin Microbiol. 2005;43(4):1684–8.
3. Aggarwal A, Perumpail RB, Tummala S, Ahmed A. Hepatitis E virus infection in the liver transplant recipients: clinical presentation and management. World J Hepatol. 2016;8(2):117–22.
4. Aggarwal R. Clinical presentation of hepatitis E. Virus Res. 2011;161(1):15–22.
5. Aggarwal R. Hepatitis E: clinical presentation in disease-endemic areas and diagnosis. Semin Liver Dis. 2013;33(1):30–40.
6. Aggarwal R, Krawczynski K. Hepatitis E: an overview and recent advances in clinical and laboratory research. J Gastroenterol Hepatol. 2000;15(1):9–20.
7. Festa S, Garbuglia AR, Baccini F, Panzuto F, Capobianchi MR, Santino I, Purchiaroni F, Orgera G, Delle Fave G, Marignani M. Acute fulminant hepatitis E virus genotype 3e infection: description of the first case in Europe. Scand J Infect Dis. 2014;46(10):727–31.
8. Guthmann JP, Klovstad H, Boccia D, Hamid N, Pinoges L, Nizou JY, Tatay M, Diaz F, Moren A, Grais RF, et al. A large outbreak of hepatitis E among a displaced population in Darfur, Sudan, 2004: the role of water treatment methods. Clin Infectious Dis. 2006;42(12):1685–91.
9. Berto A, Martelli F, Grierson S, Banks M. Hepatitis E virus in pork food chain, United Kingdom, 2009-2010. Emerg Infect Dis. 2012;18(8):1358–60.
10. Schielke A, Sachs K, Lierz M, Appel B, Jansen A, Johne R. Detection of hepatitis E virus in wild boars of rural and urban regions in Germany and whole genome characterization of an endemic strain. Virol J. 2009;6:58.
11. Fierro NA, Realpe M, Meraz-Medina T, Roman S, Panduro A. Hepatitis E virus: an ancient hidden enemy in Latin America. World J Gastroenterol. 2016;22(7):2271–83.
12. Velazquez O, Stetler HC, Avila C, Ornelas G, Alvarez C, Hadler SC, Bradley DW, Sepulveda J. Epidemic transmission of enterically transmitted non-a, non-B hepatitis in Mexico, 1986-1987. JAMA. 1990;263(24):3281–5.
13. Alvarez-Munoz MT, Torres J, Damasio L, Gomez A, Tapia-Conyer R, Munoz O. Seroepidemiology of hepatitis E virus infection in Mexican subjects 1 to 29 years of age. Arch Med Res. 1999;30(3):251–4.
14. Bernal Reyes R. Licona Solis JE: [Seroepidemiology of hepatitis E in the state of hidalgo]. Revista de Gastroenterol de Mexico. 1996;61(3):233–8.
15. Merino-Ramos T, Martin-Acebes MA, Casal J, Saiz JC, Loza-Rubio E. Prevalence of hepatitis E virus (HEV) antibodies in Mexican pigs. Food Environ Virol. 2016;
16. Walachowski S, Dorenlor V, Lefevre J, Lunazzi A, Eono F, Merbah T, Eveno E, Pavio N, Rose N. Risk factors associated with the presence of hepatitis E virus in livers and seroprevalence in slaughter-age pigs: a retrospective study of 90 swine farms in France. Epidemiol Infect. 2014;142(9):1934–44.
17. Schlosser J, Eiden M, Vina-Rodriguez A, Fast C, Dremsek P, Lange E, Ulrich RG, Groschup MH. Natural and experimental hepatitis E virus genotype 3-infection in European wild boar is transmissible to domestic pigs. Vet Res. 2014;45:121.
18. Bouwknegt M, Rutjes SA, Reusken CB, Stockhofe-Zurwieden N, Frankena K, de Jong MC, de Roda Husman AM, Poel WH. The course of hepatitis E virus infection in pigs after contact-infection and intravenous inoculation. BMC Vet Res. 2009;5:7.
19. Galiana C, Fernandez-Barredo S, Garcia A, Gomez MT, Perez-Gracia MT. Occupational exposure to hepatitis E virus (HEV) in swine workers. Am J Trop Med Hyg. 2008;78(6):1012–5.
20. Daniel WW, Cross CL. Biostatistics: a Foundation for Analysis in the health sciences, 10th edition: a Foundation for Analysis in the health sciences: New York: Wiley Global Education; 2012.
21. Drobeniuc J, Meng J, Reuter G, Greene-Montfort T, Khudyakova N, Dimitrova Z, Kamili S, Teo CG. Serologic assays specific to immunoglobulin M antibodies against hepatitis E virus: pangenotypic evaluation of performances. Clin Infect Dis. 2010;51(3):e24–7.
22. Tremeaux P, Lhomme S, Chapuy-Regaud S, Peron JM, Alric L, Kamar N, Izopet J, Abravanel F. Performance of an antigen assay for diagnosing acute hepatitis E virus genotype 3 infection. J Clin Virol. 2016;79:1–5.
23. Pischke S, Schwarze-Zander C, Bremer B, Lehmann P, Wiegand SB, Gisa A, Behrendt P, Strassburg CP, Manns MP, Wedemeyer H, et al. Hepatitis E virus Seroprevalence rate in HIV-infected patients in Germany: a comparison of two commercial assays. Intervirology. 2015;58(5):283–7.
24. Izopet J, Labrique AB, Basnyat B, Dalton HR, Kmush B, Heaney CD, Nelson KE, Ahmed ZB, Zaman K, Mansuy JM, et al. Hepatitis E virus seroprevalence in three hyperendemic areas: Nepal, Bangladesh and southwest France. J Clin Virol. 2015;70:39–42.
25. Grierson S, Heaney J, Cheney T, Morgan D, Wyllie S, Powell L, Smith D, Ijaz S, Steinbach F, Choudhury B, et al. Prevalence of hepatitis E virus infection in pigs at the time of slaughter, United Kingdom, 2013. Emerg Infect Dis. 2015;21(8):1396–401.
26. Han J, Lei Y, Liu L, Liu P, Xia J, Zhang Y, Zeng H, Wang L, Wang L, Zhuang H. SPF rabbits infected with rabbit hepatitis E virus isolate experimentally showing the chronicity of hepatitis. PLoS One. 2014;9(6):e99861.
27. Liu J, Zhang W, Shen Q, Yang S, Huang F, Li P, Guo X, Yang Z, Cui L, Zhu J, et al. Prevalence of antibody to hepatitis E virus among pet dogs in the Jiang-Zhe area of China. Scand J Infect Dis. 2009;41(4):291–5.
28. Zhao K, Liu Q, Yu R, Li Z, Li J, Zhu H, Wu X, Tan F, Wang J, Tang X. Screening of specific diagnostic peptides of swine hepatitis E virus. Virol J. 2009;6:186.

Porcine epidemic diarrhea virus (PEDV) detection and antibody response in commercial growing pigs

Jordan Bjustrom-Kraft[1], Katie Woodard[1], Luis Giménez-Lirola[1], Marisa Rotolo[1], Chong Wang[1,2], Yaxuan Sun[2], Peter Lasley[3], Jianqiang Zhang[1], David Baum[1], Phillip Gauger[1], Rodger Main[1] and Jeffrey Zimmerman[1*]

Abstract

Background: Longitudinal samples from two production sites were used to (1) describe the pattern of PEDV shedding (rRT-PCR) in individual rectal swabs, pen fecal samples, and pen oral fluids (OF); (2) describe the kinetics of PEDV antibody by ELISA (IgA, IgG) testing of pig serum and pen oral fluid samples; and (3) establish cutoffs and performance estimates for PEDV WV ELISAs (IgA, IgG). Site One was PEDV positive; Site Two was PEDV negative. On Site One, pen samples (feces and oral fluids) and pig samples (rectal swabs and sera) were collected both before and after the population was exposed to PEDV.

Results: On Site Two, pen oral fluid samples and individual pig serum samples were negative for both PEDV antibody and nucleic acid. On Site One, PEDV was detected by rRT-PCR at 6 days post exposure (DPE) in all sample types. The last rRT-PCR positives were detected in rectal swabs and oral fluids on 69 DPE. IgG and IgA were detected in oral fluids and serum samples by 13 DPE. Analysis of the PEDV serum IgG WV ELISA data showed that a sample-to-positive (S/P) cutoff of ≥ 0.80 provided a diagnostic sensitivity of 0.87 (95 % CI: 0.82, 0.91) and specificity of 0.99 (95 % CI: 0.98, 1.00). Serum IgG results declined slowly over the monitoring period, with 60 % of serum samples positive (S/P ≥ 0.80) at the final sampling on 111 DPE. Analysis of the PEDV oral fluid IgA WV ELISA found that a cutoff of S/P ≥ 0.80 provided a diagnostic sensitivity of 1.00 (95 % CI: 0.92, 1.00) and a diagnostic specificity of 1.00 (95 % CI: 0.99, 1.00). The oral fluid IgA response increased through 96 DPE and began to decline at the last sampling on 111 DPE.

Conclusions: This study showed that oral fluid-based testing could provide an easy and "animal-friendly" approach to sample collection for nucleic acid and/or antibody-based surveillance of PEDV in swine populations.

Keywords: PEDV, Virus shedding, Antibody kinetics, Oral fluids, Surveillance, IgG, IgA

Background

Porcine epidemic diarrhea virus (PEDV) is an enveloped, single-stranded, positive-sense RNA virus in the family *Coronaviridae* [1]. In susceptible herds, PEDV is characterized by the rapid onset of watery diarrhea and vomiting in pigs of all ages, with mortality approaching 100 % in suckling piglets. First identified in 1978, PEDV was not considered a serious threat to swine health until devastating outbreaks of PEDV were reported in China in 2006 in association with previously unrecognized genetic variants [2]. Thereafter, pathogenic strains producing clinical PED outbreaks were reported in Japan, Korea, Thailand, the Philippines, the Western hemisphere and subsequently Portugal and Germany [3–5]. Thus, in a relatively short time, pathogenic PEDV has become pandemic.

Since there is little possibility that PEDV will soon be eradicated, it is important to identify the means to prevent and/or control its effects: PEDV management will necessitate monitoring PEDV in swine populations. Therefore, the purpose of this study was to (1) describe the patterns of PEDV shedding and detection in growing pigs as shown by PEDV real-time reverse transcription polymerase chain reaction (rRT-PCR) testing of individual pig rectal swabs, pen fecal samples, and pen oral fluids; (2) describe PEDV

* Correspondence: jjzimm@iastate.edu
[1]Department of Veterinary Diagnostic and Production Animal Medicine, College of Veterinary Medicine, Iowa State University, 1850 Christensen Drive, Ames, IA 50011-1134, USA
Full list of author information is available at the end of the article

antibody kinetics as shown by enzyme-linked immunosorbent assay (ELISA) detection of IgA and IgG in individual pig serum and pen oral fluid samples; and (3) estimate the cutoffs and performance of the PEDV "whole virus" IgA and IgG ELISAs (WV IgA or IgG ELISA).

Methods

Experimental design

Individual pig samples (rectal swabs and/or serum) and pen samples (fecal and/or oral fluid specimens) were collected longitudinally from one PEDV-positive commercial wean-to-finish (WTF) barn in Missouri USA (Site One) and one PEDV-negative commercial WTF barn in Iowa USA (Site Two). Fecal samples and oral fluids were tested by PEDV real-time reverse-transcriptase polymerase chain reaction (rRT-PCR). Serum and oral fluid specimens were tested by two PEDV antibody WV ELISAs (IgA, IgG). Testing results were used to describe PEDV shedding, establish the performance parameters of two PEDV WV ELISAs (IgA, IgG), and characterize antibody kinetics in a commercial pig production system. This project was approved in writing both by an agent representing the livestock producer and the Iowa State University Office for Responsible Research.

Site descriptions

Site One was a 52-pen WTF barn stocked with ~800 pigs. Pens were separated by metal gates, with 26 pens on each side of the walk way. Pens were equipped with automatic feeders, bowl drinkers, and fully slatted floors. The facility was designed with negative pressure tunnel ventilation and a deep pit (2.4 m) manure handling system. Pigs were placed in the facility at the time of weaning (~3 weeks of age). Pen samples (feces and oral fluids) and pig samples (rectal swabs and serum) were collected from the same 6 pens and a convenience sample of 5 pigs in each of the 6 pens at each sampling point. Sampling began when the pigs were ~3 weeks of age and continued at ~2-week intervals for 27 weeks. At 10 weeks post-placement, i.e., when pigs were approximately 13 weeks of age, the producer exposed the pigs (replacement gilts) to PEDV by mixing PEDV-positive fecal material with water and spraying feed and the pigs' oral-nasal area with the mixture using a hand-held sprayer.

Site Two consisted of 3 identical 40-pen WTF barns, each stocked with ~900 pigs. Pens were separated by solid walls, with 20 pens on each side of the walk way. Pens were equipped with automatic feeders, bowl drinkers, and half-slatted floors. The barns were constructed with natural ventilation and deep pit (2.4 m) manure handling systems. Pigs were placed in the facility at the time of weaning (~3 weeks of age). Pen oral fluid samples were collected from 36 pens (4 pens were not stocked) in each of the 3 barns and serum samples were collected from a convenience sample of 20 pigs in 2 pens (10 pigs per pen) in each barn. Sampling began at two weeks post placement (pigs were ~5 weeks of age) and continued weekly for a total of 9 samplings. Individual pig rectal swabs and pen fecal specimens were not collected on Site Two.

Sample collection

Individual pigs were restrained and bled using 12.5 mL vacutainer tubes (Covidien, Minneapolis, MN USA) and 20 gauge x 3.81 cm (1 ½ in.) needles (Smiths Medical, Dublin, OH USA). Blood samples were centrifuged at the laboratory, aliquoted, and stored at −20 °C.

Fecal swabs were collected from individual pigs using a commercial collection and transport system (StarswabII®, Starplex® Scientific Inc., Cleveland, TN USA) and stored at −20 °C. Prior to testing, swabs were suspended in 1 mL of PBS (1X pH 7.4, Invitrogen Corporation, Carlsbad, CA USA), vortexed, and the liquid submitted for testing by PEDV rRT-PCR.

Each pen-level fecal sample consisted of a convenience sample of 3-to-5 fresh semi-solid feces from throughout the pen. Approximately equal portions of pen feces were placed in one 50 mL tube (Thermo Fisher Scientific, Waltham, MA USA) and stored at −20 °C. Prior to testing, samples were homogenized (stirred), ~1.0 g placed in 1 mL of PBS (1X pH 7.4, Invitrogen Corporation) and submitted for PEDV rRT-PCR testing.

Pen-based oral fluids were collected as described elsewhere [6]. In brief, 3-strand, 100 % cotton rope was cut with the free end at shoulder height to the animals and suspended in the pen for 20 to 30 min. Pigs actively sought out and chewed the rope, leaving the strands moistened with oral fluids. The rope was then removed from the pen and the wet portion placed in a single-use plastic bag. Oral fluids were extracted by either manual or mechanical compression (wringer) of the wet rope, after which the fluid was decanted into 50 mL centrifuge tubes (Fisher Scientific) and stored at −20 °C.

For each site, all samples were completely randomized (random.org) within specimen type and submitted for testing at the end of the collection period.

Diagnostic testing

PEDV RNA extraction and real-time reverse transcriptase PCR (rRT-PCR)

In brief, 90 μl of viral RNA was eluted from rectal swabs, fecal samples and oral fluid specimens using the Ambion® MagMAX™ viral RNA isolation kit (Life Technologies, Carlsbad CA USA) and a KingFisher® 96 magnetic particle processor (Thermo-Fisher Scientific) following the procedures provided by the manufacturers. Samples were tested for PEDV using a PEDV N gene-based rRT-PCR described in Madson et al. [7] and performed routinely at the Iowa State University-Veterinary Diagnostic Laboratory (ISU-

VDL SOP 9.5263). The forward primer sequence was 5′-CGCAAAGACTGAACCCACTAACCT-3′, the reverse primer sequence was 5′-TTGCCTCTGTTGTTACTTG GAGAT-3′, and probe sequence was 5′-FAM-TGTTG CCAT/ZEN/TACCACGACTCCTGC-Iowa Black-3′. The eluted RNA, primers, and probe were mixed with commercial reagents TaqMan® Fast Virus 1-Step Master Mix (Life Technologies) and the rRT-PCR reactions were conducted on an ABI 7500 Fast instrument (Life Technologies) in fast mode as follows: 1 cycle at 50 °C for 5 min, 1 cycle at 95 °C for 20 s, 40 cycles at 95 °C for 3 s, and 60 °C for 30 s. The results were analyzed using an automatic baseline setting with a threshold at 0.1. Quantification cycle (Cq) values < 35 were considered positive for the corresponding coronavirus. Data were reported as 'adjusted Cqs':

$$\text{Adjusted Cq} = (35 - \text{sample Cq}) \quad (1)$$

PEDV whole virus (WV) antibody ELISA

A U.S. prototype PEDV isolate (USA/NC35140/2013, [8]) was used in the PEDV WV antibody ELISA. Each batch of approximately 1000 mL of PEDV was propagated on Vero cells (ATCC CCL-81). Briefly, one 75 cm^2 flask (Thermo Fisher Scientific) of confluent Vero cells was inoculated with 3 mL of PEDV stock (1x10^5 TCID$_{50}$ per mL) followed by the addition of 50 mL of cell culture medium composed of MEM 1X (Minimum Essential Medium, Life Technologies) supplemented with 0.3 % tryptose phosphate broth, 0.02 % yeast extract, 5 ug per mL Trypsin 250 (Sigma-Aldrich, St. Louis, MO USA), plus penicillin/streptomycin (10 U per mL), gentamicin (0.05 mg per mL) and amphotericin (0.25 µg per mL) as antibiotics. After 3 to 4 days at 37 °C in a 5 % CO_2 incubator and when cytopathic effects were apparent, the contents of the flask (53 mL) were used to further expand the virus by inoculating each of 4 875 cm^2 flasks (BD Falcon, San Jose, CA) containing confluent Vero cell monolayers with 13 mL of the harvested PEDV plus 240 mL of culture medium. After 3 to 4 days of incubation and when cytopathic effects were apparent, the fluid was frozen (−80 °C), thawed, poured off, and then centrifuged at 4,000 x *g* for 15 min to remove cell debris. The virus was pelleted by ultracentrifugation at 140,992 x *g* for 3 h, after which the pellet was washed twice with sterile PBS (1X pH 7.4) to remove culture medium components. The purified virus was re-suspended in 100µl PBS (1X pH 7.4) at a 1:100 dilution of the original supernatant volume and stored at −80 °C. Following titration and optimal dilution (PBS pH 7.4), polystyrene 96-well microtitration plates (Nalge Nunc, Rochester, NY USA) were manually coated (100 µl per well) with the viral antigen solution and incubated at 4 °C overnight. After incubation, plates were washed 5 times, blocked with 300 µl per well of a solution containing 1 % bovine serum albumin (Jackson ImmunoResearch Inc., West Grove, PA USA), and incubated at 25 °C for 2 h. Plates were then dried at 37 °C for 4 h and stored at 4 °C in a sealed bag with desiccant packs. The performance of each lot of plates was standardized using a panel of reference PEDV negatives and positives. Plate lots with a coefficient of variation ≥10 % were rejected.

ELISA conditions for the detection of anti-PEDV IgA and IgG antibodies in serum and oral fluid specimens, including coating and blocking conditions, reagent concentrations, incubation times, and buffers, were identical. Serum samples were diluted 1:50 and oral fluid samples were diluted 1:2, after which plates were loaded with 100 µl of the diluted sample per well. Plates were incubated at 25 °C (serum) or 37 °C (oral fluid) for 1 h and then washed 5 times with PBS (1X pH 7.4). Positive and negative plate controls, i.e., antibody-positive and -negative experimental serum samples, were run in duplicate on each ELISA plate.

To perform the assay, 100 µl of peroxidase-conjugated goat anti-pig IgG (Fc) antibody (Bethyl Laboratories Inc., Montgomery, TX USA) diluted 1:20,000 for serum and 1:3,000 for oral fluid samples or goat anti-pig IgA (Bethyl Laboratories Inc.) diluted 1:7,000 for serum and 1:3,000 for oral fluid samples was added to each well and the plates incubated at 25 °C (serum) or 37 °C (oral fluid) for 1 h. After a washing step, the reaction was visualized by adding 100 µl of tetramethylbenzidine-hydrogen peroxide (Dako North America, Inc., Carpinteria, CA USA) substrate solution to each well. After 5 min incubation at room temperature, the reaction was stopped by the addition of 50 µl of stop solution (1 M sulfuric acid) to each well. Reactions were measured as optical density (OD) at 450 nm using an ELISA plate reader (Biotek® Instruments Inc., Winooski, VT USA) operated with commercial software (GEN5™, Biotek® Instruments Inc.). The antibody response in serum and oral fluid samples was represented as sample-to-positive (S/P) ratios calculated as:

$$\text{S/P ratio} = \frac{(\text{sample OD} - \text{negative control mean OD})}{(\text{positive control mean OD} - \text{negative control mean OD})} \quad (2)$$

Data analysis

Statistical analyses were performed using commercial statistical software (SAS® Version 9.4, SAS® Institute, Inc., Cary, NC) using test results on serum (Site One, $n = 330$; Site Two, $n = 540$), oral fluid (Site One, $n = 66$; Site 2, $n = 972$), rectal swabs (Site One, $n = 330$), and pen feces (Site One, $n = 66$). A mixed-effects repeated measures model (Proc GLIMMIX) was used to analyze the association between the detection of PEDV by rRT-PCR and the variables of interest, i.e., sample specimen (oral fluids, rectal swab, pen feces, serum) and day post exposure (DPE) using pen as a random effect. Fixed effects were considered significant at $\alpha = 0.05$. Differences in the proportion of PEDV rRT-PCR positive oral fluid, rectal swab, and pen feces was compared using the Fisher Exact Test. Point and interval estimates of the sensitivity and specificity of the PEDV WV IgG and IgA ELISAs for serum and oral fluid samples were calculated using the exact Binomial formula and confidence intervals.

Results

PEDV rRT-PCR

On Site Two, all oral fluid samples ($n = 972$) collected during the monitoring period were PEDV rRT-PCR-negative.

On Site One, PEDV was detected in individual rectal swabs, pen fecal samples, and pen oral fluids by rRT-PCR collected for 10 weeks post exposure (Fig. 1a), i.e., through 69 DPE (23 weeks of age). An analysis of the adjusted rRT-PCR Cq values showed differences in the concentration of PEDV in the three sample types over time ($p = 0.0005$). The concentration of PEDV was higher in pen fecal samples compared to rectal swabs ($p = 0.0001$) and oral fluids ($p = 0.0088$) at 6 DPE. Thereafter, no difference was detected in the concentration of virus in oral fluid and pen fecal samples through 69 DPE. In contrast, the concentration of PEDV in rectal swab samples was significantly lower than in pen fecal samples and oral fluid samples at 13, 27, and 41 DPE (15, 17, 19 weeks of age) ($p < 0.002$).

An analysis of the proportion of rRT-PCR positive samples (Fig. 1b) found differences among specimen types at 27, 41, and 55 DPE (17, 19, 21 weeks of age) (Fisher's Exact Test, $p < 0.03$). No differences were found between pen fecal samples and oral fluid samples over the monitoring period, except at 55 DPE when 6 of 6 oral fluid and 1 of 6 pen fecal samples were positive ($p = 0.015$). However, the proportion of positive oral fluid specimens was significantly greater than rectal swabs at 27, 41, and 55 DPE (17, 19, 21 weeks of age) ($p < 0.02$). Likewise, the proportion of positive pen fecal samples at 41 DPE was significantly greater than rectal swabs ($p = 0.0012$).

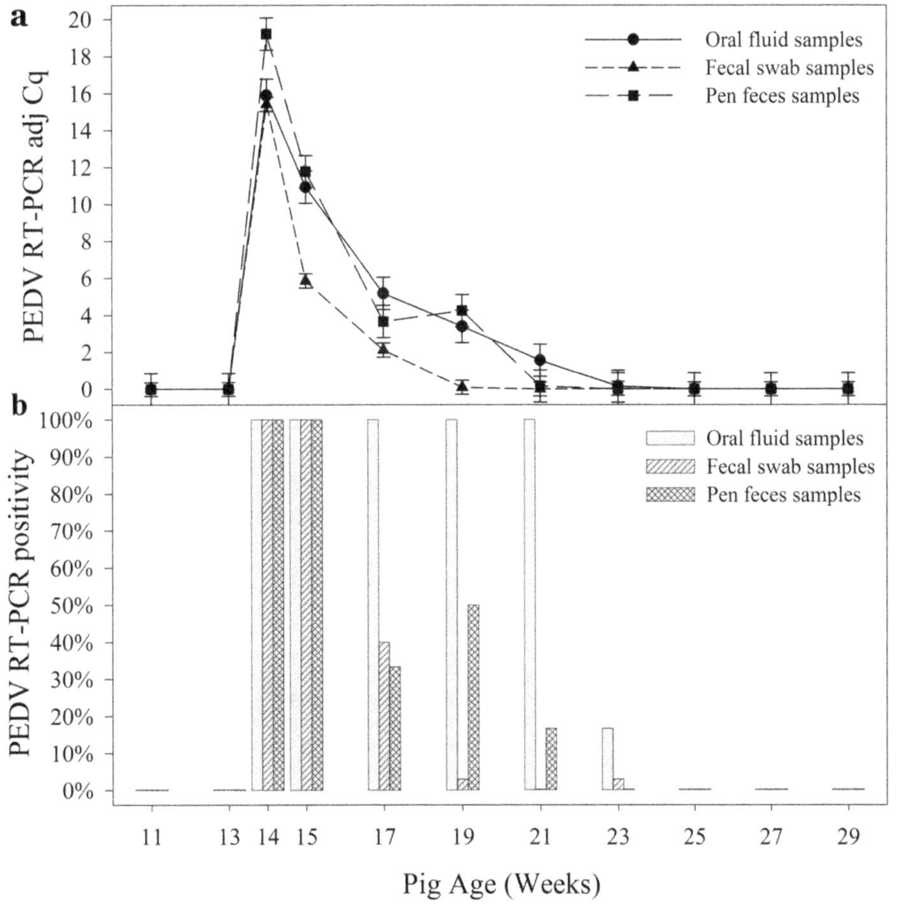

Fig. 1 Detection of porcine epidemic diarrhea virus (PEDV) in pig rectal swabs, pen-based oral fluids, and pen-based fecal specimens from Site One by rRT-PCR. At 13 weeks of age, the producer exposed the pigs to PEDV-positive fecal material mixed with water using a hand-held sprayer. **a** (above): Mean adjusted quantification cycle (Cq) (35 – sample Cq) of positive samples. **b** (below): Proportion of positive samples

PEDV whole virus (WV) antibody ELISA

On Site One, PEDV IgG and IgA were detected in all oral fluid and serum samples collected after 13 DPE (≥15 weeks of age). As shown in Figs. 2a and 3a, the oral fluid IgA S/P responses increased until 97 DPE (27 weeks of age), whereas the serum IgA response peaked at 27 DPE (17 weeks of age). Figures 2b and 3b show the percent positive oral fluid samples and serum samples, respectively, for three S/P cutoffs. Oral fluid ($n = 972$) and serum samples ($n = 540$) from Site Two were used as a source of PEDV negative samples for calculating cutoffs and performance estimates for the PEDV WV IgA and IgG ELISAs using the exact Binomial formula and confidence intervals (Table 1).

Discussion

The first objective of this study was to compare the detection of PEDV by rRT-PCR in rectal swabs, pen fecal samples, and oral fluid samples from pigs housed in commercial WTF facilities. Specifically, comparisons were made among specimens in the duration of PEDV detection, proportion of positive samples, and concentration of virus in positive samples.

PEDV was detected by rRT-PCR in rectal swabs, pen fecal samples, and oral fluid samples, with the last rRT-PCR positive rectal swabs collected at 69 DPE, pen fecal samples at 55 DPE, and oral fluid samples at 69 DPE. The fact that the cessation of PEDV detection coincided in fecal and oral fluid samples suggested that the environment did not serve as a reservoir for PEDV. Previous publications provided data with which rectal swab data could be compared, but a comprehensive search of the literature did not find previous reports on the detection of PEDV in pen feces or pen-based oral fluid samples. Madson et al. [7] detected PEDV in rectal swabs through 24 days post inoculation (DPI) in 5 of 8 pigs inoculated at 3 weeks of age with PEDV isolate US/Iowa/18984/2013. Thomas et al. [9] detected PEDV in rectal swabs for up to 21 DPI in 3-week-old pigs inoculated with PEDV isolate US/IN19338/2013. Crawford et al. [10]

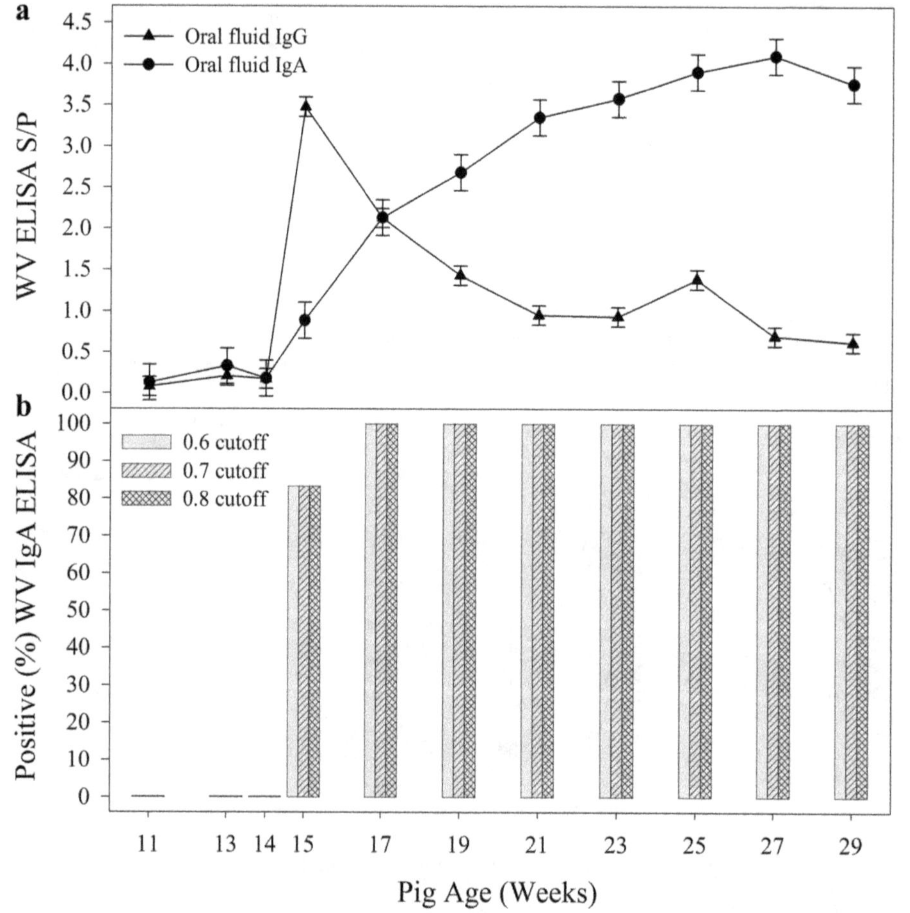

Fig. 2 PEDV Whole Virus ELISA IgG and IgA responses in oral fluid samples following exposure to PEDV at 13 weeks of age. **a** (above): Oral fluid IgG and IgA responses over time. **b** (below): Proportion of positive oral fluid IgA samples at three different S/P cutoffs

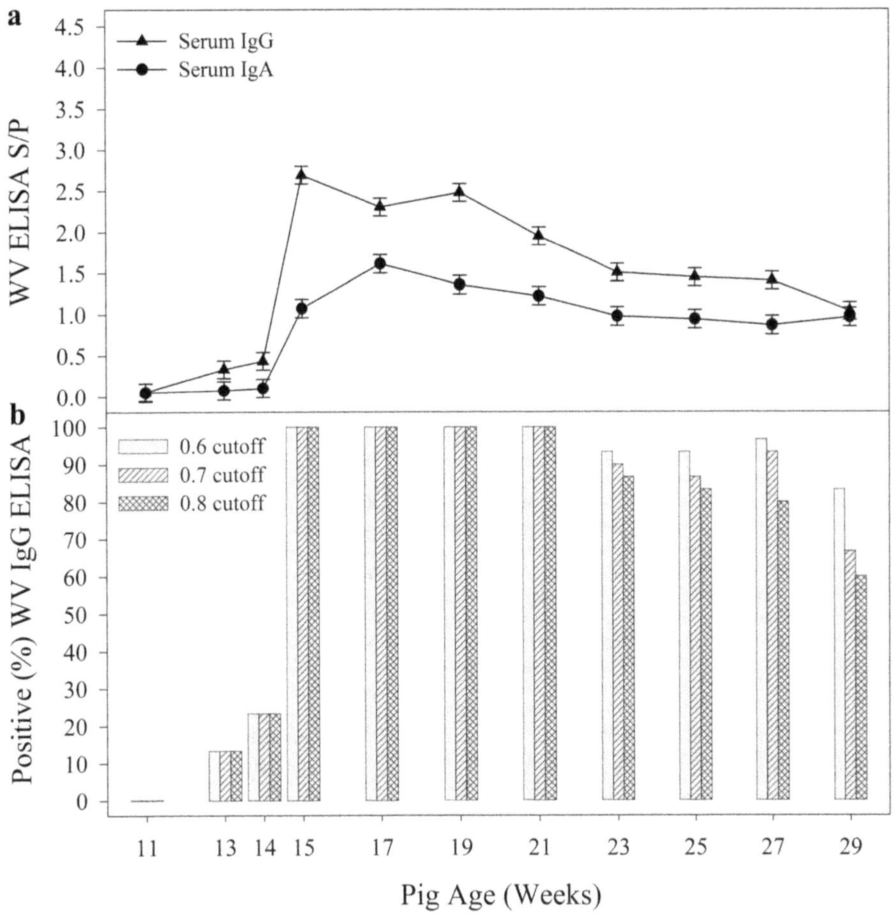

Fig. 3 PEDV Whole Virus ELISA IgG and IgA response in serum samples following exposure to PEDV at 13 weeks of age. **a** (above): Serum IgG and IgA responses over time. **b** (below): Proportion of positive serum IgG samples at three different S/P cutoffs

detected PEDV in rectal swabs for up to 42 DPI in 4-week-old pigs infected by contact with a pig inoculated with PEDV isolate US/Colorado/2013.

The concentration of virus, as measured by rRT-PCR, differed among specimen types. In particular, the concentration of PEDV nucleic acid in individual pig rectal swabs was significantly lower than oral fluid or pen-based fecal samples. The concentration of virus in PEDV rRT-PCR-positive oral fluid and pen-based fecal samples was not significantly different, except at 6 DPE.

Differences were also detected among specimen types in the proportion of positive samples by time. All oral fluid samples were rRT-PCR positive (6 of 6) through 55 DPE while the number PEDV rRT-PCR-positive pen fecal samples and rectal swabs declined to ≤ 50 % at 27 DPE and later. The lower concentration and lower rate of detection in rectal swabs could be attributed to the small volume of sample retained by the swab plus the effect of diluting each rectal swab in one mL of PBS prior to testing. The lower rate of detection in pen floor fecal samples may reflect the non-uniform distribution of positive samples within a pen. Previously, O'Connor et al. [11] reported differences in *Salmonella* concentrations at various locations within a pen, i.e., the distribution of *Salmonella* within a pen was not uniform.

Detection of PEDV by rRT-PCR using pen-based oral fluid samples has not previously been reported in the refereed literature. Using the described procedures, one oral fluid sample from a pen provided detection equal to, or better than, rectal swab samples from 5 pigs in the pen. Likewise, detection using oral fluid samples was equal to, or better than, detection using pen fecal samples. Thus, the data indicated that oral fluids were an effective and sensitive specimen for herd-level rRT-PCR-based detection of PEDV in commercial growing pig environments.

The second objective of the study was to describe PEDV serum and oral fluid IgA and IgG antibody kinetics and to estimate the performance of the PEDV "whole virus" IgA and IgG indirect ELISAs at different cutoffs.

For serum IgG and IgA, respectively, a cutoff of S/P ≥ 0.80 provided diagnostic sensitivities of 0.87 (95 %

Table 1 Porcine epidemic diarrhea virus (PEDV) whole virus (WV) ELISA sensitivity (Se) and specificity (Sp) by specimen type, antibody isotype, and sample-to-positive (S/P) ratio[a]

Oral fluid - PEDV WV IgG ELISA			Oral fluid - PEDV WV IgA ELISA		
S/P	Se (95 % CI)	Sp (95 % CI)	S/P	Se (95 % CI)	Sp (95 % CI)
0.30	1.00 (0.92, 1.00)	0.86 (0.84, 0.89)	**0.30**	1.00 (0.92, 1.00)	0.88 (0.86, 0.90)
0.40	1.00 (0.92, 1.00)	0.90 (0.88, 0.92)	**0.40**	1.00 (0.92, 1.00)	0.96 (0.94, 0.97)
0.50	0.98 (0.87, 1.00)	0.93 (0.91, 0.94)	**0.50**	1.00 (0.92, 1.00)	0.98 (0.97, 0.99)
0.60	0.88 (0.74, 0.96)	0.95 (0.93, 0.96)	**0.60**	1.00 (0.92, 1.00)	0.99 (0.99, 1.00)
0.70	0.71 (0.55, 0.84)	0.96 (0.95, 0.97)	**0.70**	1.00 (0.92, 1.00)	1.00 (0.99, 1.00)
0.80	0.69 (0.53, 0.82)	0.97 (0.96, 0.98)	**0.80**	1.00 (0.92, 1.00)	1.00 (0.99, 1.00)
Serum - PEDV WV IgG ELISA			Serum - PEDV WV IgA ELISA		
S/P	Se (95 % CI)	Sp (95 % CI)	S/P	Se (95 % CI)	Sp (95 % CI)
0.30	1.00 (0.98, 1.00)	0.95 (0.93, 0.96)	**0.30**	0.93 (0.88, 0.96)	1.00 (0.99, 1.00)
0.40	0.99 (0.96, 1.00)	0.98 (0.97, 0.99)	**0.40**	0.90 (0.86, 0.94)	1.00 (0.99, 1.00)
0.50	0.97 (0.93, 0.99)	0.99 (0.98, 1.00)	**0.50**	0.82 (0.76, 0.87)	1.00 (0.99, 1.00)
0.60	0.95 (0.91, 0.86)	0.99 (0.98, 1.00)	**0.60**	0.73 (0.67, 0.79)	1.00 (0.99, 1.00)
0.70	0.91 (0.86, 0.94)	0.99 (0.98, 1.00)	**0.70**	0.66 (0.59, 0.72)	1.00 (0.99, 1.00)
0.80	0.87 (0.82, 0.91)	0.99 (0.98, 1.00)	**0.80**	0.58 (0.51, 0.65)	1.00 (0.99, 1.00)

[a]$S/P = \frac{(\text{sample OD} - \text{negative control mean OD})}{(\text{positive control mean OD} - \text{negative control mean OD})}$

CI: 0.82, 0.91) and 0.58 (95 % CI: 0.51, 0.65) and diagnostic specificities of 0.99 (95 % CI: 0.98, 1.00) and 1.00 (95 % CI: 0.99, 1.00). Although both serum IgG and serum IgA were detected by 13 DPE, the serum IgG response provided better diagnostic performance than serum IgA (Table 1). Serum IgG results declined slowly over the monitoring period, with 60 % of serum samples positive (S/P ≥ 0.80) at the final sampling on 111 DPE. The utility of the PEDV WV serum IgA ELISA is a question for future research. In particular, research is needed to determine whether the detection of serum IgA, i.e., an antibody isotype necessarily produced by the piglet in response to infection, could be used to identify infection in the face of PEDV-specific colostral (IgG) antibody or whether serum IgA response could be used in a confirmatory assay to clarify equivocal PEDV WV IgG ELISA results.

For oral fluid IgG and IgA, respectively, a cutoff of S/P ≥ 0.80 provided diagnostic sensitivities of 0.69 (95 % CI: 0.53, 0.82) and 1.00 (95 % CI: 0.92, 1.00) and diagnostic specificities of 0.97 % (95 % CI: 0.96, 0.98) and 1.00 (95 % CI: 0.99, 1.00). Although oral fluid IgG and IgA were detected by 13 DPE, the oral fluid IgA response gave better diagnostic performance than IgG. Notably, the oral fluid IgA response increased through 96 DPE and only began to decline at the last sampling on 111 DPE.

There are no prior reports against which to directly compare the PEDV oral fluid antibody kinetics observed in the current study, but DeBuysscher and Berman [12] reported a large increase in IgA-secreting cells within the salivary glands of pigs following oral exposure to another coronavirus, transmissible gastroenteritis virus (TGEV). On the other hand, Brandtzæg [13] noted that enteric stimulation does not necessarily produce a strong salivary IgA response in humans. Because of similarities in experimental design, these data may also be compared to oral fluid IgG and IgA responses reported for porcine reproductive and respiratory syndrome virus (PRRSV) and influenza A virus (IAV) [14, 15]. Kittawornrat et al. [14] evaluated PRRSV oral fluid IgG and IgA responses using pen-based field samples and experimental oral fluid samples. Using a commercial PRRS serum antibody ELISA adapted to oral fluids, IgG was readily detected and provided a diagnostic sensitivity of 0.95 (95 % CI: 0.92, 0.97) and specificity of 1.00 (95 % CI: 0.99, 1.00). In contrast, the IgA response in oral fluid was detectable, but weak and transient. Panyasing et al. [15] evaluated influenza A virus IgG and IgA responses in oral fluids. Unlike the PRRSV response, both anti-IAV IgG and IgA were readily detected in oral fluids by ~7 DPI and throughout the study (DPI 42). These studies suggest that oral fluid IgG and IgA kinetics vary among pathogens. Thus, it will be critical to evaluate antibody isotype kinetics during the process of adapting antibody assays to the swine oral fluid matrix.

For disease surveillance in swine populations, diagnostic specificity is paramount because false positives quickly erode confidence in test results. Therefore, the investigators recommend a conservative S/P cutoff for serum and oral fluid samples, e.g., ≥ 0.80 for routine use. However, diagnostic sensitivity and specificity were presented for several PEDV WV ELISA S/P cutoffs (Table 1) to allow users to interpret results in the context of specific circumstances.

Conclusion

The purpose of surveillance is to provide timely information on pathogen exposure and immune responses in swine populations in order to optimize health and prevent disease. Well-validated, reproducible, high-throughput nucleic acid and antibody assays are necessary to achieve this purpose. This study showed that oral fluid-based testing could provide an easy and "animal-friendly" approach to nucleic acid and/or antibody-based surveillance of PEDV in swine populations. In particular, the exceptional strength and duration of the PEDV IgA antibody response in oral fluids raises the question as to its ability to serve as an indicator of protective immunity; this is a question for future research.

Abbreviations

CI, confidence interval; DPE, day post exposure; DPI, day post inoculation; ELISA, enzyme-linked immunosorbent assay; IAV, influenza A virus; IgA, immunoglobulin A; IgG, immunoglobulin G; ISU-VDL, Iowa State University Veterinary Diagnostic Laboratory; OD, optical density; PBS, phosphate-buffered saline; PED/PEDV, porcine epidemic diarrhea/PED Virus; PRRS/PRRSV, porcine reproductive and respiratory syndrome/PRRS virus; rRT-PCR, real-time reverse transcription polymerase chain reaction; S/P, sample-to-positive; TGEV, transmissible gastroenteritis virus; WTF, wean-to-finish; WV ELISA, whole virus enzyme-linked immunosorbent assay

Funding

This study was funded in part by Checkoff Dollars administered through the National Pork Board, Des Moines, Iowa (USA) and support from the Iowa State University Veterinary Diagnostic Laboratory.

Authors' contribution

JBK participated in study design, implementation of the study, analysis, and writing of the manuscript. KW participated in study design, implementation of the study. LGL developed the PEDV WV ELISA, carried out immunoassays, and helped draft the manuscript. MR participated in study design and implementation of the study. CW and YS performed statistical analyses. PL participated in the study design and implementation of the study. JQZ participated in the study design and writing. DB carried out immunoassays. PG carried out molecular studies. RM conceived of the study, participated in study design, and implementation of the study. JZ participated in study design, data analysis, and writing. All authors have read and approved the final version of the manuscript.

Competing interests

The authors declare no conflict of interest with respect to the research, authorship, or publication of this article.

Consent for publication

Not applicable.

Author details

[1]Department of Veterinary Diagnostic and Production Animal Medicine, College of Veterinary Medicine, Iowa State University, 1850 Christensen Drive, Ames, IA 50011-1134, USA. [2]Department of Statistics, College of Liberal Arts and Sciences, Iowa State University, Osborn Drive, Ames, IA 50011, USA. [3]Smithfield Hog Production Missouri, 17999 US Highway 65, Princeton, MO 64673, USA.

References

1. Saif LJ, Pensaert MB, Sestak K, Yeo S, Jung K. Coronaviruses. In: Zimmerman JJ, Karriker LA, Ramirez A, Schwartz KJ, Stevenson GW, editors. Diseases of Swine. 10th ed. Ames: Wiley and Sons; 2012. p. 501–24.
2. Chen J, Wang C, Shi H, Qiu H, Liu S, Chen X, Zhang Z, Feng L. Molecular epidemiology of porcine epidemic diarrhea virus in China. Arch Virol. 2010;155:1471–6.
3. Song D, Bongkyun P. Porcine epidemic diarrhoea virus: a comprehensive review of molecular epidemiology, diagnosis, and vaccines. Virus Genes. 2012;44:167–75.
4. Hanke D, Jenckel M, Petrov A, Ritzmann M, Stadler J, Akimkin V, Blome S, Pohlmann A, Schirrmeier H, Beer M, Höper D. Comparison of porcine epidemic diarrhea viruses from Germany and the United States, 2014. Emerg Infect Dis. 2015;21:493–6.
5. Mesquita JR, Hakze-van Der Honing R, Almeida A, Lourenço M, van der Poel WHM, Nascimento MSJ. Outbreak of porcine epidemic diarrhea virus in Portugal, 2015. Transbound Emerg Dis. 2015;62:586–8.
6. Prickett J, Simer R, Christopher-Hennings J, Yoon KJ, Evans RB, Zimmerman J. Detection of porcine reproductive and respiratory syndrome virus infection in porcine oral fluid samples: A longitudinal study under experimental conditions. J Vet Diagn Invest. 2008;20:156–63.
7. Madson DM, Magstadt DR, Arruda PHE, Hoang H, Sun D, Bower LP, Bhandari M, Burrough ER, Gauger PC, Pillatzki AE, Stevenson GW, Wilberts BL, Brodie J, Harmon KM, Wang C, Main RG, Zhang J, Yoon KJ. Pathogenesis of porcine epidemic diarrhea virus isolate (US/Iowa/18984/2013) in 3-week-old weaned pigs. Vet Microbiol. 2014;174:60–8.
8. Chen Q, Gauger PC, Stafne MR, Thomas JT, Madson DM, Huang H, Zheng Y, Li G, Zhang J. Pathogenesis comparison between the United States porcine epidemic diarrhea virus prototype and S-INDEL-variant strains in conventional neonatal piglets. J Gen Virol. 2016. doi:10.1099/jgv.0.000419.
9. Thomas JT, Chen Q, Gauger PC, Giménez-Lirola L, Sinha A, Harmon KM, Madson DM, Burrough ER, Magstadt DR, Salzbrenner HM, Welch MW, Yoon KJ, Zimmerman JJ, Zhang J. Effect of porcine epidemic diarrhea virus infectious doses on infection outcomes in naive conventional neonatal and weaned pigs. PLoS One. 2015;10(10):e0139266.
10. Crawford K, Lager K, Miller L, Opriessnig T, Gerber P, Hesse R. Evaluation of porcine epidemic diarrhea virus transmission and the immune response in growing pigs. Vet Res. 2015;46:49.
11. O'Connor AM, Gailey J, McKean JD, Hurd HS. Quantity and distribution of salmonella recovered from three swine lairage pens. J Food Protect. 2006; 69:1717–9.
12. DeBuysscher E, Berman D. Secretory immune response in intestinal mucosa and salivary gland after experimental infection of pigs with transmissible gastroenteritis virus. Am J Vet Res. 1980;41:1214–20.
13. Brandtzæg P. Secretory immunity with special reference to the oral cavity. J Oral Microbiol. 2013;5:20401.
14. Kittawornrat A, Prickett J, Wang C, Olsen C, Irwin C, Panyasing Y, Ballagi A, Rice A, Main R, Johnson J, Rademacher C, Hoogland M, Rowland R, Zimmerman J. Detection of Porcine reproductive and respiratory syndrome virus (PRRSV) antibodies in oral fluid specimens using a commercial PRRSV serum antibody enzyme-linked immunosorbent assay. J Vet Diagn Invest. 2012;24:262–9.
15. Panyasing Y, Goodell CK, Giménez-Lirola L, Kittawornrat A, Wang C, Schwartz KJ, Zimmerman JJ. Kinetics of influenza A virus nucleoprotein antibody (IgM, IgA, and IgG) in serum and oral fluid specimens from pigs infected under experimental conditions. Vaccine. 2013;2013;6210–6215.

Cholesterol of lipid rafts is a key determinant for entry and post-entry control of porcine rotavirus infection

Xiujing Dou[1†], Yang Li[1†], Junlan Han[1], Dante S. Zarlenga[2], Weijuan Zhu[1], Xiaofeng Ren[1], Na Dong[1], Xunliang Li[1*] and Guangxing Li[1*]

Abstract

Background: Lipid rafts are major structural components in plasma membranes that play critical roles in many biological processes including virus infection. However, few reports have described the relationship between lipid rafts and porcine rotavirus (PRV) infection. In this study, we investigated whether or not the locally high concentrations (3–5 fold) of cholesterol present in lipid rafts are required for PRV infection, and further examined which stages of the infection process are most affected.

Results: When cellular cholesterol was depleted by methyl-β-cyclodextrin (MβCD), PRV infectivity significantly declined in a dose-dependent manner. This inhibition was partially reversed upon reintroduction of cholesterol into the system. This was corroborated by the co-localization of PRV with a recombinant, GPI-anchored green fluorescent protein, which functioned as a marker for membranous regions high in cholesterol and indicative of lipid rafts. Changes in virus titer and western blot analyses indicated that depletion of cellular cholesterol with MβCD had no apparent effect on PRV adsorption; however, depletion of cholesterol significantly restricted entry and post-entry of PRV into the cell. Both points of inhibition were restored to near normal levels by the addition of exogenous cholesterol.

Conclusions: We conclude from these studies that membrane-based cholesterol and in particular that localized to lipid rafts, is an indispensable biomolecule for PRV infection, and that cholesterol-based control of the infection process takes place during entry and immediately post-entry into the cell.

Keywords: Porcine rotavirus (PRV), Lipid rafts, Cholesterol, Methyl-β-cyclodextrin (MβCD), Infection, Entry

Background

Porcine rotavirus (PRV) is the most important cause of severe diarrhea in newborn piglets, and results in significant economic loss to pig industry. To date, efficient drugs for preventing PRV infection have not been identified. PRV, which belongs to the genus *Rotavirus* in the family *Reoviridae*, is a non-enveloped virus formed by three concentric layers of proteins [1]. The outermost layer consists of spike-like structures comprised of an unglycosylated VP4 protein [2] and a glycoprotein VP7, which forms the smooth surface of the virus. VP7 is a calcium-binding protein that interacts with cell receptors after the initial attachment of the virus to the cell surface [3].

It remains unclear as to how non-enveloped viruses which lack an outer lipid membrane infect host cells. It is generally believed that membrane fusion is not involved in virus entry and that release of these viruses is mainly performed by cell lysis [4]. It has been proposed that non-enveloped viruses penetrate the membrane barrier, either by the formation of a pore at the cell surface, or via the endocytic pathway using clathrin-coated vesicles or caveolae [4]. Alternatively, studies with simian virus 40 (SV40) [5] and poliovirus [6] have suggested that non-enveloped viruses are transported to specific domains within the plasma membrane using a vesicular transport mechanism, followed by replication in large inclusions in

* Correspondence: 14746768@qq.com; ligx@neau.edu.cn
†Equal contributors
[1]Northeast Agricultural University, No. 59 Mucai Street, Xiangfang District, Harbin 150030, China
Full list of author information is available at the end of the article

the cell cytoplasm or viroplasm [7]. Other biochemical and structural studies have shown that the overall mechanism is similar to enveloped viruses, and that viral capsid proteins may function in a manner analogous to the membrane viral proteins [4].

In recent years, research has exposed a crucial role for lipid rafts in a variety of virus life cycles [6–8]. Lipid rafts are traditionally described as microdomains within plasma membranes that are high in cholesterol, sphingolipids, glycosyl-phosphatidylinositol (GPI)-anchored proteins, and a specific set of associated proteins often cell receptors. They are thought to provide organization to and stabilize the structure of cell membranes because the high concentration of sphingolipids and protein receptors are densely packed together with cholesterol [9]. Although they are more ordered and closely packed, they still have the ability to float freely within the membrane bilayer. The most commonly used drugs to control the formation and function of lipid drafts are nystatin and filipin which sequester cholesterol, MβCD which is used to deplete membrane-bound cholesterol, and lovastatin which inhibits cholesterol biosynthesis [8].

Recent reports have demonstrated the involvement of lipids in a variety of cellular functions such as apical cell-sorting of proteins, signal transduction, caveolae mediated endocytosis, and viral release, assembly and budding in the cell membrane. These have been well documented in human immunodeficiency virus (HIV) [9], measles virus [10], influenza virus [11–13] and rotavirus [7, 14]. Lipids have also been deemed important in intracellular trafficking of viral proteins [15–18] (e.g. echovirus types 1 and 11, Ebola [19]), and provide platforms for cell entry (e.g. SV40 [20], HIV [21–24], echovirus type 1 [25] and rhesus rotavirus (RRV) [14]). Although it has been reported that RRV depends upon lipid rafts for cell entry [14], the specific role of cholesterol in these processes of PRV remains elusive.

Herein, we explored the importance of cellular cholesterol during PRV infection of MA104 cells by demonstrating that viral protein and genomic RNA levels were reduced significantly following MβCD treatment to deplete cellular cholesterol. We further showed that viral protein and genomic RNA levels were restored by subsequently treating the cells with exogenous cholesterol. Data showing the colocalization of VP7 with recombinant, fluorescently-labeled GPI-anchored protein linked the virus predominantly to lipid rafts. In as much as cholesterol was indispensable for both PRV entry and the post-entry process, lipid rafts could be a target for development of anti-PRV strategies.

Methods

Cells, viruses, antisera and reagents

MA104 and BHK-21 cells (obtained from China Center For Type Culture Collection) were cultured in Dulbecco's Modified Eagle Medium (DMEM) (Gibco) supplemented with 10% fetal calf serum (FCS) at 37 °C under 5% CO_2. PRV (strain DN30209, isolated in a pig farm, in Heilongjiang province of China) [26] and vesicular stomatitis virus (VSV, strain Indiana, obtained from prof. Joerg Glende, University of Veterinary Medicine Hannover, Germany) were propagated on the MA104 cells and BHK-21 cells, respectively, as previously described [26, 27]. In as much as previous reports showed that VSV infection on BHK-21 is not affected by depletion of cholesterol [27], we used VSV as a negative control for our studies about relationship between lipid rafts and virus infection.

Rabbit polyclonal antibodies to VP4 and VP7 were generated in our laboratory using previously described methods [26, 28]. Anti-VSV G-protein polyclonal antibody was purchased from Abcam. An anti-β-actin monoclonal antibody was purchased from Beyotime. The secondary antibodies were purchased from BD Biosciences. Both MβCD and cholesterol were purchased from Sigma and reconstituted in DMEM and alcohol, respectively.

Virus titration

Approximately 1×10^4 MA104 or BHK-21 cells were seeded onto 96-wells plates then incubated with purified PRV or VSV (100 μL virus/well) that was serially-diluted 10-fold prior to infection. Forty-eight hours after infection, the 50% tissue culture infectious dose ($TCID_{50}$) of each well was determined according to the method of Reed and Muench by observing cytopathic effects (CPE). All experiments were conducted 5 times.

Cytotoxicity assay

Toxic effects of MβCD and cholesterol on cells were determined using the Mosmann based assay (MTT) [29]. Cells were plated onto 96-well plates and upon reaching 80% confluency, they were incubated with different concentrations of MβCD (0, 2, 4, 6, 8, 10, 15 mM) or cholesterol (0, 50, 100, 150, 200 μM) for 48 h. Mock-treated cells served as controls.

Depletion and replenishment of cholesterol from cells

For cholesterol depletion, cell monolayers were grown to 80% confluency, washed three times with cold phosphate-buffered saline (PBS), and then treated with various concentrations of MβCD ranging from 2 to 15 mM in serum-free DMEM for 30 min at 37 °C. Control cells were similarly treated but received no MβCD. All cells were subsequently washed with cold PBS. For cholesterol replenishment, washed cells were treated for 1 h at 37 °C with DMEM-soluble exogenous cholesterol at final concentrations ranging from 50 to 200 μM. Again the cells were washed extensively with PBS then subjected to virus (100 $TCID_{50}$) infection.

Indirect immunofluorescence assay (IFA)

At 24 h post-infection, all cells were washed and fixed with cold 1% paraformaldehyde for 30 min, and then balanced out by glycine 5 min. The cells were washed and permeabilized with 1% Triton X-100 for 10 min, and then incubated with 200 μL polyclonal antibody against the PRV VP7 protein or VSV-G protein at 37 °C for 45 min. After washing, the cells were incubated with an optimum dilution of fluorescein (FITC)-conjugated goat anti-rabbit IgG (H + L) (OriGene, Beijing) for 30 min at 37 °C then washed again in the dark, and examined under a fluorescence microscope (Zeiss Axiovert 200).

Co-localization of PRV VP7 and GPI-anchored protein

MA104 cells were seeded onto 24-well tissue culture plates (2×10^5 per well) and transfected using lipofectamine 2000 (Invitrogen, USA) with the pEGFP-GPI, a DNA plasmid encoding GPI-tethered to the enhanced green fluorescent protein (provided by Kai Simons, Max-Planck-Institute of Molecular Cell Biology and Genetics, Germany). At 6 h post-transfection, cells were infected with PRV (100 $TCID_{50}$) for 24 h at 37 °C. Polyclonal antibody to PRV VP7 protein was used for virus detection by IFA using a fluorescence microscope.

Real-time PCR

Real time-PCR was used to evaluate and quantify the level of viral infection following treatment. Briefly, total genomic RNA was extracted from viruses using RNA extract reagent (Fastgene, China) and cDNA was synthesized using M-MLV reverse transcriptase (Takara Bio Inc., Shiga, Japan). The cDNA was PCR amplified and the products were quantified using SYBR green as fluorescence dye (Takara Bio Inc., Shiga, Japan). The data were analyzed with ABI PRISM 7500 SDS software. Gene quantification was performed using the $2^{-\Delta\Delta CT}$ method. The primer sequences are shown in Table 1.

Western blot

The cells were harvested and lysed with cold cell lysis buffer containing 1% Triton X-100 and 1% protease inhibitor (Beyotime Institute of Biotechnology, USA). Total lysate was separated on a 12% SDS-PAGE gel then transferred to nitrocellulose membranes. The membranes were blocked with 5% non-fat dry milk in Tris-buffered saline (10 mM Tris-Cl at pH 7.5 and 150 mM NaCl) containing 0.05% Tween 20 (TBST) at 37 °C for 1 h, and then incubated with primary antibody at room temperature for 4 h. Detection was performed using horseradish peroxidase (HRP)-linked secondary antibody at room temperature for 1 h. Blots were developed using enhanced chemiluminescence detection system (Applygen, China).

Table 1 The primer sequences used for real-time PCR

Gene	Primer sequence (5′ to 3′)	
VP7	Forward	TGTCCTCTAAATACGCAGACTC
	Reverse	CTACCTGAATTACAGCGACAT
β-actin	Forward	GGCTCAGAGCAAGAGAGGTATCC
	Reverse	GGTCTCAAACATGATCTGAGTCATCT
VSV-G	Forward	TTCAAGCAGACGGTTGG
	Reverse	TGCTTCGGCATCCGTCA

Stage specificity of cholesterol effects on PRV infection

To investigate the effects of cholesterol depletion on PRV infectivity in MA104 cells, the cell monolayers were incubated with 8 mM or 15 mM MβCD for 30 min at 37 °C, then washed. Virus (100 $TCID_{50}$) was inoculated onto the cells at 4 °C where only adsorption can occur. After 2 h, the unbound virus was removed by washing and the medium replaced with DMEM. The cells were cultured until control cells exhibited complete CPE. For cholesterol replenishment, cells were pretreated with 15 mM MβCD at 37 °C for 30 min, washed, then incubated with 200 μM cholesterol for 1 h at 37 °C. The cells were then incubated with PRV at 100 $TCID_{50}$ for 2 h at 4 °C.

For studies on cell entry, the cells were mock treated or pretreated with 8 mM MβCD at 37 °C for 30 min then infected with PRV(100 $TCID_{50}$) for 1 h at 37 °C, after which remaining virus was removed by washing. The cells were kept in serum-free DMEM at 37 °C until mock treated, virus-infected cells showed complete CPE. For cholesterol replenishment, cells were pretreated with 15 mM MβCD at 37 °C for 30 min, washed and then incubated with exogenous cholesterol (200 μM) for 1 h at 37 °C.

For the post-entry study, cells were infected with PRV (100 $TCID_{50}$) for 1 h at 37 °C, and the remaining virus was removed by washing. The cells were subsequently mock treated or pretreated with 8 mM MβCD at 37 °C for 30 min, washed in cold PBS and then incubated in DMEM at 37 °C until the mock treated, virus-infected cells showed complete CPE. For cholesterol replenishment, the cells were treated as described for the cell entry studies. Western blots and virus titers were performed to assess the effects of pre- and post-treatment on virus infection.

Results

Effects of cholesterol depletion on PRV infection

To determine whether the cholesterol component of lipid rafts plays a role in PRV infection, the cholesterol level in cellular membranes of MA104 cells for PRV and BHK-21 cells for VSV, respectively, were depleted by treatment with MβCD before infecting with PRV or VSV. After 24 h, VP7 polyclonal antibody for PRV binding exhibited a dose-dependent decrease in MA104 cells pretreated with increasing concentrations of MβCD (Fig. 1a). At a concentration of 15 mM, the infection rate

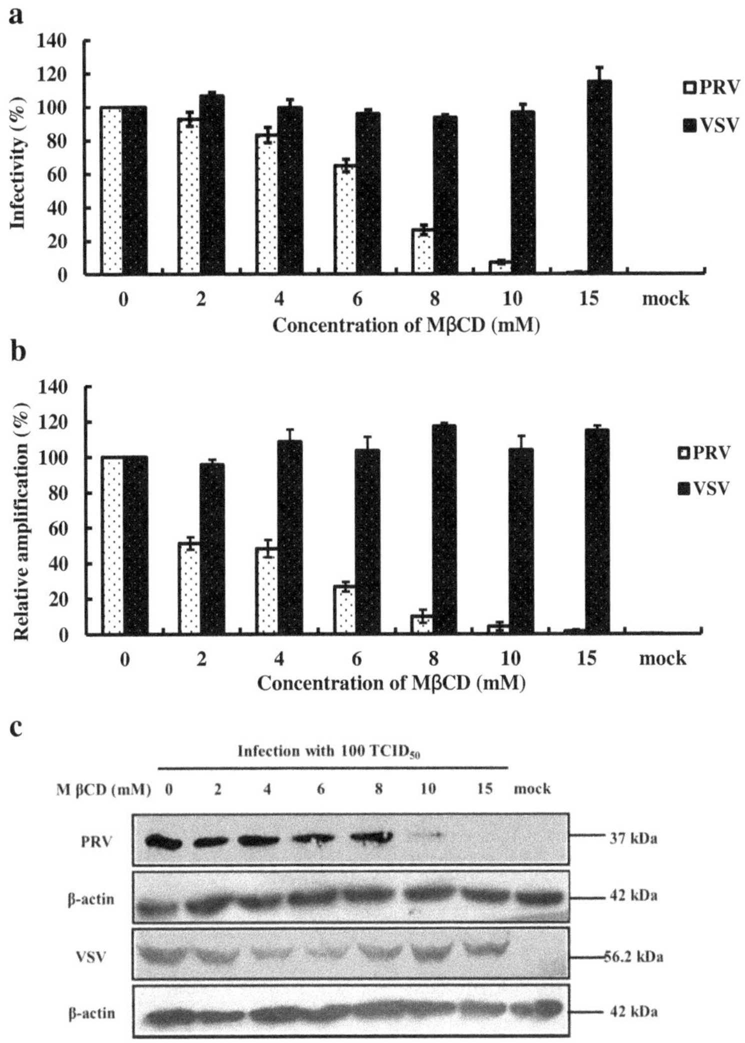

Fig. 1 PRV infection inhibited by cholesterol depletion with MβCD. MA104 cell and BHK-21 cell monolayers were treated with increasing concentrations of MβCD before virus infection. Cells were subsequently, infected with PRV or VSV (100 $TCID_{50}$) respectively, except "mock" as control without virus infection and MβCD treatment. **a** IFA data demonstrating infectivity of PRV and VSV using anti-VP7 of PRV antibodies and anti-G protein of VSV antibodies respectively. The 100% infectivity values of PRV and VSV represent average fluorescein-stained cells numbers of 100 and 240, respectively. **b** Real-time PCR data for PRV and VSV targeting the VP7 gene and G-protein. **c** Western blot analysis using antibodies to VP7 for PRV, G-protein for VSV and β-actin served as a protein loading control. Error bars indicate the standard deviations of three independent experiments

of PRV decreased by 99%. In contrast, the infection rate of cholesterol-depleted BHK-21 cells infected with the control VSV was not affected. Real-time PCR results to quantify the PRV VP7 and VSV G gene, the viral load showed a similar response in MβCD-treated cells (Fig. 1b). Western blot (Fig. 1c) also demonstrated that depletion of cholesterol reduced the level of PRV infection in a dose-dependent manner where VP7 protein expression was nearly absent from MA104 cells at 15 mM MβCD. In contrast, no significant inhibitory effects were observed in MβCD treated BHK-21 cells infected with VSV as monitored by VSV G protein levels (Fig. 1c).

Effects of cholesterol replenishment on PRV infection in cholesterol-deficient cells

The effects of PRV-infection on MA104 cells depleted of cholesterol with MβCD (15 mM) then replenished with exogenous cholesterol prior to PRV infection, are shown in Fig. 2. Virus levels were examined directly by IFA assay (Fig. 2a) and indirectly by RT-PCR (Fig. 2b). PRV infectivity as examined by IFA, increased in a dose-dependent manner and was restored to 70% of pretreatment levels (no MβCD) (Fig. 2a) with a concentration of 200 μM cholesterol. From the RT-PCR, we observed a similar, dose-dependent increase in the level of VP7 gene of PRV as the amount of exogenous cholesterol was increased

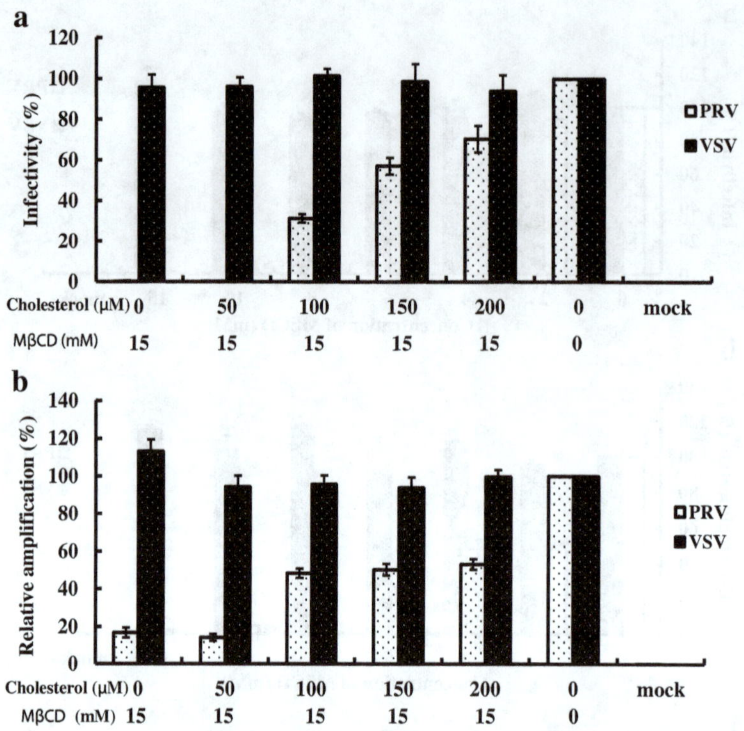

Fig. 2 The restoration of PRV-infectivity by exogenous cholesterol. MA104 cell and BHK-21 cell monolayers were treated with 15 mM MβCD before supplemented with exogenous cholesterol. Subsequently, cells were infected with PRV or VSV (100 $TCID_{50}$) respectively, except mock as control without virus infection and MβCD/ exogenous cholesterol treatment. **a** IFA data demonstrating infectivity of PRV and VSV using anti-VP7 antibodies and anti-VSV G protein antibodies respectively. The 100% infectivity values of PRV and VSV represent average fluorescein-stained cells numbers of 160 or 230, respectively; **b** Real-time PCR data for PRV and VSV targeting the VP7 and G protein gene. Error bars indicate the standard deviations of three independent experiments

(Fig. 2b), the VP7 gene expression reached 55% pretreatment levels (no MβCD).

Co-localization of PRV VP7 protein and GPI-anchored protein

GPI-proteins have a predilection for lipid rafts. MA104 cells transfected first with GPI-pEGFP then with PRV (100 $TCID_{50}$) showed a co-localization of both the recomninant GPI-protein (green) (Fig. 3a) and the PRV VP7 protein (red) (Fig. 3b) in dense regions of the cell membrane. These regions appeared yellow in merged figures (Fig. 3c). Data suggest that the PRV VP7 protein was localized in the lipid rafts of MA104 cells.

Cholesterol is not required for PRV adsorption

To determine if cholesterol is important in PRV adsorption, cholesterol-depleted cells were incubated with PRV for 24 h at 4 °C to prevent viral replication, and then assayed

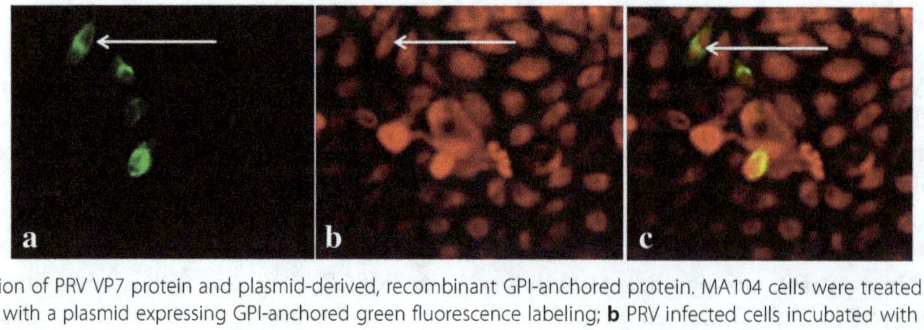

Fig. 3 Co-localization of PRV VP7 protein and plasmid-derived, recombinant GPI-anchored protein. MA104 cells were treated for IFA as follows: **a** cells transfected with a plasmid expressing GPI-anchored green fluorescence labeling; **b** PRV infected cells incubated with anti-VP7 protein antibodies and counterstained with FITC second antibody; **c** co-localization of GPI-anchored protein and PRV VP7 protein on the cell membrane (Fig. 3a and b merged). Yellow color depicts overlapping binding

for viral load by $TCID_{50}$ and western blot. As shown in Fig. 4a and b, relative to mock-infected groups, no remarkable inhibitory effects were observed by $TCID_{50}$ or western blot in the PRV-infected groups. The results mirrored those obtained with VSV (Fig. 4a and c) which is not affected by cholesterol levels. Data suggest that adsorption onto the cell membrane was not affected in cholesterol-depleted cells.

Cholesterol depletion inhibits PRV entry in a reversible manner

To study the effects of cholesterol on PRV entry, cholesterol-depleted MA104 cells were incubated with PRV at 37 °C rather than 4 °C then viral loads examined 24 h post-infection. Results show that PRV virus titers (Fig. 5a) and viral protein levels (Fig. 5b) were decreased. At a concentration of 8 mM MβCD, we observed an approximate reduction in the virus titer of 50%, relative to controls. Expression levels of PRV viral protein were also significantly reduced; however, VSV and β-actin were not changed (Fig. 5c).

The results on virus entry were reversible (Fig. 6). Cholesterol-depleted MA104 cells treated with 200 μM exogenous cholesterol for 1 h showed complete restoration of PRV virus titers relative to mock treated cells (Fig. 6a). The viral protein levels were increased significantly (Fig. 6b). Levels of VSV were not affected (Fig. 6a and c). Results suggest that stages following adsorption and most likely virus entry have a strict requirement for cholesterol.

Cholesterol depletion of MA104 cells inhibited PRV post-entry stage

To analyze post-entry stages, MA104 cells were first infected with PRV then treated with MβCD. As shown

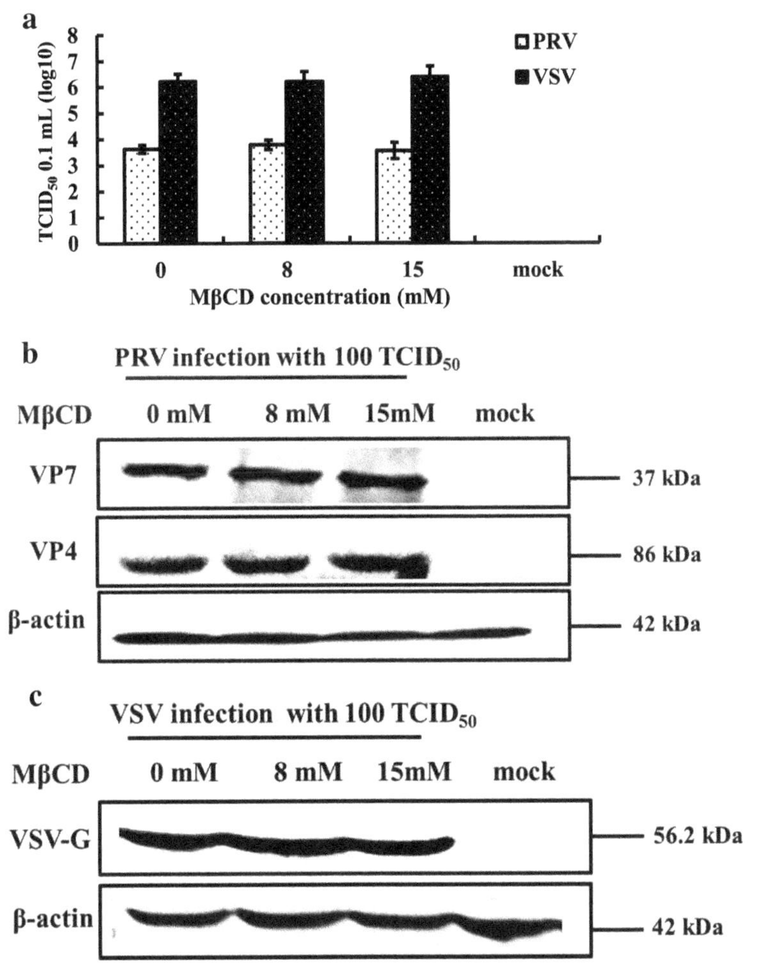

Fig. 4 Cellular cholesterol and PRV adsorption. MA104 cells (PRV) and BHK-21 cells (VSV) were either mock treated or treated with 8 mM or 15 mM MβCD for 30 min, then infected with PRV or VSV (100 $TCID_{50}$) at 4 °C for 2 h. Antibodies to the PRV VP7 or VP4 proteins and to the VSV G protein were used to screen western blots of cell homogenates and virus titers. **a** Virus titers of PRV and VSV after treatment. **b** Western blot of PRV VP7 and VP4 proteins and β-actin. **c** Western blot of VSV G protein and β-actin. Western blots depict representative experiments. Error bars (Fig. 4a) indicate the standard deviations of three independent experiments

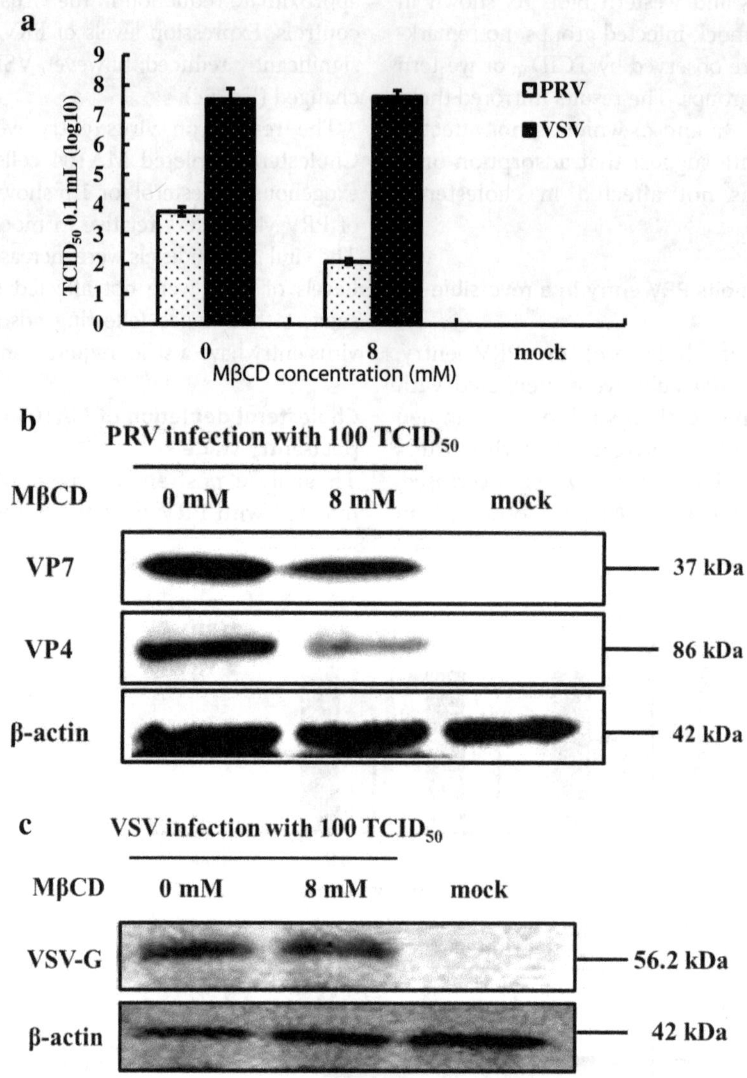

Fig. 5 Cholesterol and control of PRV entry. MA104 cells (PRV) and BHK-21 cells (VSV) were either mock treated or treated with 8 mM MβCD for 30 min then infected with PRV or VSV (100 $TCID_{50}$) for 1 h at 37 °C. Antibodies to the PRV VP7 or VP4 proteins and to the VSV G protein were used to screen western blots of cell homogenates and virus titers. **a** Virus titers of PRV and VSV after treatment. **b** Western blot of PRV VP7 and VP4 proteins and β-actin. **c** Western blot of VSV G protein and β-actin. Western blots depict representative experiments. Error bars (Fig. 5a) indicate the standard deviations of three independent experiments

in Fig. 7a, b, and c, the PRV virus titers and viral protein levels decreased relative to VSV controls, whereas replenishing exogenous cholesterol restored virus titers to pretreatment levels relative to VSV controls (Fig. 8a). The viral proteins were also increased significantly (Fig. 8b) relative to VSV controls (Fig. 8c) demonstrating that post-entry stages were also controlled by the level of cellular cholesterol.

Discussion

Lipid rafts are densely packed, floating asemblages of cholesterol, sphingolipid and mostly receptor proteins that are present within cell membranes and that function in membrane trafficking and signaling [30]. Among other things, lipid rafts play critical roles in viral entry, replication, assembly and budding, as well as in protein transport [31]. Cholesterol is a key component of lipid rafts that compartmentalize cellular processes. Further, changes in cellular cholesterol levels have been linked to alterations in the infection process of numerous viruses where the cholesterol dissipative agent, MβCD, has been used to evaluate cholesterol-enriched lipid rafts in virus infection. MβCD is a strictly surface-acting agent that rapidly removes cholesterol from the plasma membrane. Some non-enveloped viruses, such as members of *Picornaviridae* and *Reoviridae,* are assembled in the cytoplasm and released by cell lysis. However, evidence has been advanced showing that exit from infected cells can occur in the

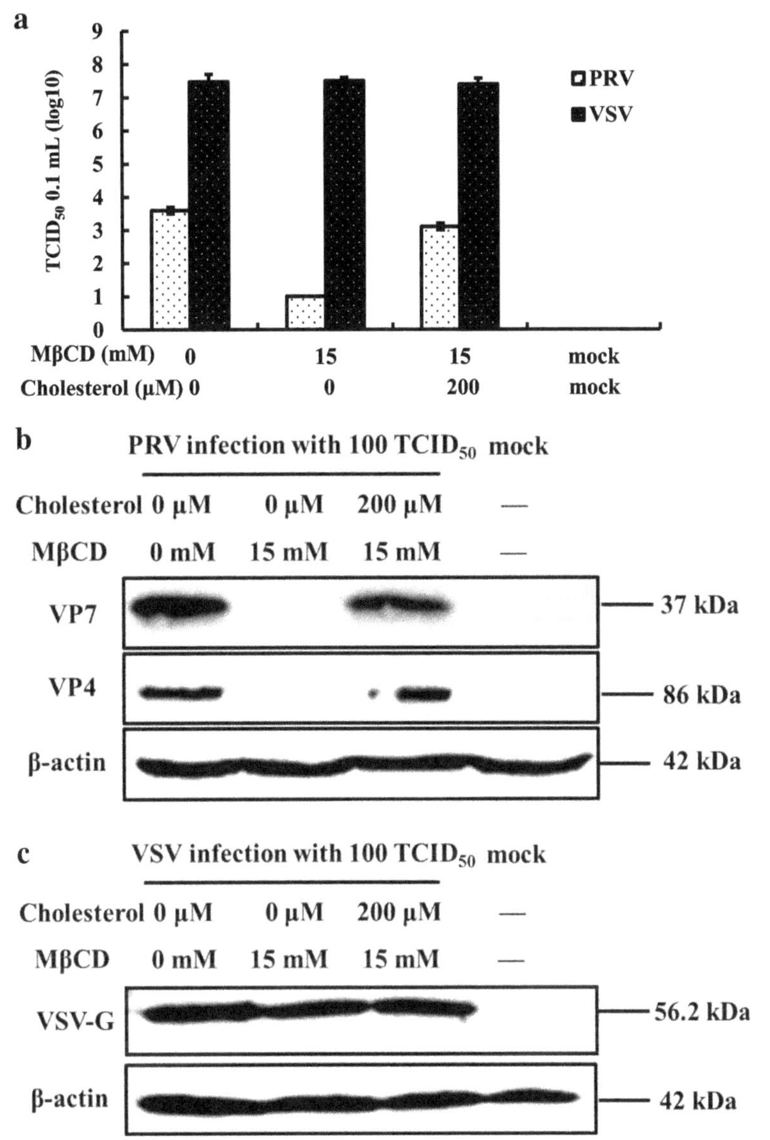

Fig. 6 Reversing the effects of MβCD on PRV entry using exogenous cholesterol. MA104 cells (PRV) and BHK-21 cells (VSV) were pretreated with 15 mM MβCD at 37 °C for 30 min, then replenished 200 μM exogenous cholesterol at 37 °C for 1 h. Treated cells were then infected with PRV or VSV (100 $TCID_{50}$), respectively, and the homogenates examined by western blot analysis and virus titers. **a** Virus titer of PRV and VSV after treatment. **b** Western blot of PRV VP7 and VP4 proteins and β-actin. **c** Western blot of VSV G protein and β-actin. Western blots depict representative experiments. Error bars (Fig. 6a) indicate the standard deviations of three independent experiments

absence of cell lysis, suggesting that alternate paths may be utilized for egress by non-enveloped viruses [4]. Other members of the non-enveloped virus, such as RRV and bluetongue virus (BTV), along with a number of enveloped viruses such as transmissible gastroenteritis virus (TGEV) [27], porcine reproductive and respiratory syndrome virus (PRRSV) [32], porcine pseudorabies virus (PrV) [33], Rift valley fever virus [34] have been shown to be sensitive to MβCD treatment of host cells. Further, RRV and BTV have been shown to interact with lipids during the progress of infection suggesting the importance of cholesterol-rich microdomains in the infection process. The entry of rotaviruses (RV) into host cells is a multistep process. Different rotavirus strains display different requirements for host cells. Some strains depend on the presence of sialic acid (SA) on the cell surface [35]. Others have demonstrated a requirement for several integrin during infection. As example, the VP4 protein of RV contains tripeptide sequence motifs for integrin α2β1 and α4β1, whereas VP7 contains ligand sites for integrin αxβ2 and α4β1 [36, 37]. In addition, heat shock protein and certain gangliosides were identified as cellular molecules associated with RV entry.

The non-enveloped PRV, is a leading etiologic cause of severe dehydrating diarrhea in piglet worldwide.

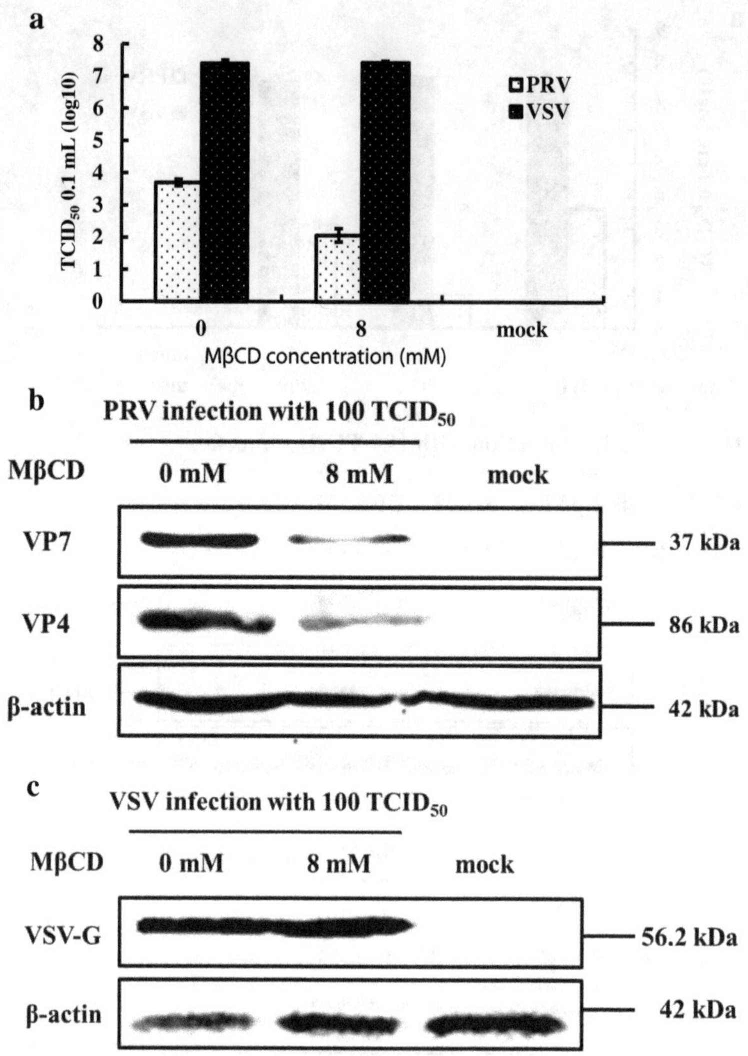

Fig. 7 Cholesterol and control of PRV post-entry. MA104 cells (PRV) and BHK-21 cells (VSV) were first infected at 37 °C for 1 h then washed to remove extra virus. Cells were then treated with 8 mM MβCD incubated at 37 °C for 24 h. Antibodies to the PRV VP7 or VP4 proteins (PRV) and to the VSV G protein (VSV) were used to screen Western blots of cell homogenates. **a** Virus titer of PRV and VSV after treatment. **b** Western blot of PRV VP7 and VP4 proteins and β-actin. **c** Western blot of VSV G protein and β-actin. Western blots depict representative experiments. Error bars (Fig. 7a) indicate the standard deviations of three independent experiments

Consequently, there is an urgent need to develop effective preventive and therapeutic strategies to combat this pathogen. Currently, it is unknown whether or not cholesterol-enriched lipid rafts which is present in the membranes of the host cells, is required for PRV infection, and if so, how it is associated with PRV infection. To address this question, cholesterol in the cellular membrane of MA104 cells was removed by MβCD treatment prior to PRV infection. Results demonstrated that lipid rafts depleted of cholesterol decreased the infectivity of PRV in a dose-dependent manner. Conversely, replenishment of cholesterol partially restored viral infection. These results are similar to those observed on RRV [14], BTV and poliovirus [6] which are also non-enveloped viruses [5, 38].

Our results collectively demonstrate that PRV infection interacts with cholesterol-enriched lipid rafts. First, direct treatment of the virus with MβCD prior to infection had no effect in the infection process (data not shown) indicating the observed effects were unrelated to interactions between the drug and the virus. Second, the concentration of MβCD and cholesterol used in this study did not generate significant adverse effects on cell viability as shown by MTT (data not shown). Third, the drug concentrations and the protocols are similar to those described in studies involving other viruses [27, 39]. Finally, co-localization studies showed that PRV VP7 protein and a recombinant GPI-anchor protein which has a predilection for lipid rafts, were localized to the lipid rafts in the plasma membranes of MA104 cells.

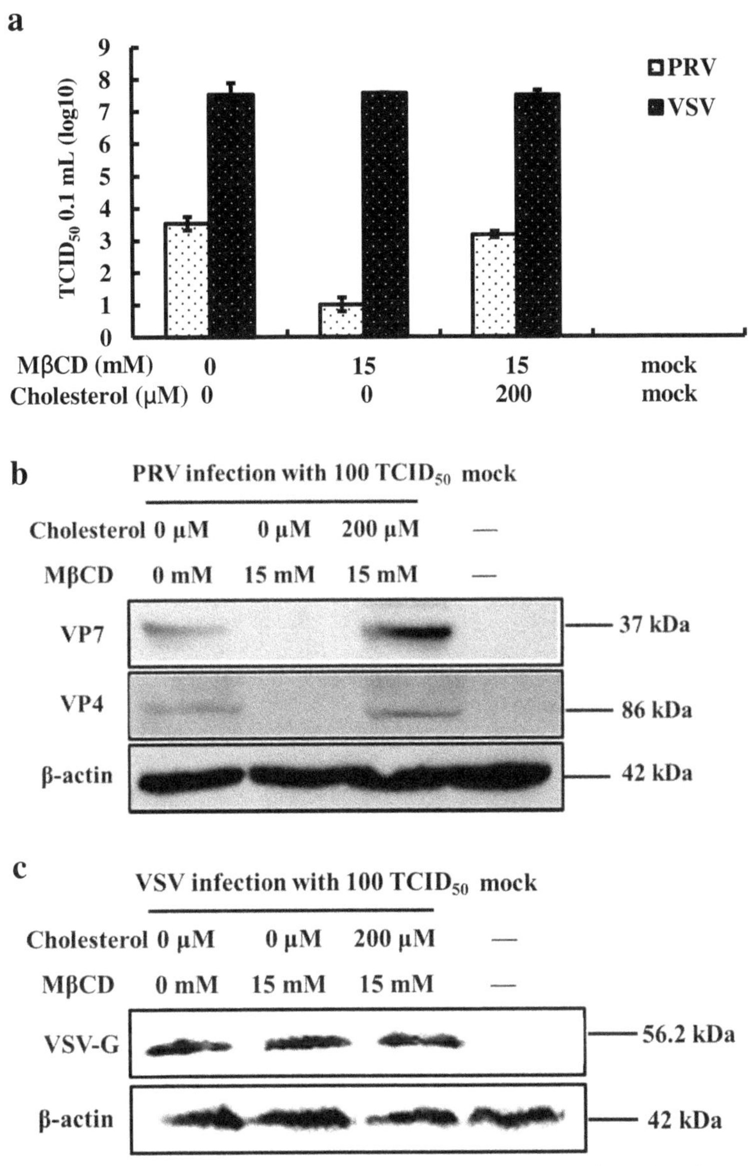

Fig. 8 Reversing the effects of MβCD on PRV post-entry using exogenous cholesterol. MA104 cells (PRV) and BHK-21 cells (VSV) that had been infected and treated with MβCD were then incubated in the presence of 200 μM exogenous cholesterol. Western blots and virus titers were performed to assess the effects of pre- and post-treatment on virus infection. **a** Virus titer of PRV and VSV after treatment. **b** Western blot of PRV VP7 and VP4 proteins and β-actin. **c** Western blot of VSV G protein and β-actin. Western blots depict representative experiments. Error bars (Fig. 8a) indicate the standard deviations of three independent experiments

Studies on the key stages of the PRV infection process requiring cholesterol have not been reported. In this study, we showed that adsorption of the virus onto the cell membrane at low temperatures was not affected by depletion of cholesterol; no significant differences were observed between MβCD-treated cells and mock cells. However, when cells were treated with MβCD prior to or after virus entry, PRV infection declined in a dose-dependent manner. The replenishing of exogenous cholesterol reversed these affects indicating that cholesterol depletion affected mechanisms involved in the entry of the virus and one or more mechanism downstream of virus entry. Similar results were also observed with the bovine rotavirus (BRV) where cholesterol depletion significantly impaired BRV entry and assembly but did not reduce BRV replication [39]. These results suggested that PRV entry may be inhibited by cholesterol depletion though disturbing lipid-raft-dependent endocytosis.

In summary, lipid rafts play vital roles in PRV infection, and plasma membrane-based cholesterol is a key determinant for entry and post-entry stages of PRV infection. By depleting plasma membrane cholesterol we were able to provide a direct link between cholesterol levels, lipid rafts and the ability of PRV to infect host cells. Future studies are needed to investigate synergistic effects between MβCD and other drugs capable of disrupting lipid rafts in porcine intestinal epithelial cell cultures.

Conclusions

Our results reveal the mechanism of PRV infection that membrane-cholesterol localized to lipid rafts is an indispensable biomolecule for PRV infection during the entry and post-entry into the cells rather than virus binding on cell surface; on the other hand, MβCD, a cellular cholesterol-depletion agent, inhibit the PRV infection on the susceptible cells, have a huge potential to develop a new anti-viral strategy.

Abbreviations

BRV: Bovine rotavirus; BTV: Bluetongue virus; CPE: Cytopathic effects; DMEM: Dulbecco's Modified Eagle Medium; FCS: Fetal calf serum; GPI: Glycosyl-phosphatidylinositol; h: Hours; HIV: Human immunodeficiency virus; HRP: Horseradish peroxidase; IFA: Indirect immunofluorescence assay; min: Minute; MTT: Mosmann based assay; MβCD: Methyl-β-cyclodextrin; PBS: Phosphate-buffered saline; PRRSV: Porcine reproductive and respiratory syndrome virus; PrV: Porcine pseudorabies virus; PRV: Porcine rotavirus; RRV: Rhesus rotavirus; SA: Sialic acid; SV40: Simian virus 40; TBST: Tris-buffered saline containing 0.05% Tween 20; $TCID_{50}$: The 50% tissue culture infectious dose; TGEV: Transmissible gastroenteritis virus; VSV: Vesicular stomatitis virus

Acknowledgements

Not Applicable.

Funding

This work was supported by the China Postdoctoral Science Foundation for the 62nd batch (2017M621), Postdoctoral Foundation in Heilongjiang Province (LBH-Z17013, LBH-Z17035), National Natural Science Foundation of China (31201911, 31300758 and 31501914), National Science & Technology Pillar Program during the Twelfth Five-year Plan Period (2013BAD12B04), and Research Fund for the Doctoral Program of Higher Education of China (Ph.D. Student Supervisor Type) of Ministry of Education of P.R. China, No. 20122325110019.

Authors' contributions

XJD and YL contributed equally to this work, and they are both co-first authors. XJD, YL participated in the design of this study, carried out all the studies, performed the statistical analysis and drafted the manuscript, XLL carried out partial infection experiments. YL, JLH and WJZ did much revision work during the major or minor revision, DSZ, XFR, ND and GXL supervised the work and edited the final version of this manuscript. All authors have read and approved the final version of the manuscript.

Consent for publication

Not applicable.

Competing interests

The authors declare that they have no competing interests.

Author details

[1]Northeast Agricultural University, No. 59 Mucai Street, Xiangfang District, Harbin 150030, China. [2]Animal Parasitic Diseases Laboratory, Agricultural Research Service, United States Department of Agriculture, Building 1180, BARC-East, Beltsville, MD 20705, USA.

References

1. Parashar UD, Hummelman EG, Bresee JS, Miller MA, Glass RI. Global illness and deaths caused by rotavirus disease in children. Emerg Infect Dis. 2003;9:565–72.
2. Desselberger U. Rotaviruses. Virus Res. 2014;190C:75–96.
3. Graham KL, Halasz P, Tan Y, Hewish MJ, Takada Y, Mackow ER, Robinson MK, Coulson BS. Integrin-using rotaviruses bind alpha2beta1 integrin alpha2 I domain via VP4 DGE sequence and recognize alphaXbeta2 and alphaVbeta3 by using VP7 during cell entry. J Virol. 2003;77:9969–78.
4. Bhattacharya B, Roy P. Role of lipids on entry and exit of bluetongue virus, a complex non-enveloped virus. Viruses. 2010;2:1218–35.
5. Clayson ET, Brando LV, Compans RW. Release of simian virus 40 virions from epithelial cells is polarized and occurs without cell lysis. J Virol. 1989;63:2278–88.
6. Danthi P, Chow M. Cholesterol removal by methyl-beta-cyclodextrin inhibits poliovirus entry. J Virol. 2004;78:33–41.
7. Cuadras MA, Greenberg HB. Rotavirus infectious particles use lipid rafts during replication for transport to the cell surface in vitro and in vivo. Virology. 2003;313:308–21.
8. Mohan KV, Muller J, Atreya CD. Defective rotavirus particle assembly in lovastatin-treated MA104 cells. Arch Virol. 2008;153:2283–90.
9. Fritz JV, Tibroni N, Keppler OT, Fackler OT. HIV-1 Vpu's lipid raft association is dispensable for counteraction of the particle release restriction imposed by CD317/Tetherin. Virology. 2012;424:33–44.
10. Robinzon S, Dafa-Berger A, Dyer MD, Paeper B, Proll SC, Teal TH, Rom S, Fishman D, Rager-Zisman B, Katze MG. Impaired cholesterol biosynthesis in a neuronal cell line persistently infected with measles virus. J Virol. 2009;83:5495–504.
11. Godefroy C, Dahmane S, Dosset P, Adam O, Nicolai MC, Ronzon F, Milhiet PE. Mimicking influenza virus fusion using supported lipid Bilayers. Langmuir. 2014;30(38):11394–400.
12. Morita M, Kuba K, Ichikawa A, Nakayama M, Katahira J, Iwamoto R, Watanebe T, Sakabe S, Daidoji T, Nakamura S, et al. The lipid mediator protectin D1 inhibits influenza virus replication and improves severe influenza. Cell. 2013;153:112–25.
13. Veit M, Engel S, Thaa B, Scolari S, Herrmann A. Lipid domain association of influenza virus proteins detected by dynamic fluorescence microscopy techniques. Cell Microbiol. 2013;15:179–89.
14. Isa P, Realpe M, Romero P, Lopez S, Arias CF. Rotavirus RRV associates with lipid membrane microdomains during cell entry. Virology. 2004;322:370–81.
15. Dansako H, Hiramoto H, Ikeda M, Wakita T, Kato N. Rab18 is required for viral assembly of hepatitis C virus through trafficking of the core protein to lipid droplets. Virology. 2014;462-463:166–74.
16. Wei Q, Zhang F, Richardson MM, Roy NH, Rodgers W, Liu Y, Fu C, Ding Y, Zhao W, Huang C, et al. CD82 restrains angiogenesis by altering lipid raft clustering and CD44 trafficking in endothelial cells. Circulation. 2014;130(17):1493–504.
17. Cuddy LK, Winick-Ng W, Rylett RJ. Regulation of the high-affinity choline transporter activity and trafficking by its association with cholesterol-rich lipid rafts. J Neurochem. 2014;128:725–40.
18. Jordy AB, Serup AK, Karstoft K, Pilegaard H, Kiens B, Jeppesen J. Insulin sensitivity is independent of lipid binding protein trafficking at the plasma membrane in human skeletal muscle: effect of a 3-day, high-fat diet. Am J Physiol Regul Integr Comp Physiol. 2014;307(9):R1136–45.
19. Bavari S, Bosio CM, Wiegand E, Ruthel G, Will AB, Geisbert TW, Hevey M, Schmaljohn C, Schmaljohn A, Aman MJ. Lipid raft microdomains: a gateway for compartmentalized trafficking of Ebola and Marburg viruses. J Exp Med. 2002;195:593–602.
20. Norkin LC, Kuksin D. The caveolae-mediated sv40 entry pathway bypasses the golgi complex en route to the endoplasmic reticulum. Virol J. 2005;2:38.
21. Van Wilgenburg B, Moore MD, James WS, Cowley SA. The productive entry pathway of HIV-1 in macrophages is dependent on endocytosis through lipid rafts containing CD4. PLoS One. 2014;9:e86071.

22. Mikulak J, Singhal PC. HIV-1 entry into human podocytes is mediated through lipid rafts. Kidney Int. 2010;77:72–3. 73-74
23. Carter GC, Bernstone L, Sangani D, Bee JW, Harder T, James W. HIV entry in macrophages is dependent on intact lipid rafts. Virology. 2009;386:192–202.
24. Campbell SM, Crowe SM, Mak J. Lipid rafts and HIV-1: from viral entry to assembly of progeny virions. J Clin Virol. 2001;22:217–27.
25. Pietiainen V, Marjomaki V, Upla P, Pelkmans L, Helenius A, Hyypia T. Echovirus 1 endocytosis into caveosomes requires lipid rafts, dynamin II, and signaling events. Mol Biol Cell. 2004;15:4911–25.
26. Zhu J, Yang Q, Cao L, Dou X, Zhao J, Zhu W, Ding F, Bu RE, Suo S, Ren Y, et al. Development of porcine rotavirus vp6 protein based ELISA for differentiation of this virus and other viruses. Virol J. 2013;10:91.
27. Ren X, Glende J, Yin J, Schwegmann-Wessels C, Herrler G. Importance of cholesterol for infection of cells by transmissible gastroenteritis virus. Virus Res. 2008;137:220–4.
28. Ren X, Dou X, Hao Y, Sun L, Wei X. Expression VP4 complete protein and polyclonal antibodies preparation or detection of porcine rotavirus DN30209 strain. J Northeast Agric Univ. 2014;45:10–7.
29. Denizot F, Lang R. Rapid colorimetric assay for cell growth and survival. Modifications to the tetrazolium dye procedure giving improved sensitivity and reliability. J Immunol Methods. 1986;89:271–7.
30. Lingwood D, Simons K. Lipid rafts as a membrane-organizing principle. Science. 2010;327:46–50.
31. Nayak DP, Hui EK. The role of lipid microdomains in virus biology. Subcell Biochem. 2004;37:443–91.
32. Huang L, Zhang YP, Yu YL, Sun MX, Li C, Chen PY, Mao X. Role of lipid rafts in porcine reproductive and respiratory syndrome virus infection in MARC-145 cells. Biochem Biophys Res Commun. 2011;414:545–50.
33. Ren X, Yin J, Li G, Herrler G. Cholesterol dependence of pseudorabies herpesvirus entry. Curr Microbiol. 2011;62:261–6.
34. Harmon B, Schudel BR, Maar D, Kozina C, Ikegami T, Tseng CT, Negrete OA. Rift Valley fever virus strain MP-12 enters mammalian host cells via caveola-mediated endocytosis. J Virol. 2012;86:12954–70.
35. Arias CF, Isa P, Guerrero CA, Mendez E, Zarate S, Lopez T, Espinosa R, Romero P, Lopez S. Molecular biology of rotavirus cell entry. Arch Med Res. 2002;33:356–61.
36. Guerrero CA, Moreno LP. Rotavirus receptor proteins Hsc70 and integrin alphavbeta3 are located in the lipid microdomains of animal intestinal cells. Acta Virol. 2012;56:63–70.
37. Hewish MJ, Takada Y, Coulson BS. Integrins alpha2beta1 and alpha4beta1 can mediate SA11 rotavirus attachment and entry into cells. J Virol. 2000;74:228–36.
38 Danthi P, Chow M. Cholesterol removal by Methyl-beta-Cyclodextrin inhibits poliovirus entry. J Virol. 2004;78(1):33–41.
39. Cui J, Fu X, Xie J, Gao M, Hong M, Chen Y, Su S, Li S. Critical role of cellular cholesterol in bovine rotavirus infection. Virol J. 2014;11:98.

Duplex fluorescence melting curve analysis as a new tool for rapid detection and differentiation of genotype I, II and Bartha-K61 vaccine strains of pseudorabies virus

Zhicheng Liu†, Chunhong Zhang†, Haiyan Shen, Junying Sun and Jianfeng Zhang*

Abstract

Background: Recently, pseudorabies (PR) outbreaks have been reported in a large number of swine herds vaccinated with the Bartha-K61 vaccine in China, the current pseudorabies virus (PRV) belonging to Genotype II is differential genetically from Bartha-K61 vaccine belonging to Genotype I. Furthermore, it has been proved that the Bartha-K61 vaccine cannot provide sufficient protection against the current PRVs in China. Therefore, the accurate and rapid identification of PRVs is essential. The objective of this study is to develop a duplex fluorescence melting curve analysis (FMCA) capable of rapid, simple, high-throughput differentiation of Chinese, European/American and Bartha-K61 vaccine strains of PRV.

Results: Primers 6F/6R and probes P1/P2, combined with three recombinant plasmids p-B (Bartha-K61), p-N (Genotype I), and p-H (Genotype II), were used to establish the Bicolor FMCA. FAM *Tm* values (probe P1) and HEX (probe P2) channels of p-B were used as reference values. *Tm* differences (ΔTm) between detected samples and reference plasmid p-B were calculated in each channel. Bartha-K61 vaccine samples had ΔTm values of ±1 °C in both FAM and HEX channels, Genotype I samples had ΔTm values of ±1 °C in the FAM channel and 4.38 ± 1 °C in the HEX channel, and Genotype II samples had ΔTm values of 6.52 ± 1 °C in the FAM channel and 4.38 ± 1 °C in the HEX channel. The minimum detection limit of the duplex FMCA was approximately 1×10^0 copies per reaction for p-B, p-N, and p-H. The duplex FMCA technique was used to detect and different 198 suspected clinical samples, of which 18 (9%) were positive for Genotype II strains and eight (4%) were positive for Bartha-K61 vaccine strains, and the results were compared with sequencing and phylogenetic analyses, which confirmed that the Bicolor FMCA worked correctly for all samples.

Conclusions: In this study, we developed a duplex FMCA of dual-labeled, self-quenched probes that was performed for rapid detection and differentiation of Genotype I, II and Bartha-K61 vaccine strains of PRV. The duplex FMCA was rapid, simple, and high-throughput, and will likely prove useful for molecular epidemiological investigations and pathogen surveillance of PRV.

Keywords: PRV, Duplex FMCA, Genotyping

* Correspondence: 13668939298@139.com

†Zhicheng Liu and Chunhong Zhang contributed equally to this work.

Institute of Animal Health, Guangdong Academy of Agricultural Sciences, Key Laboratory of Livestock Disease Prevention of Guangdong Province, Scientific Observation and Experiment Station of Veterinary Drugs and Diagnostic Techniques of Guangdong Province,Ministry of Agriculture, P.R.China, Guangzhou 510640, Guangdong, China

Background

Pseudorabies (PR), also known as Aujeszky's disease (AD), is caused by pseudorabies virus (PRV), which is also known as suid herpesvirus 1 (SuHV-1) or Aujeszky's disease virus (ADV). PR is an economically important disease in the pig industry worldwide. Swine are the only known natural host of PRV, but nearly all mammals are susceptible to infection [1]. PRV infection is characterised by neurological symptoms and death in newborn piglets, respiratory disorders in fattening pigs, and reproductive failure in pregnant pigs [2]. PR can be controlled using attenuated Bartha-based vaccines and in combination with a worldwide eradication program. However, since the latter part of 2011, PR outbreaks have been reported in a large number of swine herds vaccinated with the Bartha-K61 vaccine in China [3–8]. The Bartha-K61 vaccine did not provide full protection against the current PRVs [3, 9]. Current evidence suggests PRV can be divided into two distinct clusters, with Chinese strains belonging to genotype II and European/American strains in genotype I, which contains Bartha-K61 vaccine [10–13]. Therefore, the accurate differentiation of the PRVs is essential.

Traditionally, etiological diagnostic methods for PR include virus isolation [14], DNA hybridisation [15–17], immunofluorescence [17], loop-mediated isothermal amplification (LAMP) assay [18], real-time polymerase chain reaction (PCR) assay [19], and recombinase polymerase amplification assays (RPA) [20], none of which are able to distinguish between PRV strains. Several assays, including the LAMP assay [21], nanoparticle-assisted PCR assay [22], and two multiplex real-time PCR (qPCR) assays [23], have been developed to differentiate between wild-type (WT) PRV and gene-deleted PRV vaccines. However, these assays are unable to discriminate between WT PRV strains. Triplex real-time PCR [24] is applicable for differential detection of classical, variant and Bartha-K61 vaccine strains of PRV. However, classical PRV strains in the present study include both Chinese strains and European/American PRVs, which are evolutionarily distinct clades [10, 24].

Probe-based fluorescence melting curve analysis (FMCA) is a powerful tool for single-nucleotide polymorphism (SNP) genotyping of target sequences based on melting temperature generated by thermal denaturation of the probe-target hybrid. Recently, FMCA was used in the detection of bacterial resistance [25] and virus genotyping [26]. The aim of the present study was to develop a duplex FMCA capable of rapid, simple, high-throughput differentiation of Chinese, European/American and Bartha-K61 vaccine strains of PRV.

Results

The developed Bicolor FMCA of dual-labeled, self-quenched probes was able to discriminate 92 samples within 2 h when the template DNA was ready. This assay could identify Chinese strains (Genotype II), European/American strains (Genotype I) and Bartha-K61 vaccine strains of PRV based on *Tm* value and fluorescence type, as shown in Fig. 1b and Fig. 1c. For each sample, two *Tm* values were obtained from the FAM and HEX channels, corresponding to probes P1 and P2, respectively. P1 was designed to match Genotype II but mismatch Genotype I (including Bartha-K61 vaccine strains), while P2 was designed to match Genotype I and Genotype II but mismatch Bartha-K61 vaccine strains. As shown in Table 1, in the FAM channel, Genotype I (including Bartha-K61 vaccine strains) yielded *Tm* values of 70.41 ± 0.49 °C (0.49 °C = 3SD, n = 63), and Genotype II *Tm* values were 76.93 ± 0.48 °C (n = 32). In the HEX channel, Bartha-K61 vaccine strains gave *Tm* values of 71.62 ± 0.18 °C (n = 32), while Genotype I and Genotype II *Tm* values were 76.00 ± 0.48 °C (n = 63). In each assay, recombinant plasmids p-B (Bartha-K61 Vaccine), p-N (Genotype I), and p-H (Genotype II) were used as positive controls, and the NTC sample served as the negative control. In order to simplify data analysis, *Tm* values in FAM and HEX channels of recombinant plasmid p-B was used as reference values, and *Tm* differences (ΔTm) between detected samples and reference plasmid p-B were calculated in each channel. As shown in Table 1, *Tm* values were highly reproducible, with a maximum 3SD value of 0.49 (ΔTm = 6.52 °C, FAM channel) and 0.48 (ΔTm = 4.38 °C, HEX channel). Bartha-K61 vaccine samples had ΔTm values of ±1 °C in both the FAM and HEX channels, Genotype I samples had ΔTm values of ±1 °C in the FAM channel and 4.38 ± 1 °C in the HEX channel, and Genotype II samples had ΔTm values of 6.52 ± 1 °C in the FAM channel and 4.38 ± 1 °C in the HEX channel.

Sensitivity, specificity and reproducibility

Serial dilutions of the three recombinant plasmids p-B, p-N, and p-H ranged from 1×10^9 to 1×10^0 copies/μL when tested with the Bicolor FMCA, and fluorescence signals corresponding to melting curves were obtained between 1×10^0 and 1×10^9 copies per reaction for each plasmid. No specific signals were detected and corresponding melting curves were not obtained with the negative control (Additional file 1). Therefore, the detection limit of the Bicolor FMCA was approximately 1×10^0 copies per reaction for recombinant plasmids p-B, p-N, and p-H.

The specificity of the Bicolor FMCA was validated using DNA or cDNA samples from three PRV isolates, five other viruses known to cause similar clinical symptoms in pig, and three positive control plasmids (Fig. 2). Based on the data analysis method described above, detected samples included two Bartha-K61 vaccine samples

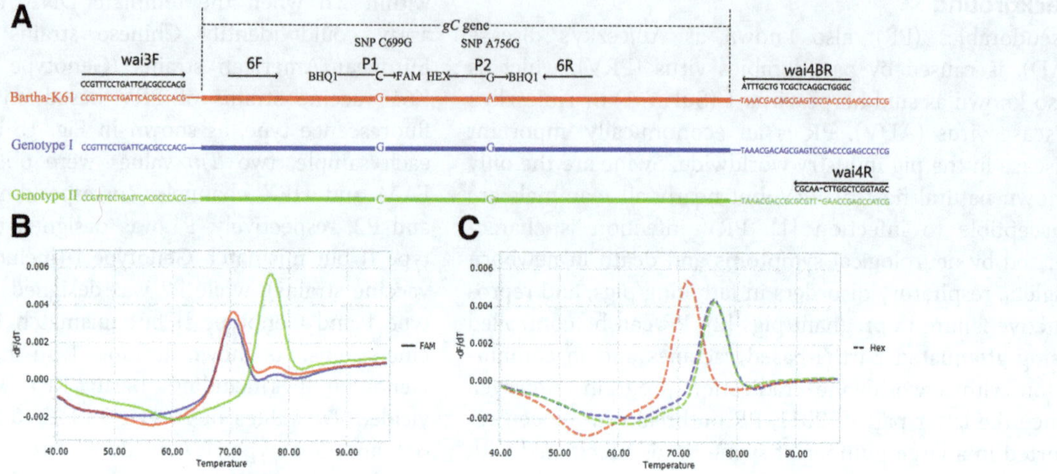

Fig. 1 Schematic illustration of the duplex FMCA method. (**a**) Relative binding positions of primers and probes along the *gC* gene of PRV. Melting peak calculation by derivative plotting -dF/dT versus temperature in the FAM channel (**b**) and the HEX channel (**c**). Red, blue, and green lines represent Bartha-K61 vaccine, European/American (Genotype I), and Chinese (Genotype II) strains, respectively

(including plasmid p-B and Bartha-K61), two Genotype I samples (including plasmid p-N and NIA3), and two Genotype II samples (including plasmid p-H and HDDJ). However, no specific melting peak was detected with other non-targeted pig viruses such as CSFV, PPV, PCV2, PRRSV, and JEV in the FAM and HEX channels. These results suggest that the designed primers and probes were highly specific and selective for their target viruses and exhibited no cross-reactivity with other viruses.

To evaluate the run-to-run reproducibility of the Bicolor FMCA, given the narrow *Tm* windows, the assay was run on different days using PRV Bartha-K61, NIA3, and HDDJ samples. Melting curve analysis for samples run on different days yielded a maximum 3SD value for *Tm* of no more than 0.5 for all melting peaks (Table 1), demonstrating the high reproducibility of this assay.

Agreement among the bicolor FMCA, sequencing and phylogenetic analysis

Of 198 suspected clinical samples were tested by the Bicolor FMCA technique, 18 (9%) were positive for Genotype II strains and eight (4%) were positive for Bartha-K61 vaccine strains (Table 2), but Genotype I strains were not detected.

To confirm that the clustering pattern resulting from the difference-melt curves of the different genotypes, the *gC* gene of each sample was sequenced and compared with consensus sequences (Additional file 2). Ten control sequences were included from the GenBank databases when sequences were aligned. Sequences of the 26 positive samples aligned well with the GenBank controls and with each other, confirming that the Bicolor FMCA worked correctly for all samples (Additional files 2 and 3). The relationship between individuals is shown in the cladogram.

To additionally confirm the eight Bartha-K61 strains, the fragment encompassing the *gE* gene was amplified by the primers gE-F and gE-R. The result showed that no fragment was amplified from the eight Bartha-K61 strains (Additional file 4). Furthermore, the eight samples were obtained from Bartha-K61–vaccinated pigs.

Table 1 Reproducibility testing of Bicolor FMCA for each positive control sample

Name	No. of times tested	*Tm* value (°C, Mean ± 3SD)	
		P1 (FAM channel)	P2 (HEX channel)
Bartha-K61	32	70.41 ± 0.49 [a,*]	71.62 ± 0.18*
NIA3	31		76.00 ± 0.48[b]
HDDJ	32	76.93 ± 0.48	

[a]*Tm* value calculated based on the number of Bartha-K61 strains and NIA3 strains tested in the FAM channel. [b]*Tm* value calculated based on the number of NIA3 strains and HDDJ strains tested in the HEX channel. *: The asterisk symbol was indicated significant difference between the melting temperature of two genotypes in same channel ($P<0.001$).

Discussion

Recently, PR outbreaks have been reported in a large number of swine herds vaccinated with the Bartha-K61 vaccine in China [3–8]. And the phylogenetic analysis based on full-length PRV sequences and based on only the *gC* gene and other genes revealed that PRV could be divided into two major genotypes, with Genotype I containing isolates from Europe, America, Australia, and Asia, and Genotype II consisting mainly of isolates from China, including classical strains such as Fa and Ea, as well as recently emerged variant strains [10–13]. Furthermore, it has been proved that the Bartha-K61 vaccine belonging to Genotype I cannot provide full

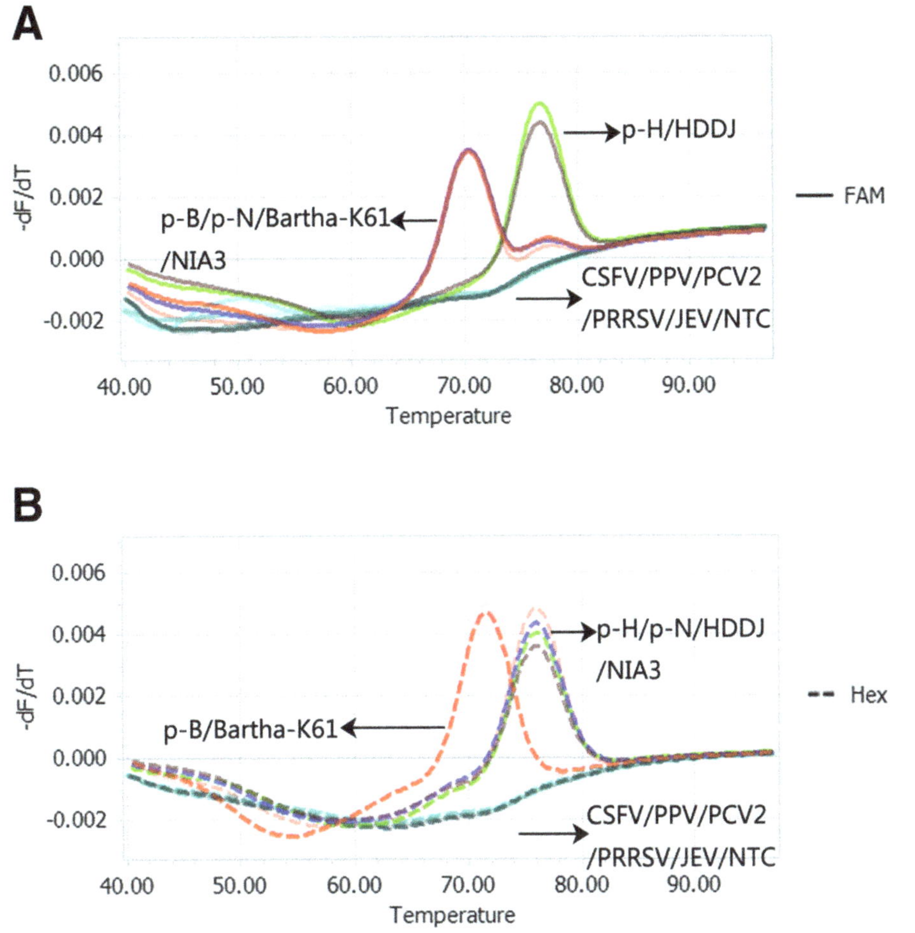

Fig. 2 Specificity of the duplex FMCA method. Melting curves obtained from duplex FMCA in the FAM channel (**a**) and the HEX channel (**b**) with 12 samples comprising 3 PRV positive samples, and five other viruses known to cause similar clinical symptoms in pig. Reference recombinant plasmids p-B (Bartha-K61 vaccine), p-N (Genotype I), and p-H (Genotype II) served as positive controls corresponding to red, blue, and green lines, and a No Template Control (NTC) served as the negative control (grey line)

protection against the current PRVs in China belonging to Genotype II [3, 9]. Therefore, it is very important to develop a method to identify pigs infected with PRV genotypes or immunized with the PRV Bartha-K61 vaccine strain.

In this study, we developed a simple and rapid method for detection and differentiation of PRV strains using a duplex FMCA approach with dual-labeled, self-quenched probes. This method proved to be easier, faster and more straightforward than conventional differentiation methods such as virus isolation combined with sequence analysis, which is often used to distinguish different strains [10].

The TaqMan probe has a random coil conformation that leads to fluorescence quenching or only weak fluorescence unless the probe is either hybridised with its target or digested. In classic TaqMan real-time PCR, generation of the fluorescence signal is based on probe degradation by the 5′-3′ exonuclease activity of DNA Taq polymerase in each round of amplification [27]. In FMCA, after PCR, a larger amount of fluorescence is emitted upon probe hybridisation with target sequences because the fluorophore is no longer in close proximity to the quencher. In this study, *TaKaRa LA Taq* DNA Polymerase combined *Taq* DNA Polymerase with 5′-3′ exonuclease activity and a DNA proofreading polymerase with 3′-5′ exonuclease activity were employed during PCR analyses. Hence, as described previously [28], the effects of hydrolysis of the probe during PCR on the melting curve profile require assessment. We compared the melting curves and melting peaks obtained from experiments in which probes were added either before or after the PCR run (Additional file 5). The results showed that the background fluorescence intensities in FAM and HEX channels increased when probes were added before the PCR run at the beginning of the melting curve analysis (Additional file 5.A and C) because some probes were digested during PCR by the 5′-3′

Table 2 *Tm* values from Bicolor FMCA of the PRV strains used in this study

Name	GenBank accession no.	*Tm* value (°C)		Δ*Tm* value (°C)[a]		Genotype	Interpretation
		P1 (FAM channel)	P2 (HEX channel)	P1 (FAM channel)	P2 (HEX channel)		
p-B	—	70.53	71.61	0	0	Genotype I (Bartha-K61)	reference control/plasmid
p-N	—	70.53	75.99	0	4.38	Genotype I	positive control/plasmid
p-H	—	76.88	75.98	6.35	4.37	Genotype II	positive control/plasmid
Bartha-K61	JF797217.1	70.50	71.59	-0.03	-0.02	Genotype I (Bartha-K61)	positive sample
NIA3	KU900059.1	70.28	75.96	-0.25	4.35	Genotype I	positive sample
HDDJ	MF434048	76.70	76.00	6.17	4.39	Genotype II	positive sample/field sample
GDGZ	MF434045	76.75	75.84	6.22	4.23	Genotype II	field sample
GDZQ	MF434042	76.93	76.20	6.4	4.59	Genotype II	field sample
GDHY	MF434044	77.13	76.21	6.6	4.6	Genotype II	field sample
GDHY2	MF434038	76.70	76.00	6.17	4.39	Genotype II	field sample
GDZQ2	MF434039	76.95	76.04	6.42	4.43	Genotype II	field sample
GDSD	MF434043	76.74	76.04	6.21	4.43	Genotype II	field sample
JXGZ	MF434047	76.67	75.97	6.14	4.36	Genotype II	field sample
JXGZ2	MF434036	76.63	75.93	6.1	4.32	Genotype II	field sample
LC	MF434047	76.69	75.98	6.16	4.37	Genotype II	field sample
HNCS	MF434046	76.51	75.81	5.98	4.20	Genotype II	field sample
GDHY8	MH053134	77.27	76.16	6.74	4.55	Genotype II	field sample
GDGZ2	MH053135	76.87	76.15	6.34	4.54	Genotype II	field sample
GDBL	MH053136	76.75	76.03	6.22	4.42	Genotype II	field sample
SXDT	MH053137	76.14	76.24	5.61	4.63	Genotype II	field sample
HNCS4	MH053138	76.99	76.08	6.46	4.47	Genotype II	field sample
GDHZ	MH053139	76.91	76.00	6.38	4.39	Genotype II	field sample
GDQY	MH053140	76.92	76.01	6.39	4.40	Genotype II	field sample
GDHY5	—[b]	70.49	71.60	-0.04	-0.01	Genotype I (Bartha-K61)	field sample
GDZQ4	—[b]	70.51	71.61	-0.02	0	Genotype I (Bartha-K61)	field sample
JXGZ4	—[b]	70.57	71.66	0.03	0.05	Genotype I (Bartha-K61)	field sample
GDSG	—[b]	70.56	71.61	0.03	0	Genotype I (Bartha-K61)	field sample
GDMM	—[b]	70.45	71.56	-0.08	-0.05	Genotype I (Bartha-K61)	field sample
GDFS	—[b]	70.71	71.61	0.18	0	Genotype I (Bartha-K61)	field sample
GDZS	—[b]	70.48	71.57	-0.05	-0.04	Genotype I (Bartha-K61)	field sample
GDQY3	—[b]	70.55	71.64	0.02	0.03	Genotype I (Bartha-K61)	field sample

[a] Δ*Tm* = *Tm* value of detected samples minus *Tm* of reference plasmid p-B in each channel. [b] The detected strains shared 100% identities in *gC* nucleotide sequence to Bartha-K61 strain (JF797217.1).

exonuclease activity of *TaKaRa LA Taq* DNA Polymerase. However, this did not affect the *Tm* value of the melting curve or the melting peak of FAM and HEX channels (Additional file 5). Additionally, this did not affect the –dF/dT value of the FAM channel when temperature equal to the *Tm* value (Additional file 5B), or slightly below the –dF/dT value of the HEX channel (Additional file 5.D). In summary, *TaKaRa LA Taq* was shown to be suitable for this assay.

In this study, the limit of detection of the Bicolor FMCA was determined to be 1×10^0 copies per reaction for recombinant plasmids p-B, p-N and p-H. Some factors contributed greatly to this. Firstly, only one pair of primers was used during the PCR process, and post-multiplex FMCA could reduce some of the nonspecific interactions if two or more pairs of primers are used [29]. Secondly, the asymmetric PCR post-multiplex FMCA was optimised in terms of the ratio of primer 6F to 6R. In order to maximise the amplified single strand used to hybridise with the probes while retaining the basic PCR reaction conditions, the ratio of primers is important, as described previously [26, 28, 30–38]. The results showed that detection by the Bicolor FMCA was highest when the ratio of primer 6F to 6R was 1:10 (0.04 μM: 0.4 μM) and probe P1 and P2 was 0.2 μM. Thirdly, the PCR amplification system containing *TaKaRa LA Taq* and GC Buffer I improved the PCR amplification efficiency significantly over the conventional PCR amplification system for the high GC content of the PRV genome.

Since the 1990s, most pig herds in China have been immunised with the Bartha-K61 vaccine, which is a live attenuated strain (Bartha, 1961) [3]. However, co-infection with more than one PRV genotype has not been widely reported, possibly due to limited differential detection methods in the past. Using the dual presence of PRV recombinant plasmids p-B and p-H as an example, we tested the ability to distinguish the two genotypes when they are simultaneously present in the same reaction. By varying their relative ratios, the results showed that levels as low as 10% (1:9) of one genotype in the presence of 90% (9:1) of the other genotype could be detected when the overall copy number was 10^8 copies per reaction (Fig. 3).

It should be pointed out that this method is only applicable for genotypes from Chinese, European/American and Bartha-K61 vaccine strains of PRV because it was developed based on SNP differences. Thus, the method is not suitable for the genotyping of PRV genetically engineered vaccine strains such as HB-98 (MF434040), HB-2000 (MF434041), and SA215 (EU719635.1) strains. Also, the method is unable to subdivide either Chinese strain into ancient and recently emerged strains, or European/American PRVs into six subgroups [10]. A more inclusive method needs to be developed in the future for this purpose.

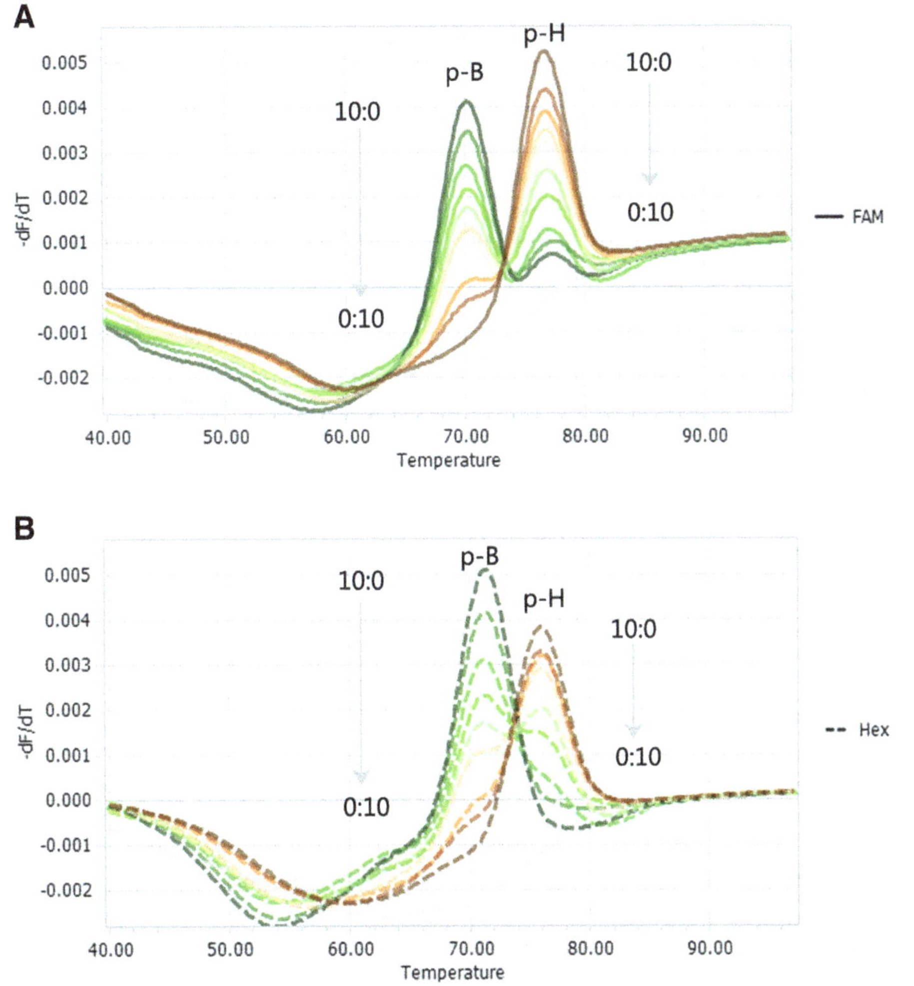

Fig. 3 Simultaneous detection of PRV Bartha-K61vaccine and Genotype II strains in mixed infections. Two co-existing genotypes were detected in the FAM channel (**a**) and the HEX channel (**b**). Melting curves of artificial plasmid templates containing p-B and p-H at various ratios (10:0, 9:1, 8:2, 7:3, 6:4, 5:5, 4:6, 3:7, 2:8, 1:9, 0:10) were tested. The overall template concentration was 10^8 copies per reaction. The NTC negative control is represented by a grey line

Conclusions

In summary, the newly developed Duplex FMCA is a specific and sensitive method for the differential detection of Chinese, European/American and Bartha-K61 vaccine strains of PRV, and will likely prove useful for molecular epidemiological investigations and pathogen surveillance of PR.

Methods

Strain collection and DNA extraction

A total of 28 PRV samples (Table 2) and five other viruses were tested in this study. Three positive strains were included to establish the Bicolor FMCA: PRV Bartha-K61 (Bartha-K61 Vaccine, Boehringer CO. LTD, Germany), NIA3 (Genotype I, the NIA3 strain), and HDDJ (Genotype II, the HDDJ strain) and other 25 field samples were isolated in our laboratory; the other five viruses are known to cause similar clinical symptoms in pigs and consisted of classical swine fever virus (CSFV) C strain (Winsun Bio, Guangzhou, China), porcine parvovirus (PPV) GD3 strain (isolated in our laboratory), porcine circovirus type 2 (PCV2) BL strain (isolated in our laboratory), porcine reproductive and porcine respiratory syndrome virus (PRRSV) GDr180 strain (Winsun Bio, Guangzhou, China), and Japanese encephalitis virus (JEV) SA14–14-2 strain (Wuhan Keqian Biology., Ltd., Wuhan, China). Viral RNA/DNA was extracted using the MiniBEST Viral RNA/DNA Extraction Kit version 4.0 (Takara, Dalian, China) according to the manufacturer's instructions.

Primer and probe design

Main primers and probes were designed to target the *gC* gene of PRV (Fig. 1a). Primers 6F (5'-GCCAACGCC TCCCTCGCCCAC-3') and 6R (5'-CGACGCACACCGCC CGGAAGG-3'), and probes P1 (BHQ1–5'-CGCCAACGG CACCGAGGTCCG<u>C</u>AGCGC-3'-FAM) and P2 (HEX-5' -TCGGCCTGAGCGCGCC<u>**G**</u>CCCGTC-3'-BHQ1; differential nucleotides are underlined) were used to establish the Bicolor FMCA. Probe P1 was designed to differentiate between Genotype II and Genotype I strains (including Bartha-K61 vaccine strains), and probe P2 was designed to distinguish Bartha-K61 vaccine strains from other strains. The single nucleotide polymorphisms (SNPs, Fig. 1a), C699G (probe P1) and A756G (probe P2), in the *gC* gene, were chose based on a sequence alignment of all available PRV *gC* gene by a BLAST search in GenBank databases from the National Center for Biotechnology Information (NCBI). The primers wai3F (5'-CCGTTTCCTGATTC ACGCCCACG-3') and wai4R (5'-CGATGGCTCGGTTC AACGC-3') and wai4BR (5'-CGGGTCGGACTCGC TGTCGTTTA-3') were used to generate recombinant plasmids, which were used to determine the limit of detection (LOD) of the assay. The primers were also used for sequencing of the gC gene. Two reverse primers wai4R and wai4BR bind to similar regions of the PRV genome, but primer wai4R is specific for Chinese strains (Genotype II), combined with primer wai3F, used to amplify a 1594-bp amplicon; while primer wai4BR is specific for European/American strains (Genotype I), combined with primer wai3F, used to amplify a 1577-bp amplicon. This experimental design could allow both PRV genotypes (I and II) to be amplified.

The primers gE-F (5'-TTGAGACCATGCGGCCCTT TCTGCT-3') and gE-R (5'- GACCGGTTCTCCCG GTATTTAAGCG-3') were used to confirm the Bartha-K61 strains detected in field samples. The primers amplified no fragment from Bartha-K61 strain, or a 1763-bp fragment encompassing the *gE* gene of PRV wild strains, respectively.

All primer and probe sequences were analysed using BLAST to confirm specificity.

Duplex real-time PCR and melting curve analysis

For each sample, 1 μL of template DNA was added to a 10 μL PCR mixture containing 1 × GC Buffer I, 400 μM of each deoxynucleoside triphosphate (dNTP), 0.04/0.4 μM primers 6F/6R, 0.2 μM probe P1/P2, and 0.5 U of TaKaRa LA Taq (Takara, Dalian, China). A No Template Control (NTC) was used as the negative control. Amplification and melting curve analysis was performed in a Roche LightCycler 96 System (Roche, Switzerland) with initial denaturation at 95 °C for 3 min, followed by amplification using 55 cycles of 95 °C for 20 s, 60 °C for 20 s, and 72 °C for 20 s. Melting curve analysis was initiated with denaturation at 95 °C for 10 s, followed by hybridisation at 40 °C for 60 s and a stepwise temperature increment from 40 °C to 97 °C at an Ramp rate of 0.13 °C/s with a duration of 1 s and five readings per °C. Fluorescence was measured at each step in both FAM and HEX channels. Melting curves were obtained by plotting the negative derivative of the fluorescence intensity with respect to temperature (−dF/dT) versus temperature (T). The *Tm* value from each probe was automatically obtained by identifying the peak of the corresponding melting curve. For best results, 11 ratios of forward primers to reverse primers (0.5:10, 1:10, 2:10, 3:10, 4:10, 5:10, 6:10, 7:10, 8:10, 9:10, 10:10) and four concentrations of two probes (0.1, 0.2, 0.3, 0.4 μM) were set. The optimization of *Tm* (s) was at a best ratio of 0.04/0.4 μM primers 6F/6R and a concentration of 0.2 μM probe P1/P2.

Analytical sensitivity

The analytical sensitivity of the Bicolor FMCA was estimated by serial dilution experiments using three recombinant plasmids p-B, p-N, and p-H. The three plasmids were generated using the pMD18-T Vector Cloning Kit (Takara, Dalian, China), and the insert fragments of the plasmids were amplified from Bartha-K61, NIA3, and HDDJ using primers wai3F/wai4R/wai4BR with the TaKaRa LA PCR Kit version 2.1, respectively. Each 25 μL PCR contained 1 × GC Buffer I, 400 μM of each deoxynucleoside triphosphate (dNTP), 0.4 μM primers wai3F/wai4R/wai4BR, 1.25 U of TaKaRa LA Taq (Takara, Dalian, China), and 2 μL of template DNA. Thermal conditions involved initial denaturation at 95 °C for 3 min, followed by amplification using 45 cycles of 95 °C for 40 s, 62 °C for 40 s, and 72 °C for 90 s. Each plasmid was 10-fold serially diluted with water to concentrations of 1×10^9 copies/μL to 1×10^0 copies/μL. The limit of detection for each genotype was determined from the lowest concentration measured by the Bicolor FMCA.

Specificity and reproducibility

In the Bicolor FMCA, primers 6F/6R and probes P1/P2 were tested for specificity using three PRV positive samples including Bartha-K61, NIA3, HDDJ, and five other viruses known to cause similar clinical symptoms in pig including CSFV C strain, PPV GD3 strain, PCV2 BL strain, PRRSV GDr180 strain, JEV SA14–14-2 strain. DNA samples from three recombinant plasmids p-B, p-N, and p-H were used as positive controls. To evaluate the reproducibility of the assay, Bicolor FMCA was performed on different days using different DNA templates of each positive control sample PRV Bartha-K61, NIA3, and HDDJ. The *Tm* value of each genotype was measured in each channel.

Screening and genotyping of clinical samples

The Bicolor FMCA was used to screen 198 suspected clinical samples received for laboratory diagnosis of PRV infection from different geographical locations in China. For confirmation of Bicolor FMCA results, each sample was rechecked by virus isolation, followed by DNA sequencing for positive samples.

The genotype of each sample was determined by sequencing using primers wai3F/wai4R/wai4BR with the PCR protocol described as above. PCR products were subjected to bi-directional sequencing (Sangon, Shanghai, China) and the results were analysed using Clustal W with BioEdit software (version 7.0.0, Tom Hall; Ibis Biosciences, Carlsbad, CA, USA). Phylogenetic analysis was performed by the neighbour-joining method with 1000 bootstrap replicates, based on the Kimura 2-parameter model, with joining comparison of the positive samples and control *gC* gene sequences using MEGA 5.2 software [39].

The Bartha-K61 strains detected in field samples was additionally confirmed based on the deleted *gE* gene by the primers gE-F and gE-R. The PCR protocol was following the amplified *gC* gene described above.

Additional files

Additional file 1: Sensitivity of the duplex FMCA method. Melting curves from duplex FMCA with recombinant control plasmids (A) p-B, (C) p-N, and (E) p-H in the FAM channel, and (B) p-B, (D) p-N, and (F) p-H in the HEX channel, ranging from 1×10^0 to 1×10^9 copies per reaction (from bottom to top). (TIF 1335 kb)

Additional file 2: Alignment of *gC* genes from the detected PRV samples used for Bicolor FMCA. Strains indicated with black discs were used for Bicolor FMCA. (TIF 1008 kb)

Additional file 3: Phylogenetic analysis (B) of *gC* genes from the detected PRV samples used for Bicolor FMCA. Strains indicated with black discs were used for Bicolor FMCA. (TIF 203 kb)

Additional file 4: The Bartha-K61 strains detected in field samples were identified by PCR. The PCR results showed no fragments were amplified from the eight Bartha-K61 strains detected in field samples using the primers gE-F and gE-R. Lane 1, DL 2000 marker; Lane 2, Bartha-K61; Lane 3, NIA3; Lane 4, HDDJ; Lane 5, NTC; Lane 6, GDHY5; Lane 7, GDZQ4; Lane 8, JXGZ4; Lane 9, GDSG; Lane 10, GDMM; Lane 11 GDFS; Lane 12, GDZS; Lane 13, GDQY3. (TIF 366 kb)

Additional file 5: Influence of probe hydrolysis on the melting curve profile. (A) Melting curves and (B) Melting peaks in the FAM channel, and (C) Melting curves and (D) Melting peaks in the HEX channel for recombinant plasmid p-H. Red and green lines indicate the addition of probes P1 and P2 before and after PCR for plasmid p-H, and blue and pink lines indicate the addition of probes P1 and P2 before and after PCR for NTC. (TIF 1001 kb)

Abbreviations

FMCA: Fluorescence melting curve analysis; PR: Pseudorabies; PRV: Pseudorabies virus; SNP: Single-nucleotide polymorphism

Acknowledgements

We thank Dr. Gali Bingga, Vocational and Technical College, Inner Mongolia Agricultural University, for assistance with discussions of the manuscript, and Dr. Jingyun Ma, College of Animal Science, South China Agricultural University, for assistance collecting samples.

Funding

This work was supported by the Science and Technology Planning Project of Guangdong Province, China [grant numbers: 2016A040403084, 2015A030401066, 2017A020208030, 2016B020234006, 2016A040403085]. The funders had no role in study design, data collection and analysis, decision to publish, or preparation of the manuscript.

Authors' contributions

ZCL, CHZ and JFZ conceived the study and wrote the paper. ZCL designed the Oligonucleotide primers and probes, ZCL and CHZ carried out this study, ZCL and JFZ analyzed the data, HYS and JYS collected the clinical samples, ZCL and JFZ revised the manuscript critically. All of the authors read and approved the final version of this manuscript.

Consent for publication

Not applicable.

Competing interests

The authors declare that they have no competing interests.

Reference

1. Mettenleiter TC. Pseudorabies virus A2 - Mahy, Brian WJ. In: Regenmortel MHW, editor. *Encyclopedia of Virology (Third Edition)*. Edn. Oxford: Academic Press; 2008. p. 341–51.
2. Beran GW, Davies EB, Arambulo PV 3rd, Will LA, Hill HT, Rock DL. Persistence of pseudorabies virus in infected swine. J Am Vet Med Assoc. 1980;176(10 Pt 1):998–1000.
3. An TQ, Peng JM, Tian ZJ, Zhao HY, Li N, Liu YM, Chen JZ, Leng CL, Sun Y, Chang D, et al. Pseudorabies virus variant in Bartha-K61-vaccinated pigs, China, 2012. Emerg Infect Dis. 2013;19(11):1749–55.
4. Wu R, Bai C, Sun J, Chang S, Zhang X. Emergence of virulent pseudorabies virus infection in northern China. J Vet Sci. 2013;14(3):363–5.
5. Yu X, Zhou Z, Hu D, Zhang Q, Han T, Li X, Gu X, Yuan L, Zhang S, Wang B, et al. Pathogenic pseudorabies virus, China, 2012. Emerg Infect Dis. 2014; 20(1):102–4.
6. Wang Y, Qiao S, Li X, Xie W, Guo J, Li Q, Liu X, Hou J, Xu Y, Wang L, et al. Molecular epidemiology of outbreak-associated pseudorabies virus (PRV) strains in Central China. Virus Genes. 2015;50(3):401–9.
7. Yang QY, Sun Z, Tan FF, Guo LH, Wang YZ, Wang J, Wang ZY, Wang LL, Li XD, Xiao Y, et al. Pathogenicity of a currently circulating Chinese variant pseudorabies virus in pigs. World journal of virology. 2016;5(1):23–30.
8. Fan J, Zeng X, Zhang G, Wu Q, Niu J, Sun B, Xie Q, Ma J. Molecular characterization and phylogenetic analysis of pseudorabies virus variants isolated from Guangdong province of southern China during 2013-2014. J Vet Sci. 2016;17(3):369–75.
9. Wang CH, Yuan J, Qin HY, Luo Y, Cong X, Li Y, Chen J, Li S, Sun Y, Qiu HJ. A novel gE-deleted pseudorabies virus (PRV) provides rapid and complete protection from lethal challenge with the PRV variant emerging in Bartha-K61-vaccinated swine population in China. Vaccine. 2014;32(27):3379–85.
10. Ye C, Zhang QZ, Tian ZJ, Zheng H, Zhao K, Liu F, Guo JC, Tong W, Jiang CG, Wang SJ, et al. Genomic characterization of emergent pseudorabies virus in China reveals marked sequence divergence: evidence for the existence of two major genotypes. Virology. 2015;483:32–43.
11. Wu XM, Chen QY, Chen RJ, Che YL, Wang LB, Wang CY, Yan S, Liu YT, Xiu JS, Zhou LJ. Pathogenicity and whole genome sequence analysis of a pseudorabies virus strain FJ-2012 isolated from Fujian, southern China. The Canadian journal of infectious diseases & medical microbiology = Journal canadien des maladies infectieuses et de la microbiologie medicale. 2017: 2017, 9073172.
12. Song C, Gao L, Bai W, Zha X, Yin G, Shu X. Molecular epidemiology of pseudorabies virus in Yunnan and the sequence analysis of its gD gene. Virus Genes. 2017;53(3):392–9.
13. Liu H, Li XT, Hu B, Deng XY, Zhang L, Lian SZ, Zhang HL, Lv S, Xue XH, Lu RG, et al. Outbreak of severe pseudorabies virus infection in pig-offal-fed farmed mink in Liaoning Province, China. Arch Virol. 2017;162(3):863–6.
14. Balasch M, Pujols J, Segales J, Pumarola M. Aujeszky's disease (pseudorabies) virus detection in cerebrospinal fluid in experimentally infected pigs. Vet Microbiol. 1998;60(2–4):99–106.
15. McFarlane RG, Thawley DG. DNA hybridization procedure to detect pseudorabies virus DNA in swine tissue. Am J Vet Res. 1985;46(5):1133–6.
16. Belak S, Rockborn G, Wierup M, Belak K, Berg M, Linne T. Aujeszky's disease in pigs diagnosed by a simple method of nucleic acid hybridization. Zentralbl Veterinarmed B. 1987;34(7):519–29.
17. Wongwatcharadumrong R, Kunavongkrit A, Neumuller M, Linne T. Comparison of virus isolation, immunofluorescence and DNA probe hybridization for detection of pseudorabies virus in experimentally infected pigs. Zentralbl Veterinarmed B. 1992;39(2):91–6.
18. En FX, Wei X, Jian L, Qin C. Loop-mediated isothermal amplification establishment for detection of pseudorabies virus. J Virol Methods. 2008; 151(1):35–9.
19. Zanella EL, Miller LC, Lager KM, Bigelow TT. Evaluation of a real-time polymerase chain reaction assay for pseudorabies virus surveillance purposes. J Vet Diagn Investig. 2012;24(4):739–45.
20. Yang Y, Qin X, Zhang W, Li Z, Zhang S, Li Y, Zhang Z. Development of an isothermal recombinase polymerase amplification assay for rapid detection of pseudorabies virus. Mol Cell Probes. 2017;33:32–5.
21. Zhang CF, Cui SJ, Zhu C. Loop-mediated isothermal amplification for rapid detection and differentiation of wild-type pseudorabies and gene-deleted virus vaccines. J Virol Methods. 2010;169(1):239–43.
22. Ma X, Cui Y, Qiu Z, Zhang B, Cui S. A nanoparticle-assisted PCR assay to improve the sensitivity for rapid detection and differentiation of wild-type pseudorabies virus and gene-deleted vaccine strains. J Virol Methods. 2013; 193(2):374–8.
23. Wernike K, Beer M, Freuling CM, Klupp B, Mettenleiter TC, Muller T, Hoffmann B. Molecular double-check strategy for the identification and characterization of Suid herpesvirus 1. J Virol Methods. 2014;209:110–5.
24. Meng XY, Luo Y, Liu Y, Shao L, Sun Y, Li Y, Li S, Ji S, Qiu HJ. A triplex real-time PCR for differential detection of classical, variant and Bartha-K61 vaccine strains of pseudorabies virus. Arch Virol. 2016;161(9):2425–30.
25. Liu Z, Zhang J, Rao S, Sun L, Zhang J, Liu R, Zheng G, Ma X, Hou S, Zhuang X, et al. Heptaplex PCR melting curve analysis for rapid detection of plasmid-mediated AmpC beta-lactamase genes. J Microbiol Methods. 2015;110:1–6.
26. Athar MA, Xu Y, Xie X, Xu Z, Ahmad V, Hayder Z, Hussain SS, Liao Y, Li Q. Rapid detection of HCV genotyping 1a, 1b, 2a, 3a, 3b and 6a in a single reaction using two-melting temperature codes by a real-time PCR-based assay. J Virol Methods. 2015;222:85–90.
27. McGuigan FE, Ralston SH. Single nucleotide polymorphism detection: allelic discrimination using TaqMan. Psychiatr Genet. 2002;12(3):133–6.
28. El Housni H, Heimann P, Parma J, Vassart G. Single-nucleotide polymorphism genotyping by melting analysis of dual-labeled probes: examples using factor V Leiden and prothrombin 20210A mutations. Clin Chem. 2003;49(10):1669–72.
29. Elnifro EM, Ashshi AM, Cooper RJ, Klapper PE, Multiplex PCR. Optimization and application in diagnostic virology. Clin Microbiol Rev. 2000;13(4):559–70.
30. Crockett AO, Wittwer CT. Fluorescein-labeled oligonucleotides for real-time pcr: using the inherent quenching of deoxyguanosine nucleotides. Anal Biochem. 2001;290(1):89–97.
31. Wittwer CT, Herrmann MG, Moss AA, Rasmussen RP. Continuous fluorescence monitoring of rapid cycle DNA amplification. Biotechniques. 1997;22(1):130–1 134-138.
32. Logan JM, Edwards KJ, Saunders NA, Stanley J. Rapid identification of campylobacter spp. by melting peak analysis of biprobes in real-time PCR. J Clin Microbiol. 2001;39(6):2227–32.
33. Howell WM, Jobs M, Brookes AJ. iFRET: an improved fluorescence system for DNA-melting analysis. Genome Res. 2002;12(9):1401–7.
34. French DJ, Archard CL, Brown T, McDowell DG. HyBeacon probes: a new tool for DNA sequence detection and allele discrimination. Mol Cell Probes. 2001;15(6):363–74.
35. Tyagi S, Kramer FR. Molecular beacons: probes that fluoresce upon hybridization. Nat Biotechnol. 1996;14(3):303–8.
36. Belousov YS, Welch RA, Sanders S, Mills A, Kulchenko A, Dempcy R, Afonina IA, Walburger DK, Glaser CL, Yadavalli S, et al. Single nucleotide polymorphism genotyping by two colour melting curve analysis using the MGB eclipse probe system in challenging sequence environment. Human genomics. 2004;1(3):209–17.
37. Ahn JJ, Kim Y, Lee SY, Hong JY, Kim GW, Hwang SY. Fluorescence melting curve analysis using self-quenching dual-labeled peptide nucleic acid probes for simultaneously identifying multiple DNA sequences. Anal Biochem. 2015;484:143–7.
38. Lukhtanov EA, Lokhov SG, Gorn VV, Podyminogin MA, Mahoney W. Novel DNA probes with low background and high hybridization-triggered fluorescence. Nucleic Acids Res. 2007;35(5):e30.
39. Tamura K, Peterson D, Peterson N, Stecher G, Nei M, Kumar S. MEGA5: molecular evolutionary genetics analysis using maximum likelihood, evolutionary distance, and Maximum Parsimony Methods. Molecular Biology and Evolution. 2011;28(10):2731–9.

19

Isolation, molecular characterization and sero-prevalence study of foot-and-mouth disease virus circulating in central Ethiopia

Mishamo Sulayeman[1*], Fufa Dawo[2], Bedaso Mammo[2], Daniel Gizaw[3] and Dereje Shegu[3]

Abstract

Background: Ethiopian livestock production and productivity is still very low due to widespread of diseases. Among the diseases, foot-and-mouth disease (FMD) is an extremely contagious and acute viral disease that causes significant economic problems in the country. A cross sectional study design was conducted from September 2015 to May 2016 to isolate and characterize FMD virus from outbreak cases; determine the sero-prevalence of antibodies against FMD virus (FMDV), and assess potential risk factors associated with sero-prevalence of the disease in selected areas of central Ethiopia. A multistage sampling technique was employed to select the study animals. Isolated viruses were characterized by antigen ELISA (IZLER, Brescia, Italy) and by genetic analysis of the sequence of the viral protein 1 (VP1). Sero-prevalence was determined using an ELISA for antibodies against non-structural proteins of FMDV based on the 3ABC proteins (ID Screen® FMD NSP Competition, ID-VET, Grabels, France). Risk factors for sero-prevalence of antibodies against FMD virus was investigated using logistic regression analysis.

Result: From outbreak investigation, 28.8% ($n = 378$) cattle showed signs and lesions suggestive of FMD and 34 samples were subjected to virus isolation. Twenty eight of these cultures exhibited cytopathic effect (CPE) and were serotyped as O, A and SAT 2 FMD viruses. One A and two SAT 2 isolates named A-ETH-19-2015, SAT 2-ETH-18-2015 and SAT 2-ETH-20-2015 were further characterized by phylogenetic analysis. The overall sero-prevalence of antibodies against non-structural proteins of FMDV was 24.2% ($n = 574$). Cattle herds with crossbreed cattle, with older cattle (> 2 years), and kept together with small ruminants had higher sero-prevalences of antibodies against FMDV ($p < 0.05$).

Conclusion: This study showed that FMD was present in the study areas. Among the associated risk factors, breed, age and herd composition were significantly associated with presence of antibodies against FMD virus. Three different serotypes (A, O and SAT 2) were responsible for the outbreaks of the disease. Genetic analysis indicated that the isolated viruses clustered differently from previous outbreaks. Thus, further molecular analyses coupled with protection potential of the existing vaccines against the isolates should be performed.

Keywords: Cattle, Central Ethiopia, FMD, Molecular characterization, Risk factors, Sero-prevalence

Background

Ethiopia has huge livestock resources that play a crucial role in the livelihoods of the majority of human the population. Animal rearing is an integral part of the agricultural sector and animals represent the major drought power (95%) for crop production. The country is believed to have the largest livestock population in Africa comprising approximately 56.7 million cattle, 29.3 million sheep and 29.1 million goats [1]. The agricultural sector constitutes about 45% of the gross domestic production (GDP), more than 90% of foreign exchange earnings, 85% of employment opportunities and most of the domestic food supply [2].

Animal diseases are currently widespread in all agro-ecological zones of the country and annual mortality rates due to diseases is estimated at 8–10% for cattle herds, and 15% and 12% for sheep and goat flocks, respectively. It is estimated that animal diseases reduce the

* Correspondence: msulayeman@gmail.com
[1]Faculty of Veterinary Medicine, Hawassa University, P.O. Box 05, Hawassa, Ethiopia
Full list of author information is available at the end of the article

production and productivity of livestock by 50 to 60% per year [3]. Among the livestock diseases hampering productivity of the sector, foot-and-mouth disease (FMD) is considered as a bottleneck for livestock production and productivity, and is prompting trade embargos for livestock and livestock products [4].

The disease is an extremely contagious and acute viral disease of all cloven-hoofed animals and is a trans-boundary disease. The disease is characterized by fever, loss of appetite, salivation, vesicular eruptions in the mouth, on the feet and teats, and sudden death of young stock [5]. The recovered animals remain in poor physical condition over long periods of time leading to economic losses for livestock industries [6, 7].

FMD is caused by FMD virus (FMDV) that has seven serotypes (O, A, C, Asia 1, SAT 1, SAT 2 and SAT 3), with distinct immunologic, antigenic and genetic properties. The seven serotypes also differ in their distribution across the globe [8, 9].

Currently, four of the seven serotypes of FMDV (O, A, SAT 1, SAT 2) are endemic in Ethiopia, while serotype C was last diagnosed in 1983 [10–14]. Studies undertaken on FMD so far revealed the existence of the disease in different parts of the country, with sero-prevalence varying from 8.18% in south Omo [15] to 44.2% selected districts of Afar Pastoral Area [10].

In Ethiopia there is no government strategy to control FMD through vaccination and/or movement control. Lack of vaccination strategies (quality, coverage and timing) and presence of free animal movement without certification are thus the main factors that could increase the spread of FMD along the cattle market chain. For the development of adequate FMD control and prevention, determining the status of FMD through serological study, virus isolation and characterization of the circulating serotypes is needed. Study areas were known with the abundance of dairy farms, thus implementing both epidemiological study and outbreak investigations are essential to generate important baseline information about the disease and circulating serotypes.

Therefore, the study was designed to isolate and molecularly characterize FMDV from outbreak cases, determine the sero-prevalence of antibodies against FMDV, and assess potential risk factors associated with sero-prevalence of the disease in central Ethiopia.

Methods

Description of the study areas

The study was conducted in three different areas, Addis Ababa (Kolfe), Arsi zone (Guna and Lude Hitosa) and East shewa zone (Adama and Boset), where FMD outbreaks occurred from September 2015 to May 2016. A cross-sectional study was also conducted to study sero-prevalence of antibodies against FMDV in and around Adama and Assela dairy farms. Detail description of the study areas with geographic and climatic parameters are presented in Table 1 and Fig. 1 [1].

Study animals

Outbreaks were reported by the district level animal health expertise to the regional veterinary laboratory centers. Then animals were sampled irrespective of age, breed and herd management system. Additionally, for the study of the presence of antibodies against FMDV, animals were sampled from households which keep dairy cattle, ranging from small individual farms to highly organized dairy farms.

Study design

Cross sectional study was implemented for both outbreak investigation and sero-prevalence study of antibodies against FMDV in the study areas. Multistage sampling technique was applied. Adama and Asella districts were purposively selected sites for sero-prevalence study of antibodies against FMDV based on their accessibility, geographical location and on the abundance of dairy farms. From each district 30% of peasant associations (PAs) were selected randomly. From each PA, 20% of privately owned herds were selected randomly to obtain primary sampling unit. Finally, individual animal from each herd were selected randomly as secondary sampling unit to attain the required sample size; the strategies differed between districts as 10% of animals were sampled in Adama herds and 20% in Asella herds. Breed, age, sex, herd composition and size, and history of sampled animals were registered as to determine risk factors for the occurrence of the disease. Sampled animals were grouped into three age categories based on their dental eruption status [6].

Sampling technique and sample size determination

Simple random sampling technique was followed to select individual animals included in the study. The sample

Table 1 Description of the study areas

Study area	Altitude	Climate	Annual rainfall	Temperature	
				Maximum	Minimum
Addis Ababa	2300 m	Sub-tropical	1180 mm	22.8 °C	10.6 °C
Arsi zone	1500 to 4245 m	Sub-tropical	2400 mm	25 °C	10 °C
East shewa zone	500 to 4307 m	Tropical	410-820 mm	30 °C	18 °C

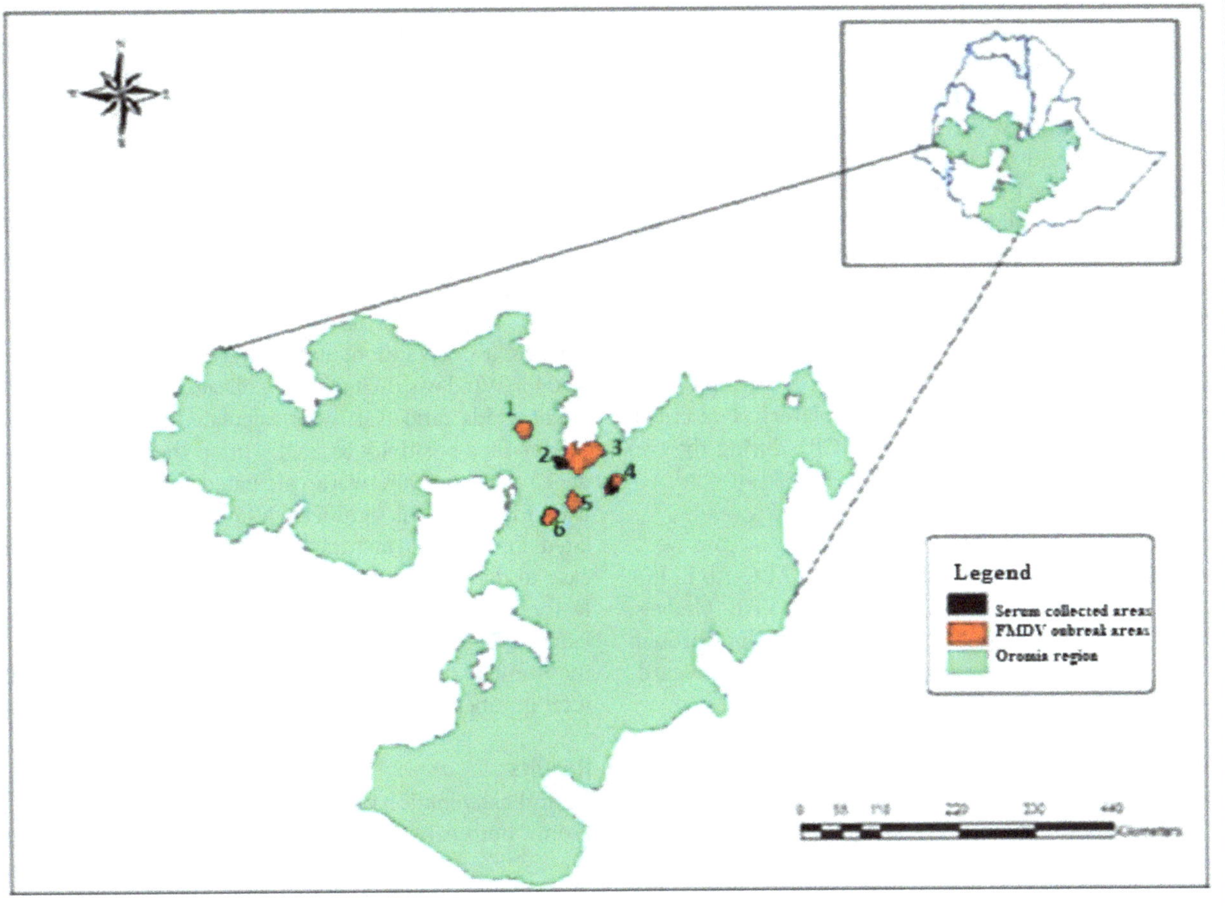

Fig. 1 Study area

size required for the study was calculated based on the following formula [16].

$$n = \frac{1.96^2 \, X \, P_{exp} X \left(1 - P_{exp}\right)}{d^2}$$

Where, n = sample size, P_{exp} = expected prevalence, and d = absolute precision.

The expected prevalence considered was 14.5% for Adama based on a previous study in the area [9], while 50% was used in Asella due to lack of previous studies. Accordingly with 95% confidence level, 5% absolute precision and expected prevalence as mentioned above, the sample size computed was 190 for Adama and 384 for Asella. Thus, the total sample size required for the study was 574 dairy cattle.

Sample collection

Tissue and oro-pharyngeal (OP) fluid samples

Epithelial tissue samples were collected from unruptured and freshly ruptured vesicles and kept in 0.04 M phosphate buffer with 50% glycerol [17]. Samples of OP fluid were collected, from apparently healthy cattle that were found in close proximity to the affected herds, by a probang cup and poured into a 20 ml bottle. Fluid samples containing cellular material was added to 5 ml tube containing about 2 ml of transport medium at sites where the samples were collected [17]. Then, the samples were labeled and kept at cold chain during transportation to NAHDIC, Sebeta, where they were kept at -80 °C until processed [18].

Blood

From each animal, 10 ml of blood was collected and kept at room temperature overnight. Then serum was separated and transferred into cryovial at Asella Regional Veterinary Laboratory and stored at – 20 °C. At the end of sampling sera were transported in cold chain to NAHDIC, Sebeta, and stored at – 20 °C [17].

FMD virus isolation

Tissue samples were ground in a small volume of tissue culture medium containing antibiotic (penicillin [1000 International Units (IU)], neomycin sulphate [100 IU], polymyxin B sulphate [50 IU], mycostatin [100 IU]) using sterile sand, pestle and mortar, and diluted in the same medium to a 10% suspension [18], which was centrifuged at 2000 rpm for 10 min and filtered through a membrane filter with a 0.22 μm pore size. About 1 ml of filtered tissue suspension was inoculated on confluent baby hamster kidney (BHK-21) (AU/PANVAC) monolayer cells grown in 25cm^2 tissue culture flask and incubated at 37 °C for 1 h for adsorption of the virus. Then cell cultures were added 8 ml of maintenance medium (2% MEM) and incubated at 37 °C and 5% CO2 in a humidified incubator. Cell cultures were examined for evidence of cytophatc effect (CPE) every 24 h for a maximum of 72 h, and CPE-positive cell cultures harvested at 85% CPE. Cell cultures without CPE after 72 h were passaged harvested and passaged onto new monolayers as described above. Samples that did not develop CPE during the two passages were considered virus negative [18, 19].

Serological diagnostic tests

The collected sera were tested by FMDV 3ABC-Ab ELISA (ID Screen® FMD NSP Competition, ID-VET, Grabels, France) for the detection of antibody to 3ABC polyprotein which is a useful indicator of past FMDV infection regardless of the serotype involved (Additional file 1).

Antigen detection ELISA

Sandwich ELISA (IZLER, Brescia, Italy) was performed on isolates with selected combinations of anti-FMDV monoclonal antibodies (MAbs). The kit was designed for serotyping of FMDV (Additional file 2).

Reverse transcription polymerase chain reaction (RT-PCR) and sequencing

CPE-positive cell culture harvests were examined for FMDV using RT-PCR and primers that amplify VP1 of FMDV and selected, representative VP1s were sequenced. All RNA extraction, RT-PCR, and sequencing were conducted in WRL for FMD, Pirbright Institute, UK [20].

Molecular evolutionary relationship

A total of one VP1 sequence of serotype A FMDV and two sequences for serotype SAT 2 FMDV were obtained, and one for each of these serotypes used for online blast search to retrieve closely related sequences from Genbank using Molecular Evolutionary Genetic Analysis software (MEGA, V 6.06) [20].

Ethical approval

Ethical approval and consent for this study was obtained from Addis Ababa University College of Veterinary Medicine and Agriculture Minutes of Animal Research Ethics and Review committee (Reference AREC001/2016). Verbal consent was also obtained from the farm managers to take samples from their cattle and for further research use of the samples.

Data management and analysis

The VP1 nucleotide sequences were aligned by using Clustal W program imbedded in the MEGA software. The alignment sequences were used to construct phylogenetic tree analysis using midpoint-rooted neighbor-joining tree and Kimura 2-parameter nucleotide substitution model using MEGA 6.06. The robustness of the tree topology was assessed with 1000 bootstrap replicates as implemented in the program.

Data generated from laboratory investigations were recorded and coded using Microsoft Excel spreadsheet (Microsoft Corporation) and analyzed using STATA version 11.0 for Windows (Stata Corp. College Station, TX, USA).

The Odds ratio (OR) was calculated for each risk factor for sero-positivity to FMD. In all the analyses, confidence levels at 95% were calculated, and a $P < 0.05$ was used for statistical significance level. The OR was calculated for the risk factors and sero-positivity of the disease to determine the degree of association between risk factors and the disease. Descriptive statistics like prevalence was used to calculate sero-positivity by dividing the number of FMDV antibodies positive animals by the total number of animals tested.

Results

Clinical examination of FMD outbreak

From outbreak investigation, 28.8% ($n = 378$) cattle showed signs and lesions suggestive of FMDV infection. The major important clinical signs observed during the outbreak investigation were salivation and lameness. Mouth lesions consisted of erosions and ulcers on tongue and dental pad, whereas foot lesions comprised erosions on the inter-digital space and the coronary bands. In severe cases the hooves of affected animals tended to separate from the coronary bands. Reluctant to move and lagging behind herds and refusal of grazing were also seen as common features of clinically affected animals.

FMD virus isolation and characterization

A total of 30 epithelial tissue and 4 OP fluid samples collected from the three study sites, were subjected to virus isolation using BHK21 cell culture. CPE characterized by a fast destruction of BHK-21 monolayer cell within 48 h was registered for 28 tissue samples only.

FMDV serotype identification and distribution

Three serotypes namely serotype A, O and SAT 2 were identified from the outbreak samples (Table 2). Different outbreaks were caused by different serotypes: in Arsi zone only serotype A was responsible for the outbreak while in East Shewa zone only serotype SAT 2 was responsible. Surprisingly, in Addis Ababa three serotypes (A, O and SAT 2) were responsible for the outbreaks observed during the study.

Table 2 FMDV serotypes and their topotype identified

Site of outbreaks			No. of samples	CPE positive	Serotype		Topotype
					Sandwich ELISA result (positive)	RT-PCR Result	
Region	Zone	District					
Oromia	Arsi	Guna	12	8	A (8)	GD[a]	Africa
		Ludehitosa	6	5	SAT 2 (5)	GD[a]	VII
	East shewa	Adama	4	4	SAT 2 (4)	GD[a]	VII
		Boset	5	4	SAT 2 (4)	NT	NT
Addis Ababa	Addis Ababa	Kolfe	7	7	O (3), A (2) & SAT 2 (2)	NT	NT
Total			34	28			

CPE Cytopathic effect, *GD* Genome detected, *ELISA* Enzyme Linked Immuno-Sorbent Assay, *NT* Not tested, *RT-PCR* Reverse transcription polymerase chain reaction
[a] One representative isolate sequenced

Molecular characterization (phylogenetic analysis)

Isolated viruses SAT2/ETH/18/2015 from Adama and SAT2/ETH/20/2015 from Ludehitosa districts were compared based on 648 nucleotide sequence of VP1. The viruses shared 99.07% genetic similarity with each other, and > 90% genetic similarity with three other SAT 2 FMDV isolates from Ethiopia (SAT2/ETH/15/2015, SAT2/ETH/10/2015 and SAT2/ETH/14/2015 from Sidama (SNNPR), Awi (Amahara) and North Shoa (Oromia), respectively. These five SAT 2 FMDVs were homologous, geographically clustered and formed a single genetic lineage called topotype VII and genotype Alx-12. The genetic relationship of the isolates with the other SAT 2 serotypes is displayed on phylogenetic tree (Fig. 2).

One representative serotype A isolated from Guna District, Arsi zone of Oromia region, during the study period was also compared with other countries FMD serotype A isolate sequences. The isolated serotype A in the current study falls into African topotype and genotype IV. The genetic relationship of the isolates with the other A serotypes is displayed on phylogenetic tree (Fig. 3).

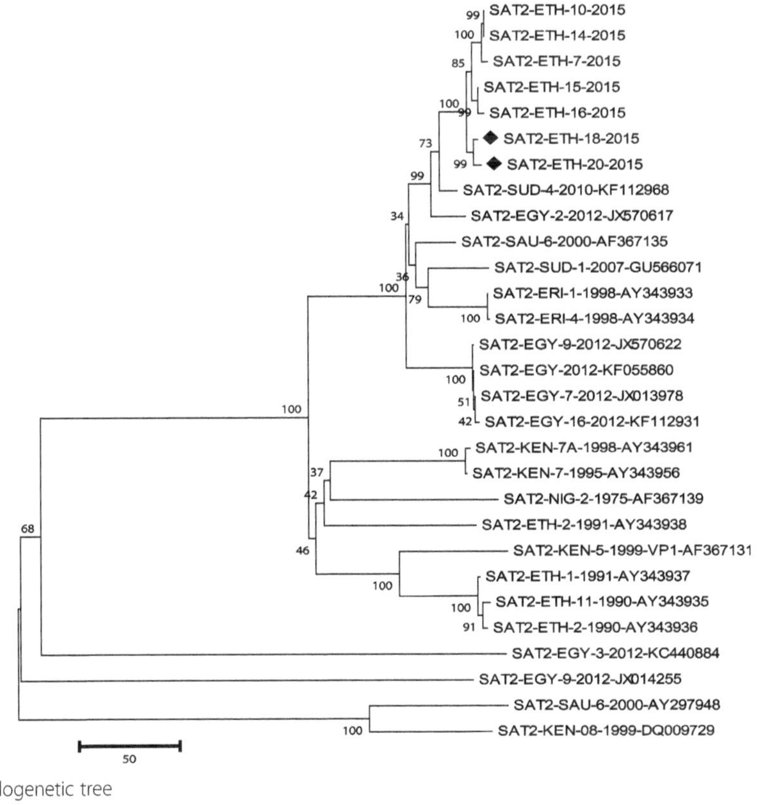

Fig. 2 Serotype SAT 2 phylogenetic tree

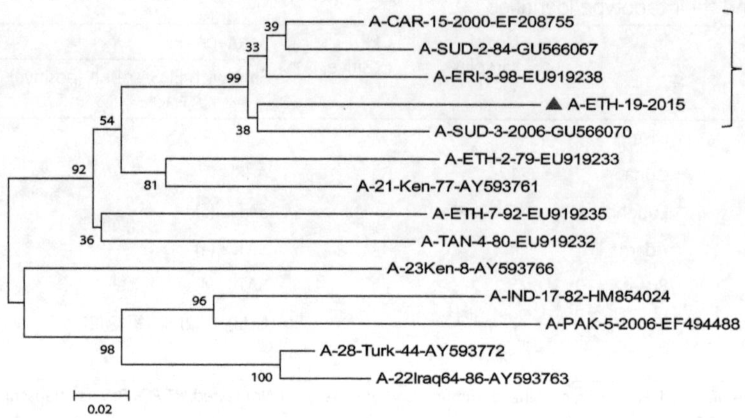

Fig. 3 Serotype A phylogenetic tree

Sero-prevalence of antibodies against FMDV

From the total of 574 sera collected from dairy animals and tested by 3ABC-Ab ELISA, 24.22% ($n = 139$) were found positive. The higher sero-prevalence was observed in and around Adama town compared to Asella (Table 3) but the difference was not statistically significant ($p > 0.05$).

Sero-prevalence in relation to host intrinsic risk factors

Sero-prevalence of antibodies against FMDV among different age groups

Sero-prevalence of antibodies against FMDV were compared berween different age groups of dairy cattle. An increasing sero-prevalence trend was observed with increasing age (Fig. 4) and the difference was statistically significant among age groups ($\chi 2 = 37.43$; $P < 0.001$).

Sero-prevalence of antibodies against FMDV between sex groups

The sero-prevalence of antibodies against FMDV was 25.26% in females and 18.95% in males (Table 4), but this difference was not statistically significant ($P > 0.05$).

Sero-prevalence of antibodies against FMDV in different cattle breeds

Interestingly, sero-prevalence of antibodies against FMDV differed significantly ($\chi 2 = 14.02$; $P < 0.05$) between local (12.69%, $n = 134$) and crossbred (27,73%, $n = 440$) cattle.

Table 3 Sero-prevalence of antibodies against FMDV in dairy cattle in and around Adama and Asella towns

Origin	Sera tested	Test (+) (%)	95%CI	χ^2	*p*-value
Adama	190	51 (26.8)	0.20–0.33	1.06	0.304
Asella	384	88 (22.9)	0.18–0.27		
Total	574	139 (24.2)	0.20–0.27		

(+) Positive, *CI* Confidence Interval

Sero-prevalence of antibodies against FMDV in relation to host extrinsic risk factors

Sero-prevalence of antibodies against FMDV in relation to herd size

Sero-positivity and herd size seems to have positive relationship in that an increasing sero-prevalence of antibodies against FMDV was observed as herd size increases (Table 5); but the difference was not statistically significant ($P > 0.05$).

Sero-prevalence of antibodies against FMDV in relation to animal composition and management system

Significantly higher sero-prevalence of antibodies against FMDV was recorded in cattle kept together with small ruminants than those that were not ($P < 0.05$) (Table 6). Animals managed semi-intensively were more likely to have antibodies against FMDV than animals under intensive management (Table 6) but the prevalence was not significantly different ($P > 0.05$).

Logistic regression analysis

The univariable and multivariable logistic regression analysis included effects of breed, history of herd contact with small ruminants, and age of animals (Tables 7 and 8). Univariable logistic regression revealed cross-bred cattle were 2.64 times more likely to have antibodies against FMDV than local breeds. The risk of having antibodies against FMDV was increased (odds ratio (OR) = 1.54) when herds of cattle and small ruminant were kept together compared to herd of cattle kept alone. Animals greater than 3 years old were found 8.14 times more likely to be sero-positive of antibodies against FMDV than young animals (those found below 2 years old).

Discussions

During outbreak investigation, 28.8% ($n = 378$) cattle showed signs and lesions suggestive of FMD. In agreement with this finding, Negussie et al. [21] reported 28.2%

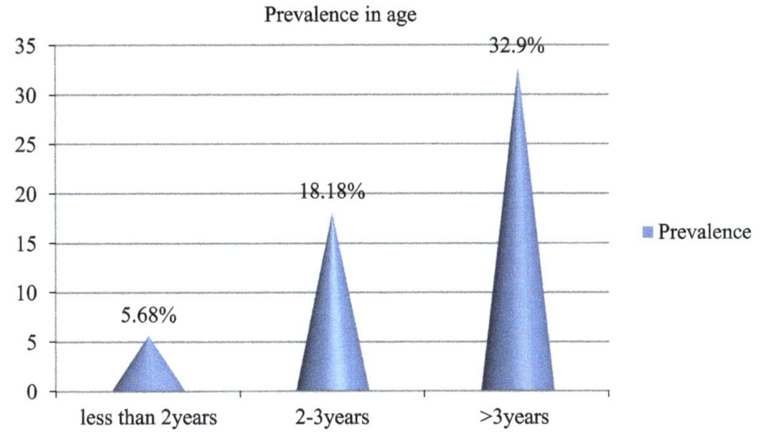

Fig. 4 Sero-prevalence of antibodies against FMDV among different age groups in dairy cattle in and around Adama and Asella towns

clinically sick animals after conducting a number of outbreak investigations in different parts of the country.

In current study, three serotypes (A, O, and SAT 2) of FMD viruses were isolated. Serotype O was isolated from the samples collected from Kolfe district (Addis Ababa). This result is in line with previous serotype O FMDV outbreaks in Ethiopia [9, 13] and the most prevalent serotype worldwide [22].

Serotype A was isolated from the samples collected from Kolfe and Guna district of Addis Ababa and Arsi zone, respectively. Previously serotype A was reported from bovine samples collected from Hadiya and Yabello areas [23, 24]; similarly from samples collected from different outbreak areas of Ethiopia [24].

Serotype A identified from Guna District was clustered to genotype IV of African topotype. This genotype was not reported before from this area and more detailed analysis need to be conducted using advanced software's. This is in support of the previous findings that reported serotype A FMDV belonged to African topotype [19] and all viruses from Ethiopia belonged to the African topotype [25].

Serotype SAT 2 FMD viruses were identified from cattle found in Ludehitosa district (Arsi zone), Adama and Boset district (East shewa zone) and Kolfe district (Addis Ababa). Previously serotype SAT 2 was isolated and reported from cattle in Addis Ababa [9], Borana pastoral area [13] and Benshangul-Gumz [9]. Serotype SAT 2 FMDV has previously been reported from many sub-Saharan African countries [26–28] suggesting endemicity of the serotype in these countries.

The presently identified SAT 2 serotype was clustered to topotype VII. This is in agreement with the findings of [9], who reported that SAT 2 viruses circulating in Ethiopia belonged to topotype VII along with the Sudanese isolates. This indicate that SAT 2 was introduced to the present study districts; the possible way of entry of the virus might be related to communal resource utilization and free movement of animals across the regions because SAT 2 is endemic to different regions of the country [9, 13] and neighboring African countries like Sudan republic [18, 29, 30]. The present isolates seem to be different from previously published isolates as they cluster differently on the tree. Further detailed genetic analysis like genetic distance determination is needed to have more insight about these viruses.

The FMDVs causing 2015 outbreaks in Ethiopia were not closely related to previous Ethiopian isolates. These new introductions are likely to have happened through uncontrolled trans-boundary movements of animals, which constitute a significant risk for virus crossing the border in both directions. This is due to lack of strong animal movement regulation across the border and the ability of the virus to transmit with the wind. This explanation is supported by a previous study which conclude closely related viruses could either be from the

Table 4 Sero-prevalence of antibodies against FMDV between sex groups in dairy attle in and around Adama and Asella towns

Sex	Sera tested	Test (+) (%)	95% CI	χ2	*p*-value
Female	479	121 (25.3)	0.21–0.29	1.80	0.179
Male	95	18 (19)	0.09–0.38		
Total	574	139 (24.1)	0.21–0.28		

(+) Positive, *CI* Confidence Interval

Table 5 Sero-prevalence of antibodies against FMDV in relation to herd size in dairy cattle in and around Adama and Asella towns

Herd size	Sera tested	Test (+) (%)	95%CI	χ2	*p*-value
Small	438	98 (22.4)	0.18–0.26	4.76	0.092
Medium	77	20 (26)	0.16–0.36		
Large	59	21 (35.6)	0.23–0.48		

(+) Positive, *CI* Confidence Interval

Table 6 Sero-prevalence of antibodies against FMDV in relation to animal composition and management in dairy cattle in and around Adama and Asella towns

Risk factors	Tested	Test (+) (%)	95% CI	χ2	p-value
Animal composition					
Only cattle	422	93 (22)	0.18–0.26	3.99	0.040
Cattle and small ruminants	152	46 (30.7)	0.23–0.38		
Management					
Intensive	254	55 (21.7)	0.17–0.27		
Semi-intensive	320	84 (26.3)	0.21–0.31	1.64	0.200

(+) Positive, *CI* Confidence Interval

same outbreak or from the other oubreaks due to closely related viruses [29].

The overall sero-prevalence of antibodies against FMDV was 24.22%, which agreed with the overall sero-prevalence of 26.5% found in an Ethiopian pastoral area [12]. Compared to the present findings lower prevalence of 5.6% [21], 8.01% [31] and 9% [23] were reported from different parts of Ethiopia. On the other hand relatively higher sero-prevalence was previously reported from Eastern zone of Tigray with 41.5%; followed by the Guji zone of Oromia and Yeka district of Addis Ababa city, with 32.7% and 30%, respectively [25].

The sero-prevalence of antibodies against FMDV was significantly higher when cattle and small ruminants were kept together. Previous study conducted in four selected Districts of Gambella Regional State reported a similar effect [23]. In Sub-Saharan Africa [30], similar high sero-prevalence of FMD where communal farming of cattle, sheep and goats occur, indicated a high sero-prevalence of antibodies against the virus infection associated with sheep and goats in the absence of clinical signs. This suggests that small ruminants have an important role in the epidemiology of FMD as they can serve as potential carriers and transmitters of the disease [32].

Sero-prevalence of antibodies against FMDV increased with increasing herd size. This may be attributed to crowding of animals that can facilitate frequency of direct contact and hence enhances chances of transmission.

Table 7 Univariable logistic regression analysis of potential FMD risk factors in dairy cattle in and around Adama and Asella towns

Explanatory variable	Variable categories	OR	95% CI	P-value
Breed	Cross vs. local	2.64	1.52–6.67	0.001
Cattle composition	Kept with small ruminants vs. without	1.54	1.01–2.33	0.046
Age	Old vs. young	8.14	3.20–20.70	0.000
	Adult vs. young	3.69	1.38–9.83	0.009

OR odds ratio, vs. versus, *CI* confidence; old > 3 years, adult 2–3 years, young < 2 years old

Table 8 Multi-variable logistic regression analysis of potential risk factors for dairy cattle sero-positivity in and around Adama and Asella towns

Explanatory variable	OR	SE	95% CI	P-value
Breed	2.79	0.81	1.59–4.92	0.000
Animal composition	1.54	0.34	0.99–2.38	0.048
Age	2.55	0.44	1.81–3.58	0.000

OR odds ratio, *SE* standard error, *CI* confidence interval

A study conducted around South Omo Zone and Borana pastoral area reported a similar effect [15, 33].

Significantly higher sero-prevalence of antibodies against FMDV in old and adult animals than in young observed in the current study was in agreement with the previous reports of [8] in Borena pastoral area and [33] Awbere and Babille districts of Jijiga zone. This effect can be a result of cumulative exposures over time, but is also to some extent caused by the persistence of antibodies against FMDV for extended periods of time [27]. Aged animals might have acquired the infection from multiple serotypes, and could have produced antibodies against those serotypes. Relatively low sero-prevalence in animal groups below 2 years old might be indicative of the existence of passive maternal immunity and low frequency of exposure [10, 33].

Higher sero-prevalence of antibodies against FMDV in cross-bred cattle might be associated with the genetic difference among cattle breeds. These indicated that cross-breeds may be more susceptible to FMDV endemic in Ethiopia, as is also reported Sub-Saharan Africa [34].

The presence of this disease in the country is a major obstacle to the development of livestock resource because of its adverse effects on production and their product exports. In Ethiopia, factors such as the presence of high numbers of susceptible domestic animals, herd composition or the involvement of multiple hosts (cattle, sheep and goats), herd size and individual animal age variability, lack of prophylactic vaccination, absence of regulation for prohibition of animal movement, high contact of animals at marketing and common grazing place as well as at watering points could contribute to the occurrence of FMD and create the difficulty in controlling the outbreaks.

Conclusion

FMD is prevalent in the study Districts as shown clinically, serologically, virologically and by molecular characterization and reported to be endemic in Ethiopia. During the study period serotype A, O and SAT 2 were identified, with highest prevalence of serotype SAT 2. Serotype SAT 2 and A isolated in Ethiopia were genotype Alx-12, topotype VII and genotype IV, African topotype, respectively. But these molecularly characterized serotypes seem to be emerging viruses as they cluster differently from the previously reported FMD viruses from Ethiopia.

An extensive regular surveillance, serotyping of the outbreak isolates, regular vaccination and movement control should be implemented. Also it is important to continue characterization of circulating FMDV and to match field isolates to vaccine strains to support the control of the disease by vaccination.

Additional files

Additional file 1: Serological diagnostic tests procedures. Procedures and principles of the test during the study were discussed in detail. (DOCX 12 kb)

Additional file 2: Antigen detection ELISA procedures. Antigen detection ELISA procedures and result interpretation during the study were discussed in detail. (DOCX 13 kb)

Abbreviations

BM: Bedaso Mammo; CI: Confidence interval; CPE: Cytopathic effect; DG: Daniel Gizaw; DS: Dereje Shegu; ELISA: Enzyme-linked immunosorbent assay; FD: Fufa Dawo; FMD: Foot-and-mouth disease; FMDV: Foot-and-mouth disease virus; GDP: Gross domestic production; MAb: Monoclonal antibodies; MS: Mishamo Sulayeman; NAHDIC: National animal health diagnostic and investigation centre; OR: Odd ratio; PA: Peasant association; PA: Peasant association; PBS: Phosphate-buffered saline; SAT: Southern African territories; WRL: World reference laboratory

Acknowledgements

We are very much grateful to Ayelech Muluneh, Membere Kidane, Aynalem Fente and Genet Bogale, all staff of National Animal Health Diagnostic and Investigation Center (NAHDIC) for their positive cooperation and technical assistance during the laboratory work. We would like to extend our thanks to Demeke Sebhat and Abebe Garuma for their excellent support during sample collection from dairy farms and outbreak areas. Finally, the authors would like to thank WRL-FMD at Pirbright for sequencing the isolates.

Funding

The cost of this research work was covered by NAHDIC.

Authors' contributions

MS: Contributed to conception of the research idea, designing and data collection, data analysis, interpretation of data, writing and editing of the manuscript. FD: Contributed to the study concept, interpretation of data, editing or reviewing of the manuscript. BM: Contributed to conception of the research idea. All authors read and approved the final manuscript. DG: Contributed to the data analysis, interpretation of data, writing and editing of the manuscript. DS: Contributed to data analysis (as Laboratory analyst).

Consent for publication

Not applicable.

Competing interests

The authors declare that they have no competing interests.

Author details

[1]Faculty of Veterinary Medicine, Hawassa University, P.O. Box 05, Hawassa, Ethiopia. [2]College of Veterinary Medicine, Addis Ababa University, P.O.Box 34, Debre Zeyit, Ethiopia. [3]National Animal Health Diagnostics and Investigation Center, P.O.Box 04, Sebeta, Ethiopia.

References

1. CSA. Federal Democratic Republic of Ethiopia. Central Statistical Agency, Agricultural Sample Survey Report on Livestock and Livestock Characteristics. Volume II, 2014/15. Addis Ababa, Ethiopia.
2. CSA. Central Statistical Authority, Federal Democratic Republic of Ethiopia, Central Statically investigation, statically Abstract; 2009.
3. Ganeshkumar B. Economic Impact of Foot-and-Mouth Disease in India, Scientific Developments and Technical Challenges in the Progressive Control of Foot-and-Mouth Disease in South Asia, New Delhi, India. Glob. Res. Alli. 2012;13:5.
4. Mansley LM, Donaldson AI, Thrusfield MV, Honhold N. Destructive tension: mathematics versus experience – the progress and control of the foot and mouth disease epidemic. Rev sci-entifique et tech. 2011;30:483–98.
5. Quinn PJ, Markey BK, Carter ME, Donnelly WJ, Leonard FC. Veterinary microbiology and microbial disease: Blackwell Science Ltd, A Blackwell publishing company; 2005. p. 402–7.
6. Berecha B, Gelagay A, Moses K, Yasmin J, Esayas G. Study on seroprevalence, risk factors, and economic impact of foot-and-mouth disease in Borena pastoral and agro-pastoral system, southern Ethiopia. Trop Anim Health Prod. 2011;43:759–66.
7. Land O'Lakes Inc. The next stage in dairy development for Ethiopia dairy value chains. In: End markets and food security cooperative agreement 663-A-00- 05- 00431-00. Addis Ababa, Ethiopia: Land O'Lakes Inc.; 2010.
8. Rufael T, Catley A, Bogale A, Sahle M, Shiferaw Y. Foot and mouth disease in the Borana pastoral system, southern Ethiopia and implications for livelihoods and international trade. Trop Anim Health Prod. 2008;40:29–38.
9. Ayelet G, Mahapatra M, Gelaye E, Egziabher GB, Rufeal T, Sahle M, Ferris NP, Wadsworth J, Hutchings HG, Knowles JN. Genetic characterization of foot and mouth disease viruses, Ethiopia, 1981-2007. J Emer Infec Dis. 2009;15(9):1–40.
10. Jenbere S, Etana M, Negussie H. Study on the risk factors of foot and mouth disease in selected districts of afar pastoral area. Northeast Ethiopia J Anim Vet Adv. 2011;10(11):1368–72.
11. Admassu B, Getinet K, Shite A, Mohammed S. Review on foot and mouth disease: distribution and economic significance in Ethiopia: Acad. J of Anim Dis. 2015;4(3):160–9.
12. Samuel A, Knowles N. Foot and mouth disease type O viruses exhibit genetically and geographically distinct evolutionary lineages (topotypes). J Gen Virol. 2001;82:609–21.
13. Gelaye E, Beyene B, Ayelet G. Foot and mouth disease virus serotype identified in Ethiopia. Ethiopian Vet J. 2005;9:75–9.
14. Mitiku T, Garedew L, Zemene M, Dagnaw M, Admassu B, Getaneh G. A review on foot and mouth disease and its current status in Ethiopia. Res. 2016;8(8):2.
15. Wondwossen A, Tariku S. The status of FMD in Ethiopia: a growing concern. Eth Vet Epid Newsletter. 2000;1(2):1–5.
16. Thrusfield M. Veterinary epidemiology. 2nd ed. UK: Blackwell science Ltd; 2005. p. 189–91.
17. OIE. Manual of diagnostic tests and vaccines for terrestrial animals (mammals, birds and bees), vol. I. 5th ed. Paris: Office international des Epizooties (OIE); 2004. p. 111–28.
18. OIE. Manual of Diagnostic Tests and Vaccines for Terrestrial Manual: 7th edition, volume I. Version adopted by the World Assembly of Delegates of the OIE, Paris, France; 2012. p. 1401-05.
19. Ding YZ, Chen J, Zhang JH, Zhou LN, Ma L, Zhang Y. An overview of control strategy and diagnostic technology for foot-and-mouth disease in China. Virol J. 2013;10:78.
20. Ahmed HA, Salem SA, Habashi AR, Arafa AA, Aggour MG, Salem GH, Gaber AS, Selem O, Abdelkader SH, Knowles NJ, Madi M, Valdazo-Gonza'lez, Wadsworth J, Hutchings GH, Mioulet V, Hammond JM, King DP. Emergence of foot-and-mouth disease virus SAT 2 in Egypt during. Transbound Emerg Dis. 2012;59:476–81.

21. Negussie H, Moses KN, Yami M, Ayelet G, Jenberie T. Outbreak investigations and genetic characterization of foot-and-mouth disease virus in Ethiopia. Trop Anim Health Prod. 2011;43:235–43.
22. Kitching P, Hammond J, Jeggo M, Charleston B, Paton D, Rodriguez L, Heckert R. Global FMD control-is it an option? Vaccine. 2007;25:5660–4.
23. Beyene B, Tolosa T, Rufael T, Hailu B, Teklue T. Sero-prevalence and associated risk factors of Foot and mouth disease in selected districts of western Ethiopia. Rev. Sci. Tech. Off. Int. Epiz. 2015;34(3):21–25.
24. Gelaye E, Ayelet G, G/Egziaber B, Zeleke A. A study on foot and mouth disease (FMD) virus serotypes circulating in Ethiopia. Debre Zeit: National Veterinary Institute; 2007. p. 116–25.
25. Ayelet G, Gelaye E, Negussie H, Asmare K. Study on the epidemiology of foot and mouth disease in Ethiopia. Rev Sci Tech Off Int Epiz. 2012; 31(3):789–98.
26. Bastos AD, Haydon DT, Forsberg R, Knowels NJ, Anderson EC, Bengis RG, Nel LH, Thomson GR. Genetic hetrogenecity of SAT1 type foot and mouth disease virusese in southern Africa. Arch Virol. 2001;146:1537–51.
27. Sangare O. Molecular epidemiology of foot and mouth disease virus in West Africa. Pretoria: PhD Thesis. University of Pretoria; 2005.
28. FAO. Focus on foot and mouth disease: Situation worldwide and major epidemiological events in 2005–2006, EMPRES, issue No. 1, Pp 1–11. FMD Homepage - Maps. 2006: http://www.wrlfmd.org/maps/fmd%2000-2006.pdf.
29. Knowles NJ, Samuel AR. Molecular epidemiology of foot-and mouth disease virus. Virus Res. 2003;91:65–80. https://doi.org/10.1016/ S0168-1702(02)00260-5.
30. Vosloo W, Bastos AD, Sangare O, Hargreaves SK, Thomson GR. Review of the status and control of foot and mouth disease in sub-Saharan Africa. Rev Sci Tech Off Int Epizt. 2002;21:437–49.
31. Bayissa B. Foot and mouth disease sero-prevalence and implications in Borana pastoral and agro pastoral systems, southern Ethiopia: FVM, AAU, Debre-Zeit: MSc, Ethiopia. MSc Thesis; 2009.
32. Ayelet G, Soressa M, Sisay T, Belay A, Gelaye E, Jemberea S, Skjerve E, Asmare K. FMD virus isolates: the candidate strains for polyvalent vaccine development in Ethiopia. Acta Trop. 2013;126:244–8.
33. Mohamoud A, Tessema E, Degefu H. Sero-prevalence of bovine foot and mouth disease (FMD) in Awbere and Babille districts of Jijiga zone, Somalia regional state, eastern Ethiopia. African J Microbio Res. 2011;5(21):3559–63.
34. Sahle M, Dwarka RM, Venter EH, Vosloo W. Comparison of SAT-1 foot and mouth disease virus isolates obtained from East Africa between 1971 and 2000 with viruses from the rest of sub-Saharan Africa. Arch Virol. 2007;152:797–804.

20

Risk factors for recurrence of FMD outbreaks in Iran: a case-control study in a highly endemic area

Kayhan Ilbeigi[1*], Saied Bokaie[2], Sina Aghasharif[1], Ricardo J. Soares Magalhães[3,4] and Mohamad Rashtibaf[5]

Abstract

Background: Foot-and-mouth disease (FMD) is an acute viral disease of cloven-hoofed animals with high economic impact. FMD remains endemic in Iran particularly in the livestock-dense province of Khorasan Razavi in northeastern Iran where FMD outbreaks continuously occur. In this study, we aimed to quantify risk factors for the recurrence of FMD outbreaks in Iran by analyzing a time-series of FMD outbreak data from the province of Khorasan Razavi.

Results: This study used FMD outbreak data collected from 2012 to 2014. Data were collected by local offices of the Iranian Animal Disease Department and the veterinarian of the veterinary council of the Khorasan Razavi province. An outbreak investigation questionnaire was delivered to 127 farms, including 46 case farms (FMD-infected) and 81 control farms (FMD-free). To quantify and compare the odds of exposure to a risk factor in FMD-infected farms versus FMD-free farms, logistic regression models were built using SPSS software version 16.
Our results of multivariable logistic regression indicate that hygienic status of the farm (OR = 11.83; CI = 3.38–41.43), FMD vaccination status (OR = 0.06; CI = 0.01–0.68), transportation of livestock (OR = 0.40; CI = 0.163–0.981) and inhibition of livestock dealers' entry into the farm (OR = 0.36; CI = 0.12–1.09) were identified as important risk factors for farm-level FMD infection.

Conclusion: This study generated much needed evidence on a set of modifiable risk factors for the recurrence of FMD outbreaks in the high risk province of Khorasan Razavi. This information can be used to improve existing national FMD control program and suggest new guidelines to prevent FMD outbreaks in the country.

Keywords: Foot-and-mouth disease, Risk factors, Case-control study, Logistic regression analysis

Background

Foot-and-mouth disease (FMD) is considered one of the highly contagious viral diseases affecting all cloven-hoofed animals. Among these animals, cattle are the main species affected, however, other species such as sheep, goats, pigs and so forth are also susceptible [1]. Pyrexia, lethargy, lameness and extra salivation with vesicles and erosions in the mouth, on the teats and on the feet are the typical clinical signs of FMD [2, 3]. The causative virus can be transmitted from infected animals to other susceptible animals by direct contact, fomites, animal products, contaminated surfaces and through the air [4]. Although the mortality rate of FMD is less than 5%, the importance of the disease is due to its negative effects on the marketing of animals and animal products, impacting on the national economy and return to trade of animals and the livestock industry [5].

The FMD virus belongs to the genus Aphthovirus, family Picornaviridae and has seven different serotypes including, A,C,O,SAT1,SAT2,SAT3 and Asia1 [6]. Three of the seven FMD serotypes (A,O and Asia1) have been circulating in Iran since 2011 [7–9].

Control of FMD in endemic regions such as Iran is mainly focused on mass vaccination of all susceptible livestock with a tetravalent vaccine [10] identification and testing of animals, establishment of protection and surveillance zones and enforcement of quarantine and

* Correspondence: keyhan.ilbeigi@gmail.com
[1]Department of Clinical Sciences, Faculty of Veterinary Medicine, Islamic Azad University of Garmsar, Garmsar, Iran
Full list of author information is available at the end of the article

biosecurity (Iranian Veterinary Organization). Despite the implementation of the national FMD control program, Iran is still faced with a number of challenges with respect to FMD status in that several outbreaks are still reported nationally. One of the worse affected areas in Iran is the province of Khorasan Razavi where 119 outbreaks of clinical FMD declared in 2012, 55 outbreaks in 2013 and 123 outbreaks in 2014 (GISVET database, IVO). This resulted in an annual FMD incidence rate between 0.73 and 4.63% of epidemiological-units. According to these statistics, we can claim that FMD virus transmission may have gone unnoticed in this endemic situation and with variable preventive measures. FMD vaccination is administered routinely by IVO in the province using a non-purified tetravalent vaccine containing serotypes A, Asia 1 and two strains of serotype O, which were produced locally in Razi institute (Tehran, Iran). Since 2011, current vaccination protocol by the IVO declares that vaccination needs to be applied three times a year for cattle in Khorasan Razavi as well as the country.

Usage of real-time case-control studies is uncommon in animal disease outbreaks and the majority of recent knowledge on FMD transmission originated from experimental studies and simulation modelling rather than field data [11, 12]. Previous studies investigating risk factors for FMD recurrence have identified various risk factors such as low effectiveness of the used vaccine [13, 14], long periods between vaccination and infection [14], proximity to borders [15], exposure to infected wild animals [16, 17], movement of infected animals [18–20] and lack of suitable biosecurity [19, 21, 22]. However, for the province of Khorasan Razavi very little is known about the determinants associated with the recurrence of FMD outbreaks in the region; this will help to distinguish why certain herds or farms in the region are at a higher risk of having FMD than others [23, 24].

This study is the first to investigate risk factors for the recurrence of FMD outbreaks in northeastern Iran. In this study we aimed to analyse FMD outbreak data for a three-year period (2012–2014) in the Khorasan Razavi province (northeastern Iran) to quantify the risk factors for FMD infection in order to inform evidence-based disease control recommendations to prevent future outbreaks.

Methods

Study population

To identify risk factors for recurrent FMD outbreaks between 2012 and 2014 in the Khorasan Razavi province, a case-control study was designed targeting all 138 farms (including 49,366 cattle) in the province. However, 11 farms declined to participate. A total of 127 farms (GISVET database, Iranian Veterinary Organization) were included in the investigation. The investigations were performed as part of the control measures applied by the Iranian Veterinary Organization in order to prevent further FMD outbreaks and were carried out based on the ethical standards agreed by the IVO for outbreak investigations. Khorasan Razavi province, which is a 119,000 km^2 area close to the borders with Afghanistan and Turkmenistan, has one of the highest population density of cattle farms in Iran (Fig. 1). In 2014, there were an estimated 300,000 cattle and 7.4 million small ruminants in Khorasan Razavi province, which 80% of livestock accommodated in epidemiological-units including villages, commercial dairy herds and commercial mixed herds (combination of sheep, goats, beef and or dairy). The remaining part of livestock was distributed in nomadic herds. Holstein Friesians are the breed of dairy cattle in Khorasan Razavi province.

Case definition for case and control farms

Classification of case farms was based on the appearance of clinical signs of FMD as observed by the herdsmen and the attending veterinarian in one or more animals and laboratory confirmation by polymerase chain reaction (PCR) by the IVO. Control farms were defined as those which the herdsmen and the attending veterinarian did not observe clinical signs compatible with FMD and a negative laboratory result by PCR. As a result, out of 127 farms a total of 46 case farms and 81 control farms were included in the study. The case and control farms were matched based on herd size; 35 case farms were matched with two control farms while the remaining 11 case farms were matched with one control farm. That is because we could not find suitable control farms for those 11 case farms based on herd size.

Data collection

Risk factor data were collected for each case and control farm by means of a questionnaire composed of 13 questions on particular risk factors associated with FMD transmission which were organized into 4 sections: 1) general farm information, 2) movement of people, 3) movement of vehicles and 4) general farm management. Questions included in the risk factor questionnaire were designed based on the potential risk factors recognized by IVO in previous FMD outbreaks in Iran [unpublished observations, Mohamad Rashtibaf]. We evaluated the hygiene status of the farms by asking specific questions in the general farm management section in the questionnaire to consider the implementation of quarantine (i.e. separating infected animals from others, restriction movements of staff, veterinarians and vehicles) and biosecurity guidelines (i.e. presence of main gate, physical barrier to livestock area, wheel wash, boot dips, farm-specific clothing, clothes-changing area and so forth).

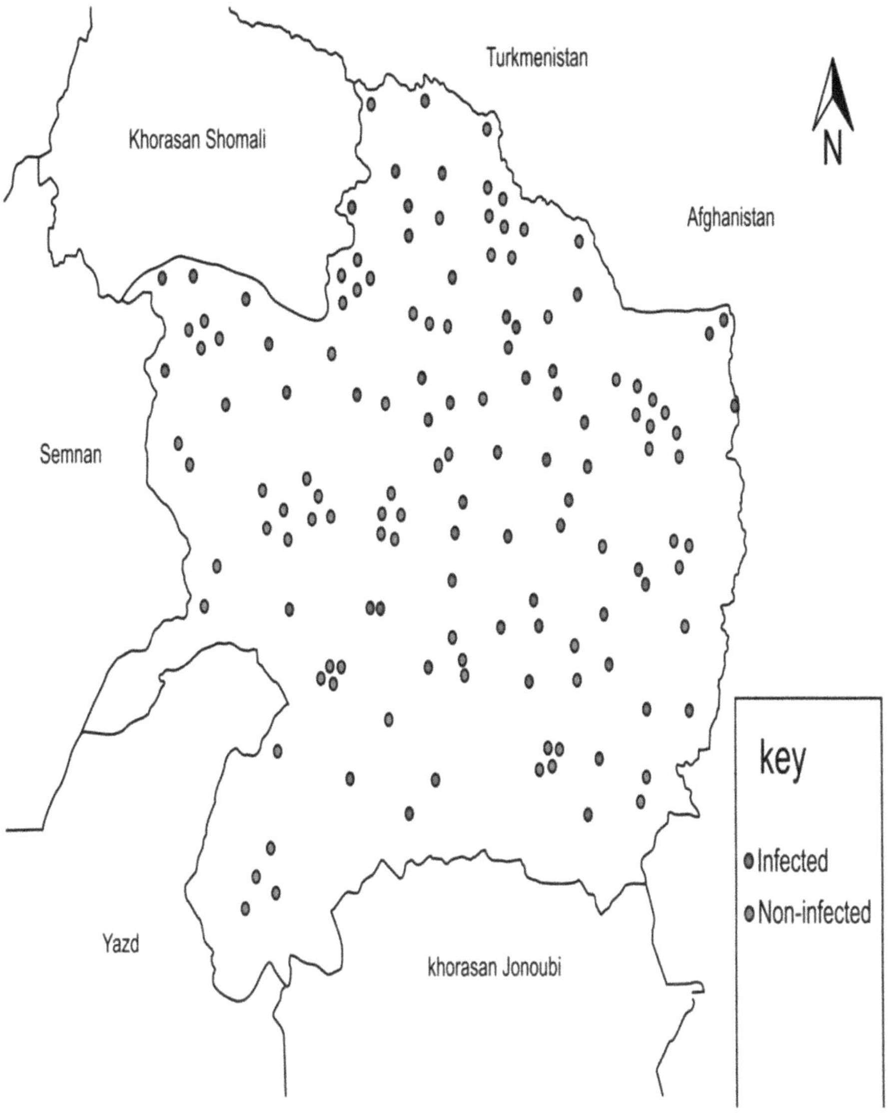

Fig. 1 Map of Khorasan Razavi, northeastern of Iran. The infected farms are displayed by red dots and non-infected farms are showed by grey dots. The vaccinated areas included both infected and non-infected farms

Data were collected from case and control farms by personnel from the province animal disease department and veterinarians of the Veterinary Council of the province by visiting each farm and interviewing the farm manager. Incomplete information was followed up by subsequent telephone interviews of the farm manager.

Statistical analyses

The statistical analysis was conducted in two phases: firstly, all variables were examined by univariable analysis using a chi-squared or Fisher's exact test; variables with p-value ≤ 0.15 in the univariable analysis were considered for the multivariable model [25]. Correlation between candidate variables for multivariable analysis were tested using the phi coefficient. Phi coefficient is a measure of association between two binary variables and is applicable to categorical variables. Among variables, those variables that were highly correlated (phi coefficient > 0.4), were selected for the multivariable analysis.

Secondly, following univariable variable screening, a conditional multivariable logistic regression model was built. To select the final multivariable model, a backward stepwise elimination approach was applied using $p < 0.05$ for variable retention. Confounding and effect modification between variables in the final model were evaluated. For the presence of confounding we evaluated the impact of removing a non-significant variable on the measure of disease association of other variables; if the odds ratio of a variable changed by 10%, after removal of a non-significant variable, we considered the latter as a confounder and retained in the multivariable model. For effect modification, we used – 2 log likelihood test from logistic regression to test the statistical significant of potential effect modifiers and calculate the estimators of exposure-disease association according to the level of significant effect modifiers. All statistical analyses were performed using SPSS version 17.0 (SPSS Inc., Chicago, IL, USA).

Results

Risk factors for FMD emergence

Results of univariable analyses on cattle farms in this area are shown in Table 1. Among 13 variables, a total of six explanatory variables ($p < 0.15$) were selected for the multivariable analysis: 'hygienic status of the farm', 'vaccination', 'transportation of livestock', 'feed transport vehicles visited the farm', 'inhibition of livestock dealers' entry in the farm', and 'the number of people involved in the livestock market' as protective factors (Table 2). The final model was checked for goodness-of-fit using Hosmer-Lemeshow statistics [26]. Based on results of multivariable logistic regression, four factors, including hygienic status of the farm (OR = 11.83; CI = 3.375–41.43), FMD full course vaccination (OR = 0.06; CI = 0.005–0.684), transportation of livestock (OR = 0.40; CI = 0.163–0.981) and inhibition of livestock dealers' entry into the farm (OR = 0.362; CI = 0.12–1.093) were identified as important factors influencing the occurrence of FMD.

Discussion

This study is one of the few studies on FMD outbreaks in Iran and the first one in northeastern Iran which evaluates risk factors for FMD infection. Apart from our study, there is only one study on FMD risk factors in northwestern Iran (West Azerbaijan) which is a serological cross-sectional study, and investigates prevalence

Table 1 Results of univariable analysis for risk factors associated with FMD outbreaks

Variable	Category	Frequency		Odds ratio	%95 Confidence interval	*P* value
		Case	Control			
Type of livestock units	Traditional	38	69	0.826	0.311–2.197	0.702
	Dairy cattle farms	8	12			
Hygienic status of the farm	Suitable	19	8	6.421	2.517–16.383	< 0.001
	Not suitable	27	27			
Vaccination (every 4 months)	Yes	29	75	0.203	0.25–1.676	0.098
	No	17	6			
Rappel Vaccination	Yes	31	52	0.868	0.403–1.866	0.435
	No	15	29			
Transportation of livestock	Yes	29	26	0.227	0.130–0.592	0.001
	No	17	55			
Feed transport vehicles visited The farm	Yes	26	35	0.0585	0.282–1.215	0.149
	No	20	46			
Entrance of manure unloading vehicles	Yes	21	41	0.800	0.359–1.782	0.585
	No	32	60			
Entrance of Vehicles carrying Milk	Yes	30	50	0.860	0.405–1.829	0.695
	No	16	31			
Entrance of vaccinator groups	Yes	28	40	0.627	0.301–1.308	0.212
	No	18	41			
Entrance of artificial insemination groups	Yes	22	36	0.873	0.422–1.803	0.713
	No	24	45			
Inhibition of livestock dealers' entry into the farm	Yes	27	23	0.279	0.130–0.597	0.001
	No	19	58			
Farm owners associated with livestock market	Yes	37	43	0.275	0.118–0.643	0.002
	No	9	38			
People associated with milk collection, artificial insemination and manure collection	Yes	38	69	1.211	0.455–3.22	0.702
	No	8	12			

Table 2 Results of conditional multivariable analysis for risk factors associated with FMD outbreaks in Khorasan Razavi, Iran

Variable	Odds ratio	%95 Confidence interval	*P* value
Hygiene status of the farm	11.826	3.375–41. 434	< 0.001
Vaccination (every 4 months)	0.060	0.005–0.684	0.023
Transportation of livestock	0.400	0.163–0.981	0.045
Inhibition of livestock dealers' entry into the farm	0.310	0.118–1.093	0.017

of antibodies to non-structural proteins in young cattle showing FMD infection to assess potential risk factors for FMD outbreaks [19]. FMD outbreaks still occur annually in Iran despite the application of FMD control measures including, routine vaccination of livestock (i.e. cattle and small ruminants), the usage of emergency vaccination and post-movement quarantine based on the IVO protocol. In endemic countries, FMD outbreaks are frequently underreported in regard to level of economic and political development of the country [27]. This case-control study was carried out in order to investigate risk factors associated with the recurrence of FMD outbreaks in cattle farms located in the Khorasan Razavi province (northeastern Iran), an area in Iran heavily impacted by FMD outbreaks. The results of the current study which analysed data from 46 case and 81 control farms within the Khorasan Razavi province advance the knowledge base yielded by other field epidemiological investigations, and establish principles to inform evidence-based farm-level surveillance and control operations in the future.

Our results demonstrate that the hygiene status of the farms' play an important role in FMD transmission in that the odds of lack of biosecurity in FMD-infected farms was 11 times greater than in non-infected farms. This finding is in line with recent evidence from other nearby countries. For example, an outbreak in four regions of Bhutan in 2009, it was considered that raising awareness of farmers is required to implement simple biosecurity procedures in FMD endemic villages in order to reduce the spread of the virus to other areas [22]. Recent outbreaks in West Azerbaijan (northwestern Iran) indicated that FMD prevention could not be achieved by vaccination alone in the endemic situations such as Iran [19]. Therefore, additional control measures like strict application of biosecurity and quarantine measures through monitoring professionals (veterinary practitioners, vaccinators, milk-collectors, inseminators) are required [19].

The most important factor in the long-range geographical spread of FMD in endemic areas is the movement of infected livestock through traditional or informal networks of livestock trade [18, 20, 28, 29]. In our study we demonstrated that 'transportation of livestock' is a crucial risk factor for FMD spread (OR = 0.40, CI = 16.3–981). Cattle are transported to different regions of Iran by dealers and herdsmen without any pre-movement testing; hence, the FMDV would be transmitted from infected cattle to the other susceptible livestock easily. In a similar study which was conducted in West Azerbaijan (northwestern Iran), more than 60% of herdsmen claimed that they traded livestock locally and distantly; moreover, this common trade is a social pass time for farmers throughout Iran which increases the risk of FMDV transmission. Therefore, limitation of animals' movement has become the first priority of the veterinary services and stakeholders in Iran [19]. In fact, the IVO has recruited some veterinarians in the livestock markets in order to prevent excessive livestock movements.

Another risk factor influencing the occurrence of FMD in Iran is the movement of people strange to the farm, particularly those that have frequent contact with livestock such as dealer, traders, and middle men [29]. Dealers are people who trade animals and move regularly between farms and markets without any permission all over Iran (i.e. Khorasan Razavi province) and producers commonly move cattle from one market to another in search of better prices. Dealers transfer animals between farms and markets and can introduce the FMDV through infected animals and fomites [30]. In this situation, animals are kept for at least 1 to 3 days in the markets which result in the transmission of FMDV from infected to susceptible livestock.

According to the FMD vaccination protocol of Razi Institute (Tehran, Iran), cattle should be vaccinated three times a year. However, the results of our study in Khorasan Razavi province, indicate that some cattle in our study population had only been vaccinated once or twice at most. Therefore, a long period between vaccination and infection occur for herds that are not vaccinated according to the vaccination protocol [19]. Indeed our results confirm that the odds of lack of compliance in FMD vaccination (every 4 months) was greater in FMD-infected farms compared to non-infected farms suggesting that reducing the susceptibility of farms through full compliance with FMD vaccination is an important mitigating factor for the recurrence of outbreaks in the region. This finding could be partly explained by the fact that a few epi-units effectively received three annual vaccine rounds prior to the study. A possible explanation for this is the limited production capacity of vaccines in some years [19]. Previous studies indicate that timing and number of vaccine rounds are an important factor against FMD outbreaks [14]. During a FMD outbreak in Israel, a study was carried out on beef farms and illustrated a time period more than 6 months between adult vaccination and FMDV infection resulted in low protective effectiveness of vaccine and those farms were affected by FMD virus when the outbreak occurred [31].

The findings of this study need to be interpreted in light of a few limitations. First, it is known that case-control studies are based on questionnaires. To minimize the failures through collecting data by questionnaires in our study, the obtained data were validated by paper-based records and field veterinarians as well as GISVET database of Iranian Veterinary Organization. Second, case-control studies include detection of infection origin, identification of risk factors and aid case findings and control during an outbreak; however, such studies present no information about cause and effect [32–35].

Conclusions

Our findings enabled an insight into risk factors for the recurrence of FMD outbreaks in Iran and have generated potential recommendations for farmers. The identified risk factors from this study may contribute to the risk-based strategy plan in Iran, as part of the Progressive Control Pathway for FMD control. Continuous efforts including further follow-up studies should be undertaken to evaluate the efficacy of strategies that aim to tackle the risk factors identified in this study.

Abbreviations

FMD: Foot-and-mouth disease; GIS: Geographical Information System; IVO: Iranian Veterinary Organization; PCR: Polymerase Chain Reaction

Acknowledgements

We would like to thank the herdsmen for their cooperation and the Iranian Veterinary Organization for their support to this study.

Author's contributions

SB and KI designed the study. MR, KI and SA led the data collection. SB performed all data handling and analysis. RSM, MR, KI and SA supported the data analysis performed by SB. SA and KI drafted the manuscript. RSM revised the manuscript critically for important intellectual and content. All authors were given the opportunity to review and comment on the manuscript. All authors read and approved the final manuscript.

Consent for publication

Not applicable.

Competing interests

The author Ricardo J. Soares Magalhães is a member of the editorial board (Associate Editor) of this journal. The authors declare that they have no competing interests.

Author details

[1]Department of Clinical Sciences, Faculty of Veterinary Medicine, Islamic Azad University of Garmsar, Garmsar, Iran. [2]Department of Food Hygiene and Quality Control, Faculty of Veterinary Medicine, University of Tehran, Tehran, Iran. [3]UQ Spatial Epidemiology Laboratory, School of Veterinary Science, The University of Queensland, Gatton, Australia. [4]Children's Health and Environment Program, Child Health Research Centre, The University of Queensland, Brisbane, Australia. [5]Iranian Veterinary Organization, Provincial Department of Surveillance and Disease Control, Khorasan Razavi, Islamic Republic of Iran.

References

1. Radostits OM, Gay CC, Hinchcliff KW, Constable PD. Veterinary medicine E-book: a textbook of the diseases of cattle, horses, sheep pigs and goats. 10th edition, Chapter 21, Part 2. Elsevier Health Sci; 2006. p. 1223-1230.
2. Defra. Foot and mouth disease ageing of lesions. London: Defra Publications; 2005. http://webarchive.nationalarchives.gov.uk/20130402160224/http://archive.defra.gov.uk/foodfarm/farmanimal/diseases/atoz/fmd/about/clinicalsigns/index.htm.
3. Kitching RP, Alexandersen S. Clinical variation in foot and mouth disease: pigs. Rev Sci Tech. 2002;21:513–8.
4. Alexandersen S, Mowat N. Foot-and-mouth disease: host range and pathogenesis. Curr Top Microbiol Immunol. 2005;288:9–42.
5. Longjam N, Deb R, Sarmah A, Tayo T, Awachat V, Saxena V. A brief review on diagnosis of foot-and-mouth disease of livestock: conventional to molecular tools. Vet Med Int. 2011:905768–85.
6. Belsham GJ. Distinctive features of foot-and-mouth disease virus, a member of the picornavirus family; aspects of virus protein synthesis, protein processing and structure. Prog Biophys Mol Biol. 1993;60:241–60.
7. FAO, 2013a. World Reference Laboratory for FMD, FMD alerts, http://www.wrlfmd.org/fmd_alerts/asia_1_2011.htm (Accessed 10.10.2013) and http://www.wrlfmd.org/fmd_genotyping/2011/WRLFMD-2011-00003%20Asia1%20Pakistan%202010-2011.pdf. Accessed 13 Oct 2013.
8. FAO, 2013b. World Reference Laboratory for FMD, reports on Iran. http://www.wrlfmd.org/fmd_genotyping/me/irn.htm. Accessed 13 Oct 2013.
9. Zibaei M, Kianizadeh M, Keivanfar H, Rabani M, Hematzadeh F, Bokaei S. Identification of the foot and mouth disease foci from susceptible foci in Khorasan Razavi province. J Vet Res. 2007;62:151–5.
10. Singh SN. Foot and mouth disease control strategies global frame work. Int J Life Sci Pharma Res. 2011;1(1):63–70.
11. Cottam EM, Wadsworth J, Shaw AE, Rowlands RJ, Goatley L, Mann S. Transmission pathways of foot-and-mouth disease virus in the United Kingdom in 2007. PLoS Pathog. 2008;4:e1000050.
12. Schiley D, Burgin L, Gloster J. Predicting infection risk of airborne foot-and-mouth disease. J R Soc Interface. 2009;6:574.
13. Woolhouse ME, Haydon DT, Pearson A, Kitching RP. Failure of vaccination to prevent outbreaks of foot-and-mouth disease. Epi demiol Infect. 1996;116:363–71.
14. Elnekave E, Li Y, Zamir L, Even-Tov B, Hamblin P, Gelman B, Hammond J, Klement E. The field effectiveness of routine and emergency vaccination with an inactivated vaccine against foot and mouth disease. Vaccine. 2013;31:879–85.
15. Allepuz A, Stevenson M, Kivaria F, Berkvens D, Casal J, Picado A. Risk factors for foot-and-mouth disease in Tanzania, 2001-2006. Transbound Emerg Dis. 2015;62(2):127–36.
16. Shimshony A. Foot and mouth disease in the mountain gazelle in Israel. Rev Sci Tech Off Int Epizoot. 1988;7:917–23.
17. Thomson GR, Vosloo W, Bastos AD. Foot and mouth disease in wildlife. Virus Res. 2003;91:145–61.
18. Rweyemamu M, Roeder P, Mackay D, Sumption K, Brownlie J, Leforban Y, Valarcher JF, Knowles NJ, Saraiva V. Epidemiological patterns of foot-andmouth disease worldwide. Transbound Emerg Dis. 2008;55:57–72.

19. Emami J, Rasouli N, McLaws M, Bartels CJM. Risk factors for infection with foot-and-mouth disease virus in a cattle population vaccinated with a non-purified vaccine in Iran. Prev Vet Med. 2015;119:114–22.
20. Ayebazibwe C, Tjornehoj K, Mwiine FN, Muwanika VB, Okurut ARA, Siegismund HR, Alexandersen S. Pattern risk factors and characteristics of reported and perceived foot-and-mouth disease (FMD) in Uganda. Trop Anim Health Prod. 2010;42:1547–59.
21. Ellis-Iversen J, Smith RP, Gibbens JC, Sharpe CE, Dominguez M. Cook AJ (2011) risk factors for transmission of foot-and-mouth disease during an outbreak in southern England in 2007. Vet Rec. 2011;168:128.
22. Dukpa K, Robertson ID, Edwards JR, Ellis TM, Tsherin P, Rinzin K, Dahal N. Risk factors for foot-and-mouth disease in sedentary livestock herds in selected villages in four regions of Bhutan. N Z Vet J. 2011b;59:51–8.
23. Cleland PC, Baldock FC, Chamnanpood P, Gleeson LJ. Village-level risk factors for foot-and-mouth disease in northern Thailand. Prev Vet Med. 1996;26:253–61.
24. Bronsvoort BM, Nfon C, Hamman SM, Tanya VN, Kitching RP, Morgan KL. Risk factors for herdsman-reported foot-and-mouth disease in the Adamawa Province of Cameroon. Prev Vet Med. 2004;66:127–39.
25. Dohoo IR, Martin W, Stryhn HE. Veterinary epidemiologic research. In: Charlottetown. Canada: AVC Inc; 2003.
26. Hosmer DW, Lemeshow S. Applied logistic regression. New York, USA: Johns: Wiley & Sons; 1989.
27. Sumption K, Rweyemamu M, Wint W. Incidence and distribution of foot-and-mouth disease in Asia, Africa and South America. Combining expert opinion, official disease information and livestock populations to assist risk assessment. Transbound Emerg Dis. 2008;55(55):5–13.
28. Christley RM, Robinson SE, Lysons R. French NP (2005) network analysis of cattle movement in Great Britain. Proc Soc Vet Epidemiol Prev Med. 2005:234–43.
29. Qrtiz-Pelaez A, Pfeiffer DU, Soares-Magalhaes RJ, Guitian FJ. Use of social network analysis to characterize the pattern of animal movements in the initial phases of the 2001 foot and mouth disease (FMD) epidemic in the UK. Prev Vet Med. 2006;76(1):40–55.
30. Lindholm A, Hewitt E, Toress P, Lasso M, Echeverria C, Shaw J, Hernandez J. Epidemiologic aspects of a foot-and-mouth disease epidemic in cattle in Ecuador. Intern J Appl Res Vet Med. 2007;5(1)
31. Elnekave E, Zamir L, Hamd F, Tov BE, Klement E. Risk factors of foot and mouth disease outbreaks in grazing beef cattle herds. Prev Vet Med. 2015;120(2):236–40.
32. Muroga N, Kobayashi S, Nishida T, Hayama Y, Kawano T, Yamamoto T. Tsutsui T (2013) risk factors for the transmission of foot-and-mouth disease during the 2010 outbreak in Japan: a case–control study. BMC Vet Res. 2013;9:150.
33. Ethelberg S, Lisby M, Vestergaard LS, Enemark HL, Olsen KE, Stensvold CR, Nielsen HV, Porsbo LJ, Plesner AM, Molbak K. A foodborne outbreak of cryptosporidium Hominis infection. Epidemiol Infect. 2009a;137:348–56.
34. Ethelberg S, Smith B, Torpdahl M, Lisby M, Boel J, Jensen T, Nielsen EM, Molbak K. Outbreak of non-O157 Shiga toxin-producing Escherichia coliinfection from consumption of beef sausage. Clin Infect Dis. 2009b;48:e78–81.
35. Whittaker PJ, Sopwith W, Quigley C, Gillespie I, Willshaw GA, Lycett C, Surman-Lee S, Baxter D, Adak GK, Seyed Q. A national outbreak of verotoxin-producing Escherichia coli O157 associated with consumption of lemon-and-coriander chicken wraps from a supermarket chain. Epidemiol Infect. 2009;137:375–82.

Overcoming species barriers: an outbreak of *Lagovirus europaeus* GI.2/RHDV2 in an isolated population of mountain hares (*Lepus timidus*)

Aleksija S. Neimanis[1,2*], Harri Ahola[3], Ulrika Larsson Pettersson[1], Ana M. Lopes[4,5], Joana Abrantes[4], Siamak Zohari[3], Pedro J. Esteves[4,6,7] and Dolores Gavier-Widén[1,2]

Abstract

Background: Prior to 2010, the lagoviruses that cause rabbit hemorrhagic disease (RHD) in European rabbits (*Oryctolagus cuniculus*) and European brown hare syndrome (EBHS) in hares (*Lepus* spp.) were generally genus-specific. However, in 2010, rabbit hemorrhagic disease virus 2 (RHDV2), also known as *Lagovirus europaeus* GI.2, emerged and had the distinguishing ability to cause disease in both rabbits and certain hare species. The mountain hare (*Lepus timidus*) is native to Sweden and is susceptible to European brown hare syndrome virus (EBHSV), also called *Lagovirus europaeus* GII.1. While most mountain hare populations are found on the mainland, isolated populations also exist on islands. Here we investigate a mortality event in mountain hares on the small island of Hallands Väderö where other leporid species, including rabbits, are absent.

Results: Post-mortem and microscopic examination of three mountain hare carcasses collected from early November 2016 to mid-March 2017 revealed acute hepatic necrosis consistent with pathogenic lagovirus infection. Using immunohistochemistry, lagoviral capsid antigen was visualized within lesions, both in hepatocytes and macrophages. Genotyping and immunotyping of the virus independently confirmed infection with *L. europaeus* GI. 2, not GII.1. Phylogenetic analyses of the *vp60* gene grouped mountain hare strains together with a rabbit strain from an outbreak of GI.2 in July 2016, collected approximately 50 km away on the mainland.

Conclusions: This is the first documented infection of GI.2 in mountain hares and further expands the host range of GI.2. Lesions and tissue distribution mimic those of GII.1 in mountain hares. The virus was most likely initially introduced from a concurrent, large-scale GI.2 outbreak in rabbits on the adjacent mainland, providing another example of how readily this virus can spread. The mortality event in mountain hares lasted for at least 4.5 months in the absence of rabbits, which would have required virus circulation among mountain hares, environmental persistence and/or multiple introductions. This marks the fourth *Lepus* species that can succumb to GI.2 infection, suggesting that susceptibility to GI.2 may be common in *Lepus* species. Measures to minimize the spread of GI.2 to vulnerable *Lepus* populations therefore are prudent.

Keywords: Rabbit hemorrhagic disease, *Lagovirus europaeus* GI.2, RHDV2, *Lepus timidus*, Hare, Virus, Wildlife, Hepatitis

* Correspondence: aleksija.neimanis@sva.se

[1]Department of Pathology and Wildlife Diseases, National Veterinary Institute (SVA), 751 89 Uppsala, Sweden

[2]Department of Biomedical Sciences and Veterinary Public Health, Swedish University of Agricultural Sciences (SLU), Box 7028, 750 07 Uppsala, Sweden

Full list of author information is available at the end of the article

Background

Pathogenic lagoviruses (Family *Caliciviridae*) cause hepatitis in leporids. The disease is referred to as rabbit hemorrhagic disease (RHD) or European brown hare syndrome (EBHS) depending on whether it affects rabbits or hares. Viruses identified prior to 2010 are generally considered to be genus-specific and do not cause clinical disease in animals less than five weeks of age. Disease caused by rabbit hemorrhagic disease virus (RHDV) and its antigenic variant (RHDVa), also collectively known as *Lagovirus europaeus* GI.1 [1], is almost exclusively confined to domestic and wild European rabbits (*Oryctolagus cuniculus*). Similarly, European brown hares (*Lepus europaeus*) and other hare species including mountain hares (*Lepus timidus*) are susceptible to EBHS virus (EBHSV) [2], also called *Lagovirus europaeus* GII.1 [1], but not to GI.1 viruses. However, in 2010, RHDV2 or RHDVb, also known as *L. europaeus* GI.2 [1], emerged in France [3]. Differing significantly from the previously detected viruses, GI.2 has a broader age and host range. GI.2 can cause clinical disease and death in rabbits as young as 11 days old [4]. In addition to infecting rabbits, GI.2 can also cause EBHS-like disease in the Sardinian Cape hare (*Lepus capensis mediterraneus*) [5], the Italian hare (*Lepus corsicanus*) [6] and the European brown hare [7–9].

The mountain hare (*Lepus timidus*) is an arctic/subarctic species that inhabits the tundra and taiga habitats of northern Europe and Asia [10]. While listed as a species of least concern globally [11], certain regions in Europe and Russia have been experiencing gradual population declines [12]. This species is particularly prone to dramatic population crashes on islands [13]. In Sweden, the mountain hare is a native species and it historically ranged throughout the country. Isolated populations of mountain hares also exist on many small Swedish islands because of relatively recent introductions [10]. While populations in the north are robust, mountain hare range and density have decreased in south and central Sweden since the beginning of the twentieth century, and mountain hares have completely disappeared from the far south [12]. Postulated reasons for the decline include negative impacts from introduced European brown hares (*Lepus europaeus*), predation pressure, competition with other herbivores, or landscape change [12]. While competitive exclusion by, and hybridization with, brown hares are considered primary candidates for the decline of southern mountain hare populations in Sweden, disease-mediated competition through, for example, GII.1 or *Francisella tularensis* may also play a role [12]. Although GII.1 can infect and cause disease in both European brown hares and mountain hares, documented cases of EBHS in Sweden are geographically restricted to the range of European brown hares. Confirmed cases in mountain hares have only occurred in the southern half of the country where the ranges of European brown and mountain hares overlap [14, 15]. This suggests that the virus circulates mainly in European brown hares and that mountain hares may be spillover hosts [14].

In the early autumn of 2016, managers of a small island nature reserve off the Swedish west coast began to find carcasses of mountain hares. Here we describe an outbreak of a pathogenic lagovirus in this island population of mountain hares and provide evidence for the further expansion of GI.2 host range. The outbreak occurred on an island without rabbits or European brown hares and we explore the epidemiological circumstances of the outbreak, describe the pathology in mountain hares, investigate the molecular epidemiology of GI.2, and discuss the implications of disease introductions for isolated wildlife populations.

Methods

Study site

Hallands Väderö (N 56° 26.6′, E 12° 33.7′) is a small, 310 ha island 3 km off the southwest coast of Sweden, accessible only by boat (Fig. 1). It is a nature reserve with no permanent residents living on the island, but is host to approximately 50,000 visitors per year, primarily in the summer months. The island is also home to an introduced, managed mountain hare population and organized hunts are typically held 1–2 times per year. The earliest documented introduction of hares occurred in 1857 from Godska Sandön, a Swedish island in the Baltic Sea, and numerous restocking events have occurred since then [16]. There are no European brown hares or wild rabbits on the island, making the mountain hare the only leporid species present.

Animals

In September 2016, managers of Hallands Väderö began finding mountain hare carcasses. Remains of approximately 15 animals were noted from September to December 2016. In the beginning of November 2016, the first dead hare (animal 2147) was collected, frozen and transported to the National Veterinary Institute (SVA), Uppsala, Sweden for necropsy on November 17. Two other dead hares found at the beginning of December 2016 (animal 2381) and middle of March 2017 (animal 1208) were frozen and transported to SVA for examination on December 19, 2016 and March 29, 2017, respectively (Table 1).

All three animals showed characteristic features of *Lepus timidus*. Compared to *Lepus europaeus*, they were smaller, had shorter ears and front limbs and the forehead was rounder [10]. The pelage was in varying stages of moulting from grey-brown to grey-white (Fig. 2). The

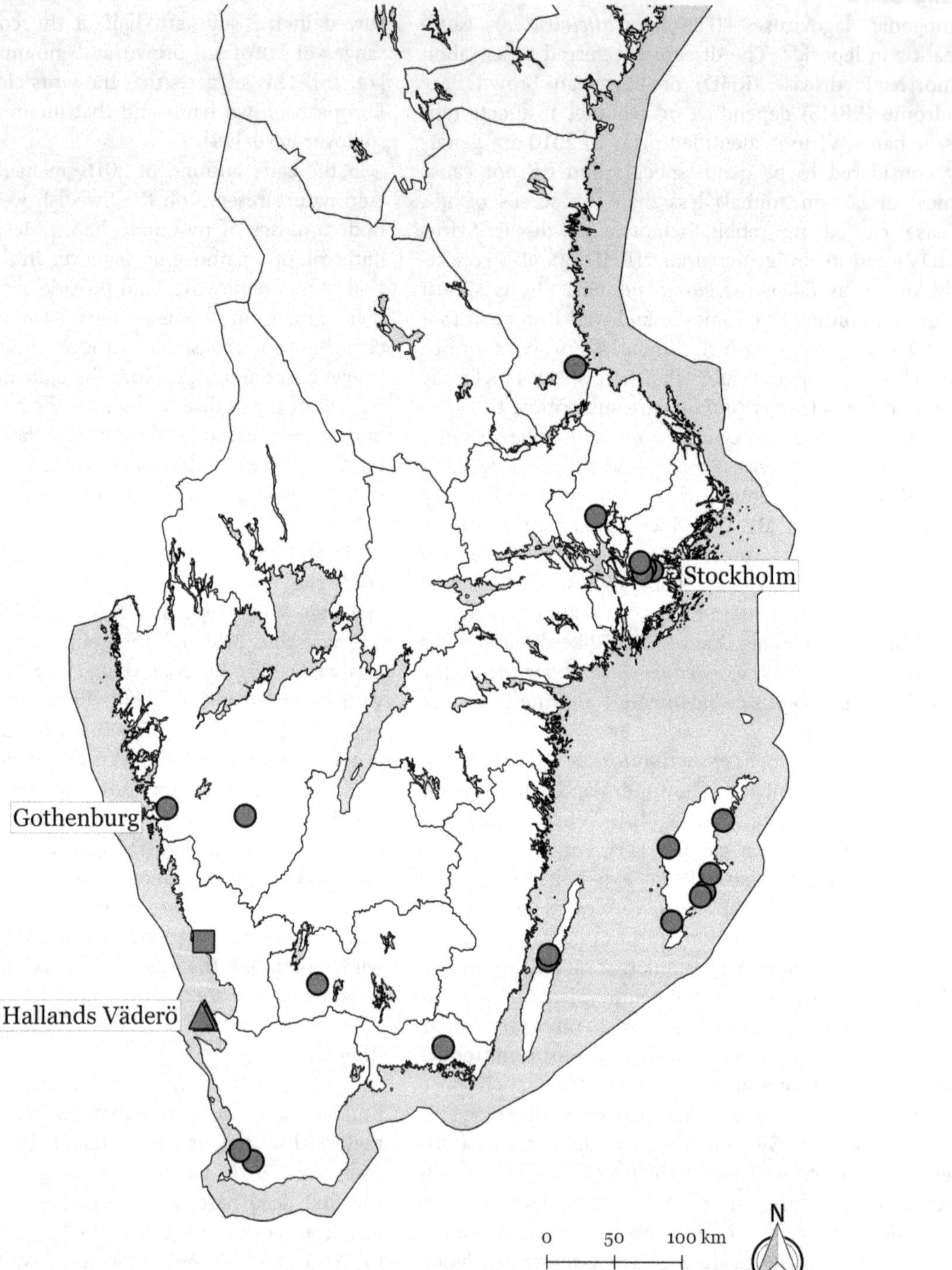

Fig. 1 A map of the southern Sweden depicting cases of *Lagovirus europaeus* G1.2/RHDV2/b infection from which the *vp60* gene sequences originated. The three mountain hares from Hallands Väderö (2147, 2381 and 1208) are represented by a triangle (▲), the rabbit from Falkenberg (1251) is depicted by a square (■) and other rabbits are shown with a circle (●).

animal found in November had the greatest proportion of brown in its pelage and the animal in March was almost completely grey-white. To confirm species identity, molecular analyses were also carried out on liver samples of two of the hares (2147 and 1208). DNA was extracted with the EasySpin Genomic DNA Minipreps Tissue Kit (Citomed, Portugal) following manufacturer's instructions. When considered together, the nuclear

Table 1 Mountain hares (*Lepus timidus*) found dead or hunted on Hallands Väderö, Sweden

Hare identification number	Found dead (D) or hunted (H)	Date collected	Sex[a]	Age[b]	Body condition
2147	D	November 2016	F	Y	Poor
2381	D	December 2016	F	A	Normal
1208	D	March 2017	M	U	Emaciated
123	H	January 14, 2017	M	NE	Normal
124	H	January 14, 2017	M	NE	Normal
126	H	January 14, 2017	M	NE	Normal
127	H	January 14, 2017	F	A	Normal
2539	H	September 21, 2017	NE	NE	Normal
2540	H	September 21, 2017	NE	NE	Normal

[a] *F* female, *M* male, *NE* not examined
[b] *Y* young of year, *A* adult, *U* unable to determine *NE*, not examined

genes uncoupling protein 2 (*upc2*) and immunoglobulin heavy constant gamma (*ighg*) and the mitochondrial gene cytochrome b (*cytb*) distinguish *L. timidus* from the other leporid species. Amplification of these markers was carried out using the primers described in [17, 18]; PCR conditions are available upon request. After purification, PCR products were sequenced on an automatic sequencer ABI PRISM 310 Genetic Analyzer (PE Applied Biosystems, USA) using the amplification primers. Sequences were submitted to the publicly available GenBank database (https://www.ncbi.nlm.nih.gov/genbank) under the accession numbers MH107277–82. Genetic distances between the sequences of 2147 and 1208 and other lagomorphs were calculated for each gene in MEGA6 [19] using the following parameters: p-distance method, 500 replicates, pairwise deletion.

Management of the mountain hare population on Hallands Väderö included a hunt in January and September 2017. Sampling of these hunted animals provided an opportunity to screen for evidence of GI.2 infection in these apparently healthy animals during (n = 4, January) and after ($n = 2$, September) the outbreak. Fresh liver and duodenum samples were collected from animals hunted in January 2017 and frozen at −20 °C. Formalin-fixed tissues from these animals included liver, spleen, duodenum, jejunum, ileum, sacculus rotundus and cecal appendix. In September 2017, fresh and formalin-fixed liver were collected.

Post-mortem and microscopic examination and bacteriology

All three fallen animals were examined by necropsy. Nutritional condition was determined according to the following criteria: emaciated (visible muscle atrophy, absence of visible fat stores), poor (scant to no visible internal fat stores, but no visible muscle atrophy), normal (at a minimum, fat stores visible in mesentery and around kidneys). A suite of internal organs including liver, spleen, lung, kidney, bone marrow, brain, small intestine, colon, heart, trachea, salivary gland, nasal

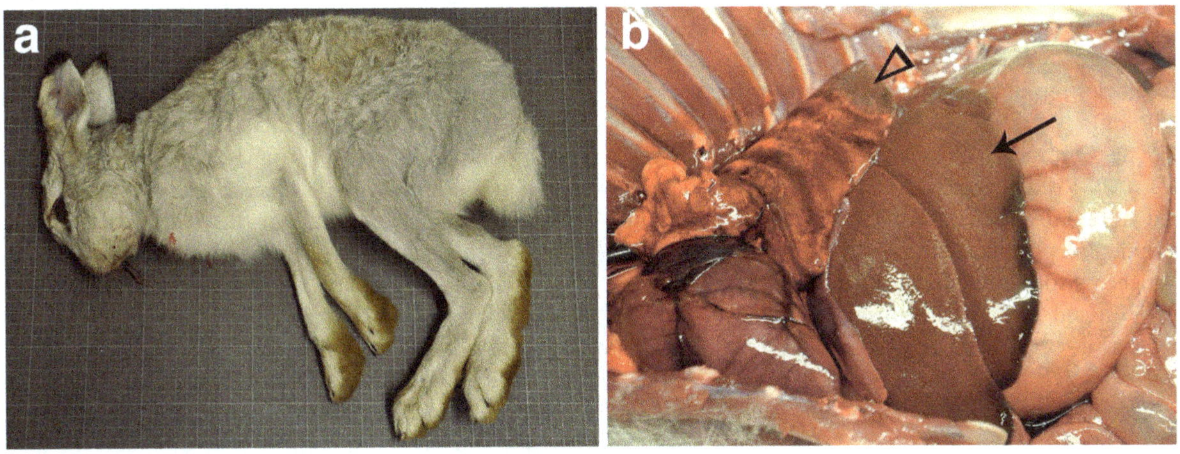

Fig. 2 A mountain hare (*Lepus timidus*) that died of Lagovirus europaeus GI.2/RHDV2/b infection on the island of Hallands Vädero, Sweden. **a** Characteristic external features include a grey-white winter pelage. **b** Post-mortem findings. The liver shows pallor and enhanced reticular pattern (arrow). Distal lung lobes are consolidated because of nematode parasitism (arrowhead)

mucosa and skin were fixed in 10% neutrally buffered formalin for microscopic examination. Not all tissues were collected from all animals. Liver was frozen at – 20 °C and – 70 °C for additional analyses.

Formalin-fixed tissues from the found dead and hunted hares were processed and embedded in paraffin for microscopic examination. Sections 3 to 4 µm thick were stained with Mayer's hematoxylin and eosin [20]. Liver sections also were stained with von Kossa to visualize calcium deposits [21].

Even though no organisms were seen microscopically, the mild to moderate heterophilic infiltration observed in the liver of 2147 prompted the submission of liver from this animal to the Department of Microbiology, National Veterinary Institute, Uppsala, Sweden for routine aerobic bacterial culture. Samples were inoculated onto blood agar plates containing 5% horse blood and bromocresol purple lactose agar plates and held at 37 °C under aerobic conditions. Plates were inspected for growth at 24 and 48 h after inoculation.

Immunohistochemistry

Immunohistochemistry was used to detect the presence of lagovirus antigen in the formalin-fixed and paraffin-embedded tissues using a panlagovirus antibody cocktail of 3H6 + 6G2 IgG1 mouse monoclonal antibodies [22] kindly provided by the OIE Reference Laboratory for RHD, Brescia, Italy. Immunohistochemical staining was performed on liver, spleen, lung, bone marrow and kidney from the three fallen hares and on the liver and small intestine of hares hunted in January. Methods, antibodies and reagents are described in detail in Neimanis et al. [23] with the following modifications. After treatment with hydrogen peroxide, sections were treated with proteinase K (Dako Proteinase K, Agilent Technologies Sweden AB, Kista, Sweden) for six minutes to demask antigens. Visualization of bound antibodies was facilitated with either the chromagen diaminobenzidine (DAB) (Dako Liquid DAB+ Substrate Chromagen System, Agilent Technologies Sweden AB, Kista, Sweden) or the chromagen 3-amino-9-ethylcarbazole (AEC) (Dako AEC+ High Sensitivity Substrate Chromagen, Agilent Technologies Sweden AB, Kista, Sweden). The liver from a rabbit confirmed to be infected with GI.2 by PCR, sequencing and immunological characterization [24] and/or the liver from a European brown hare confirmed to be infected with GII.1 by nested PCR [25] was used as the positive tissue control while the liver from a healthy rabbit and/or European brown hare (negative for lagoviruses by PCR) served as the negative tissue control.

Immunological virus typing

Liver samples from all three fallen hares were submitted to the OIE Reference Laboratory for RHD in Brescia, Italy for immunological typing of the lagovirus. Briefly, typing analysis was performed using the sandwich ELISA described in the OIE Terrestrial Manual for RHD (2016) [26]. Four pools of monoclonal antibodies specific for GI.1b-d/RHDV [22], GI.1a/RHDVa [27], GI.2/RHDV2 [5] and GII.1/EBHSV [15] were used. Samples (10% liver homogenates) were tested at the dilution 1/5 and 1/30 and classified as positive when the OD of the sample exceeded that of the negative control by at least 0.15 at dilution 1/5. A more detailed description of the methods is provided in Neimanis et al. [24].

Genotyping and phylogenetic analyses

Based on gross and microscopic findings typical for pathogenic lagovirus infection in the three hares found dead, various molecular analyses were carried out on liver samples to confirm the presence of a lagovirus and to genotype the virus. For hares 1208 and 2147, samples were first analyzed for the presence of GI and GII.1 with two nested PCRs using primers and methods as described in Bascuñana et al. [25]. In both cases, GI but not GII.1 RNA was detected. Because this nested PCR does not differentiate between GI.1 and GI.2 viruses [24], liver samples from these two hares and from 2381 were analyzed by GI.2-specific RT-qPCR as described in Neimanis et al. [24]. To screen for the presence of GI.2, liver samples from all six hunted hares were also analyzed by this same GI.2-specific RT-qPCR.

For samples found to contain GI.2 RNA by RT-qPCR, sequencing of the entire *vp60* gene following methods in Neimanis et al. [24] was carried out. In 2016 and 2017, a concurrent, widespread outbreak of GI.2 occurred in wild and domestic rabbits in the southern half of Sweden [24]. To gain insight into the origins of GI.2 in mountain hares on Hallands Väderö, the entire *vp60* gene was also sequenced from the livers of ten additional rabbits known to have died from GI.2 infection for phylogenetic comparison with hare strains. Rabbit samples were selected to represent the broad spatial and temporal range of the outbreak. Locations from where these 10 rabbits, the three fallen mountain hares and an additional 11 rabbits previously reported with GI.2 in Sweden [24] originated are presented in Fig. 1. All *vp60* gene sequences generated in this study were deposited in GenBank under accession numbers MH341501–13.

To identify homologous sequences in GenBank, a Basic Local Alignment Search Tool (BLAST, http://www.ncbi.nlm.nih.gov/BLAST/) was used on the *vp60* gene sequences from the three fallen hares. Additionally, evolutionary relationships between the mountain hare viruses and other lagoviruses were explored. Sequences were aligned using the Clustal W algorithm before building phylogenetic trees using MEGA6: Molecular Evolutionary Genetics Analysis [19]. The best-fit nucleotide substitution model (GTR + G + I) was determined with the same software. The final alignment included *vp60* gene sequences generated for this study (from the three mountain hares and 10 rabbits) and publicly available GI.2 sequences from Europe and Australia, including 11 previously published sequences from Sweden from 2013 to 2016 [24]. GI.1, GI.4 and GII.1 sequences, as well as MRCV (a lagovirus with variable pathogenicity [28]) and other sequences not assigned to a genotype, were included in the analysis, producing a final dataset of $n = 364$. A list of all sequences used is provided as supplementary material in Additional file 1. Trees were built using the Maximum likelihood (ML) method and statistical support for the nodes was estimated using 2000 bootstrap replicates.

Results

Sex, age and nutritional condition of the mountain hares are presented in Table 1. Body condition of the fallen hares ranged from normal to emaciated whereas the hunted hares were all in normal nutritional condition. Age was not assessed for the majority of the hunted animals and sex was not determined for animals hunted in September 2017.

Hares found dead

Molecular species identification

The obtained sequences for *ucp2*, *ighg*-hinge and *cytb* were visually inspected and aligned with publicly available sequences for lagomorphs. Only species with information for at least two markers were considered. Genetic distances indicate that our samples are closest to three hare species *L. timidus*, *L. arcticus* and *L. othus* and clearly distinct from the European brown hare. Despite the lack of resolution, we confirm the species as being *L. timidus*, which is consistent with the morphological characterization and species geographic range (*L. arcticus* inhabits the coastal regions of Greenland, northern Quebec, northern Manitoba, Arctic islands and western Newfoundland; *L. othus* ranges from west to southwest Alaska). The three arctic hare species (*L. timidus*, *L. arcticus* and *L. othus*) are closely related and their status as independent species has been critically discussed [29, 30].

Gross pathology

All three animals found dead and examined by necropsy had subtle to moderate liver lesions in which the liver was mildly to moderately discoloured (light brown to orange-pink), had an accentuated lobular pattern in the parenchyma, and was friable (Fig. 2). All three animals also displayed mild to moderate pulmonary congestion and multifocal to coalescing hemorrhage and/or edema. There was mild to moderate splenomegaly in all animals and the spleen was discoloured dark red in hares 2147 and 2381. All animals had soft, unformed feces in the rectum and in 2381, the cecal appendix and sacculus rotundus were diffusely dark red. There was mild to moderate consolidation of the distal margins of the caudal lung lobes consistent with nematode infestation in all animals (Fig. 2) and few to more frequent 1×2 mm beige, oblong foci consistent with coccidial organisms were seen in the small intestine of hares 2147 and 1208.

Microscopic pathology

All fallen hares had been previously frozen and were moderately to severely autolyzed. However, liver lesions could still be detected. All animals displayed acute necrosis and/or apoptosis of individual hepatocytes characterized by hypereosinophilic, hyaline cytoplasm, cell shrinkage, rounding up and dissociation from the hepatic plate (Fig. 3). Affected hepatocytes were observed throughout the lobule. In hares 2147 and 1208, small scattered, focal areas of lytic necrosis were also seen. Additionally, dark grey-basophilic, irregular intracytoplasmic granules confirmed to be mineral using von Kossa histochemical stain were observed in scattered (2147) to frequent (1208) hepatocytes (Fig. 3). In all hares, mildly to moderately increased numbers of inflammatory cells, most consistent with heterophils, were observed in sinusoids and occasionally surrounding individual hepatocytes (Fig. 3). There also was mild (2147 and 1208) to moderate (2381) microvesiculation of hepatocytes consistent with lipid. Hare 2381 had a mild trematode infestation evidenced by scattered trematode eggs observed within larger bile ducts.

Microscopic examination of the lungs and small intestine confirmed granulomatous pneumonia from lungworm infection and intestinal coccidiosis, respectively. Autolysis precluded further interpretation of other tissues.

Immunohistochemistry

Viral antigen was detected in the liver of all three fallen hares (Fig. 3). In 2147 and 2381, the antigen was primarily confined to hepatocytes as fine intracytoplasmic stippling or concentrated at the cell membrane, although occasional intranuclear staining also was seen (Fig. 3). In 1208, staining frequently was seen within the cytoplasm of both hepatocytes and Kupffer cells (Fig. 3), and very rarely within hepatocellular nuclei. Immunostaining was not detected in the negative controls.

Immunohistochemical evaluation of the spleen of 2147 and 2381 was hindered by autolysis and artifact. However, within the spleen of 1208, viral antigen was clearly and coarsely clumped within the cytoplasm of macrophages (Fig. 3). Poor tissue quality precluded interpretation of immunohistochemistry for remaining tissues.

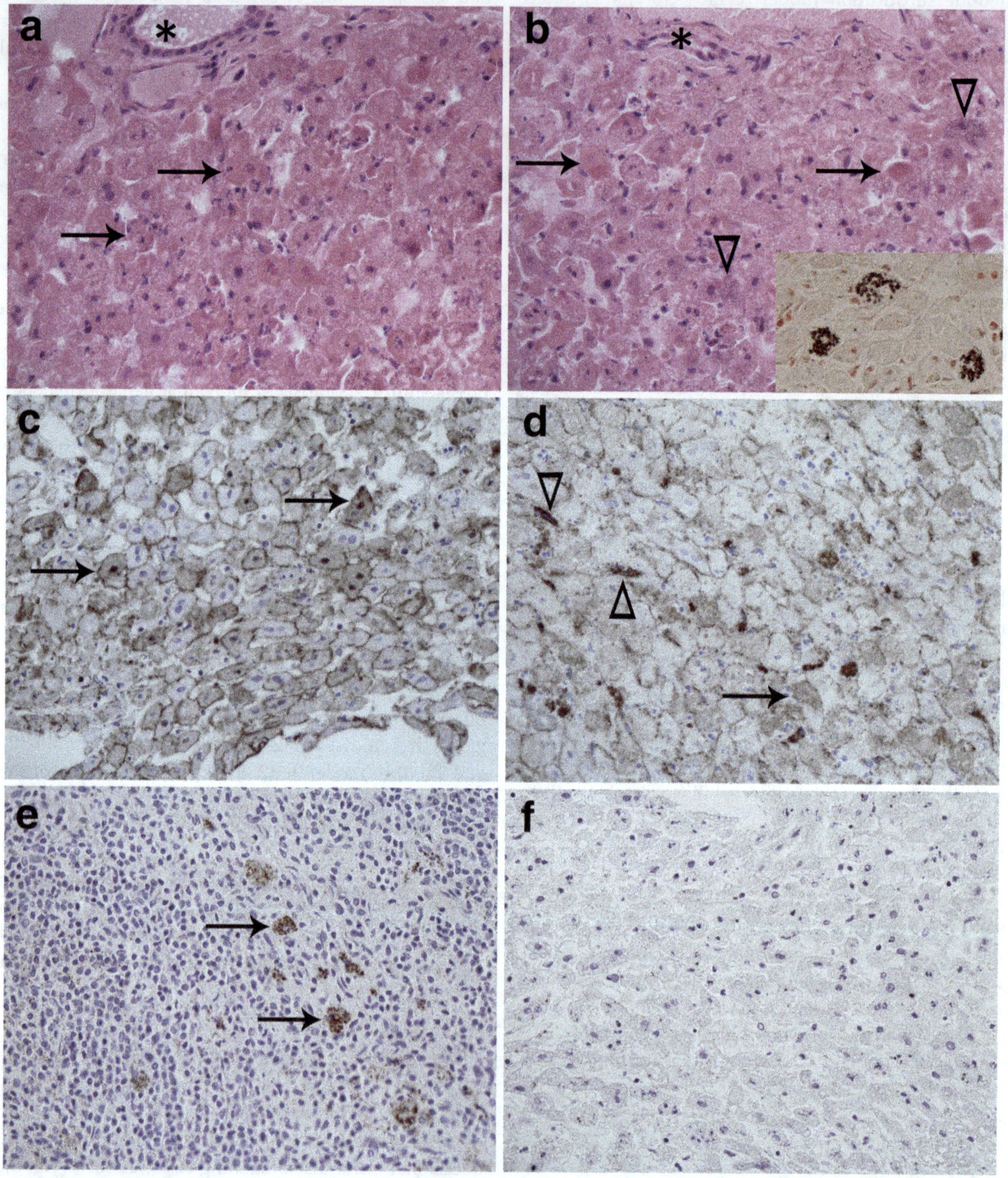

Fig. 3 Microscopic lesions and viral antigen localization in mountain hares (*Lepus timidus*) that died of *Lagovirus europaeus* GI.2/RHDV2/b infection. **a** Acute hepatocellular apoptosis and necrosis. Dead cells are denoted with an arrow and they frequently are surrounded by heterophils. The portal region is denoted by an asterisk. **b** Acute hepatocellular apoptosis and necrosis (arrows). Arrowhead denote hepatocellular calcification and the asterisk marks the portal area. Insert: von Kossa histochemical stain with calcium granules stained black. **c** Immunohistochemical visualization of viral capsid antigen (brown) in the liver of hare 2147. Arrows denote hepatocytes with both intracytoplasmic and intranuclear staining. **d** Immunohistochemical visualization of viral capsid antigen (brown) in the liver of hare 1208. Intracytoplasmic staining of hepatocytes (arrow) and Kupffer cells (arrowhead). **e** Immunohistochemical visualization of viral capsid antigen (brown) in the spleen of hare 1208. Arrows indicate intracytoplasmic staining of macrophages in the red pulp. **f** Negative immunoglobulin control of the liver of 1208

Bacteriology

No bacterial infection was identified in the liver of hare 2147.

Hunted hares

Pathology and immunohistochemistry

No significant lesions were observed grossly in the hunted hares. Microscopically, no lesions consistent with pathogenic lagoviruses were seen in the liver. In hares 126 and 127, hilar bile ducts contained cross-sections of adult trematodes and/or thick-walled yellow-brown trematode eggs that were accompanied by mild to moderate periductal eosinophilic and lymphoplasmacytic inflammation. Small intestine only was available for examination in hares hunted in January 2017. Although scattered intraluminal nematodes were observed in hares 124, 126 and 127, the intestinal tissue was unremarkable.

No viral antigen was detected in the liver or small intestine of hares hunted in January 2017 and immunohistochemistry was not performed on the two hares hunted in September 2017.

Immunological virus typing

In all three fallen hares, the lagovirus in the liver was identified as GI.2 by the specific pool of MAbs directed against GI.2. Results for the other pools of MAbs specific for GI.1b-d, GI.1a and GII.1 were negative. Additionally, the high OD values registered at the dilution of 1/30 are consistent with acute lagovirus infection and cause of the death of the hares.

Molecular detection and phylogenetic analysis

A 127-base pair fragment from the *vp60* capsid gene of GI.2 was amplified in large quantities in the liver of all three hares that were found dead. The threshold cycle values ranged from 15.24 to 15.96. RT-qPCR did not detect GI.2 in any of the livers of the six hunted hares. Complete *vp60* gene sequences were determined for all

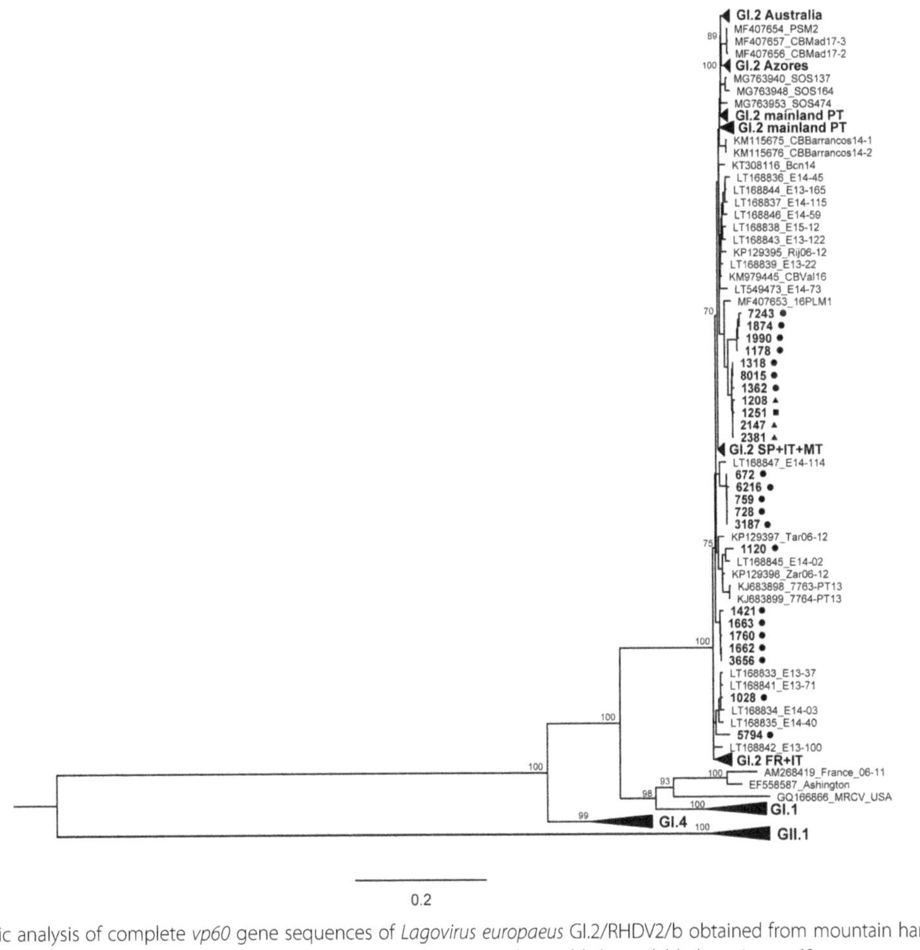

Fig. 4 Phylogenetic analysis of complete *vp60* gene sequences of *Lagovirus europaeus* GI.2/RHDV2/b obtained from mountain hares (*Lepus timidus*) and European rabbits (*Oryctolagus cuniculus*) in Sweden in relation to other publicly available lagovirus *vp60* gene sequences. The tree was generated in MEGA6 [19] using the Maximum Likelihood method and GTR + G + I nucleotide substitution model. Bootstrap values ≤70% (of 2000 replicates) are indicated at the nodes. A complete list of GenBank accession numbers used in the analysis is provided in Additional file 1

three fallen hares and 10 rabbits that died of RHD in other areas of Sweden in 2016 (Genbank accession numbers MH341501–13).

A BLAST comparison of the *vp60* gene sequences from the three mountain hares with publicly available sequences revealed the closest identity with GI.2. More specifically, they showed a maximum identity of 98% at the nucleotide level to the 16PLM1 isolate (GenBank accession number MF407653), a non-recombinant GI.2 strain from La Palma, Canary Islands, Spain, collected in 2016 [31] (comparison performed March 20, 2018). Phylogenetic analyses grouped all three mountain hare strains together, along with other strains collected in 2016–2017 for this study (Fig. 4). Strain 1251 came from a GI.2 outbreak in rabbits in Falkenberg and was collected at the end of July 2016 on the adjacent mainland approximately 50 km away (Fig. 1). The other three strains that clustered near the hare strains (1318, 8015 and 1362) came from GI.2 outbreaks in southern mainland Sweden in July and August 2016.

Discussion

The detection of lagoviral antigen associated with lesions of acute hepatitis, coupled with immunotyping and molecular detection of GI.2 in the liver, conclusively show that all three fallen mountain hares on Hallands Väderö died of acute viral hepatitis caused by GI.2. This is significant because, prior to this study, mountain hares were only known to be susceptible to GII.1, the pathogenic lagovirus of hares causing EBHS. The gross and microscopic pathology caused by GI.2 in mountain hares and tissue distribution of viral antigen mimics that of GII.1 infection in this species. Consistent gross lesions include a lighter coloured and friable liver, a dark red, congested and often enlarged spleen and pulmonary congestion and edema. Microscopically, periportal to massive hepatic necrosis has been described for GII.1 infections in mountain hares [32], and in this study, necrosis was classified as massive. Other lesions in these three hares that are consistent with GII.1 infections include areas of lytic necrosis, inflammation, hepatocellular fatty degeneration and mineralization of hepatocytes. Interestingly, mineralization seems to be a phenomenon of lagoviral hepatitis in hares, irrespective of the causative virus, and is not a feature commonly associated with RHD [33]. Viral antigen in the cytoplasm and nuclei of hepatocytes and cytoplasm of Kupffer cells was described both for GII.1 [31] and GI.2 in mountain hares (this study). Gross and microscopic lesions can still be considered characteristic of infection with a pathogenic lagovirus, but further analyses are required to identify the lagovirus responsible. Just as for other hare species that succumb to GI.2 infection, EBHS is no longer an adequate name for lagoviral hepatitis in mountain hares and we support the proposal by Le Gall-Reculé et al. [9] for a new name. While 'hare hemorrhagic disease' makes reference to the equivalent disease in rabbits (RHD), hemorrhage and disseminated intravascular coagulation (DIC) are not prominent features of pathogenic lagovirus infections in hares ([32, 34], this study). We therefore support hare lagovirus disease or hare lagoviral hepatitis as an alternate name for viral hepatitides of hares caused by different pathogenic lagoviruses.

This outbreak of GI.2 in mountain hares is also significant because it represents an expansion of GI.2 host range. GI.2 differs notably from previously described GI viruses because of its broader host range. Clinical disease from GI.1 viruses is almost exclusively restricted to the European rabbit, with the exception of GI.1 infection described in two Iberian hares (*Lepus granatensis*) [35]. In contrast, GI.2 can be pathogenic for European rabbits, but also for the Sardinian Cape hare [5], the Italian hare [6], the European brown hare [7–9] and now the mountain hare. Certain hare species are proposed to be more susceptible to GI.2 infection than others [6] and this may reflect different species-specific host factors such as glycan expression for viral attachment [36]. However, the epidemiological context may also play a role. For example, the broad and rapid dispersion of GI.2 in rabbits in France and Sardinia when compared to mainland Italy is thought to be related to the widespread presence of wild rabbits in the former areas versus sparse and patchily distributed wild rabbit populations in continental Italy [3]. Sporadic infection of European brown hares with GI.2 in mainland Italy [7] compared to large-scale outbreaks of GI.2 in European brown hares in France [9] may also reflect differences in the presence and densities of sympatric wild rabbits and thus environmental virus loads. To date, although mountain hares range throughout much of Sweden, GI.2 infection has only been detected in mountain hares on the small island of Hallands Väderö. It is unclear if all mountain hares are equally susceptible or if this particular mountain hare population was somehow predisposed to GI.2 infection. Genetic isolation, concurrent parasitic infections (found in all three dead hares and in three of four hunted hares that were examined microscopically) and the poor nutritional condition (seen in two of the three dead hares and observed in hares hunted in October 2016, B. Gunnarsson, pers. comm) may have made this population of animals more prone to GI.2 infection. Elucidation of the susceptibility of other mountain hare populations to GI.2 requires further field and/or experimental research.

Epidemiological and molecular data from the majority of previously reported GI.2 outbreaks in hares support a link to concurrent local or regional outbreaks in European rabbits [5, 6, 8, 9]. Outbreaks typically were connected in time and/or space with outbreaks in rabbits and, when data were available, the GI.2 virus in affected hares was most closely related to those strains locally circulating in rabbits [6, 9]. This suggests that while hares are susceptible to infection, they require spillover of GI.2 from the primary maintenance host, the rabbit, to initiate new outbreaks in hares. The findings presented here provide further support for this hypothesis. Although there are no rabbits on the island from which initial spillover of infection could have originated, there was a concurrent, widespread outbreak of GI.2 in wild and domestic rabbits in the southern half of Sweden in 2016 and 2017, including the adjacent mainland. The GI.2 *vp60* gene sequences from mountain hares grouped together with a sequence collected from an outbreak in rabbits at the end of July 2016 on the adjacent mainland in Falkenberg (Fig. 1), approximately 50 km away. The other *vp60* gene sequences from Sweden represent outbreaks of GI.2 in rabbits that were more distant from the outbreak on Hallands Väderö in time and/or space (Fig. 1).

Pathogenic GI viruses can be readily transmitted indirectly via contaminated material and transfer can be facilitated by insects, scavengers and people [37]. The exact mode of virus introduction onto Hallands Väderö is not known, but introduction by the 50,000 people who visit the island every year, by insects or by scavenging birds are all possibilities. Once the virus arrived on the island, GI.2 circulated for at least 4.5 months based on necropsy findings, and six months based on observations of dead hares in the field, all in the absence of rabbits. GI.2 was either introduced once to the island and then persisted for the duration of the outbreak or it was repeatedly introduced. *VP60* gene sequences of all three hares group very closely together, with only one, synonymous nucleotide substitution between the two hares found dead in 2016 and four synonymous and one non-synonymous nucleotide substitutions in the hare found dead in 2017. This lends support to a single, rather than multiple, introduction, but sequencing of the whole genome of these hares and additional rabbit samples followed by spatial and temporal analyses are needed to further substantiate this hypothesis. GI viruses are hardy and can persist in the environment for months in organic material [38]. GI.2 may have circulated within the mountain hare population during the outbreak in the absence of rabbits and/or the introduced virus may have persisted in the environment (e.g. in feces or hare carcasses), causing re-infections of hares over the period of the outbreak. Therefore, the ability of mountain hares to serve as competent maintenance hosts for GI.2 in the absence of other leporids presently is unknown and requires additional investigation.

Mountain hare populations are declining in the southern half of Sweden, coinciding geographically with where they are sympatric with brown hares [12]. Disease-mediated competition from brown hares through, for example, GII.1, has been proposed as a possible contributing factor [12]. It is now clear that mountain hares can also succumb to GI.2 infection. Wild rabbit distribution also overlaps with areas where mountain hares are in decline. The arrival of GI.2 to Sweden and subsequent large-scale epizootics in rabbits may now pose an additional threat to sympatric mountain hares. The impact of GI.2 on isolated island populations of mountain hares may be even more significant. Island populations of mountain hares are particularly vulnerable to population crashes [13]. Factors responsible for crashes such as food availability are often multifactorial and declines are often set off by a stochastic event [13]. While extreme weather and appearance of a predator have been cited as stochastic events, we propose that the sudden introduction of GI.2 could exert the same effect and trigger a decline. Continued monitoring of the hare population on Hallands Väderö is needed to assess the longer-term significance of GI.2 introduction for this population. No evidence of GI.2 infection was found in six hares hunted in January and September 2017 and, with the exception of a juvenile that died of intestinal coccidiosis, no further reports of dead hares from the island have been received to date. GI.2 has spread quickly and widely throughout Europe and beyond, and, as evidenced by this outbreak, the virus can be introduced to islands and circulate among hares in the absence of rabbits. Awareness of this potential risk coupled with actions that minimize unintended introductions of GI.2 by humans through, for example, contaminated footwear, can help mitigate exposure of other island populations of mountain hares to GI.2.

Conclusions

We demonstrate for the first time that GI.2 can infect and cause mortality in mountain hares. These findings add a new species to the host range of GI.2. Further investigation of the mechanisms responsible for the expanded host range of GI.2 compared to GI.1 viruses could provide valuable insight into host species jumps. Lesions and virus tissue distribution of GI.2 infection in mountain hares mimic those of GII.1 infection, therefore typing of the virus must be performed to identify the lagovirus responsible for a given mortality event. The mortality event in mountain hares lasted at least 4.5 months in the absence of rabbits, but because environmental persistence and multiple introductions cannot be excluded, further research is required to determine if mountain hares are competent reservoir hosts. Phylogenetic analyses support virus introduction from a concurrent, large-scale GI.2 outbreak in rabbits on the adjacent mainland and demonstrates the relative ease with which GI.2 can spread. Finally, mountain hares represent the fourth *Lepus* species that is susceptible to GI.2. This raises the possibility that most or even all

Lepus species may be susceptible. Not only should incidents of morbidity and mortality in other *Lepus* species sympatric with wild European rabbits or in contact with domestic rabbits be evaluated with respect to GI.2, but exposure to European rabbits should be minimized for vulnerable *Lepus* species and populations.

Abbreviations

BLAST: Basic Local Alignment Search Tool; EBHS: European brown hare syndrome; EBHSV: European brown hare syndrome virus; MAb: Monoclonal antibody; ML: Maximum likelihood; OD: Optical density; PCR: Polymerase chain reaction),; RHD: Rabbit hemorrhagic disease; RHDV: Rabbit hemorrhagic disease virus; RT-qPCR: Reverse transcription quantitative polymerase chain reaction

Acknowledgements

The authors thank Bo Gunnarsson for submission of the dead hares, Caroline Bröjer, Holly Cedervind, Bertil Malmsten and Carl-Gustav Thulin for help with sample and data collection and Linda Svensson for assistance with Fig. 1. Lorenzo Capucci, OIE Reference laboratory for RHD, generously provided the monoclonal antibodies used in the immunohistochemistry and performed the immunotyping.

Funding

Funding was provided by the Swedish Environmental Protection Agency, and the Research Council FORMAS (contract 221–2014-1841) as part of the ECALEP research consortium funded by the EU Animal Health and Welfare ERA-Net (ANIHWA). Fundação para a Ciência e Tecnologia (FCT) supported the Post-doctoral grant of Ana M. Lopes (SFRH/BPD/115211/2016) and the FCT Investigator grants of Joana Abrantes (IF/01396/2013) and Pedro J. Esteves (IF/00376/2015). The funding bodies had no role in the design of the study, in the collection, analysis and interpretation of the data or in the writing of the manuscript.

Author's contributions

AN conceived the study, AN, HA and ULP acquired the samples and data and performed the laboratory work, AN, HA, AL, JA, SZ, PE and DGW analyzed and interpreted the data, AN wrote the paper, HA, ULP, AL, JA, SZ, PE and DGW revised the paper and all authors approved the final manuscript.

Consent for publication

Not applicable.

Competing interests

The authors declare they have no competing interests.

Author details

[1]Department of Pathology and Wildlife Diseases, National Veterinary Institute (SVA), 751 89 Uppsala, Sweden. [2]Department of Biomedical Sciences and Veterinary Public Health, Swedish University of Agricultural Sciences (SLU), Box 7028, 750 07 Uppsala, Sweden. [3]Department of[4]Microbiology, National Veterinary Institute (SVA), 751 89 Uppsala, Sweden. CIBIO/InBio, Centro de Investigação em Biodiversidade e Recursos Genéticos, Universidade do Porto, Campus Agrário de Vairão, 4485-661 Vairão, Portugal. [5]Department of Anatomy and Unit for Multidisciplinary Research in Biomedicine (UMIB), Institute of Biomedical Sciences Abel Salazar (ICBAS), University of Porto, Porto, Portugal. [6]Departamento de Biologia, Faculdade de Ciências, Universidade do Porto, R. Campo Alegre s/n, 4169-007 Porto, Portugal. [7]Instituto de Investigação e Formação Avançada em Ciências e Tecnologias da Saúde (CESPU), Gandra, Portugal.

References

1. Le Pendu J, Abrantes J, Bertagnoli S, Guitton JS, Le Gall-Reculé G, Lopes AM, Marchandeau S, Alda F, Almeida T, Célio AP, Bárcena J, Burmakina G, Blanco E, Calvete C, Cavadini P, Cooke B, Dalton K, Delibes Mateos M, Deptula W, Eden JS, Wang F, Ferreira CC, Ferreira P, Foronda P, Gonçalves D, Gavier-Widén D, Hall R, Hukowska-Szematowicz B, Kerr P, Kovaliski J, Lavazza A, Mahar J, Malogolovkin A, Marques RM, Marques S, Martin-Alonso A, Monterroso P, Moreno S, Mutze G, Neimanis A, Niedzwiedzka-Rystwej P, Peacock D, Parra F, Rocchi M, Rouco C, Ruvoën-Clouet N, Silva E, Silvério D, Strive T, Thompson G, Tokarz-Deptula B, Esteves P. Proposal for a unified classification system and nomenclature of lagoviruses. J Gen Virol. 2017; 98(7):1658–66. https://doi.org/10.1099/jgv.0.000840.
2. Gavier-Widén D, Mörner T. Epidemiology and diagnosis of the European brown hare syndrome in Scandinavian countries: a review. Rev Sci Tech. 1991;10(2):453–8.
3. Le Gall-Reculé G, Lavazza A, Marchandeau S, Bertagnoli S, Zwingelstein F, Cavadini P, Martinelli N, Lombardi G, Guerin J-L, Lemaitre E, Decors A, Boucher S, Le Normand B, Capucci L. Emergence of a new lagovirus related to rabbit haemorrhagic disease virus. Vet Res. 2013;44. https://doi.org/10.1186/1297-9716-44-81.
4. Dalton KP, Nicieza I, Abrantes J, Esteves PJ, Parra F. Spread of new variant RHDV in domestic rabbits on the Iberian Peninsula. Vet Microbiol. 2014; 169(1–2):67–73. https://doi.org/10.1016/j.vetmic.2013.12.015.
5. Puggioni G, Cavadini P, Maestrale C, Scivoli R, Botti G, Ligios C, Le Gall-Reculé G, Lavazza A, Capucci L. The new French 2010 rabbit hemorrhagic disease virus causes an RHD-like disease in the Sardinian cape hare (Lepus capensis mediterraneus). Vet Res. 2013;44. https://doi.org/10.1186/1297-9716-44-96.
6. Camarda A, Pugliese N, Cavadini P, Circella E, Capucci L, Caroli A, Legretto M, Mallia E, Lavazza A. Detection of the new emerging rabbit haemorrhagic disease type 2 virus (RHDV2) in Sicily from rabbit (Oryctolagus cuniculus) and Italian hare (Lepus corsicanus). Res Vet Sci. 2014;97(3):642–5. https://doi.org/10.1016/j.rvsc.2014.10.008.
7. Velarde R, Cavadini P, Neimanis A, Cabezon O, Chiari M, Gaffuri A, Lavin S, Grilli G, Gavier-Widén D, Lavazza A, Capucci L. Spillover events of infection of brown hares (*Lepus europaeus*) with rabbit haemorrhagic disease type 2 virus (RHDV2) caused sporadic cases of an European brown hare syndrome-like disease in Italy and Spain. Transbound Emerg Dis. 2017;64(6):1750–61. https://doi.org/10.1111/tbed.12562.
8. Hall RN, Peacock DE, Kovaliski J, Mahar JE, Mourant R, Piper M, Strive T. Detection of RHDV2 in European brown hares (Lepus europaeus) in Australia. Vet Rec. 2017;180(5):121. https://doi.org/10.1136/vr.104034.
9. Le Gall-Reculé G, Lemaitre E, Bertagnoli S, Hubert C, Top S, Decors A, Marchandeau S, Guitton J-S (2017) Large-scale lagovirus disease outbreaks in European brown hares (Lepus europaeus) in France caused by RHDV2 strains spatially shared with rabbits (Oryctolagus cuniculus). Vet Res 48 (1): 70. doi:https://doi.org/10.1186/s13567-017-0473-y.
10. Angerbjorn A, Flux JEC. Lepus timidus. Mamm Species. 1995;(495):1, 1–1.
11. IUCN (2008) *Lepus timidus*. http://www.iucnredlist.org/details/11791/0. Accessed 6 May 2018.
12. Thulin C-G. The distribution of mountain hares Lepus timidus in Europe: a challenge from brown hares L. europaeus? Mammal Rev. 2003;33(1):29–42. https://doi.org/10.1046/j.1365-2907.2003.00008.x.
13. Angerbjörn A. Proximate causes of mountain hare population crashes: a review. Finn Game Res. 1983;41:29–38.
14. Gavier-Widén D, Mörner T. Descriptive epizootiological study of European brown hare syndrome in Sweden. J Wildl Dis. 1993;29(1):15–20.
15. Lopes AM, Capucci L, Gavier-Widén D, Le Gall-Reculé G, Brocchi E, Barbieri I, Quemener A, Le Pendu J, Geoghegan JL, Holmes EC, Esteves PJ, Abrantes J. Molecular evolution and antigenic variation of European brown hare

syndrome virus (EBHSV). Virology. 2014;468:104–12. https://doi.org/10.1016/j.virol.2014.08.002.
16. Isacson C-G. Hallands Väderö och jakten på ön. In: Isacson international AB. Sweden: Gothenburg; 1993.
17. Melo-Ferreira J, Alves PC, Freitas H, Ferrand N, Boursot P. The genomic legacy from the extinct *Lepus timidus* to the three hare species of Iberia: contrast between mtDNA, sex chromosomes and autosomes. Mol Ecol. 2009;18:2643–58.
18. Pinheiro A, Woof JM, Almeida T, Abrantes J, Alves PC, Gortázar C, Esteves PJ. Leporid immunoglobulin G shows evidence of strong selective pressure on the hinge and CH3 domains. Open Biol. 2014;4(9):140088. https://doi.org/10.1098/rsob.140088.
19. Tamura K, Stecher G, Peterson D, Filipski A, Kumar S. MEGA6: molecular evolutionary genetics analysis version 6.0. Mol Biol Evol. 2013;30:2725–9.
20. Bancroft JD, Cook HC. Manual of histological techniques. London, England: Churchill Livingstone; 1984.
21. Lillie RD. Histopathologic technic and practical histochemistry. 3rd ed. New York: Blakiston Division, McGraw-Hill; 1965.
22. Capucci L, Frigoli G, Rønshold L, Lavazza A, Brocchi E, Rossi C. Antigenicity of the rabbit hemorrhagic disease virus studied by its reactivity with monoclonal antibodies. Virus Res. 1995;37:221–38.
23. Neimanis A, Larsson Pettersson U, Huang N, Gavier-Widén D, Strive T. Elucidation of the pathology and tissue distribution of *Lagovirus europaeus* GI.2/RHDV2 (rabbit haemorrhagic disease virus 2) in young and adult rabbits (*Oryctolagus cuniculus*). Vet Res. 2018;49:46. https://doi.org/10.1186/s13567-018-0540-z.
24. Neimanis AS, Ahola H, Zohari S, Larsson Pettersson U, Bröjer C, Capucci L, Gavier-Widén D. Arrival of rabbit haemorrhagic disease virus 2 to northern Europe: emergence and outbreaks in wild and domestic rabbits (Oryctolagus cuniculus) in Sweden. Transbound Emerg Dis. 2017. https://doi.org/10.1111/tbed.12650.
25. Bascuñana CR, Nowotny N, Belak S. Detection and differentiation of rabbit hemorrhagic disease and European brown hare syndrome viruses by amplification of *vp60* genomic sequences from fresh and fixed tissue specimens. J Clin Microbiol. 1997;35(10):2492–5.
26. OIE Rabbit Haemorrhagic Disease.https://www.oie.int/fileadmin/Home/eng/Health_standards/tahm/2.06.02_RHD.pdf. 2016. Accessed 6 May 2018.
27. McIntosh MT, Behan SC, Mohamed FM, Lu Z, Moran KE, Burrage TG, Neilan JG, Ward GB, Botti G, Capucci L, Metwally SA. A pandemic strain of calicivirus threatens rabbit industries in the Americas. Virol J. 2007;4. https://doi.org/10.1186/1743-422x-4-96.
28. Bergin IL, Wise AG, Bolin SR, Mullaney TP, Kiupel M, Maes RK. Novel Calicivirus identified in rabbits, Michigan, USA. Emerg Infect Dis. 2009;15(12):1955–62. https://doi.org/10.3201/eid1512.090839.
29. Waltari E, Cook JA. Hares on ice: phylogeography and historical demographics of Lepus arcticus, L. othus, and L. timidus (Mammalia: Lagomorpha). Mol Ecol. 2005;14(10):3005–16. https://doi.org/10.1111/j.1365-294X.2005.02625.x.
30. Alves PC, Melo-Ferreira J, Freitas H, Boursot P. The ubiquitous mountain hare mitochondria: multiple introgressive hybridization in hares, genus *Lepus*. Philos Trans R Soc Lond Ser B Biol Sci. 2008;363(1505):2831–9.
31. Lopes AM, Blanco-Aguiar J, Martin-Alonso A, Leitao M, Foronda P, Mendes M, Goncalves D, Abrantes J, Esteves PJ. Full genome sequences are key to disclose RHDV2 emergence in the Macaronesian islands. Virus Genes. 2018;54(1):1–4. https://doi.org/10.1007/s11262-017-1523-2.
32. Gavier-Widén D. Morphological and immunohistochemical characterization of the hepatic lesions associated with European brown hare syndrome. Vet Pathol. 1994;31(3):327–34.
33. Marcato PS, Benazzi C, Vecchi G, Galeotti M, Della Salda L, Sarli G, Lucidi P. Clinical and pathological features of viral haemorrhagic disease of rabbits and the European brown hare syndrome. Rev Sci Tech. 1991;10(2):371–92.
34. Fuchs A, Weissenbock H. Comparative histopathological study of rabbit haemorrhagic disease (RHD) and European brown hare syndrome (EBHS). J Comp Pathol. 1992;107(1):103–13.
35. Lopes AM, Marques S, Silva E, Magalhaes MJ, Pinheiro A, Alves PC, Jl P, Esteves PJ, Thompson G, Abrantes J. Detection of RHDV strains in the Iberian hare (*Lepus granatensis*): earliest evidence of rabbit lagovirus cross-species infection. Vet Res. 2014;45:94.
36. Lopes AM, Breiman A, Lora M, le Moullac-Vaidye B, Galanina O, Nyström K, Marchandeau S, Le Gall-Reculé G, Strive T, Neimanis A, Bovin NV, Ruvoën-Clouet EPJ, Abrantes J, Le Pendu J. Host specific glycans are correlated with susceptibility to infection by lagoviruses, but not with their virulence. J Virol. 2018;92:e01759–17. https://doi.org/10.1128/JVI.01759-17.
37. Abrantes J, van der Loo W, Le Pendu J, Esteves PJ. Rabbit haemorrhagic disease (RHD) and rabbit haemorrhagic disease virus (RHDV): a review. Vet Res. 2012;43. https://doi.org/10.1186/1297-9716-43-12.
38. Henning J, Meers J, Davies PR, Morris RS. Survival of rabbit haemorrhagic disease virus (RHDV) in the environment. Epidemiol Infect. 2005;133(4):719–30. https://doi.org/10.1017/s0950268805003766.

22

A cross-sectional study to identify a set of risk factors for caprine herpesvirus 1 infection

S. Bertolini[1*], A. Rosamilia[2], C. Caruso[1], C. Maurella[1], F. Ingravalle[1], A. Quasso[3], P. L. Acutis[1], M. Pitti[4], L. Masoero[1] and G. Ru[1]

Abstract

Background: Caprine herpesvirus 1 (CpHV-1) causes neonatal mortality and reproductive failure in goats. Despite its impact on herd reproductive performance, few studies have investigated the risk factors associated with CpHV-1 infection. The aim of this cross-sectional study was to identify potential herd- and host-level risk factors associated with CpHV-1 prevalence in a goat population with heterogeneous seropositivity for CpHV-1.

Results: Blood samples and individual data from 4542 goats were collected from 255 herds in Piedmont, Italy. Enzyme-linked immunosorbent assay (ELISA) and serum neutralization tests were carried out to detect antibodies against CpHV-1. A mixed-effects model was applied to identify any statistical association between CpHV-1 seropositivity and a set of putative host-level and herd-level risk factors. A total of 630 samples tested were found positive by ELISA (prevalence = 13.9%; 95% confidence interval (CI) 12.9–14.9). Of the 255 tested herds, 85 were classified as positive for the presence of at least one gB-positive animal (herd prevalence 33.3%, 95% CI 27.5–39.2), with a within-herd prevalence between 0.7 and 100% (Q1 = 17.6%; median = 32.3%; Q3 = 50%) (Q = quartiles). The prevalence ratios showed a statistical association with the following risk factors: breeds other than Saanen, older age, larger herd size, meat and extensive herds, and co-existence of CAEV-infected animals.

Conclusions: Results from this cross sectional study may help to elucidate the natural history of the infection and inform targeted strategies to control a disease with a potentially important impact on animal health and goat farming economy.

Background

Caprine herpesvirus 1 (CpHV-1), an alphaherpesvirus antigenically closely related to bovine herpesvirus type 1 (BoHV-1), causes systemic disease and neonatal mortality in 1- or 2-week old kids [1] and reproductive failure in adult goats. A serological testing is often inconclusive due to the antigenic similarity of ruminant alphaherpesviruses related to BoHV-1 [2]. The percentage of nucleotide sequence identity for gB gene among different herpesviruses is indeed greater than 78% [3].

Even though BoHV-1 virus does not play a major role in small ruminants, both the natural infection in goat by Tolari *and coll.*, (1990) [4] and the susceptibility to experimental infection by Six *an coll.* (2001) [5] have been reported. Therefore ad hoc diagnostic strategies have been developed to discriminate the two viruses based on combination of ELISA tests [6–8].

CpHV-1 infects animals through the genital [9–11] or the respiratory mucosa [11] and establishes latent infection in sacral or trigeminal ganglia depending on the route of infection and the following spread through the body [12]. Although CpHV-1 infection is usually subclinical in adult goats, it can be responsible for different disorders including respiratory diseases, fever and leukopenia [10], vulvovaginitis [13, 14], balanoposthitis [15], and neonatal mortality. Abortions can be induced by the infection of pregnant goats at 3–4 months of gestation [16–19]. Severe disease may occur in neonatal kids characterized by pyrexia, conjunctivitis, oculonasal discharge, dyspnea, ulcerative and

* Correspondence: silvia.bertolini@izsto.it
[1]Istituto Zooprofilattico Sperimentale del Piemonte, Liguria e Valle d'Aosta, Turin, Italy
Full list of author information is available at the end of the article

necrotic lesions throughout the enteric tract and high morbidity and mortality [20–22].

First isolated in the 1970s in California [22] and Switzerland [21] from young kids with severe generalised infection, CpHV-1 has been found worldwide since then in symptomatic animals from New Zealand [23], Australia [14, 15], Norway [24], and Greece [25]. More recently, CpHV-1 was isolated during an outbreak of infectious pustular vulvovaginitis in goats [13]. In Italy, it was first isolated from latently infected goats in 1996 [26]. Serological surveys indicate a worldwide distribution of CpHV-1 infection [14, 21, 22, 27, 28] and a widespread prevalence in Mediterranean countries where goats play an important economic role, with rates of more than 50% reported for Greece [25] and France [29], 36–43% for southern Italy [30, 31], and 21% for Spain [32].

In general, it is not clear if clinical disease outbreaks may go unreported or if the infection is lowly pathogenic: where prevalence is high unexplained abortions and reproductive disorder, such as infertility and return to estrus, might be associated with undiagnosed infections [33–35] and might cause substantial economic loss, especially in countries with many goat herds [20, 27, 32, 34, 36]. Despite its impact on herd reproductive performance, few studies have investigated the risk factors associated with CpHV-1 infection. To date, the use of natural mating, the herd size and the animal age have been reported as risk factor significantly positively associated with CpHV-1 prevalence [28, 33]. The aim of this cross-sectional study was to identify potential herd- and host-level risk factors associated with CpHV- prevalence in a goat population with heterogeneous seropositivity for CpHV-1.

Results

A total of 630 out of 4542 caprine blood samples tested positive in the BoHV-1 gB blocking ELISA (prevalence 13.9%, 95% confidence interval (CI) 12.9–14.9); 5.5% of the positives ($n = 35$) tested positive also in the BoHV-1 gE blocking ELISA. On subsequent testing in the serum neutralization assay, all the 630 samples were classified as positive for CpHV-1 because of higher titers detected for this virus as compared with the titers for BoHV-1, by a factor of four dilutions. Of the 255 tested herds, 85 were classified as positive for the presence of at least one gB-positive animal (herd prevalence 33.3%, 95% CI 27.5–39.2), with a within-herd prevalence between 0.7 and 100% (Q1 = 17.6%; median = 32.3%; Q3 = 50%) (Q = quartiles).

Tables 1 and 2 show the results of the univariate analysis for host- and herd-risk factors, respectively. The prevalence ratios show a significant statistical association for all risk factors but sex. Both herd size and age showed a statistically linear dose-response trend with risk of infection. Table 3 presents the results of a multivariable mixed-effects Poisson regression model. Despite adjustment for confounding, all variables were still statistically associated with CpHV-1 infection except the presence of co-inhabitant cattle. This variable was therefore omitted in the last model.

The goodness of fit of this model was better than that of a fixed effects model, as shown by the Akaike information criterion (AIC) values of 1683.8 and 1811.4, respectively, showing a significant herd random effect. In the final model, a total of 2879 records was considered because of missing data related to the presence of caprine arthritis and encephalitis virus (CAEV) infection in the herds (689 records). The latter variable was omitted in a further model including 3568 records; however, as compared with the previous one, the effect of all risk factors was still statistically significant (in particular meat/mixed goats showed a prevalence ratio of 12.2, 95% CI 1.9–78.9 and goats kept in extensive herds a prevalence ratio of 3.5, 95% CI 1.6–7.3).

Table 1 Association between CpHV-1 seropositivity and potential host-level risk factors as estimated by univariate analysis for caprine herpesvirus-1 infection in Piedmont (Italy). $N = 4542$ (PR = prevalence ratio)

Risk factor	Exposure level	No. of tested animals	No. of positive animals	Prevalence (%)	PR (95% CI)	*P*-values
Sex	Female	3762	581	15.4	Referent	
	Male	244	35	14.3	0.93 (0.66–1.3)	0.671
Breed	Saanen	629	9	1.4	Referent	
	Chamoisee	784	45	5.7	4.0 (2.0–8.2)	0.000
	Alpine	629	88	14.0	9.8 (4.9–19.4)	0.000
	All others	1901	466	24.5	17.1 (8.9–33.1)	0.000
Age*	1. (2–16 months)	914	47	5.1	Referent	
	2. (17–31 months)	913	80	8.8	1.7 (1.2–2.4)	0.004
	3. (32–56 months)	916	196	21.4	4.2 (3.0–5.7)	0.000
	4 (> 56 months)	917	265	28.9	5.6 (4.1–7.7)	0.000

*extension of the Wilcoxon rank-sum test for the age variable = 15.5, *P* value = 0.000

Table 2 Association between CpHV-1 seropositivity and potential herd-level risk factors as estimated by univariate analysis for caprine herpesvirus-1 infection in Piedmont (Italy). N = 4542 (PR = prevalence ratio)

Risk factor	Exposure level	No. tested animals	No. positive animals	Prevalence (%)	PR (95% CI)	*P*-values
Presence of CAEV-infected goats	No	1610	57	3.5	Referent	
	Yes	2132	428	20.1	5.7 (4.3–7.5)	0.000
Breeding type	Dairy	859	8	0.93	Referent	
	Meat/mixed	3581	613	17.1	18.4 (9.2–36.9)	0.000
Management type	Confined	1753	104	5.9	Referent	
	Extensive	2665	505	18.8	3.2 (2.6–3.9)	0.000
Herd size (no. of animals)*	1 (< 9 goats)	506	50	9.9	Referent	
	2 (9–21 goats)	777	99	12.7	1.3 (0.91–1.8)	0.143
	3 (> 21 goats)	3259	481	14.8	1.5 (1.1–2.0)	0.007
Presence of co-inhabitant cattle	No	2221	158	7.1	Referent	
	Yes	2321	472	20.3	2.9 (2.4–3.4)	0.000

*extension of the Wilcoxon rank-sum test for the herd size variable = 3.11; *P* value = 0.002

Discussion

This is the first study to seek associations between host- and herd-risk factors and CpHV-1 infection in Italian goats. The excess risk associated with several of these factors (breeds other than Saanen, older age, larger herd size, meat and extensive herds, and co-existence of CAEV-infected animals) was quantified by fitting a multivariable mixed-effects model that takes into account both the potential confounding effect of combined risk factors and the aggregation of animals in herds (herd random effect). While the risk factors examined here were similar to those known for bovine herpesvirus infections, CpHV-1 infection was also associated with two additional factors: meat/mixed breeding type and co-presence of CAEV-infected animals in the goat herds.

The association of the infection with herd size and age has been reported also in a recent study [33]. The effect of aging on the risk may be explained by prolonged exposure to the virus over time, with age acting as a surrogate measure of cumulative exposure. This holds true also for life-long seropositivity in BHV-1 infection [37–41]. As suggested by previous studies in cattle, the

Table 3 The combined effect of risk factors according to the multivariable mixed-effects Poisson regression model for caprine herpesvirus-1 infection in Piedmont (Italy). *N* = 2879 (PR = prevalence ratio)

Risk factor	Exposure level	PR (95% CI)	*P*-values
Breed	Saanen	Referent	
	Chamoisee	2.9 (1.0–8.7)	0.053
	Alpine	4.2 (1.4–12.5)	0.009
	All others	4.4 (1.6–12.1)	0.005
Age	1 (2–16 months)	Referent	
	2 (17–31 months)	1.5 (1.0–2.2)	0.073
	3 (32–56 months)	2.9 (1.9–4.4)	0.000
	4 (> 56 months)	3.6 (2.3–5.5)	0.000
Breeding type	Dairy	Referent	
	Meat/mixed	11.5 (1.2–113.8)	0.037
Management type	Confined	1.0	
	Extensive	8.7 (2.8–27.2)	0.000
Herd size (n. of animals)	1 (< 9 goats)	Referent	
	2 (9–21 goats)	1.4 (0.7–3.0)	0.323
	3 (> 21 goats)	2.7 (1.4–5.3)	0.003
Presence of CAEV-infected goats	No	Referent	
	Yes	5.4 (2.3–12.8)	0.000

Likelihood-ratio test (mixed-effects model vs. fixed-effects model): *P*-value = 0.000

excess risk was also associated with herd size because larger herds are more likely to have cases since they have more animals at risk and more contacts with other herds through visits by animal handlers (e.g., veterinarians, farmers, inseminators) [37, 42–45]. The potential role of the number and frequency of new animal purchases could not be assessed because such data are, unfortunately, not recorded in the National Animal Registry system for sheep and goats. Finally, the smaller number of susceptible animals in small herds may limit the maintenance of infections over time [38].

The association with extensive running of a herd may, again, reflect a higher probability of transmission through contacts between susceptible and infected goats in situations where the farmer has less direct control over animal movement and behaviour. In contrast, the greater control typical of dairy goat herd management appears to confer dairy herds a protective effect, as seen even after having adjusted for breed. Generally, dairy farmers pay more attention to such health-related practices as selection of purchased animals and compliance with quarantine regulations and biosecurity standards. In meat herds the productive life of the animals is shorter and productivity is prioritized.

Moreover, the calculated risk for breed further confirms this observation. Most goats are reared for cheese production. Specifically, the Saanen breed is typically reared for the sale of fresh goat milk, which imposes stricter adherence to good biosecurity practices (pasture, reproduction, etc.) by dairy goat farms than farms where mixed breeds are reared. A greater or lesser susceptibility by breed cannot be excluded, however.

The strong association between the risk of herpesvirus and the presence of CAEV-infected animals highlights a potential for an epidemiological link between the two infections. Previous studies have found an association between bovine herpesvirus infection and other infectious diseases [38, 46] and showed that infectious diseases share common risk factors [45]. We cannot exclude that the presence of CAEV infection, which is frequently contracted in the first months of life without manifesting clinical symptoms [47, 48] may predispose infected animals to contracting other infectious diseases, and may also increase the probability of herpesvirus infection. Small ruminant lentivirus (SRLVs) does not infect lymphocytes, however, and immunodeficiency is not a significant feature in SRLV disease [49].

Finally, we think that the external validity of the results was not put at risk by the way the data has been collected: our cross-sectional dataset was not based merely on convenience sampling as the large majority of the sampled herds had been randomly recruited in the frame of the national brucellosis plan.

Conclusions

What the study does suggest is that the type of herd most at risk for CpHV-1 infection is a large one, extensively reared, of the meat or mixed breeding type, and with CAEV co-infection and in which the eldest animals are more likely to be infected. Because most of these risk factors are common to several infectious diseases, veterinary services should promote effective prevention strategies that increase adherence to biosecurity standards and good herd management practices. Better knowledge of the risk factors for CpHV1 infection is needed. Our results may help to elucidate the natural history of the infection and inform targeted strategies to control a disease with a potentially important impact on animal health and goat farming economy.

Methods

Sample collection

This cross-sectional study was conducted in Piedmont, Italy's second largest region in geographical area after Sicily, located in the northwest corner of the country where it borders with France and Switzerland. According to the latest National Animal Registry Office figures (as of 31/08/2013), the total regional goat population is 72,900 distributed across 7028 herds.

A total of 255 goat herds were sampled for this project from May 2008 to December 2010. These herds were comprised of 199 herds (78.0%) sampled as part of the national plan for brucellosis prevention (81 of these herds were also on the CAE eradication and monitoring program); 14 herds (5.5%) on the CAE programme but not part of the brucellosis programme; and 42 herds (16.5%) sampled for non-specified reasons. On these farms, a total of 4542 animals were blood sampled; individual animal data (sex, age and breed) was also collected. The herd size ranged from 1 to 143 animals (Q1–3; median = 8; Q3 = 21).

As an age requirement for being part of this study, only animals over two months of age were recruited. Information at the herd-level (breeding type, management type, herd size, etc.) was downloaded from the official database of the National Animal Registry system which is provided by the veterinary officers of the Ministry of Health through routine annual censuses.

Serological testing for CpHV-1

The same approach as that described by Thiry et al. (2008) was applied to detect antibodies to CpHV-1 using an ELISA that has a specificity of 100% and a sensitivity of 93.5%.

Elisa

BoHV-1 is serologically related to CpHV-1 [2]. CpHV-1 antibodies are known to cross-react with BoHV-1 antigens.

A BoHV-1 ELISA was used following the approach suggested by Thiry et al. (2008). The serum samples were tested to detect antibodies to the highly conserved gB of alphaherpesviruses by means of a commercially available ELISA (Herdchek Anti-IBR gB, Idexx, Germany) following the manufacturer's recommendations.

In order to rule out that the CpV-1 positivity might be due to BoHV-1, the samples testing positive for gB antibodies were also tested for gE antibodies using a BoHV-1 blocking ELISA (Herdchek Anti-IBR gE, Idexx). This combination with BoHV-1 gE blocking ELISA allows to distinguish between CpHV-1 and BoHV-1. This was demonstrated by Thiry et al. (2008), where CpHV-1-infected goats are determined seropositive by BoHV-1 gB blocking ELISA and seronegative by BoHV-1 gE blocking ELISA. We used a gB blocking ELISA different from that Thiry et al. used, but the overall performance of the diagnostic techniques are similar.

Samples showing an inhibition of < 45%, 45%–55%, and > 55% were classified as negative, doubtful, and positive, respectively. The serum samples classified as doubtful were subsequently analysed in a second round; those resulting doubtful on two tests were classified as CpHV-1 positive.

Serum neutralization assay

Since in some cases goats may still be gE positive although infected by CpHV-1 [34], serum samples found positive in both ELISAs ($n = 35$) were subsequently tested using a cross-serum neutralization assay to detect antibodies to both the goat and the bovine viruses. Serum neutralization assays were carried out according to the procedure described in the Manual of Diagnostic Test and Vaccines for Terrestrial Animals [50]. Briefly, serum samples were heated to 56 °C for 30 min. Serial twofold dilutions of each serum sample were incubated at 37 °C for 2 h in the presence of 100 TCID50/cell of CpHV-1 Ba-1 strain [26] or 24 h in the presence of 100 TCID50/cell of BoHV-1 [50]. Each virus-serum dilution was then dispensed into 96 wells on microtiter plates containing Madin-Darby bovine kidney (MDBK) cells grown and incubated at 37 °C. The plates were read 3 days later. The titer of each serum is expressed as the highest dilution that neutralized the virus.

Statistical analysis

Goat-level prevalence of CpHV-1 and within-herd prevalence were computed as the percentage of goat cases and relative 95% CI. We carried out a preliminary univariate analysis to identify any statistical association between CpHV-1 seropositivity (dependent variable) and potential risk factors: the respective prevalence in the exposed and the non-exposed animals was used to obtain prevalence ratios and relative 95% CI. When the 95% CI of the prevalence ratios did not include the null value (PR = 1), the findings were considered statistically significant.

Animal characteristics (sex, breed, and age) were used as host-level factors; herd-level factors were breeding type (dairy/meat/mixed), management type (extensive/confined), herd size, presence of CAEV-infected goats and of co-inhabitant cattle. As mentioned above, the herd-level data were obtained through a record linkage technique based on official herd identifiers to link our database with the National Animal Registry system. The databases and the data processes for statistical analysis were created with Stata Software 11.1 (Stata Corp, College Station, TX). Age and herd size were categorized into classes based on quartiles (first and second quartiles were conflated in a single category for herd size). The prevalence ratios were then estimated separately for each stratum using the lowest category as the reference. An extension of the Wilcoxon rank-sum test was used to evaluate trends in the prevalence ratios across strata of increasing age and herd size. For the "breed" variable, the less numerous breeds were grouped into a single class. Taking into account the cross-sectional study design and the clustering due to herds, we fit a mixed-effects Poisson regression model ($N = 2879$) with robust variance using the xtpoisson command to obtain adjusted prevalence ratios [51]. All variables that were statistically associated with CpHV-1 infection at the univariate analysis were then entered as independent variables, including "herd" as a random-effect variable. Finally, the AIC was applied to compare the mixed versus the fixed-effect models [52]. Due to the large proportion of missing values affecting the variable "presence of CAEV-infected goats", a model omitting the variable was also fitted ($N = 3568$) in order to increase the number of total observations included in the analysis.

As all samples collected during the mentioned time window were considered for analysis, a prior calculation of the statistical power when comparing two independent proportions (i.e. in animals from the referent group and exposure level group) was carried out before the statistical analysis using WinPepi (version 11.65, http://www.brixtonhealth.com/pepi4windows.html): given a 95% significance level, thanks to the large available sample sizes (i.e. 2879 or 3568 goats respectively in the two final models), a 80% power could easily obtained to detect prevalence ratios between 1.5 and 2.

Abbreviations

AIC: Akaike information criterion; BoHV-1: Bovine herpesvirus type 1; CAE: Caprine arthritis encephalitis; CAEV: Caprine arthritis and encephalitis virus; CI: Confidence interval; CpHV-1: Caprine herpesvirus 1; gB: Glycoprotein B; gE: Glycoprotein E; PR: Prevalence ratio; Q: Quartiles; SRLVs: Small ruminant lentivirus

Acknowledgements

Not applicable

Funding
This research was supported by the Ministry of Health.

Authors' contributions
SB, GR, CM: conceived the study, participated in its design and data analysis, and drafted the manuscript. AR: participated in the study design, carried out the laboratory analysis and drafted the manuscript. CC, PLA, MP, LM: participated in the study design, carried out the laboratory analysis and reviewed the paper. FI assisted in the data analysis and reviewed the paper. AQ collected the samples and reviewed the paper. All authors read and approved the final manuscript.

Ethics approval and consent to participate
Blood samples were collected by the veterinary officers of the Regional Veterinary Services in the frame of approved national and regional animal disease plans. The veterinary officers daily operate on animal farms complying with the animal welfare procedures. When the study started (2008), in Italy there wasn't any requirement for a research being approved by an institutional ethics committee or Institutional Animal Care and Use Committee. The goat owners were informed and they were consenting about the inclusion of their animal blood samples for research purposes.

Consent for publication
Not applicable

Competing interests
None of the authors of this paper has a financial or personal relationship with other people or organizations that could inappropriately influence or bias the content of the paper.

Author details
[1]Istituto Zooprofilattico Sperimentale del Piemonte, Liguria e Valle d'Aosta, Turin, Italy. [2]Istituto Zooprofilattico Sperimentale dell'Abruzzo e del Molise G. Caporale, Teramo, Italy. [3]Local Health Unit AT, Asti, Italy. [4]Local Health Unit TO4, Turin, Italy.

References

1. Van der Lugt JJ, Randles JL. Systemic herpesvirus infection in neonatal goats. J S Afr Vet Assoc. 1993;64:169–71.
2. Thiry J, Keuser V, Muylkens B, Meurens F, Gogev S, Vanderplasschen A, Thiry E. Ruminant alphaherpesviruses related to bovine herpesvirus 1. Vet Res. 2006;37:169–90.
3. Griffin AM. The nucleotide sequence of the glycoprotein gB gene of infectious laryngotracheitis virus: analysis and evolutionary relationship to the homologous gene from other herpesviruses. J Gen Virol. 1991; 72(Pt 2):393–8.
4. Tolari F, White H, Nixon P. Isolation and reactivation of bovid herpesvirus 1 in goats. Microbiologica. 1990;13:67–71.
5. Six A, Banks M, Engels M, Ros Bascuñana C, Ackermann M. Latency and reactivation of bovine herpesvirus 1 (BHV-1) in goats and of caprine herpesvirus 1 (CapHV-1) in calves. Arch Virol. 2001;146:1325–35.
6. Nogarol C, Bertolotti L, De Carlo E, Masoero L, Caruso C, Profiti M, Martucciello A, Galiero G, Cordioli P, Lelli D, Nardelli S, Ingravalle F, Rosati S. Expression and antigenic characterization of bubaline herpesvirus 1(BuHV1) glycoprotein E and its potential application in theepidemiology and control of alphaherpesvirus infections in Mediterranean water buffalo. J Virol Methods. 2014;207:16–21.
7. Bertolotti L, Rosamilia A, Profiti M, Brocchi E, Masoero L, Franceschi V, Tempesta M, Donofrio G, Rosati S. Characterization of caprine herpesvirus 1 (CpHV1) glycoprotein E and glycoprotein I ectodomains expressed in mammalian cells. Vet Microbiol. 2013;164:222–8.
8. Thiry J, Widén F, Grégoire F, Linden A, Belák S, Thiry E. Isolation and characterisation of a ruminant alphaherpesvirus closely related to bovine herpesvirus 1 in a free-ranging red deer. BMC Vet Res. 2007;28:3–26.
9. Tempesta M, Buonavoglia D, Sagazio P, Pratelli A, Buonavoglia C. Natural reactivation of caprine herpesvirus 1 in latently infected goats. Vet Rec. 1998;143:200. https://doi.org/10.1136/vr.143.7.200.
10. Tempesta M, Pratelli A, Corrente M, Buonavoglia C. A preliminary study on the pathogenicity of a strain of caprine Herpesvirus-1. Comp Immunol Microbiol Infect Dis. 1999;22:137–43. https://doi.org/10.1016/S0147-9571(98)00029-0.
11. Tempesta M, Greco G, Camero M, Bozzo G, Guarda F, Buonavoglia C. Virological and histological findings in goats infected by caprine herpesvirus 1. New Microbiol. 2002;25:281–4.
12. Tempesta M, Pratelli A, Greco G, Martella V, Buonavoglia C. Detection of caprine herpesvirus 1 in sacral ganglia of latently infected goats by PCR. J Clin Microbiol. 1999;37:1598–9.
13. Piper KL, Fitzgerald CJ, Ficorilli N, Studdert MJ. Isolation of caprine herpesvirus 1 from a major outbreak of infectious pustular vulvovaginitis in goats. Aust Vet J. 2008;86:136–8.
14. Grewal AS, Wells R. Vulvovaginitis of goats due to a herpesvirus. Aust Vet J. 1986;63:79–82.
15. Tarigan S, Webb RF, Kirkland D. Caprine herpesvirus from balanoposthitis. Aust Vet J. 1987;64:321.
16. Papanastasopoulou M, Koptopoulos G, Lekkas S, Papadopoulos O, Ludwig H. An experimental study on the pathogenicity of the caprine herpesvirus type 1 (CHV-1) comp. Immunol Microbiol Infect Dis. 1991;14:47–53. https://doi.org/10.1016/0147-9571(91)90040-K.
17. Williams NM, Vickers ML, Tramontin RR, Petrites-Murphy MB, Allen GP. Multiple abortions associated with caprine herpesvirus infection in a goat herd. J Am Vet Med Assoc. 1997;211:89–91.
18. Tempesta M, Camero M, Sciorsci RL, Greco G, Minoia R, Martella V, Pratelli A, Buonavoglia C. Experimental infection of goats at different stages of pregnancy with caprine herpesvirus 1. Comp Immunol Microbiol Infect Dis. 2004;27:25–32. https://doi.org/10.1016/S0147-9571(03)00012-2.
19. McCoy MH, Montgomery DL, Bratanich AC, Cavender J, Scharko PB, Vickers ML. Serologic and reproductive findings after a Herpesvirus-1 abortion storm in goats. J Am Vet Med Assoc. 2007;231:1236–9. https://doi.org/10.2460/javma.231.8.1236.
20. Roperto F, Pratelli A, Guarino G, Ambrosio V, Tempesta M, Galati P, Iovane G, Buonavoglia C. Natural caprine herpesvirus 1 (CpHV-1) infection in kids. J Comp Pathol. 2000;122:298–302.
21. Mettler F, Engels M, Wild P, Bivetti A. Herpesvirus infection in kids in Switzerland. Schweiz Arch Tierheilkund. 1979;121:655–62.
22. Saito JK, Gribble DH, Berrios PE, Knight HD, McKercher DG. A new herpesvirus isolate from goats: preliminary report. Am J Vet Res. 1974;35:847–8.
23. Horner GW, Hunter R, Day AM. An outbreak of vulvovaginitis in goats caused by a caprine herpesvirus. N Z Vet J. 1982;30:150–2.
24. Kao M, Leiskau T, Koptopoulos G, Papadopoulos O, Horner OW, Hyllseth B, Fadel M, Gedi AH, Straub OC, Ludwig H. Goat herpesvirus infections: a survey on specific antibodies in different countries survey on specific antibodies. In: Thiry E, Sapliki J, Pastoret PP, editors. Immunity to herpesvirus infections of domestic animals. Commission of the European Communities; 1985. p. 93–7.
25. Koptopoulos G, Papanastasopoulou M, Papadopoulos O, Ludwig H. The epizootiology of caprine herpesvirus (BHV-6) infections in goat populations in Greece. Comp Immunol Microbiol Infect Dis. 1988;11: 199–205.
26. Buonavoglia C, Tempesta M, Cavalli A, Voigt V, Buonavoglia D, Conserva A, Corrente M. Reactivation of caprine herpesvirus 1 in latently infected goats. Comp Immunol Microbiol Infect Dis. 1996;19:275–81.
27. Chénier S, Montpetit C, Hélie P. Caprine herpesvirus-1 abortion storm in a goat herd in Quebec. Can Vet J. 2004;45:241–3.
28. Silva ML, Pituco EM, Nogueira AH, Martins MS, Lima MS, de Azevedo SS. Serological evidence and risk factors associated with caprine herpesvirus 1 in dairy goat flocks in a semiarid region of northeastern Brazil. J Vet Diagn Investig. 2013;25:125–8.
29. Thiry J, Keuser V, Schynts F, Chartier C, Tempesta M, Espejo-Serrano J, Saegerman C, Thiry E. Evaluation de la prévalence sérologique de l'infection

à herpésvirus caprin 1 dans le sud-ouest de l'Europe. Epidèmiol et Santé Anim. 2006;49:55–8.

30. Guercio A, Greco A, Iannizzotto G, Di Marco V, Todaro M. Valutazione della diffusione di anticorpi anti Herpes Virus della capra in allevamenti caprini della Sicilia. Atti della Società Italiana di Patologia Allevamento Ovini e Caprini. 1998;12:138–42.
31. Tempesta M, Cavalli A, Voigt V, Buonavoglia D. Presenza di anticorpi per Caprine herpesvirus 1 (CapHV-1) in allevamenti caprini dell'Italia meridionale. Atti della Società Italiana di Patologia e Allevamento Ovini e Caprini. 1994;11:121–2.
32. Keuser V, Espejo-Serrano J, Schynts F, Georgin JP, Thiry E. Isolation of caprine herpesvirus type 1 in Spain. Vet Rec. 2004;154:395–9.
33. Suavet F, Champion JL, Bartolini L, Bernou M, Alzieu JP, Brugidou R, Darnatigues S, Reynaud G, Perrin C, Adam G, Thiéry R, Duquesne V. First description of infection of caprine herpesvirus 1 (CpHV-1) in goats in mainland France. Pathogens. 2016;5(1):17.
34. Thiry J, Saegerman C, Chartier C, Mercier P, Keuser V, Thiry E. Serological evidence of caprine herpesvirus 1 infection in Mediterranean France. Vet Microbiol. 2008;128:261–8.
35. Keuser V, Gogev S, Schynts F, Thiry E. Demonstration of generalized infection with caprine herpesvirus 1 diagnosed in an aborted caprine fetus by PCR. Vet Res Commun. 2002;26:221–6.
36. Marinaro M, Rezza G, Del Giudice G, Colao V, Tarsitano E, Camero M, Losurdo M, Buonavoglia C, Tempesta M. A caprine herpesvirus 1 vaccine adjuvanted with MF59™ protects against vaginal infection and interferes with the establishment of latency in goats. PLoS One. 2012;7:4.
37. Boelaert F, Speybroeck N, de Kruif A, Aerts M, Burzykowski T, Molenberghs G, Berkvens DL. Risk factors for bovine herpesvirus-1 seropositivity. Prev Vet Med. 2005;69:285–95.
38. Carbonero A, Saa LR, Jara DV, García-Bocanegra I, Arenas A, Borge C, Perea A. Seroprevalence and risk factors associated to bovine herpesvirus 1 (BHV -1) infection in non-vaccinated dairy and dual purpose cattle herds in Ecuador. Prev Vet Med. 2011;100:84–8.
39. Kadohira M, McDermott JJ, Shoukri MM, Thorburn MA. Assessing infections at multiple levels of aggregation. Prev Vet Med. 1997;29:161–77.
40. Van Wuijckhuise LW, Bosch J, Franken P, Hage H, Verhoeff J, Zimmer G. The prevalence of infectious bovine rhinotracheitis (IBR) in the Netherlands, vol. 7. The Netherlands: Proceedings of the Dutch Society for Veterinary Epidemiology and Econimics, Boxtel; 1993. p. 15.
41. Woodbine KA, Medley GF, Moore SJ, Ramirez-Villaescusa AM, Mason S, Green LE. A four year longitudinal sero-epidemiological study of bovine herpesvirus type-1 (BHV-1) in adult cattle in 107 unvaccinated herds in south West England. BMC Vet Res. 2009;5:5.
42. McDermott JJ, Kadohira M, O'Callaghan CJ, Shoukri MM. A comparison of different models for assessing variations in the sero-prevalence of infectious bovine rhinotracheitis by farm, area and district in Kenya. Prev Vet Med. 1997;32:219–34.
43. Solis-Calderon JJS-CV, Segura-Correa JC, Alvarado-Islas A. Seroprevalence of and risk factors for infectious bovine rhinotracheitis in beef cattle herds of Yucatan. Mexico Prev Vet Med. 2003;57:199–208.
44. Speybroeck N, Boelaert F, Renard D, Burzykowski T, Mintiens K, Molenberghs G, Berkvens DL. Design-based analysis of surveys: a bovine herpesvirus 1 case study. Epid Infect. 2003;131:991–1002.
45. Van Wuijckhuise L, Bosch J, Franken P, Frankena K, Elbers AR. Epidemiological characteristics of bovine herpesvirus 1 infections determined by bulk milk testing of all Dutch dairy herds. Vet Record. 1998;142:181–4.
46. Raaperi K, Bougeard S, Aleksejev A, Orro T, Viltrop A. Association of herd BRSV and BHV-1 seroprevalence with respiratory disease and reproductive performance in adult dairy cattle. Acta Vet Scand. 2012;54:4.
47. Blacklaws BA, Berriatua E, Torsteinsdottir S, Watt NJ, de Andres D, Klein D, Harkiss GD. Transmission of small ruminant lentiviruses. Vet Microbiol. 2004; 101:199–208.
48. Leitner G, Krifucks O, Weisblit L, Lavi Y, Bernstein S, Merin U. The effect of caprine arthritis encephalitis virus infection on production in goats. Vet J. 2010;183:328–31.
49. Patel JR, Heldens JG, Bakonyi T, Rusvai M. Important mammalian veterinary viral immuno diseases and their control. Vaccine. 2012;30:1767–81.
50. OIE. Manual of Diagnostic Tests and Vaccines for Terrestrial Animals. 2016. http://www.oie.int/en/international-standard-setting/terrestrial-manual/access-online/. Accessed 27 Feb 2017.
51. Lee J, Tan CS, Chia KS. A practical guide for multivariate analysis of dichotomous outcomes. Ann Acad Med Singap. 2009;38:714–9.
52. Hill G. Model checking and comparison. In data analysis using regression and multilevel/hierarchical models. Cambridge University Press. 2007:513–27.

23

Protection induced by a glycoprotein E-deleted bovine herpesvirus type 1 marker strain used either as an inactivated or live attenuated vaccine in cattle

Sonia Alejandra Romera[1,7,8*†], Mariana Puntel[2†], Valeria Quattrocchi[1], Paula Del Médico Zajac[1], Patricia Zamorano[1,7,8], Javier Blanco Viera[3], Consuelo Carrillo[4], Shafiqul Chowdhury[5], Manuel V Borca[6] and Ana M Sadir[1,7,8]

Abstract

Background: Bovine herpesvirus type 1 (BoHV-1) is the causative agent of respiratory and genital tract infections; causing a high economic loss in all continents. Use of marker vaccines in IBR eradication programs is widely accepted since it allows for protection of the animals against the disease while adding the possibility of differentiating vaccinated from infected animals.
The aim of the present study was the development and evaluation of safety and efficacy of a glycoprotein E-deleted (gE-) BoHV-1 marker vaccine strain (BoHV-1ΔgEβgal) generated by homologous recombination, replacing the viral gE gene with the β-galactosidase (βgal) gene.

Results: *In vitro* growth kinetics of the BoHV-1ΔgEβgal virus was similar to BoHV-1 LA. The immune response triggered by the new recombinant strain in cattle was characterized both as live attenuated vaccine (LAV) and as an inactivated vaccine. BoHV-1ΔgEβgal was highly immunogenic in both formulations, inducing specific humoral and cellular immune responses. Antibody titers found in animals vaccinated with the inactivated vaccine based on BoHV-1ΔgEβgal was similar to the titers found for the control vaccine (BoHV-1 LA). In the same way, titers of inactivated vaccine groups were significantly higher than any of the LAV immunized groups, independently of the inoculation route ($p < 0.001$). Levels of IFN-γ were significantly higher ($p < 0.001$) in those animals that received the LAV compared to those that received the inactivated vaccine. BoHV-1ΔgEβgal exhibited an evident attenuation when administered as a LAV; no virus was detected in nasal secretions of vaccinated or sentinel animals during the post-vaccination period. BoHV-1ΔgEβgal, when used in either formulation, elicited an efficient immune response that protected animals against challenge with virulent wild-type BoHV-1. Also, the deletion of the gE gene served as an immunological marker to differentiate vaccinated animals from infected animals. All animals vaccinated with the BoHV-1ΔgE βgal strain were protected against disease after challenge and shed significantly less virus than control calves, regardless of the route and formulation they were inoculated.

Conclusions: Based on its attenuation, immunogenicity and protective effect after challenge, BoHV-1ΔgEβgal virus is an efficient and safe vaccine candidate when used either as inactivated or as live attenuated forms.

Keywords: BoHV-1ΔgEβgal, BoHV-1 marker vaccine, Inactivated/live attenuated vaccine, Bovines

* Correspondence: aromera@cnia.inta.gov.ar
[†]Equal contributors
[1]Instituto de Virología Instituto de Virología, Centro de Investigaciones en Ciencias Veterinarias (CICV), Instituto Nacional de Tecnología Agropecuaria (INTA), Castelar, CC77, 1708 Morón, Argentina
[7]Universidad del Salvador, Buenos Aires, Argentina
Full list of author information is available at the end of the article

Background

Bovine herpesvirus-1 (BoHV-1) is an important pathogen of cattle and responsible for a wide variety of clinical diseases, including conjunctivitis and upper respiratory tract infection known as infectious bovine rhinotracheitis (IBR), reproductive tract lesions, abortion in pregnant cows, and systemic infection in the newborn [1-3]. In addition, BoHV-1 has been recognized as an important component of the bovine respiratory disease (BRD) complex [1,4]. The BoHV-1 infection in cattle is responsible for considerable economic losses due to decreased milk production, weight loss and abortion.

The virus genome consists of a linear double-stranded DNA molecule of about 135.3 kb that encodes for approximately 70 proteins [5]. Twelve of them (gB, gC, gD, gE, gG, gI, gH, gK, gL, gM, UL49.5 and Us9) are envelope proteins, of which the first ten are glycosylated [5]. Envelope glycoproteins gE and gI form complexes and gE is involved in viral intercellular spread (cell-to-cell spread). BoHV-1 gE open reading frame (ORF) is predicted to contain 575 amino acid (aa) residues with a 28 aa cleavable signal sequence. The structure of glicoprotein E (gE) corresponds to a type I transmembrane glycoproteins. The glycoprotein contains three distinct domains: a 387 aa long hydrophilic extracellular domain (ecto-domain), a 33 aa long hydrophobic transmembrane domain and a 125 aa long highly charged cytoplasmic domain/tegument domain. The mature gE is phosphorylated and glycosylated with an apparent molecular mass of about 92 kD.

Attenuated live viruses or inactivated virions are used widely as vaccines to control the disease. Thus, BoHV-1-specific antibodies can be found in bovines on all continents; its prevalence varies greatly depending on herd size and management. Classical vaccines complicate serological diagnosis and determination of the true prevalence of infection. Marker and conventional vaccines can prevent disease but not latent infection. Due to the current restrictions in international trade for products derived from seropositive animals a number of European countries have eradicated BoHV-1 with very high costs involved. In countries with a high prevalence of infection, including the United States, the control of IBR is associated with the immunization of cattle with marker vaccines. In this context, the ability to differentiate infected from vaccinated animals (DIVA) has become critical issue. Gene-deleted marker vaccines offer the advantage of deletion of specific viral genes that are non-essential for viral replication [6,7] while inducing a substantial protein-specific immune response. Currently, vaccines used in BoHV-1 control programs utilize highly attenuated BoHV-1 strains marked by a deletion of the gE gene [8]. Glycoprotein E is considered a virulence factor of all known members of the subfamily *Alphaherpesvirinae* [9-11].

Live and killed gE-deleted marker vaccines are now widely used in Europe, in combination with gE-based diagnostic tests to monitor cattle. The gE-deleted mutants generated thus far include derivations of herpes simplex virus (HSV), pseudorabies virus, equine herpesvirus 1 and BoHV-1; these were shown to be attenuated in mice, swine, foals and calves, respectively [8,9,12,13]. Notably, expression of gE and gI is required for full pathogenic potential in animals but is not required for growth in tissue culture [14], thus allowing for it replication in cell culture. In infected animals, gE is required for anterograde neuronal spread and neurovirulence. Accordingly, an interesting safety feature that comes from using LAV based on gE-deleted viruses is that the virus cannot spread in an anterograde direction from sensory neurons in trigeminal ganglia to respiratory mucosa. Furthermore, gE induces specific antibodies both in the context of inactivated vaccines or as infectious virus, thus facilitating serological differentiation of animals immunized with a gE-deleted marker vaccine from infected cattle [7]. Safety and efficacy of both the live and the inactivated gE-deleted vaccines that are available have been tested thoroughly [15-22].

In this report, we present data regarding the development of a gE-deleted and βgal expressing BoHV-1 (BoHV-1ΔgEβgal) strain and its use as either an inactivated immunogen or as an LAV in cattle. Our results demonstrate that BoHV-1ΔgEβgal virus is an efficient vaccine candidate when used either as inactivated or as live attenuated form.

Methods

Virus and cells

BoHV-1 Los Angeles (LA) (American Type Culture Collection, VR-188) and BoHV-1ΔgEβgal strains were propagated in Madin Darby Bovine Kidney (MDBK) cells grown in Eagle's Minimal Essential Medium (MEM), supplemented with 10% fetal bovine serum (FBS).

Construction of the recombinant plasmid

Virus DNA was extracted from cell-free supernatant virus preparations following a standard phenol/chloroform procedure using sodium dodecyl sulfate (SDS) and proteinase K lysis, phenol/ether extraction, and ethanol precipitation [23]. Discrete flanking regions corresponding to gE gene were amplified by PCR from this material. Primer sequences were based on the published BoHV-1 glycoprotein E (gE) gene sequences [GenBank Accession Number NC 001847]. Primers were designed to add restriction sites in order to facilitate further cloning. The left flanking region of gE (L fragment) was obtained using primers gE1 (5′-GCGAGCAGCGGGAGCGGGGCC-3′),; and gE2(5′-GGGCGGATCCGTGGGTTGCA-3′), which introduced a Sal I and a Bam HI sites, respectively. The right flanking region of gE (R fragment) was amplify using primers gE3(5′- AGCTTGGATCCCGGCCGCA CC- 3′) and gE4 (5′- CCTCAGAATTCGGGGTCTC GG- 3′), which introduced a Bam Hi and an EcoR I sites to amplified fragment, respectively.

DNA fragments corresponding to the left (L) and right (R) gE flanking regions obtained by PCR were digested with the appropriate enzymes and cloned sequentially into the pUC19 vector (Clontech). First, the L product (734 bp long, corresponding to position 120956 to 121714 of the BoHV-1 genome) was cloned between the SalI and BamHI sites (recombinant plasmid pUCL), and then the R product (632 bp long, corresponding to position 123375 to 124008 of the BoHV-1 genome) was cloned between the BamHI and EcoRI sites (recombinant plasmid pUCLR), using a BamHI site that linked both L and R fragments. The blunt 4.5 kb fragment, which contains the bacterial β-gal gene under the control of the human cytomegalovirus immediate early promoter (HCMV-IE), was inserted into the blunted BamHI site of pUCLR. The resulting gE-deletion/β-gal insertion plasmid (pUCLRβ-gal) carried a deletion of 1,640 bp of BoHV-1 DNA, and the insertion of the β-gal gene controlled by the human cytomegalovirus immediate early promoter. In pUCLRβ-gal, the β-gal gene is flanked by virus-specific sequences required for recombination with the viral DNA: a 734 bp upstream sequence (L) containing part of the gE promoter and the first 23 bp of the coding sequence, a 632 bp downstream sequence (R) containing the last 67 bp at the 3′ extreme, and the complete ORF of the US9 gene (474 bp). Identity of both fragments corresponding to L and R were confirmed by sequencing (Fmol, Promega) (data not shown).

Generation of recombinant BoHV-1 gE-deleted βgal (BoHV-1ΔgEβgal) virus

To generate the BoHV-1 gE-deleted recombinant virus, MDBK cells were co-transfected with a ScaI linearized pUCLRβ-gal plasmid DNA together with a full-length DNA derived from BoHV-1 LA strain. Briefly, a mixture of 2 μg of parental BoHV-1 LA DNA, 0.2 μg of ScaI linearized pUCLRβgal vector and 16 μl of Lipofectamine (Gibco BRL, Life Technologies) was added onto a 60% confluent MDBK cell monolayergrown in a 6-well plate, and then incubated for 8 hours at 37°C in a CO_2-controlled atmosphere. A media change was then performed using MEM containing 5% FBS and the plates were incubated for 16 hours in the same conditions described above. Each transfected cell monolayer was trypsinized and transferred to a 25 cm^2 flask containing 5% FBS MEM and incubated until cytopathic effects (CPE) were observed. To determine the dilution of the inoculum for the Bluo-gal screening assay, the co-transfection products were titrated by plaque forming units (PFU) and frozen until the screening assay was performed.

Purification of the recombinant virus

Co-transfection products were examined for their β-gal expression by histochemical staining of infected cells. The recombinant viruses able to form blue plaques in the presence of the β-galactosidase substrate (halogenated indolyl-β-D-galactoside) were plaque purified five times under an agar overlay [24]. Recombinant viruses expressing β-gal activity were selected by the appearance of blue plaques.

Molecular characterization of the recombinant virus

The recombinant virus was further characterized by PCR (gE-specific primers: gE7: 5′-CGCCCGTCTTT CTCCCAG-3′ and gE8: 5′-GCGGGACGAGGAGAGG GA-3′) and by Southern blot analysis targeting a part of the gE ORF. Lack of gE protein expression in BoHV-1ΔgEβgal infected cell lysates done by Western blot.

Southern blot hybridization

Genomic DNA extracted from purified wild-type and recombinant BoHV-1 viruses were digested with HindIII and the corresponding fragments were separated by electrophoresis in a 0.6% agarose TBE gel, then transferred to a nitrocellulose membrane (Zprobe, Bio-Rad). [25]. The membrane bearing the immobilized DNA fragments was blocked with 2x SSC solution and fixed by heating at 80°C for 30 minutes. Hybridization was performed separately with three specific probes (L, R, y gE) previously obtained by PCR and labeled with 32S (Prime-a-Gene Labeling System, Promega).

gE-specific immunoblot analyses

Polyacrylamide gel electrophoresis in the presence of SDS (SDS-PAGE) and additional immunoblot analyses were performed using mock and virus-infected cells. Briefly, either mock (non-infected MDBK cells) and virus-infected cells were concentrated by ultracentrifugation at 12,000 g for 1 h at 47°C, resuspended in sample buffer (50 mM Tris–HCl, pH 7.5, 1 mM PMSF, 8 M urea, 1% SDS, 2 mM DTT and 2% β-Mercaptoethanol), boiled for 10 minutes, separated by gel electrophoresis in 12.5% polyacrylamide gels and blotted on to Immobilon P membranes (Millipore). Membranes were blocked overnight in phosphate buffered saline and 0.05% Tween 20 (PBST) containing 5% skim milk (all subsequent steps were performed using this buffer). Then, they were incubated for 2 hours at 37°C with the corresponding monoclonal antibodies: anti-gE, MAb3 (kindly provided by Dr. J.T. Van Oirschot from the Institute of Animal Science and Health, Lelystad, Netherlands), or anti-gD (kindly provided by Dr. L.A. Babiuk from the Vaccine and Infectious Disease Organization, University of Saskatchewan, Saskatoon, Saskatchewan, Canada). After three washes with PBST, membranes were incubated with peroxidase-labeled anti-mouse IgG rabbit antiserum (KLP Inc) for 1 hour at 37°C. After washing three times, antibody binding was visualized by chemiluminescence (Renaissance kit, NEN Life Science) after exposure to an X-ray film (CurixOrto ST-G2, AGFA).

Virus growth kinetics

The growth kinetics of the BoHV-1ΔgEβgal strain in MDBK cells was compared to that of the parental BoHV-1 LA strain. A series of replicate cultures of MDBK cells were infected separately with a MOI of 0.1 per cell of recombinant BoHV-1ΔgEβgal or the parental BoHV-1 LA strain. Infected cultures were harvested at successive post-infection intervals and frozen in aliquots until titration. Virus titration was performed by the end-point dilution method of Reed & Muench, in three independent repetitions.

Inactivated vaccine formulation

BoHV-1 LA or BoHV-1ΔgEβgal were propagated according to the conditions described earlier [26]. Preparations were inactivated by treatment with 1% (v/v) 0.1 M binary bromoethylenimine (BEI) for 25 h at 37°C. One volume of inactivated virus suspension was mixed with one volume of INTA mineral oil adjuvant (formulated with Arlacel C, Markol 52 and Tween 80), to produce a water-in mineral oil emulsion according to Smitssart *et al.* [27].

Vaccination experiments

The animal experiments reported in this manuscript have been performed following internationally recognized guidelines with the approval of the Institutional Committee for Care and Use of Experimental Animals, CICUAE-CICVyA. INTA, Argentina.

Vaccination experiments were performed using 12 to 18 month-old Holando and Angus × Hereford calves with undetectable BoHV-1 serum antibodies (evaluated by ELISA and virus neutralization tests).

All challenge experiments using virulent BoHV-1 LA, and inoculations using attenuated BoHV-1ΔgEβgal (dose: $10^{8.25}$ $TCID_{50}$/mL) were performed in a type II biosafety animal facility.

Viral challenge was performed using 2 ml virulent BoHV-1 LA ($10^{7.5}$ $TCID_{50}$/ml) into each nostril, by intranasal inoculation (IN) with an ultrasonic nebulizer (ELECTROLAB AP-300).

Evaluation of BoHV-1ΔgEβgal as either inactivated and attenuated vaccines

Table 1 shows the experimental design describing number of animals, vaccination date and route, date of challenge, date of BoHV-1 specific antibodies determination, BoHV-1 excretion in nasal fluids, date of lymphoproliferative response.

Safety assessment for BoHV-1ΔgEβgal as a life attenuated vaccine

The safety test was performed in pregnant cows. Five pregnant cows (being in the third to sixth month of pregnancy) were IV infected with attenuated BoHV-1ΔgEβgal virus (4 ml of the viral suspension with a titer of $10^{8.25}$ $TCID_{50}$/ml). Animals were clinically observed until they gave birth and serologically evaluated until 370 dpv. Likewise, newborn calves were also evaluated in regards to their clinical and immune conditions, as well as the virus shedding.

Detection of virus neutralizing antibodies

Virus neutralization (VN) was performed using primary fetal bovine testis (FBT) cell cultures in 96-well microtiter plates using the constant virus-variable serum method [26,27]. Each dilution was tested in four wells containing FBT cell monolayers an adsorbed for 1 hour, the unabsorbed virus was removed and MEM with 5% FBS, was added. Plates were then incubated for 3 days at 37°C and the number of wells and serum dilution showing cytopathic effect was scored. Log10 of the reciprocal value of the highest serum dilution in which CPE was prevented was considered the virus neutralization titer.

Detection of anti-BoHV-1 and anti-gEantibodies in serum

Total antibodies against BoHV-1 in bovine serum were measured by an indirect ELISA as described elsewhere [28]. Titers for bovine sera were expressed as Log10 of the reciprocal of the highest serum dilution which gives readings of absorbance greater or equal to 40% of the positive control measuring at an OD of 405 nm. Detection of gE-specific antibodies was performed using a commercial ELISA for BoHV-1 that allows for the detection of gE-specific antibodies (HerdChek Anti-IBR gE/IDEXX Laboratories), according to the manufacturer's directions.

Detection of IgG1/IgA antibodies in nasal swabs

The mucosal immune response was determined using a specific ELISA for the detection of IgG1 and IgA. Briefly, nasal swabs were collected and frozen at −80°C. The antigen was prepared as described before (Romera *et al.*, [26]).

BoHV-1-specific lymphoproliferation assay

Whole blood samples were collected by venipuncture in syringes containing heparin. Lymphocyte-enriched cells were isolated from the buffy coat as described elsewhere [26] by centrifugation on Lymphoprep (Nycomed Pharma A.S.). Cells were washed twice in RPMI + 5% FBS. UV light-inactivated suspensions of virus-infected MDBK cells (5 μg/ml) and control MDBK cells were used as antigens. The corresponding inactivated antigen was added to a 100 μl volume of medium containing 2×10^5 lymphocytes,

Table 1 Experimental design

Experiment	Vaccine	# animals	Vaccination time (dpv) [route, vol.]	Challenge (dpv)	BoHV-1 antibodies (dpv)	BoHV-1 sheeding (dpv/dpc)	LPT (dpv/dpc)
inactivated BoHV-1ΔgEβgal vaccine	BoHV-1ΔgEβgal	5	0, 21 [SC, 3 ml]	186	0, 14, 21, 30, 67, 150 and 186	0, 3, 5, 7, 8, 10, 12, 14, 17 and 22 dpc	7,72 dpv
	BoHV-1LA	5	0, 21 [SC, 3 ml]	186			
	mock	6		186			
attenuated BoHV-1ΔgEβgal vaccine	BoHV-1ΔgEβgal	5	Group 1: 0 [IN, 4 ml]	42	0, 7, 19, 34 and 42	1 to 42dpv	7,30 dpc
		5	Group 2: 0 [IM, 4 ml]	42		and	
	Sentinel	5	Group 4			3, 5, 7, 8, 10, 12, 14, 17 and 22 dpc	
	Mock	5	Group 5	42			
attenuated BoHV-1ΔgEβgal vaccine SAFETY	BoHV-1ΔgEβgal	5	Group 3: 0 [IV, 4 ml]		along 370		

SC: subcutaneous, dpv: days post-vaccination; dpc: days post-challenge.
During the next 42 days post- vaccination with attenuated BoHV-1ΔgEβgal, viral excretion was controlled, as well as clinical signs such as loss of appetite, lesions of nasal, ocular and oral mucosae and discharge from the nose or eyes and rectal temperature. General clinical status was evaluated and recorded using a rating system (ranging from 0 = asymptomatic to 3 = severe symptoms). Nasal swabs were scored as follows: 0 = absent, 1 = slightly serous, 2 = severely serous, 3 = seromucous, 4 = mucopurulent.

performed in triplicate in a 96-well plate format. One microgram of the mitogen Concavalin A (Sigma, St Louis, USA) was added to the positive control wells. The lymphocyte cultures were incubated for 4 days at 37°C in a humidified atmosphere containing 5% CO_2. Twenty hours before harvesting, 4 μCi of [3H] tymidine was added to each well. Cell proliferation was measured as [3H] tymidine uptake in a scintillation counter (LKB, Wallac, 1219 Rackbeta) and results were obtained as counts per minute (CPM). The values are the mean of the triplicate values and are expressed as stimulation index (SI), where SI = mean CPM of antigen-stimulated lymphocytes/mean CPM of MDBK-stimulated lymphocytes). A threshold value of SI = 3 was established.

Interferon Gamma assay

The capacity of mononuclear cells to secrete interferon γ (IFNγ) in response to a specific *in vitro* stimulation with inactivated BoHV-1 viral antigen was evaluated by a indirect sandwich ELISA. Briefly, 1.5 × 10^6 mononuclear cells were diluted in 100 μl of RPMI 10% FBS per well, in sterile microplates of 96 "U" bottom wells. The supernatant was added on Immulon II microplates, previously sensitized ON with anti bovine IFNγ monoclonal antibody (mAbs), and blocked with PBST 0.1% BSA. A reference curve was performed using IFNγ standard at known concentrations. Detection of the captured IFNγ was done using a rabbit anti-bovine IFNγ serum, diluted in 0.1% PBST-BSA. In order to improve the sensibility of the assay, plates were later incubated with biotin-labeled rat anti-rabbit IgG and developed using disodium p-nitrophenyl phosphate (PPN) as substrate. Optical densities (OD) at A_{405} were measured 25 minutes after the addition of the substrate.

Statistical analysis

Comparison of the vaccine profiles obtained throughout the experimental period was performed using an analysis of variance (ANOVA) for repeated measures with the Greenhouse and Geisser correction of the significance levels (fixed at 5%). The post-ANOVA comparisons were performed using the Bonferroni test with the same level of significance. All the statistical calculations were performed using the SAS program (release 6.04), following the G.M.L. procedure [29].

Results

Construction of a gE deletion vector

The gE gene of BoHV-1 is located between BoHV-1 genome nucleotide positions 121714 and 123440, within the US region (Figure 1a), similarly to other alphaherpesviruses. The BoHV-1 gE gene is flanked upstream by the gI (US7) gene and downstream by the BoHV-1 homologue of the herpes simplex virus (HSV-1) US9 gene [30,31] (Figure 1b). Based on the position of the gE ORF, a gE deletion recombinant vector, pΔgEβgal, was constructed and composed of two DNA fragments flanking the gE coding region (pUCLRβgal), created by PCR amplification of viral DNA from the BoHV-1 LA parental strain (Figure 1d). The upstream flanking fragment is a SalI/BamHI 734 bp region (L) covering from position 120956 to 121714 of the BoHV-1 genome while the downstream fragment is a BamHI/EcoRI 632 bp region (R) covering from position 123375 to 124008 of the BoHV-1 genome (Figure 1c). The

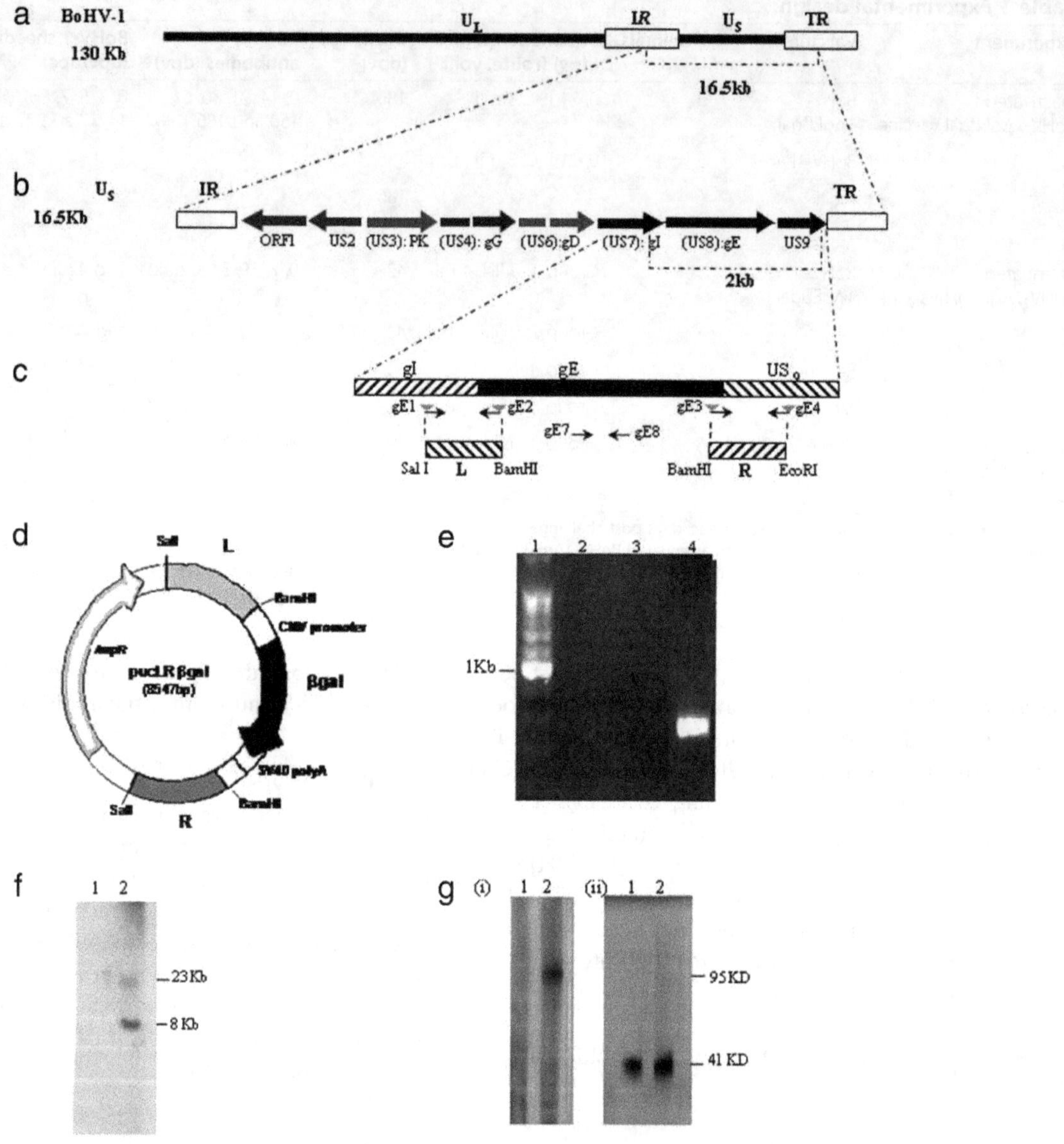

Figure 1 Molecular structure of BoHV-1ΔgEβgal virus. (a) Target region for the gE deletion in BoHV-1 genome. **(b)** gE ORF (US8) is flanked by gI (US7) and US9 genes. **(c)** Primers gE1 and gE2 were designed to amplify the left (L) fragment, and primers gE3 and gE4 were designed to amplify the right (R) fragment. The sequences of primers gE2, gE3 and gE4 were designed in order to create the depicted restriction sites to facilitate the cloning strategy. **(d)** pUCLRβgal recombination vector diagram restriction sites used for cloning and relative position of the elements decribed are shown **(e)** Confirmation gE-specific deletion by PCR. Lanes 2–4 primers specific to the gE sequence (gE7 and gE8) were used. Different templates were used for each lane shown: Lane 2 negative control (ultrapure sterile water); lane 3 BoHV-1ΔgEβgal DNA; lane 4 parental BoHV-1 LA DNA; lanes 1 molecular weight marker (100pb, Promega). **(f)** Molecular characterization of the recombinant BoHV-1ΔgEβgal strain. Southern blot analysis for gE gene. Viral DNA from BoHV-1ΔgEβgal (lane 1) and from parental BoHV-1 LA strain (lane 2) were digested with HindIII restriction enzyme, separated by 0.6% agarose gel electrophoresis, blotted to a membrane and probed with the gE probe. **(g)** Western blot for gE protein. Concentrated virus (BoHV-1ΔgEβgal, lane 1; and parental BoHV-1 LA, lane 2) was separated by electrophoresis in a 12% SDS-PAGE, blotted to a membrane and incubated with specific serum. Panel (i) gE-specific monoclonal antibody, panel (ii) gD-specific monoclonal antibody.

βgal marker gene was inserted into the BamHI site of the construct.

Development of a BoHV-1 gE-deleted virus mutant (BoHV-1ΔgEβgal)

To generate the gE deletion mutant virus, the recombinant vector pUCLRβgal was co-transfected with BoHV-1 LA DNA into MDBK cells. The first screening was based on βgal expression. Selected viruses (blue plaque +) were further evaluated by PCR amplification using specific primers for gE regions (Figure 1e). The intended gE gene deletion and insertion of the βgal gene at the gE locus was further confirmed by Southern blot analysis with a gE-specific probe (Figure 1f). The absence of the 1639 bp gE fragment and the presence of a recombinant βgal fragment with the anticipated size of 4.5 kb demonstrated that the intended recombination had taken place in a site-specific manner. Western blot analysis using a BoHV-1 gE-specific MAb3 confirmed the deletion of the gE protein in the BoHV-1ΔgEβgal virus while a 92- to 95-kd BoHV-1 gE product was detected in BoHV-1 cell extracts (Figure 1g). The L and R fragments of BoHV-1ΔgEβgal were sequenced. No difference with wt virus were found.

Growth properties of the BoHV-1gE deletion mutant virus, BoHV-1ΔgEβgal, were compared with the BoHV-1 LA strain in a multistep growth curve performed using MDBK cell cultures infected at a MOI of 0.1. Virus yields were determined by titration performed using MDBK cells. No significant differences were detected between the titers achieved with wt BoHV-1 strain and the gE-deleted strain (Figure 2).

Assessment of BoHV-1ΔgEβgal virus as an inactivated vaccine

Animals (n = 5/group) were subcutaneously vaccinated at days 0 and 21 with either a vaccine formulated with BoHV-1ΔgEβgal or wild-type BoHV-1 LA strain. At 186 dpv, the two vaccinated groups and a mock-vaccinated group (n = 6) were IN challenged with $10^{7.5}$ $TCID_{50}$/ml virulent BoHV-1 LA strain by aerosol exposure.

Total BoHV-1-specific antibody responses in animals immunized with the BoHV-1ΔgEβgal inactivated vaccine did not differ significantly from those of bovines vaccinated with BoHV-1 LA virus (Figure 3b). Antibody titers were first detected at 14 dpv, with highest levels reached at 30 dpv (approximately 4.0) in both vaccinated groups.

Similarly, neutralizing antibodies were first detected in vaccinated bovines at 30 dpv, (titers of 2.04 and 1.8 for BoHV-1ΔgEβgal-immunized and BoHV-1 LA-immunized groups, respectively). The neutralizing antibody titers before challenge ranged between 1.2 and 1.1 (Figure 3a). No significant differences were found in the responses elicited by BoHV-1ΔgEβgal and BoHV-1 LA as inactivated antigens. Nasal swabs were analyzed for isotype profiles of the virus-specific antibody responses at the time of challenge. We found that 5/5 animals vaccinated with BoHV-1 and 4/5 animals vaccinated with BoHV-1ΔgEβgal exhibited anti-BoHV-1 IgG1 antibodies in nasal swabs (titer = 1.6), while no IgA antibodies were detected in the same samples (data not shown).

Assessment of the gE-specific antibody response could be effectively utilized to differentiate animals vaccinated with inactivated BoHV-1ΔgEβgal, inactivated BoHV-1 LA, as well as those infected with BoHV-1 LA virus. At 14 dpv, groups that were BoHV-1ΔgEβgal-vaccinated, mock-vaccinated, or sentinel animals were found to be negative for gE-specific antibodies. However, these animals developed anti-gE antibodies by 216 dpv, 30 days after challenge. Additionally, gE-specific antibodies were

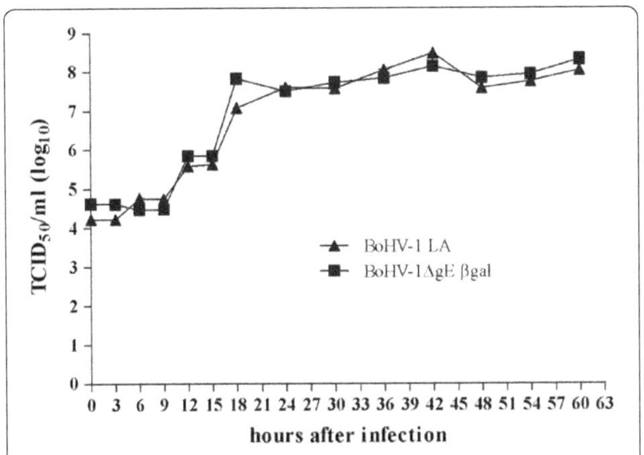

Figure 2 Growth kinetics of the BoHV-1ΔgEβgal virus. MDBK cells were infected at a MOI of 0.1 with either BoHV-1ΔgEβgal or BoHV-1 LA virus strains. Viral replication was checked every 3 hours during a period of 60 hours pi. Virus titrations were performed in duplicate for each time point on MDBK cells. Titers are expressed as $TCID_{50}$/ml. Each data point represents the mean of the titers obtained.

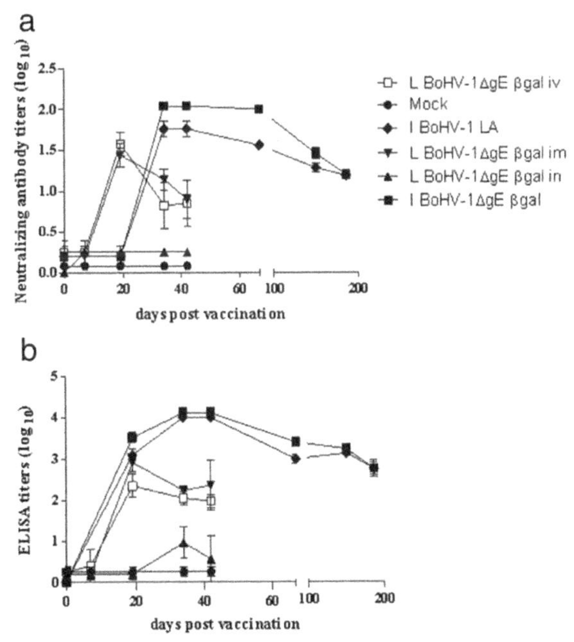

Figure 3 Antibody response to BoHV-1 observed in vaccinated cattle. BoHV-1-specific antibody response detected by ELISA **(b)** or virus neutralization assay **(a)** in animals vaccinated either with inactivated (I) or live attenuated vaccine (L) formulated with BoHV-1ΔgEβgal or BoHV-1 LA viruses. Live attenuated vaccines were administered by intranasal (in), intramuscular (im) or intravenous (iv) route. Neutralizing antibody titers are expressed as log10 of the reciprocal value of the serum dilution giving protection to CPE. Averages and SEM of the titers obtained for each group are shown for each time point. Antibody titers measured by ELISA are expressed as log10 of the reciprocal value of the serum dilution giving an A405 of 40% of the positive control. Each point represents the mean titer and SEM of five animals.

detected in animals vaccinated with inactivated BoHV-1 LA strain at 14 dpv and were also positive by the end of the experimental period (data not shown).

Cellular immune responses, detected by LPT and IFNγ production specific to BoHV-1 are shown in Figure 4. Animals produced a positive LPT (SI ≥ 3) in the BoHV-1ΔgEβgal group while a LPT response >3 was detected for one of the BoHV-1 LA-vaccinated animals. No significant differences were found in the responses elicited by BoHV-1ΔgEβgal versus BoHV-1 LA when administered as inactivated antigens, and none of the bovines belonging to the sentinel or mock-vaccinated groups showed positive reactions throughout the duration of the experiment (Figure 4a). Only low levels of IFNγ could be detected in the inactivated-vaccinated group during the evaluated period (Figure 4b).

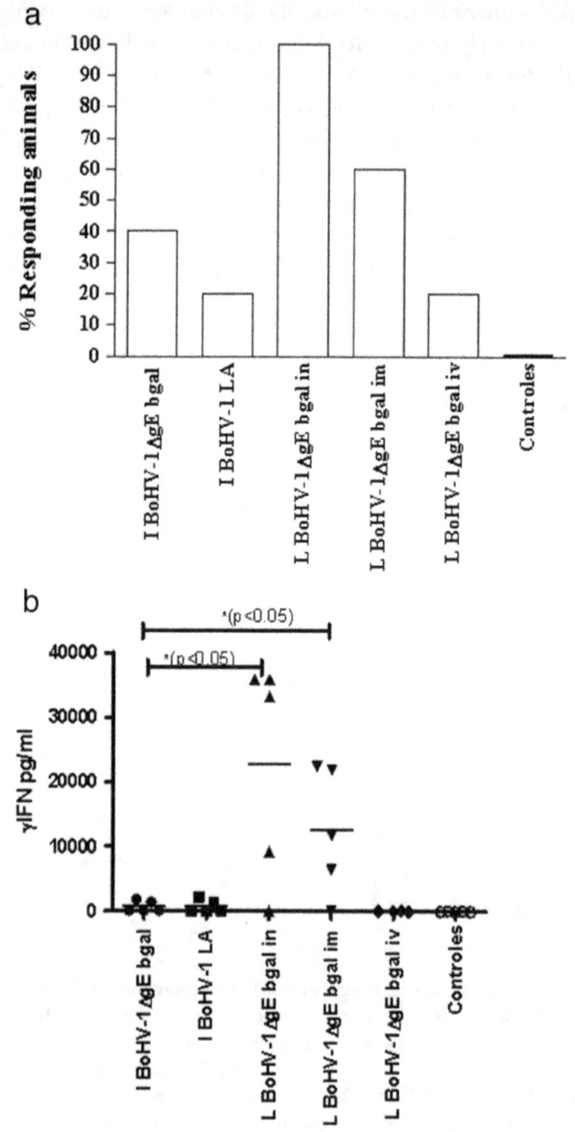

Figure 4 Cellular response to BoHV-1 observed in vaccinated cattle. Cellular immune response at 7 dpv detected by (a) Lymphocyte proliferation test (LPT). Values are expressed as the percentage of animals in each treatment group exhibiting significant (LPT response >3) lymphocyte proliferation after vaccination at 7 dpv. **(b)** IFNγ at 7dpv. Values are expressed as pg/ml. References in this figure are as described in Figure 3.

Clinical monitoring of animals was performed daily, starting the day of vaccination until the end of the post-challenge observational period. No animals exhibited signs of BoHV-1 disease after vaccination. Bilateral nasal serous discharge was detected in the BoHV-1ΔgEβgal group at 2 days post-challenge (dpc) and for 11 days virus shedding was detected, with a maximum mean titer of 1.3 $TCID_{50}$/ml at 8 dpc. In the BoHV-1 LA group, nasal discharge was mucous or serous. Virus shedding in mock-vaccinated animals peaked at 8 dpc (6.1 $TCID_{50}$/ml) and serous to mucous nasal discharge lasted approximately 2 weeks. The protective responses were statistically different ($p < 0.001$) between vaccinated vs. mock-vaccinated animals, while no significant differences were found between animals vaccinated either BoHV-1ΔgEβgal or BoHV-1 LA.

Assessment of efficacy BoHV-1ΔgEβgal virus as a live attenuated vaccine

Animals involved in this assessment were randomly allotted into five groups of five cattle each. Groups 1, 2 and 3 received 4 ml of $10^{8.25}$ $TCID_{50}$/ml of BoHV-1ΔgEβgal virus by the IN, IM and IV routes, respectively. Group 4, the sentinel group, did not receive vaccine or challenge virus, but was housed with vaccinated animals beginning at 3 dpv, to evaluate horizontal transmission. Group 5 consisted of mock-vaccinated calves.

BoHV-1ΔgEβgal virus was shown to be attenuated. All animals vaccinated with BoHV-1ΔgEβgal, regardless of the inoculation route, exhibited minimal clinical symptoms of infection, with serous rhinitis as the only observed indicator of disease. No apathy, depression or loss of appetite was observed in these calves and their body temperatures never exceeded 40°C. Additionally, no detectable BoHV-1ΔgEβgal virus was found in the nasal or ocular secretions of the vaccinated calves. Only two animals belonging to the IN group shed virus, with viral titers of 1.5 $TCID_{50}$/ml at 3 dpv, likely due to the existence of residual virus from the vaccination. No virus shedding was detected in the sentinel animals.

Analysis of the antibody response in animals vaccinated with BoHV-1ΔgEβgal indicated that detection of antibodies, measured by ELISA, started at 19 dpv in those vaccinated either IM or IV, while those vaccinated IN began exhibiting detectable antibody responses at 34 dpv, with significantly lower titers ($p < 0.001$) compared to the IM- and IV-vaccinated groups. On the day of challenge (42 dpv), the average antibody titers were 0.7 (±1.2) in the IN-vaccinated group and 2.36 (±1.2) and

2.05 (±0.3) in the IM- and IV-vaccinated groups respectively (Figure 3b). After challenge, antibody levels increase for all groups, reaching their maximal levels at 56 dpv with values of 3.7 (±0.3) for the IN-vaccinated group and 3.88 (±0.26) for the IM-vaccinated group (data not shown). While in the mock-vaccinated group animals displayed average antibody titers of 3.04 (±0.29) at 30 dpc, no antibodies were detected during the entire post-vaccination period in the sentinel group. Antibody responses were statistically different ($p < 0.001$) between IM/IV- vs. IN-vaccinated groups, and between vaccinated vs. mock-vaccinated animals, while no significant differences were found between animals vaccinated either IM or IV.

In agreement to the presence of total BoHV-1 antibodies, detection of virus neutralizing antibodies (VN) started at 19 dpv in animals vaccinated IM and IV. Titers found for IM and IV groups were significantly higher than in the IN-vaccinated group ($p < 0.001$). No VN titers were detected in the IN-vaccinated, mock-vaccinated or sentinel groups (Figure 3a).

At 14 dpv, all three groups of animals vaccinated with BoHV-1ΔgEβgal were found negative for presence of gE specific antibodies. After challenge with BoHV-1 LA strain, only animals from two vaccinated groups (IN and IM) turned to be positive for the presence of gE-specific antibodies.

The BoHV-1 specific T lymphocyte stimulation was evaluated using the LPT. At 7 dpv, the percentages of calves with a positive response to the LPT assay depended on the infection route. In the BoHV-1ΔgEβgal IN group, all calves produced a positive LPT response, while 60% and 20% of the IM- and IV-vaccinated groups were positive responders, respectively (Figure 4a). At 72 dpv (30 dpc), a positive response was seen in 80% of the calves in the IN-vaccinated group, and in 40% of the IM-vaccinated group (data not shown). The results of IFNγ production were in agreement with the data obtained with the LPT. When the production of IFNγ was evaluated at 7 dpv the calves that received the vaccine by IN spray demonstrated greater levels of IFNγ compared to those which received the IM vaccine (Figure 4b). The levels of IFN-γ were significantly higher ($p < 0.05$) in those animals that received the live virus vaccine by IM and IN routes, than those receiving the inactivated virus vaccine. Surprisingly, no detectable INF-γ response was found for the group vaccinated via IV.

Virus shedding titers during the post-challenge period of BoHV-1ΔgEβgal-vaccinated animals were significantly lower ($p < 0.001$) than in mock-vaccinated animals. Virus shedding of animals vaccinated via IN- and or IM showed maximum individual titers of approximately $10^{5.5}$ $TCID_{50}$/ml. Mock-vaccinated calves shed virus for a period of 13 days and exhibited high individual titers ($10^{6.6}$ $TCID_{50}$/ml) (Figure 5a).

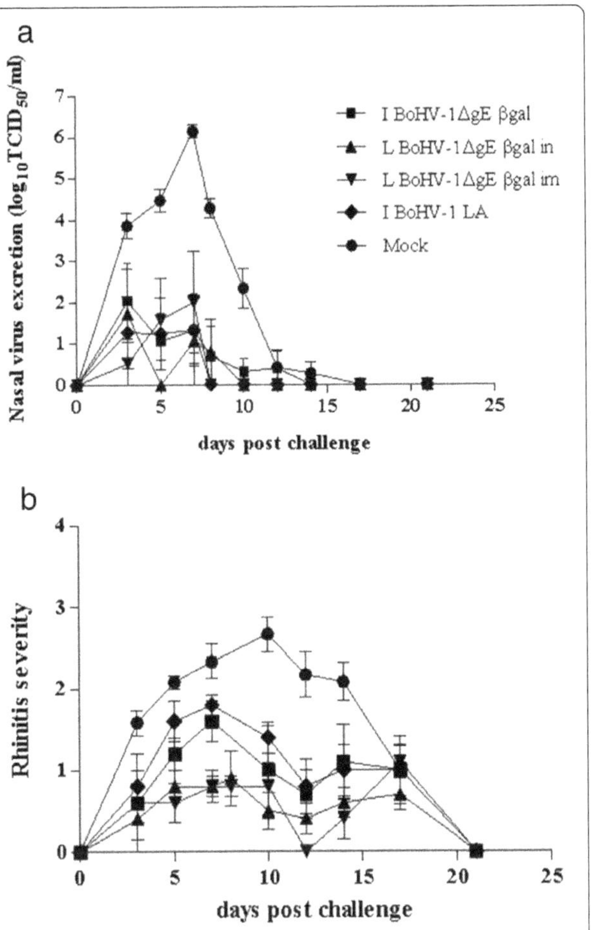

Figure 5 Values of virus shedding (a) and rhinitis severity (b) in vaccinated cattle after challenge. Virus shedding titers are expressed as log10 TCID50 per ml nasal fluid. **(b)** Each point in the graph is a average and SEM of the score taken in all the animals of each group. Rhinitis severity is score as follows: 0, absence; 1, slightly serous; 2, severely serous; 3, seromucous; 4, mucopurulent. References in this figure are as described in Figure 3.

Clinical analysis of the mock-vaccinated animals demonstrated the presence of symptoms, characterized by bilateral serous rhinitis observed at 2 dpc that increased in severity, as manifested by severe seromucous rhinitis (score 2–4) by 8–11 dpc, returning to normal by 22 dpc. All vaccinated animals, regardless of the route of inoculation, displayed significantly less severe symptoms, suffering slight serous rhinitis (score 1 to 2) or absence of rhinitis (score 0) ($p < 0.001$) in comparison with the mock-vaccinated group (Figure 5b). No apathy or loss of appetite was registered in the vaccinated animals.

Safety of BoHV-1ΔgEβgal LAV in pregnant animals

The pregnant cows that received the BoHV-1ΔgE-βgal virus by the IV route did not present abortions and all reached labor successfully. Animals only presented a transient and slight symptom manifestation of after the inoculation, without loss of appetite, depression or rise of body temperature. All the births reached term and none of the newborn calves showed detectable viral titers in their nasal secretions. Since their ninth day of life, we were able to detect in blood serum a titer of 1.6 of specific antibodies against BoHV-1 indicating the absorption of specific immunoglobulins from the maternal colostrum. BoHV-1ΔgE-βgal was shown to be completely innocuous not causing adverse collateral effects abortions/mummifications. Pregnant cows showed BoHV-1 specific antibody titers (≥ 1.6) until day 370 pv (data not shown). In addition, the LAV inoculated by IV route (group 3) induced long term immunity, since antibodies were detected during up to 370 days after a single immunization.

Discussion

We describe here the development of a βgal-expressing gE-mutated BoHV-1 strain (BoHV-1ΔgEβgal). We characterized the use of BoHV-1ΔgEβgal as an immunogen in the formulation of both inactivated and LAV against BoHV-1. It is shown that BoHV-1ΔgEβgal, when used in either formulation, elicits an efficient immune response that protects animals against challenge with virulent wild-type BoHV-1. Importantly, antibody responses induced by BoHV-1ΔgEβgal virus (inactivated or live) can be serologically distinguished from those induced by wild-type virus, even at long term time-points after being exposed to infectious virus (30 dpc).

The viral gE ORF in BoHV-1ΔgEβgal was completely removed with the exception of the first 23 bp in its 5′ end and the last 67 bp in its 3′ end, and the β-gal gene was inserted in its place. Thus, BoHV-1ΔgEβgal differs from the mutant virus previously described by van Engelenburg *et al.*, which carries a deletion of the complete gE gene based on the Lam strain [9]; from the mutant described by Rebordosa *et al.* [10] and from the recombinant strain developed by Chowdhury *et al.* that contains 372 of the 575 aa of gE [32].

The βgal marker gene was chosen to be incorporated in the genome in order to facilitate the identification of the virus both for selection of recombinant clones and for the potential use in identification of the agent in samples derived from vaccinated animals. Removing the whole gE ORF constitutes a safety feature of the novel BoHV-1ΔgEβgal strain which also resulted in virulence attenuation. Due to the length of the insert, the addition of a βgal expressing cassette (4.5 kb) reduces to the minimum the probability of reversion to wild type forms of the BoHV-1.

Despite efforts made to generate a revertant, we were not able to obtain one from BoHV-1ΔgEβgal. Thus, the parental strain BoHV-1 LA was used as control for all vaccination experiments.

The vaccination schedule followed for testing efficacy for the inactivated vaccines was based on the official schedule of vaccination using inactivated vaccines against IBR disease (National Sanitary Service, SENASA). The official schedule mentioned involves first vaccination and a booster immunization after 21 days. It is known that 6 months after immunization with an inactivated BoHV-1 vaccine, virus-specific antibodies drop to a minimum value. In order to work with the maximum astringency, the calves were maintained and monitored during 6 months until challenge. On the other hand, manipulation of animals immunized using a LAV is considered a biohazard by the official authorities (National Advisory Commission of Agronomic Biotechnology, CONABIA). Thus, the experiments should be performed in closure and only after obtaining the corresponding authorization. For that, animals were maintained in a Type II biosafety facility. The experiment lasted the minimum period of time (42 days) enough for the vaccinated animals to develop a detectable immune response of a similar level to the one found in the field.

Inactivated BoHV-1ΔgEβgal displayed similar virus shedding period and titers as those recorded for the wild-type-based inactivated vaccine. These results are comparable to those communicated by Bosch *et al.* [21] and Kaashoek *et al.* [16] and ourselves [26]. A thorough evaluation of the specific BoHV-1 humoral and cellular immune responses demonstrates the antigenic integrity of the glycoprotein E-deleted bovine herpesvirus type 1 strain. Importantly, BoHV-1ΔgEβgal-vaccinated bovines were easily differentiated from BoHV-1 LA-vaccinated animals, mock-vaccinated and BoHV-1-challenged animals, indicating the efficacy of inactivated BoHV-1ΔgEβgal as a marker vaccine.

BoHV-1ΔgEβgal as a LAV was highly immunogenic, inducing a humoral immune response comparable to those induced by previous BoHV-1 attenuated vaccines [2,11,15,18,32,33].

Significantly, BoHV-1ΔgEβgal induced an antibody response that could easily be differentiated from that elicited by parental wild-type BoHV-1 LA virus. During the post-vaccination period of both inactivated and LAV BoHV-1ΔgEβgal studies, no anti-gE antibodies were detected until after challenge with the wild-type BoHV-1 virus, thus demonstrating its suitability as a DIVA marker vaccine.

The aim of the present work was to evaluate safety in terms of vertical or horizontal spreading of a novel BoHV-1 marker strain. Thus, an extremely high dose of BoHV-1ΔgEβgal was used for immunization. The minimum immunogenic and protective dose for its use in a commercial vaccine will be determined in future experiments. Live BoHV-1ΔgEβgal exhibits a noticeable attenuation, no virus was detected in nasal secretions during the post-vaccination period. This performance was better than other BoHV-1 recombinant strains containing gE deletions [2,32,33], which showed virus shedding from 10^4 to 10^6 $TCID_{50}$/ml in a period from 6 to 8 days post-immunization. In order be considered safe, a LAV should not perpetuate in the cattle population [34]. Strube *et al.* reported that although the gE-deleted IBR vaccine strain Difivac® may be shed by immunized animals, it has a limited ability to pass from animal to animal [35]. In our study, although a high dose of virus was used to inoculate the animals ($10^{8.25}$ $TCID_{50}$/ml), no BoHV-1ΔgEβgal was recovered from the nasal secretions of vaccinated or sentinel animals although both groups cohabitated up to the 42 dpv. Furthermore, BoHV-1ΔgEβgal IV immunized pregnant cows did not transmit the recombinant virus to their newborns.

The IV route of inoculation is usually considered the most aggressive immunization or infection method during pregnancy, since it represents a direct access of any pathogen or drug to critical organs (ie, spleen, liver, lungs), and thus is the route of choice to test drug safety. Safety assays performed in pregnant cows demonstrated that vertical spreading of BoHV-1ΔgEβgal was null and newborn calves born to infected mothers showed detectable levels of anti-BoHV-1 maternal antibodies by day 9 after birth.

Two important features should be considered when comparing our results to those from Mars *et al.* their mutant virus did not carry a deletion of the complete gE ORF and cattle used in that study were 4 weeks-old calves [34]. Similar results were reported by van der Poel *et al.* using a BoHV-1ΔgE strain inoculated intramuscularly [36]. Once in the animals, BoHV-1ΔgEβgal showed absence of horizontal and vertical spreading most probably related to the low replication levels of the recombinant strain, although this should be clarified by future pathogenicity, latency and reactivation experiments.

Protection against challenge induced by the recombinant virus was evaluated in terms of reduction of clinical disease and, most importantly, reduction of shedding of challenge virus. Only half of the IM- or IN-vaccinated and challenged animals excreted virus, with titer values of $10^{2.6}$ to $10^{5.5}$ $TCID_{50}$/ml during a 2 day period. The levels of excreted virus in a post-challenge period were similar to those reported by other authors [2,11,15,17,18,33,35]. Even though animals vaccinated with inactivated BoHV-1ΔgEβgal showed higher VN titers than those immunized with live attenuated virus (IM or IN routes), no differences were found on virus shedding following BoHV-1 viral challenge. Remarkably, despite the fact that no detectable VN titers were found in circulating blood, the animals vaccinated by intranasal route with BoHV-1ΔgEβgal virus were protected against challenge. This result may probably related to the local induction of virus-specific immunity, as mentioned for individuals immunized with the inactivated BoHV-1ΔgEβgal virus, but needs to be further confirmed.

As a whole, our results showed that the BoHV-1ΔgEβgal may be used both as an inactivated immunogen or as a LAV against BoHV-1 infection in cattle. This recombinant virus elicited an efficient immune response with both strategies, which can protect animals from challenge with virulent wild-type BoHV-1 and may be serologically differentiated from that induced by wild-type virus. Safety assays demonstrated that BoHV-1ΔgEβgal was not horizontally or vertically transmitted when administered as a LAV, even when very high doses were utilized. The minimum immunogenic and protective dose for its use in a commercial vaccine will be determined in future experiments.

Conclusion

The BoHV-1ΔgEβgal strain is completely safe in terms of transmission to unvaccinated animals or environmental dissemination; BoHV-1ΔgEβgal is absolutely innocuous in pregnant cows and behaves as an attenuated BoHV1 strain in calves. Also, BoHV-1ΔgEβgal is protective against viral challenge and acts as an efficacious marker vaccine, since no antibodies were detected against gE protein during the post-vaccination period. Therefore, the new vaccine strain described here provides a useful combination of safety, attenuation, immunogenicity and DIVA capability.

Competing interests

The authors declare that there are no competing interests.

Authors' contributions

SR, MP and AS designed the experiments, analyzed the data. SR, MP and MB drafted the manuscript together. SR and MP performed the experiments. PDM, VQ, PZ and JBV helped with *in vivo* experiments. MB, SC and CC participated in the interpretation of data and preparation of the manuscript draft. All authors read and approved the final manuscript.

Acknowledgements

Special thanks to Dr. F. Maliandi for his constant support during the project. This research was supported by grant BID 802 OC-AR PMT/PIT nº 053 from SECYT- INTA-San Jorge Bagó, Argentina. We particularly thank Melanie Prarat and Dr. Mariano Perez Filgueira for the editing of the manuscript.

Author details

[1]Instituto de Virología Instituto de Virología, Centro de Investigaciones en Ciencias Veterinarias (CICV), Instituto Nacional de Tecnología Agropecuaria (INTA), Castelar, CC77, 1708 Morón, Argentina. [2]Fundacion Instituto Leloir-IIBBA, CONICET, Av. Patricias Argentinas 435, 1405 CABA, Argentina. [3]Instituto de Patobiología-CICVyA, INTA, Castelar CC77, 1708 Morón, Argentina. [4]Plum Island Animal Disease Center, APHIS, USDA, Greenport, NY 11944 USA. [5]Department of Pathobiological Sciences, School of Veterinary Medicine, Louisiana State University, Baton Rouge, LA 70803 USA. [6]Plum Island Animal Disease Center, ARS, USDA, Greenport, NY 11944 USA. [7]Universidad del Salvador, Buenos Aires, Argentina. [8]CONICET, Buenos Aires, Argentina.

References

1. Jones C, Chowdhury S: **A review of the biology of bovine herpesvirus type 1 (BHV-1), its role as a cofactor in the bovine respiratory disease complex and development of improved vaccines.** *Anim Health Res Rev/ Conference of Research Workers in Animal Diseases* 2007, **8**(2):187–205.
2. Kaashoek MJ, van Engelenburg FA, Moerman A, Gielkens AL, Rijsewijk FA, van Oirschot JT: **Virulence and immunogenicity in calves of thymidine kinase- and glycoprotein E-negative bovine herpesvirus 1 mutants.** *Vet Microbiol* 1996, **48**(1–2):143–153.
3. Tikoo SK, Campos M, Babiuk LA: **Bovine herpesvirus 1 (BHV-1): biology, pathogenesis, and control.** *Adv Virus Res* 1995, **45**:191–223.
4. Ellis JA: **Update on viral pathogenesis in BRD.** *Anim Health Res Rev/ Conference of Research Workers in Animal Diseases* 2009, **10**(2):149–153.
5. Muylkens B, Thiry J, Kirten P, Schynts F, Thiry E: **Bovine herpesvirus 1 infection and infectious bovine rhinotracheitis.** *Vet Res* 2007, **38**(2):181–209.
6. Babiuk LA, van Drunen L, van den Hurk S, Tikoo SK, Lewis PJ, Liang X: **Novel viral vaccines for livestock.** *Vet Immunol Immunopathol* 1996, **54**(1–4):355–363.
7. van Oirschot JT, Kaashoek MJ, Rijsewijk FA: **Advances in the development and evaluation of bovine herpesvirus 1 vaccines.** *Vet Microbiol* 1996, **53**(1–2):43–54.
8. Muylkens B, Meurens F, Schynts F, Farnir F, Pourchet A, Bardiau M, Gogev S, Thiry J, Cuisenaire A, Vanderplasschen A, *et al*: **Intraspecific bovine herpesvirus 1 recombinants carrying glycoprotein E deletion as a vaccine marker are virulent in cattle.** *J Gen Virol* 2006, **87**(Pt 8):2149–2154.
9. van Engelenburg FA, Kaashoek MJ, Rijsewijk FA, van den Burg L, Moerman A, Gielkens AL, van Oirschot JT: **A glycoprotein E deletion mutant of bovine herpesvirus 1 is avirulent in calves.** *J Gen Virol* 1994, **75**(Pt 9):2311–2318.
10. Rebordosa X, Pinol J, Perez-Pons JA, Lloberas J, Naval J, Serra-Hartmann X, Espuna E, Querol E: **Glycoprotein E of bovine herpesvirus type 1 is involved in virus transmission by direct cell-to-cell spread.** *Virus Res* 1996, **45**(1):59–68.
11. Kaashoek MJ, Rijsewijk FA, Ruuls RC, Keil GM, Thiry E, Pastoret PP, Van Oirschot JT: **Virulence, immunogenicity and reactivation of bovine herpesvirus 1 mutants with a deletion in the gC, gG, gI, gE, or in both the gI and gE gene.** *Vaccine* 1998, **16**(8):802–809.
12. Jacobs L, Kimman TG: **Epitope-specific antibody response against glycoprotein E of pseudorabies virus.** *Clin Diagn Lab Immunol* 1994, **1**(5):500–505.
13. Dingwell KS, Brunetti CR, Hendricks RL, Tang Q, Tang M, Rainbow AJ, Johnson DC: **Herpes simplex virus glycoproteins E and I facilitate cell-to-cell spread in vivo and across junctions of cultured cells.** *J Virol* 1994, **68**(2):834–845.
14. Rijsewijk FAM, Kaashoek MJ, Madic J, Paal H, Ruuls R, van Engelenburg F, van Oirschot JT: **In vivo and in vitro role of the non-essential glycoprotein gC, gG, gI and gE of bovine herpesvirus 1.** In *Proccedings of the symposium on IBR and other Rumiant Herpesvirus infections (abstract).* Liege Belgium: European Society for Veterinary Virology; 1995:27.
15. Kaashoek MJ, Moerman A, Madic J, Rijsewijk FA, Quak J, Gielkens AL, van Oirschot JT: **A conventionally attenuated glycoprotein E-negative strain of bovine herpesvirus type 1 is an efficacious and safe vaccine.** *Vaccine* 1994, **12**(5):439–444.
16. Kaashoek MJ, Moerman A, Madic J, Weerdmeester K, Maris-Veldhuis M, Rijsewijk FA, van Oirschot JT: **An inactivated vaccine based on a glycoprotein E-negative strain of bovine herpesvirus 1 induces protective immunity and allows serological differentiation.** *Vaccine* 1995, **13**(4):342–346.
17. Strube W, Auer S, Block W, Heinen E, Kretzdorn D, Rodenbach C, Schmeer N: **A gE deleted infectious bovine rhinotracheitis marker vaccine for use in improved bovine herpesvirus 1 control programs.** *Vet Microbiol* 1996, **53**(1–2):181–189.
18. Bosch JC, Kaashoek MJ, Kroese AH, van Oirschot JT: **An attenuated bovine herpesvirus 1 marker vaccine induces a better protection than two inactivated marker vaccines.** *Vet Microbiol* 1996, **52**(3–4):223–234.
19. Bosch JC, Kaashoek MJ, van Oirschot JT: **Inactivated bovine herpesvirus 1 marker vaccines are more efficacious in reducing virus excretion after reactivation than a live marker vaccine.** *Vaccine* 1997, **15**(14):1512–1517.
20. Bosch JC, De Jong MCM, Van Bree J, Van Oirschot JT: **Quantification of transmission of bovine herpesvirus 1 in cattle vaccinated with marker vaccines.** In *Bovine herpesvirus 1 marker vaccines: tools for eradication?* PhD-thesis. the Netherlands: Utrecht University; 1997:54–65.
21. Bosch JC, De Jong MC, Franken P: **An inactivated gE-negative marker vaccine and an experimental gD-subunit vaccine reduce the incidence of bovine herpesvirus 1 infections in the field.** *Vaccine* 1998, **16**(2–3):265–271.
22. Kerkhofs P, Renjifo X, Toussaint JF, Letellier C, Vanopdenbosch E, Wellemans G: **Enhancement of the immune response and virological protection of calves against bovine herpesvirus type 1 with an inactivated gE-deleted vaccine.** *Vet Rec* 2003, **152**(22):681–686.
23. Chowdhury SI, Kubin G, Ludwig H: **Equine herpesvirus type 1 (EHV-1) induced abortions and paralysis in a Lipizzaner stud: a contribution to the classification of equine herpesviruses.** *Arch Virol* 1986, **90**(3–4):273–288.
24. Chowdhury SI: **Construction and characterization of an attenuated bovine herpesvirus type 1 (BHV-1) recombinant virus.** *Vet Microbiol* 1996, **52**(1–2):13–23.
25. Southern EM: **Detection of specific sequences among DNA fragments separated by gel electrophoresis.** *J Mol Biol* 1975, **98**(3):503–517.
26. Romera SA, Hilgers LA, Puntel M, Zamorano PI, Alcon VL, Dus Santos MJ, Blanco Viera J, Borca MV, Sadir AM: **Adjuvant effects of sulfolipo-cyclodextrin in a squalane-in-water and water-in-mineral oil emulsions for BHV-1 vaccines in cattle.** *Vaccine* 2000, **19**(1):132–141.
27. Smitsaart EN, Bratanich AC, Ruiz M, Sardi S, Blancoviera FJ, Leon E, Gonzalez O, Pugliese M, Schudel A, Schudel AA: **Comportamiento inmunogénico de vacunas inactivadas polivalentes para herpesvirus bovino1.** *Rev Med Vet (Bs As)* 1987, **3**:148–154.
28. Parreño V, Romero SA, Makek L, Rodriguez D, Malacari D, Maidana S, Compaired D, Combessies G, Vena MM, Garaicoechea L, *et al*: **Validation of an indirect ELISA to detect antibodies against BoHV-1 in bovine and guinea-pig serum samples using ISO/IEC 17025 standards.** *J Virol Methods* 2010, **169**(1):143–153.
29. SAS Institute Inc: *SAS/STAT User's guide, Release 6.04.* Cary, NC 27512, USA: SAS Institute; 1988.
30. Rebordosa X, Pinol J, Perez-Pons JA, Lloberas J, Naval J, Querol E: **Mapping, cloning and sequencing of a glycoprotein-encoding gene from bovine herpesvirus type 1 homologous to the gE gene from HSV-1.** *Gene* 1994, **149**(2):203–209.
31. Leung-Tack P, Audonnet JC, Riviere M: **The complete DNA sequence and the genetic organization of the short unique region (US) of the bovine herpesvirus type 1 (ST strain).** *Virology* 1994, **199**(2):409–421.
32. Chowdhury SI, Ross CS, Lee BJ, Hall V, Chu HJ: **Construction and characterization of a glycoprotein E gene-deleted bovine herpesvirus type 1 recombinant.** *Am J Vet Res* 1999, **60**(2):227–232.
33. Belknap EB, Walters LM, Kelling C, Ayers VK, Norris J, McMillen J, Hayhow C, Cochran M, Reddy DN, Wright J, *et al*: **Immunogenicity and protective efficacy of a gE, gG and US2 gene-deleted bovine herpesvirus-1 (BHV-1) vaccine.** *Vaccine* 1999, **17**(18):2297–2305.
34. Mars MH, de Jong MC, van Oirschot JT: **A gE-negative BHV1 vaccine virus strain cannot perpetuate in cattle populations.** *Vaccine* 2000, **18**:2120–2124.
35. Strube W, Abar B, Bergle RD, Block W, Heinen E, Kretzdorn D, Rodenbach C, Schmeer N: **Safety aspects in the development of an infectious bovine rhinotracheitis marker vaccine.** *Dev Biol Stand* 1995, **84**:75–81.
36. van der Poel WH, Hage JJ: **[Spread of an intramuscularly administered live gE-negative BHV1 marker vaccine in 2 cattle farms].** *Tijdschr Diergeneeskd* 1998, **123**(4):109–111.

24

Long-distance aerial dispersal modelling of *Culicoides* biting midges

Debbie Eagles[1,2*], Lorna Melville[3], Richard Weir[3], Steven Davis[3], Glenn Bellis[4], Myron P Zalucki[2], Peter J Walker[1] and Peter A Durr[1]

Abstract

Background: Previous studies investigating long-distance, wind-borne dispersal of *Culicoides* have utilised outbreaks of clinical disease (passive surveillance) to assess the relationship between incursion and dispersal event. In this study, species of exotic *Culicoides* and isolates of novel bluetongue viruses, collected as part of an active arbovirus surveillance program, were used for the first time to assess dispersal into an endemic region.

Results: A plausible dispersal event was determined for five of the six cases examined. These include exotic *Culicoides* specimens for which a possible dispersal event was identified within the range of two days – three weeks prior to their collection and novel bluetongue viruses for which a dispersal event was identified between one week and two months prior to their detection in cattle. The source location varied, but ranged from Lombok, in eastern Indonesia, to Timor-Leste and southern Papua New Guinea.

Conclusions: Where bluetongue virus is endemic, the concurrent use of an atmospheric dispersal model alongside existing arbovirus and *Culicoides* surveillance may help guide the strategic use of limited surveillance resources as well as contribute to continued model validation and refinement. Further, the value of active surveillance systems in evaluating models for long-distance dispersal is highlighted, particularly in endemic regions where knowledge of background virus and vector status is beneficial.

Keywords: Culicoides, Bluetongue, Atmospheric dispersal modelling, Surveillance

Background

Culicoides (Diptera: Ceratopogonidae) are small, haematophagous insects present on all continents except Antarctica. Whilst their movements for host seeking, feeding and breeding are usually over distances of less than 2 km [1], they can be dispersed up to hundreds of kilometres by the wind [2]. This so-called long-distance dispersal is particularly important because *Culicoides* are vectors for a range of pathogens, including viruses, bacteria and protozoa, some of which cause disease in humans or animals [3]. It is for this reason that their long-distance movements have been extensively modelled, particularly with respect to transmission of livestock diseases.

One such disease of ruminant livestock is bluetongue disease (BT), caused by the arbovirus of the same name. Bluetongue virus (BTV), for which certain *Culicoides* species are the only confirmed vectors, is endemic in many tropical and sub-tropical regions of the world. Whilst disease outbreaks in these regions are rare, infection of susceptible ruminants in non-endemic regions often results in clinical disease, particularly in sheep [4]. Modelling of the long-distance dispersal of *Culicoides* vectors has predominantly focussed on such outbreaks of disease, in cases where dispersal of infected vectors is considered the most plausible route of virus transmission [5-8]. Recently, the pathways of dispersal of *Culicoides* into northern Australia, from eastern Indonesia, Timor-Leste and Papua New Guinea (PNG) have been modelled [9,10].

* Correspondence: Debbie.eagles@csiro.au
[1]CSIRO Animal, Food and Health Sciences, 5 Portarlington Rd, 3220 Geelong, Victoria, Australia
[2]School of Biological Sciences, The University of Queensland, 4072 Brisbane, Queensland, Australia
Full list of author information is available at the end of the article

Eagles *et al.*'s [10] analysis differed from previous analyses of long-distance *Culicoides* movement, in that retrospective assessment of a 15 year period was used to establish the likely spatio-temporal patterns of their dispersal within a BTV-endemic region.

Whilst aerial collections [11-14] have provided some evidence supporting the concept of long-distance dispersal of *Culicoides*, confirmation of their exact pathways of windborne movement is not currently possible [6]. For larger insects such as moths, migration pathways can be directly monitored using entomological radars [15,16] and, where applicable, these results can be used to validate predictive models [17]. Such radars are not yet sensitive enough to detect and distinguish *Culicoides*, which measure 1–3 mm in length [18]. Artificial tagging and recapturing can also be used to directly assess dispersal events [19]. Whilst *Culicoides* have been successfully tagged and recaptured, this has been attempted only for short vegetative flights, and even in these studies the recapture rates were very low (<0.5-2.1%) [1,20]. The primary evidence for *Culicoides* dispersal has been outbreaks of *Culicoides*-borne disease in non-endemic regions. In these cases, the date of onset of clinical signs, the implausibility of other means of virus introduction and the BTV status in possible source regions have been used, together with model outputs to build a case for the most likely dispersal pathways. More recently, genetic data have been used as evidence for the movement of haematophagous insects across long distances. Chapman *et al.* [21] demonstrated gene flow between mosquito populations from PNG and northern Australia, indicating the frequent movement of mosquitoes across the Torres Strait. Although genetic tools have yet to be explored for populations of Australian species of *Culicoides*, phylogeographical analyses have been used to demonstrate multiple incursions of *C. imicola* Kieffer into the northern Mediterranean basin from northern Africa [22].

In a BTV-endemic region, in the absence of clinical disease, the concept of evaluating predicted dispersal pathways is seemingly more difficult. However, by utilising the results of routine surveillance an independent assessment of the model is possible. In Australia, BTV is endemic in the north, where it does not currently cause clinical disease [23]. Despite this, the threat of incursion of a more pathogenic BTV, in addition to the ongoing requirement for monitoring to inform the implementation of live animal export protocols, necessitates regular, Australia-wide surveillance for BTV and its *Culicoides* vectors [24,25]. One specific objective of this surveillance is to provide early warning of incursions of exotic BTVs and *Culicoides* into the north [26]. In 2007, the first novel serotype detected in Australia for over 20 years, BTV-7, was isolated from sentinel cattle in the Northern Territory [27]. BTV-2 was detected for the first time the following year, in the same location [28]. Between 2009 and 2012, single specimens of exotic *Culicoides* species were collected in traps across northern Australia on four occasions (Bellis *et al.*, in prep).

Here we use all cases of novel BTV and exotic *Culicoides* detections in northern Australia since 2007 to evaluate the model of *Culicoides* movement established in the previous studies [10]. These incursions, and their associated pathways of dispersal, can be considered as supportive of the previous model's results. However, we also propose that such models cannot be fully 'validated' on surveillance (either active or passive) alone, but that surveillance and dispersal models can be used together to indicate likely patterns and pathways of dispersal, and to highlight areas requiring further research and surveillance.

Methods

The collections

All of the exotic *Culicoides* were identified in routine collections conducted by the National Arbovirus Monitoring Program (NAMP), except the two detections in the Torres Strait that were detected through the Australian Department of Agriculture's Northern Australia Quarantine Strategy (NAQS) program (Figure 1, Table 1) [29]. These collections make use of green LED light traps [30], generally set for 2–3 consecutive nights. All specimens are identified to species level [31] based on morphological characteristics.

Each of the novel BTVs were identified in routine collections from a NAMP sentinel herd at Beatrice Hill, approximately 50 km SE of Darwin (Figure 1). Blood was collected from each of the cattle for virus isolation on a weekly basis and serology on the same cattle was conducted monthly [27]. Sampling of animals was conducted under Charles Darwin University Animal Ethics Committee approval, Project A11033. Virus isolation was conducted in two parallel systems [32].

Collections of both vectors and viruses were made at a number of other NAMP sites in northern Western Australia (WA), Queensland (QLD) and the Northern Territory (NT) during the period in which these incursions took place (2007–2012) (Figure 1).

Dispersal windows

A hypothesised 'dispersal window' during which the incursion event was most likely to have occurred was determined for each detection (Table 1). For the exotic *Culicoides* collected, the duration of the dispersal window equated to the maximum lifespan of an adult insect, based on the assumption that the collected specimen itself was dispersed and collected. The length of the adult lifespan was set at 21 days, based on previous studies [18].

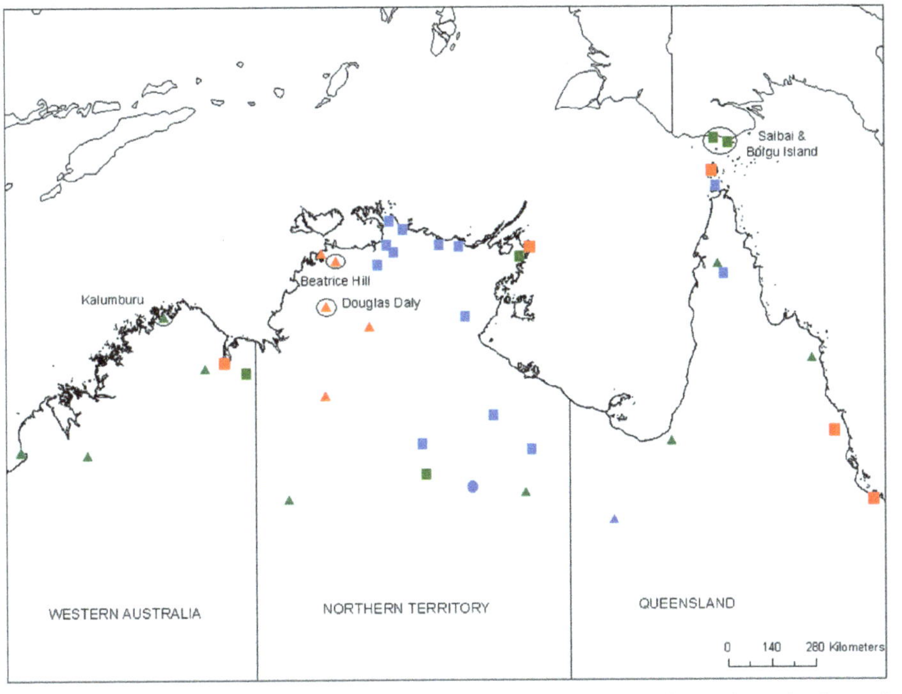

Figure 1 Map of northern Australia showing all sentinel herd and vector collection sites used during the evaluation period (2007–2012). Symbol shape represents the collections conducted at that site (circle – sentinel herd only, square – entomology only, triangle – both), colour represents the frequency of collections (red – regular (10-12/year), green – irregular (5-9/year), blue – rarely (4/year). Sites at which novel virus or exotic *Culicoides* have been collected, as listed in Table 1, are named and circled.

The dispersal window for the novel BTVs was set as all dates between the previous December up to two days prior to the collection date. The latter is to allow for the minimum period for detection of virus in the blood, which coincides with the incubation period (time between infection and onset of clinical signs, where present). The incubation period is host species and virus dependent, ranging from 2–8 days [33]. December was chosen as the start of the dispersal window as, based on previous studies, this appears to be the start of the seasonal incursion risk period [10].

The model

Within the dispersal windows likely dates of incursion were explored utilising the Hybrid Single Particle Lagrangian Integrated Trajectory Model (HYSPLIT) (Version 4), an atmospheric dispersion model (ADM). This model has previously been described [10] and elsewhere in more technical detail [34]. The model was used in particle mode for dispersion, which allows for transport of particles with mean wind and a random component to account for turbulence. The maximum allowable altitude was 1000 m, meaning that *Culicoides* particles transported beyond this height were no longer available to the model. Both 'dry' (gravitational) and 'wet' (rainfall) deposition were permitted.

Twenty hour back-trajectories were generated at 6-hourly intervals for the period under assessment (Figure 2). The clustering component of the HYSPLIT model was used to aggregate like-trajectories, as described in Eagles *et al.* [10]. Based on the direction and distance of the

Table 1 Collection dates, dispersal windows and likely dispersal dates (see text for details) for each of the *Culicoides* and BTV isolates

Species/Isolate	Collection date (site)	Previous collection at this site	Hypothesised dispersal window	Plausible dispersal dates
C. nudipalpis	22-24 Mar 2012 (Kalumburu)	22-24 Feb 2012	1-24 Mar	14-16 Mar
C. flavipunctatus	4-8 Nov 2010 (Saibai Is)	5-8 Oct 2012	14 Oct – 8 Nov	15-17 Oct
C. palpifer, C. flavipunctatus	5 May 2009 (Douglas Daly)	7-8 Apr 2009	14 April – 5 May	None
C. orientalis	24-27 Mar 2009 (Boigu Is)	23-26 Feb 2009	3 - 27 Mar	3-13 Mar, 17–22 Mar
BTV-2	10 Jan 2008 (Beatrice Hill)	3 Jan 2008	1 Dec 07–8 Jan	3-4 Jan
BTV-7	15 Mar 2007 (Beatrice Hill)	8 Mar 2007	1 Dec 06–13 Mar	14-16 Jan, 3–5 Mar

clustered trajectories, the potential source area was defined for each incursion and within this area, putative point source locations were specified. In the model *Culicoides* were 'released' from each of the putative source sites, at dusk and dawn on every date on which a dispersal event appeared possible, based on the back-trajectory results. A total of 1000 particles (representing *Culicoides*) were 'released' over a 3 hour period. The flight/dispersal time was set at 20 hours, based on previous studies which suggest dispersal up to this period may be possible [2]. Figures were generated in ArcGIS Desktop 10.1.

Meteorological input

The meteorological dataset used as input for the model was the Global Data Assimilation System (GDAS), available at three hour intervals with a global resolution of 1 degree latitude/longitude (approximately 100 km^2) [35]. The GDAS data is considered suitable for determining pathways of dispersal over long distances.

Results

An associated dispersal period and source region was determined for five of the six investigated incursions (Table 1, Figures 2, 3). Below we present the findings for each incursion.

Case 1: *C. nudipalpis* Delfinado, Kalumburu, 22–24 March 2012

Collections were made on the nights 22–24 March 2012 at a site near Kalumburu, on the northern coastline of WA [23]. The previous collection at this site was made on 22–24 February 2012. Almost 8000 *Culicoides* were collected in March (compared to fewer than 1000 in February), and all were identified to species level. *Culicoides austropalpalis* Lee & Reye was the most abundant species, with large numbers of *C. bundyensis* Lee & Reye and *C. brevitarsis* Kieffer (all established species) also collected. A single specimen was morphologically identified as the exotic species *C. nudipalpis*. Subsequent collections at Kalumburu did not yield further specimens of this species, although almost 4000 *Culicoides* were collected and identified in the following six months (Luke Halling, Senior Entomologist, NAQS, pers comm.).

The dispersal window was defined as 1–24 March and seven putative source sites were assessed, ranging from Denpasar, Bali in the west to West Timor in the east. From 14–16 March dispersal was possible to Kalumburu from as far west as Lombok and as far east as West Timor (Figure 2). *Culicoides nudipalpis* is known from all of these islands [36,37]. Whilst molecular analysis of Indonesian specimens of *C. nudipalpis* has not been possible, the WA specimen has been shown to be 99.6% similar to *C. nudipalpis* from neighbouring Timor-Leste, based on analysis of the cytochrome oxidase I (COI) gene (Bellis *et al.*, in prep).

Case 2: *C. flavipunctatus* Kitaoka, Saibai Island, 4–8 November 2010

A single female specimen of *C. flavipunctatus* was collected on Saibai Island in the Torres Strait in November 2010 [38]. The previous collection at this site was on 5–8 October 2010. At its northern most point, Saibai Island is less than 4 km from the PNG mainland. Despite this short distance, vegetative movements over an expanse of water would seem unlikely, although transport on vessels cannot be categorically ruled out.

The dispersal window was set at 15 October – 8 November. Based on 20 hour back-trajectories, dispersal is most likely to have occurred in the period 15–17 October, from southern PNG. Dispersal between the PNG mainland and Saibai Island may have occurred in less than one hour on 15 October 2010 (Figure 3A).

Case 3: *C. palpifer* Das Gupta & Ghosh and *C. flavipunctatus*, Douglas Daly, 5 May 2009

One female specimen each of *C. palpifer* and *C. flavipunctatus* were collected at Douglas Daly in NT in May 2009 [39]. The previous collection at this site was on 7–8 April 2009. There were no dates within the dispersal window (15

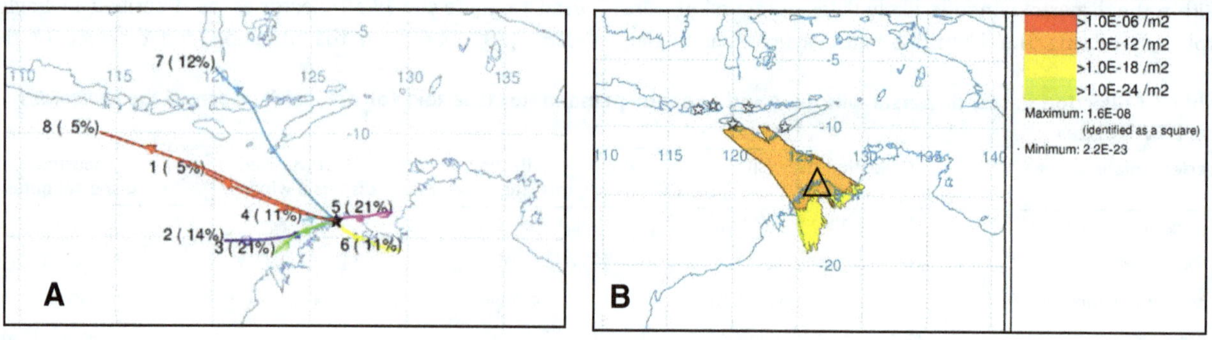

Figure 2 Method of assessment of dispersal pathways. A. Clustered back-trajectories from the incursion site. **B.** Source region defined and putative source sites selected (stars). Dispersal from the source sites at dusk and dawn assessed. Dispersal to Kalumburu (triangle) on 16 March 2012 is shown in this figure. The relative numbers of dispersed *Culicoides* are represented by the colours in the dispersal figure.

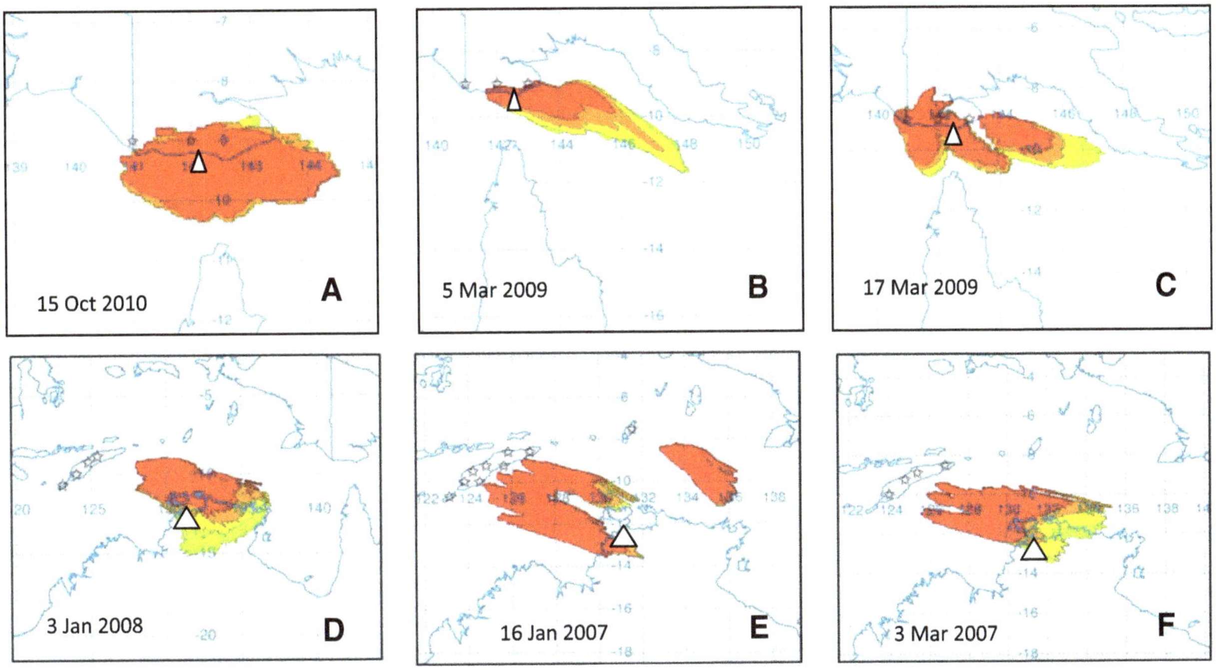

Figure 3 Representative dispersal events for *C. flavipunctatus* collected on Saibai Island (A), *C. orientalis* collected on Boigu Island (B, C), BTV-2 collected at Beatrice Hill (D), BTV-7 (E, F) collected at Beatrice Hill. The stars represent the putative source sites and the white triangle represents the collection site. The relative numbers of dispersed *Culicoides* are represented by the colours in the dispersal figure, with red the greatest number, followed by orange, yellow and light green.

April – 5 May) in which dispersal to the approximate site – or anywhere in NT - appeared possible from Timor-Leste, Indonesia or PNG. Both species (*C. palpifer* and *C. flavipunctatus*) are considered endemic across the region, having been collected across the Indonesian archipelago from West Java to West Papua [40].

In order to further explore this case, a number of alternative possibilities were investigated. Firstly the flight duration in the model was increased to 30 hours. Again, no likely dispersal dates or source sites were identified. To allow for the possibility that both collected specimens may have been part of newly established populations, as opposed to the actual dispersed individuals, the dispersal window was extended to include the entire 'high risk' period (December-March) prior to the collection, as well as the start of April. Dispersal to the vicinity of the collection site did not appear likely during this period. Dispersal to more northern sites in NT did appear possible in December 2007, January and February 2008 (Figure 4).

Case 4: *C. orientalis* Macfie, Boigu Is, 24–27 March 2009

A single specimen of *C. orientalis* was collected on Boigu Island in the Torres Strait in March 2009 [39]. The previous collection on at this site was on 23–26 February 2009. This island is in less than 4 km from the PNG mainland.

Dispersal from the southern PNG mainland appears to have been possible on a number of occasions within the dispersal window (between the dates of 2–13 and 17–22 March). As with the incursion on Saibai Island, dispersal is likely to have occurred in less than 20 hours (Figure 3B, C).

Case 5: BTV-2, Beatrice Hill, 10 January 2008

The first BTV-2 detected in Australia was from a sentinel cow at Beatrice Hill on 10 January 2008 [39]. By May 2008, more than half of the sentinel herd were positive for BTV-2. The virus was also detected in samples from cattle at Douglas Daly in the same season.

The modelling indicates that dispersal to the vicinity of the collection site could have occurred one week (3–4 January) prior to sample collection, from a site within West Timor (Figure 3D). Recent full genome analysis of the prototype Australian BTV-2 showed that eight of the ten genome segments were more closely related to Asian than Australian viruses [28], supporting the conclusion that this virus is a recent introduction. Surveys of ruminants for BTV antibodies in Indonesia in the 1990s detected serological reactors to BTV-2, suggesting exposure to this serotype [41] and in the source region.

Case 6: BTV-7, Beatrice Hill, 15 March 2007

Australia's first isolate of BTV-7 came from a blood sample collected on 15 March 2007 from a sentinel cow at

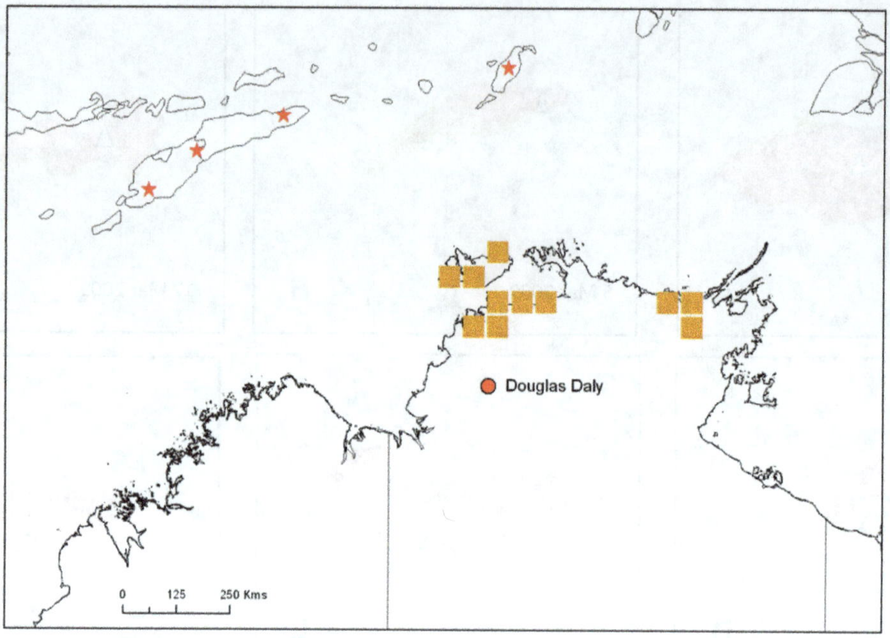

Figure 4 Dispersal to northern NT in December 2008-February 2009, prior to the collection of two exotic specimens (Case 3) at Douglas Daly (red circle). The orange squares represent grid cells to which dispersal in the model appears possible during these months; red stars represent the putative source sites.

Beatrice Hill [27]. The previous sample collection from this herd was on 8 March 2007, one week earlier. BTV-7 was subsequently detected in another three of the 24 sentinel cattle between 19 April and 28 June 2007 but was not detected in any other NT sentinel herd in that season [27]. The next detection of BTV-7 was in 2010.

A potential dispersal event occurred approximately two weeks (3–5 March) prior to sample collection (Figure 3F), from sites across West Timor and Timor-Leste, as well as two months (14–16 Jan) prior (Figure 3E), from the same source region. BTV-7 has previously been isolated from cattle in Indonesia [42].

Discussion

To date, all previous aerial dispersal modelling of *Culicoides* has been in the context of emergency animal disease outbreaks. In this study we have used, for the first time, results of routine ('active') arbovirus surveillance to strengthen predictions made by an ADM of *Culicoides* long-distance dispersal in a non-disease context. A likely or possible source and period of incursion was identified for five of the six cases evaluated. In each of these cases, modelling indicated that dispersal could possibly have originated from within the previously predicted source region spanning the Indonesian archipelago east of Lombok across to southern PNG and including the island of Timor. Of these five incursions, all but one was likely to have occurred in either January or March, within the previously described 'high risk' period of dispersal [10] for *Culicoides* into Australia. The incursion outside of this period and the case which could not be resolved using the model are discussed below.

The detection of *C. flavipunctatus* on Saibai Island in October is outside of the 'high risk' period of December-March proposed by Eagles *et al.* [10]. However, that study assessed dispersal into mainland Australia, approximately 150 km further south of Sabai Island and it is conceivable that dispersal events are both more frequent and across a broader 'season' for the short distance between southern PNG and the islands of the Torres Strait. It is likely that secondary dispersal from these islands into mainland Australia is restricted to the previously determined 'high risk' period. This distinction may be important if an exotic species of *Culicoides* or novel virus becomes established on one of the islands.

In the case of the specimens collected at Douglas Daly (Case 3), no site of origin from outside Australia (given their exotic status) or date of incursion could be determined. This makes it an important case to explore further in relation to the sensitivity of the surveillance system and the input parameters to the model. The *Culicoides* 'flight' duration in this study was set at 20 hours and dispersal to five out of six sites appears possible within this timeframe. However, it has previously been shown that this input parameter is the one to which the model system is most sensitive [10]. Whilst dispersal beyond 20 hours may be possible, the Douglas Daly case was re-evaluated in the model with a 30 hour dispersal duration (results not shown) with still no identification of a likely source site outside of Australia. Based on previous studies [9,10], a dispersal duration of longer than this seems highly unlikely, but this may be an important area for further research. Secondly, consecutive dispersal events where a single insect arrives at one site in Australia then subsequently moves to a different site and enters a trap may be possible and, again, this is an area where future studies could assist with ongoing model validation and confidence in model predictions. A constraint with the model set-up that may have contributed to the inability to identify a dispersal event for this case is the low resolution of the meteorological data, although over the long distances evaluated this is less likely to have an impact.

Additionally, the sensitivity of the light trap network as a surveillance system for exotic *Culicoides* species must be considered, with the implication that the detected specimens may have been part of an already established population. Although the network of traps in northern Australia is extensive (Figure 1) there are a range of factors that can affect the sensitivity of vector surveillance, including trap- and species-specific factors, meteorological conditions at time of trapping and proximity of traps to established *Culicoides* populations [30,43,44]. Interestingly, the Douglas Daly specimens were collected outside of the previously described 'high risk' incursion period, but they have not been collected at any site within the NAMP network since their first detection and it appears unlikely either species has established in Australia.

In both cases of novel virus detection presented in this paper a possible incursion date was identified within the ten days prior to sample collection. This time is considered sufficient for a dispersed (infected) vector to find, bite and infect a mammalian host and for the minimum incubation period to be met in that host. It is also concurs with the period between likely dispersal event and onset of clinical signs in a BTV outbreak in Sweden [6]. In the case of BTV-7, a dispersal event may also have occurred two months prior to its detection. Given the highly variable biological nature of BTV viruses [25] including variation in infection rates and virus persistence [32], it is difficult to determine which of the two identified dispersal events was the more likely incursion event.

The question arises, can detections in sentinel herds and vector traps (forms of 'active' surveillance) be used equally well for model appraisal as outbreak data (a form of "passive" surveillance), which has been so heavily relied upon previously for assessment of *Culicoides* dispersal? Due to the number of sentinel herds, the frequency of testing, and the use of supplementary sero-surveys, the sensitivity for virus detection is reportedly high [32]. Collection of vectors, by one method only (trapping), is perhaps less sensitive, although it is likely that if a dispersed species becomes established it will ultimately be detected. The sensitivity of passive surveillance, which is reliant on the onset of clinical signs, is also not infallible. Incursion of BTV into a non-endemic zone typically results in infection of susceptible ruminants, but even in these areas infection can occur in the absence of clinical signs of disease. Whilst BTV-8, first detected in Europe in 2006, caused clinical disease in cattle, the presentation of clinical signs in this species is rare, and they are generally considered a silent reservoir for the virus. Even with BTV-8, morbidity in cattle was significantly lower than in sheep, and in infected herds in the Netherlands, only 2.5% of cattle developed clinical signs [45]. Thus, it is possible that the exact date of incursion may not be identified in all cases, dependent on the livestock present at the arrival site, the susceptibility of these to expression of clinical disease and the disease reporting and surveillance mechanisms in place. The importance of this has also previously been noted by Agren [5] and is highlighted in the case of BTV-8 detection in cattle in Norway, based on bulk milk testing rather than clinical signs [6].

As mentioned in the introduction, rigorous 'validation' of these models by use of entomological radars or mark/recapture techniques is currently not feasible. The concept of model evaluation has been extensively discussed and debated in the ecological sciences [46] and has recently been reviewed with respect to epidemiological models in veterinary science [47]. Model evaluation should be considered as following a continuum or spectrum, starting with initial technical verification, followed by acceptance of the model concepts. An example of the latter for dispersal models may include that the insect of interest has been caught at altitude or is able to fly for many hours in laboratory conditions. This is followed by validation, for example by assessment against field data, as shown here, or, as mentioned previously, use of radars or mark/recapture techniques. Validation may also include comparison against other models ('relative validation') and sensitivity analysis, which can show to which parameters a model is most sensitive [47]. All these steps lead toward either operational use (as is the aim for many models) and/or the point where a model can be considered "an adequate respresentation of the real system" [46,47] (Figure 5).

Where there is no "conclusive" evidence to validate a model, multiple pieces of information may be combined to support (or otherwise) the model results. With specific respect to insect incursions, Kim [48] proposed a multidisciplinary approach to determining the source of boll weevils collected in an eradication zone. The approach incorporated the results of a model for wind dispersal, along with genetic population analyses of boll weevils caught in the eradication zone and at proposed source sites, and profile analysis of pollen collected on/in the insects [48]. In doing so, they suggested that the application of a multidisciplinary approach increased their confidence in elucidating the source of the incursion.

In two cases presented in this paper – one virus, one vector - genetic analysis of the collected specimen and comparison with conspecific Australian and regional material equivalents [28] (Bellis *et al.*, in prep) supports the suggestion that these are (recent) incursions. Clearly, more substantive genetic analysis of both viruses and vectors within the region is necessary to pinpoint the specific sources of *Culicoides* and the viruses they transmit. If such information were available, a similar multidisciplinary approach as used for boll weevils could be applied to *Culicoides* dispersal – combining field data (such as onset of clinical signs in disease outbreaks or collections from sentinel/vector sites), serological status of surrounding herds, analysis of wind dispersal in an ADM and genomic (population genetics and/or specific marker) analysis.

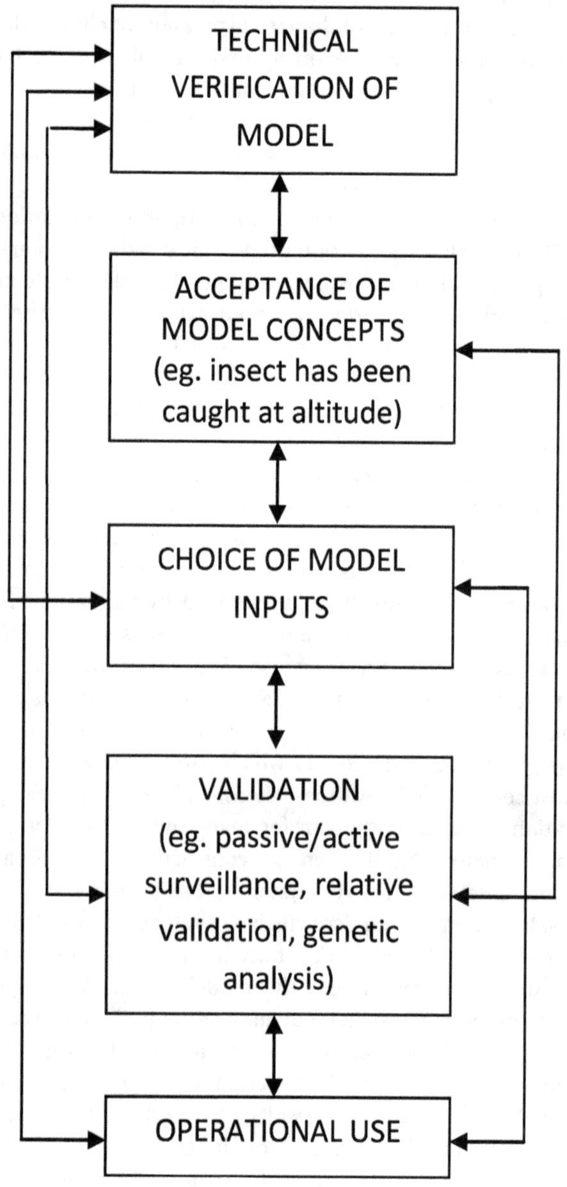

Figure 5 Steps in model evaluation as they pertain to insect vector dispersal models, adapted from Reeves *et al.*, [47].

Finally, comparison between incursion detections (both virus and vector) and predictions by the model of the possible frequency of such events are indicative of an "over-prediction" of events by the model. During the period from January 2007-March 2010 there were four detected incursions in total (two virus, two vector), yet in Eagles *et al.*'s [10] previous analysis fourteen possible dispersal events were predicted from the entire source region into Australia. The discrepancy is likely due to a combination of factors, most notably the requirement of more than "just a dispersal event" to occur for successful incursion and detection. Dispersed *Culicoides* must survive long enough on arrival to be caught in a trap or, for successful BTV transmission, to bite a susceptible host. For BTV transmission to occur also requires the vector to be infected at origin – itself dependent on BTV circulation in ruminants at source. Thus, the model framework presented in the previous paper [10], and substantiated here with incursion data, should be considered as indicating the spatial and temporal nature of *dispersal*, and the *relative* frequency of such dispersal from specific source sites, and to arrival regions. As noted above, if the sensitivity of surveillance is not perfect, then some dispersal events predicted by the model – resulting in incursion of vector with or without virus – may not be detected. Additionally, in this paper only novel *serotypes* of BTV and exotic species of *Culicoides* have been investigated. Incursions of BTVs of the same serotype or species of *Culicoides* as those already established in Australia may be expected to occur. Evidence for this comes from the detection of novel *genotypes* of the virus (based on sequencing of segment 3 of the genome) in northern Australia [49]. Subsequent detections of new genotype/serotype combinations may also be incursion events but due to the propensity for genome segment reassortment in BTVs, they cannot be distinguished from reassortments of endemically circulating viruses.

Conclusions

This study has shown that active surveillance can be used in collaboration with results of an ADM to assess the spatial and temporal nature of *Culicoides* dispersal into an endemic region. Previously, retrospective use of such models has primarily been in response to the presentation of clinically affected animals in outbreaks of disease. Where BTV is already endemic, the concurrent use of an ADM alongside existing BTV and *Culicoides* surveillance may help guide the strategic use of limited surveillance resources as well as contribute to continued model validation and refinement. The same methodology can be applied to other arboviruses with windborne vectors and their relevant surveillance systems.

Competing interests

The authors declare that they have no competing interests.

Authors' contributions

Conceived and designed the experiments: DE, MPZ, PJW, PAD. Conducted modelling: DE. Contributed data for case study: LM, RW, SD, GB. Wrote the paper: DE. All authors contributed to editing, and read and approved the final manuscript.

Acknowledgements

We thank Drs. Peter Daniels and David Williams for critical review of the manuscript. We acknowledge all contributors of the National Arbovirus Monitoring program and the Northern Australian Quarantine Strategy for access to surveillance data and scientific advice and to the staff of the Berrimah Veterinary Laboratory and the Australian Animal Health Laboratory for testing of the virus samples. Debbie Eagles conducted this work as part of her doctoral studies which were funded by the Australian Biosecurity Cooperative Research Centre.

Author details

[1]CSIRO Animal, Food and Health Sciences, 5 Portarlington Rd, 3220 Geelong, Victoria, Australia. [2]School of Biological Sciences, The University of Queensland, 4072 Brisbane, Queensland, Australia. [3]Department of Primary Industry and Fisheries, Berrimah Veterinary Laboratories, GPO Box 3000, 0801 Darwin, Northern Territory, Australia. [4]Department of Agriculture, Northern Australia Quarantine Strategy, PO Box 37846, 0821 Winnellie, Northern Territory, Australia.

References

1. Lillie TH, Marquardt WC, Jones RH: **The flight range of *Culicoides variipennis* (Diptera, Ceratopogonidae).** *Can Entomol* 1981, **113**:419–426.
2. Sellers RF, Pedgley DE, Tucker MR: **Possible spread of African horse sickness on the wind.** *J Hyg (Lond)* 1977, **79**:279–298.
3. Mellor P, Carpenter S, White D: **Bluetongue virus in the insect host.** In *Bluetongue. Volume 3.* Firstth edition. Edited by Mellor P, Baylis M, Mertens P. Paris: Elsevier: Biology of Animal Infections; 2009:483.
4. Maclachlan NJ: **The pathogenesis and immunology of bluetongue virus infection of ruminants.** *Comp Immunol Microb* 1994, **17**:197–206.
5. Agren ECC, Burgin L, Sternberg Lewerin S, Gloster J, Elvander M: **Possible means of introduction of bluetongue virus serotype 8 (BTV-8) to Sweden in August 2008: comparison of results from two models for atmospheric transport of the *Culicoides* vector.** *Vet Rec* 2010, **167**:484–488.
6. Burgin LE, Gloster J, Sanders C, Mellor PS, Gubbins S, Carpenter S: **Investigating incursions of bluetongue virus using a model of long-distance *Culicoides* biting midge dispersal.** *Transbound Emerg Dis* 2012, **60**:263–272.
7. Garcia-Lastra R, Leginagoikoa I, Plazaola JM, Ocabo B, Aduriz G, Nunes T, Juste RA: **Bluetongue virus serotype 1 outbreak in the Basque Country (Northern Spain) 2007–2008. Data support a primary vector windborne transport.** *PLoS ONE* 2012, **7**:e34421.
8. Gloster J, Burgin L, Witham C, Athanassiadou M, Mellor PS: **Bluetongue in the United Kingdom and northern Europe in 2007 and key issues for 2008.** *Vet Rec* 2008, **162**:298–302.
9. Eagles D, Deveson T, Walker PJ, Zalucki MP, Durr P: **Evaluation of long-distance dispersal of *Culicoides* midges into northern Australia using a migration model.** *Med Vet Entomol* 2012, **26**:334–340.
10. Eagles D, Walker PJ, Zalucki MP, Durr PA: **Modelling spatio-temporal patterns of long-distance Culicoides dispersal into northern Australia.** *Prev Vet Med* 2013, **110**:312–322.
11. Hardy AC, Cheng L: **Studies in the distribution of insects by aerial currents. 3. Insect drift over the sea.** *Ecol Entomol* 1986, **11**:283–290.
12. Johansen CA, Farrow RA, Morrisen A, Foley P, Bellis G, Van Den Hurk AF, Montgomery B, Mackenzie JS, Ritchie SA: **Collection of wind-borne haematophagous insects in the Torres Strait, Australia.** *Med Vet Entomol* 2003, **17**:102–109.
13. Sanders CJ, Gubbins S, Mellor PS, Barber J, Golding N, Harrup LE, Carpenter ST: **Investigation of diel activity of *Culicoides* biting midges (Diptera: Ceratopogonidae) in the United Kingdom by using a vehicle-mounted trap.** *J Med Entomol* 2012, **49**:757–765.
14. Sanders CJ, Selby R, Carpenter S, Reynolds DR: **High-altitude flight of *Culicoides* biting midges.** *Vet Rec* 2011, **169**:208.
15. Chapman JW, Drake VA, Reynolds DR: **Recent insights from radar studies of insect flight.** *Ann Rev Entomol* 2011, **56**:337–356.
16. Reynolds DR, Chapman JW, Harrington R: *The migration of insect vectors of plant and animal viruses.* Elsevier, Waltham, MA, USA: Academic Press; 2006.
17. Leskinen M, Markkula I, Koistinen J, Pylkko P, Ooperi S, Siljamo P, Ojanen H, Raiskio S, Tiilikkala K: **Pest insect immigration warning by an atmospheric dispersion model, weather radars and traps.** *J App Ent* 2011, **135**:55–67.
18. Mellor PS, Boorman J, Baylis M: ***Culicoides* biting midges: Their role as arbovirus vectors.** *Annu Rev Entomol* 2000, **45**:307–340.
19. Pedgley DE: **Windborne spread of insect-transmitted diseases of animals and man.** *Philos Trans R Soc Lond B Biol Sci* 1983, **302**:463–470.
20. Kirkeby C, Bodker R, Stockmarr A, Lind P, Heegaard PMH: **Quantifying Dispersal of European Culicoides (Diptera: Ceratopogonidae) Vectors between Farms Using a Novel Mark-Release-Recapture Technique.** *PLoS ONE* 2013, **8**(4):1.
21. Chapman HF, Hughes JM, Ritchie SA, Kay BH: **Population Structure and Dispersal of the Freshwater Mosquitoes Culex annulirostris and Culex palpalis (Diptera: Culicidae) in Papua New Guinea and Northern Australia.** *J Med Entomol* 2003, **40**:165–169.
22. Nolan DV, Dallas JF, Piertney SB, Mordue Luntz AJ: **Incursion and range expansion in the bluetongue vector Culicoides imicola in the Mediterranean basin: a phylogeographic analysis.** *Med Vet Entomol* 2008, **22**:340–351.
23. Animal Health Australia, 2013: *National Arbovirus Monitoring Program 2011–2012 Annual Report.* 2013. http://www.animalhealthaustralia.com.au/programs/disease-surveillance/national-arbovirus-monitoring-program/namp-archived-reports/ (accessed 1 February 2013.
24. Animal Health Australia: *National Arbovirus Monitoring Program.* 2013. http://www.animalhealthaustralia.com.au/programs/disease-surveillance/national-arbovirus-monitoring-program/ (accessed 1 February 2013).
25. Melville LF: **Bluetongue surveillance methods in an endemic area: Australia.** *Veter Ital Ser* 2004, **40**:184–187.
26. Animal Health Australia, 2011: *National Arbovirus Monitoring Program 2009–2010 Annual Report.* 2013. http://www.animalhealthaustralia.com.au/programs/disease-surveillance/national-arbovirus-monitoring-program/namp-archived-reports/ (accessed 1 February 2013).
27. Melville L, Davis S, Hunt N, Weir R, Harmsen M, Walsh S: **Isolation of bluetongue serotype 7 from sentinel cattle in the Northern Territory.** In *Arbovirus Research in Australia Tenth Symposium; Coffs Harbour.* Edited by Ryan PA, Aaskov JG, Russell R. Australia: QIMR; 2008:99–101.
28. Boyle DB, Bulach DM, Amos-Ritchie R, Adams MM, Walker PJ, Weir R: **Genomic sequences of Australian bluetongue virus prototype serotypes reveal global relationships and possible routes of entry into Australia.** *J Virol* 2012, **86**:6724–6731.
29. Animal Health Australia, 2001: *The history of bluetongue, Akabane and ephemeral fever viruses and their vectors in Australia 1975–1999.* 2013. http://www.animalhealthaustralia.com.au/ (accessed 1 February 2013).
30. Bishop AL, Bellis GA, McKenzie HJ, Spohr LJ, Worrall RJ, Harris AM, Melville L: **Light trapping of biting midges *Culicoides* spp. (Diptera: Ceratopogonidae) with green light-emitting diodes.** *Aust J Entomol* 2006, **45**:202–205.
31. Kirkland PD, Ellis T, Melville LF, Johnson SJ: **Australian National Arbovirus Monitoring Program - a model for studying bluetongue epidemiology in China.** In *Proceedings of the First Southeast Asia and Pacific Regional Bluetongue Symposium; Kunming, China.* Edited by St George TD, Kegao P. Kunming, China: ACIAR; 1995:95–99.
32. Melville L, Hunt N, Weir R, Davis S, Harmsen M: **Results of a decade of virus monitoring of sentinel cattle in the Northern Territory (1994–2004).** In *Arbovirus Research in Australia Ninth Symposium; Noosa Lakes.* Edited by Ryan PA, Aaskov JG. St George TD, Dale PE: QIMR; 2005:240–245.
33. Animal Health Australia, 2008: *Disease Strategy: Bluetongue (Version 3.0) Australian Veterinary Emergency Plan (AUSVETPLAN).* 2013. http://www.animalhealthaustralia.com.au/ (accessed 1 February 2013.).
34. Draxler RR, Hess GD: **An overview of the HYSPLIT_4 modelling system for trajectories, dispersion and deposition.** *Aust Meteorol Mag* 1998, **47**:295–308.

35. NOAA: *HYSPLIT - Hybrid Single Particle Lagrangian Integrated Trajectory Model.* 2011. http://www.arl.noaa.gov/HYSPLIT_info.php (accessed 9 January 2012).
36. Sukarsih, Sendow I, Bahri S, Pearce M, Daniels PW: ***Culicoides* survey in Indonesia.** *Aciar Proc* 1995, 123–128.
37. Bellis G, Melville L, Walsh S: **Preliminary assessment of the vector capacity of *Culicoides nupipalpis* and *C. orientalis* for Bluetongue virus.** In *Arbovirus Research in Australia Ninth Symposium; Noosa Lakes.* Edited by Ryan PA, Aaskov JG. St George TD, Dale PE: QIMR; 2005:28–32.
38. Animal Health Australia: *National Arbovirus Monitoring Program 2010–2011 Annual Report.* 2012. http://www.animalhealthaustralia.com.au/programs/disease-surveillance/national-arbovirus-monitoring-program/namp-archived-reports/ (accessed 1 February 2013).
39. Animal Health Australia: *National Arbovirus Monitoring Program 2008–2009 Annual Report.* 2009. http://www.animalhealthaustralia.com.au/programs/disease-surveillance/national-arbovirus-monitoring-program/namp-archived-reports/ (accessed 1 February 2013).
40. Sukarsih, Daniels PW, Sendow I, Soleha E: **Longitudinal studies of *Culicoides* associated with livestock in Indonesia.** In *Arbovirus Research in Australia Sixth Symposium; Brisbane.* Edited by Uren MF, Kay BH. Indonesia: CSIRO, QIMR; 1993:203–209.
41. Daniels P, Sendow I, Pritchard LI, Sukarsih, Eaton BT: **Regional overview of bluetongue viruses in South-East Asia: viruses, vectors and surveillance.** In *Bluetongue, Proceedings of the Third International Symposium; Taormina.* Edited by Maclachlan J, Pearson JE. South-East Asia: Veterinaria Italiana; 2004:94–100.
42. Sendow I, Daniels P, Soleha E, Hunt N, Ronohardjo P: **Isolation of bluetongue viral serotypes 7 and 9 from healthy sentinel cattle in west Java, Indonesia.** *Aust Vet J* 1991, **68:**405–406.
43. Bellis GA, Melville LF, Hunt NT, Hearnden MN: **Temporal activity of biting midges (Diptera : Ceratopogonidae) on cattle near Darwin, Northern Territory, Australia.** In *Bluetongue - Proceedings of the Third International Symposium; Taormina.* Edited by Maclachlan J, Pearson JE. ; 2004:324–328.
44. Carpenter S, Szmaragd C, Barber J, Labuschagne K, Gubbins S, Mellor P: **An assessment of *Culicoides* surveillance techniques in northern Europe: have we underestimated a potential bluetongue virus vector?** *J Appl Ecol* 2008, **45:**1237–1245.
45. Elbers AR, Backx A, Mintiens K, Gerbier G, Staubach C, Hendrickx G, van der Spek A: **Field observations during the bluetongue serotype 8 epidemic in 2006. II. Morbidity and mortality rate, case fatality and clinical recovery in sheep and cattle in the Netherlands.** *Prev Vet Med* 2008, **87:**31–40.
46. Rykiel EJ: **Testing ecological models: The meaning of validation.** *Ecol Model* 1996, **90:**229–244.
47. Reeves A, Salman MD, Hill AE: **Approaches for evaluating veterinary epidemiological models: verification, validation and limitations.** *Rev Sci Tech Oie* 2011, **30:**499–512.
48. Kim KS, Jones GD, Westbrook JK, Sappington TW: **Multidisciplinary fingerprints: forensic reconstruction of an insect reinvasion.** *J R Soc Interface* 2010, **7:**677–686.
49. Pritchard LI, Sendow I, Lunt R, Hassan SH, Kattenbelt J, Gould AR, Daniels PW, Eaton BT: **Genetic diversity of bluetongue viruses in south east Asia.** *Virus Res* 2004, **101:**193–201.

Management of the slowly emerging zoonosis, Hendra virus, by private veterinarians in Queensland, Australia

Diana H Mendez[1*], Jenny Kelly[2,3], Petra Buttner[4], Madeleine Nowak[2] and Rick Speare[1,4]

Abstract

Background: Veterinary infection control for the management of Hendra virus (HeV), an emerging zoonosis in Australia, remained suboptimal until 2010 despite 71.4% (5/7) of humans infected with HeV being veterinary personnel or assisting a veterinarian, three of whom died before 2009. The aim of this study was to identify the perceived barriers to veterinary infection control and HeV management in private veterinary practice in Queensland, where the majority of HeV outbreaks have occurred in Australia.

Results: Most participants agreed that a number of key factors had contributed to the slow uptake of adequate infection control measures for the management of HeV amongst private veterinarians: a work culture characterised by suboptimal infection control standards and misconceptions about zoonotic risks; a lack of leadership and support from government authorities; the difficulties of managing biosecurity and public health issues from a private workforce perspective; and the slow pattern of emergence of HeV. By 2010, some infection control and HeV management changes had been implemented. Participants interviewed agreed that further improvements remained necessary; but also cautioned that this was a complex process which would require time.

Conclusion: Private veterinarians and government authorities prior to 2009 were unprepared to handle new slowly emerging zoonoses, which may explain their mismanagement of HeV. Slowly emerging zoonoses may be of low public health significance but of high significance for specialised groups such as veterinarians. Private veterinarians, who are expected to fulfil an active biosecurity and public health role in the frontline management of such emerging zoonoses, need government agencies to better recognise their contribution, to consult with the veterinary profession when devising guidelines for the management of zoonoses and to provide them with greater leadership and support. We propose that specific infection control guidelines for the management of slowly emerging zoonoses in private veterinary settings need to be developed.

Keywords: Veterinarians, Emerging infectious disease, Zoonoses, Hendra virus, Infection control, Management, Behavioural change, Queensland

Background

Hendra virus (HeV) is amongst a plethora of zoonoses emerging as new infectious threats to animal as well as human health [1]. HeV first emerged in 1994 in Brisbane, Queensland, Australia [2,3]. HeV is a paramyxovirus carried by pteropid bats with low infectivity to other susceptible species [4,5]. However, the virus can sporadically spillover from its natural reservoir to horses with secondary spillover to humans in some instances. HeV has high fatality rates in both species, 75% and 57% respectively [6]. Humans can become infected with HeV when exposed to blood and bodily fluids from an infected horse [2,3,7-11]. In 2011, a dog became infected with HeV but did not develop any clinical signs prior to being sacrificed [12]. Since 1994 there have been a relatively low number (49) of self-limiting outbreaks along the eastern coast of Australia between northern New South Wales and Far North Queensland [6]. These outbreaks resulted in the deaths of 90 horses and a total of three non-fatal and four fatal human infections [6]. So

* Correspondence: Diana.Mendez@jcu.edu.au
[1]College of Public Health, Medical and Veterinary Sciences, James Cook University, Townsville, QLD 4811, Australia
Full list of author information is available at the end of the article

far, all human HeV cases have occurred between August 1994 and September 2009 in Queensland [6].

HeV infection in humans can be prevented by avoiding contact with infected horses or avoiding exposure to infected substances by implementing infection control (IC) measures such as using personal protective equipment (PPE) [13]. Administration of monoclonal antibodies during the incubation period has been shown to prevent experimentally induced HeV disease in ferrets and non-human primate models and this has also been used in humans exposed to HeV as an experimental prophylaxis [14]. A vaccine for horses became available in late 2012 and was promoted for the protection of horse populations from HeV and humans from secondary spillover [15,16].

Since the emergence of HeV the veterinary profession has paid the highest price with the death of two veterinarians, a veterinary assistant and the non-fatal infection of a veterinarian and a veterinary nurse [2,3,6-11]. As a result of these HeV-related deaths, Federal and State governments and professional agencies initiated an IC and HeV management campaign targeted at equine veterinary practices. Despite the early information campaigns about HeV related risks and risk mitigation strategies targeting private veterinarians, the last two human cases of HeV occurred as late as 2008 and 2009 and proved fatal for two veterinarians, one of whom had recently attended a HeV management workshop [6,9-11]. Additionally, an Australian study conducted in early 2010 by a State government agency showed that IC and HeV management practices in private equine veterinary clinics were still sub-optimal particularly when carrying out high risk procedures (such as dental procedures, endoscopy of the upper respiratory or urinary tracts or endotracheal intubation) with high likelihood of exposure to oral, respiratory and urogenital bodily fluids from a healthy or a sick horse [17]. As a result, government authorities and veterinary professional agencies questioned why private veterinarians were still becoming infected with HeV. In mid to late 2010, in an attempt to promote changes in HeV management and related IC behaviours, the Queensland government sent a new comprehensive HeV management information package to all private veterinarians registered in Queensland (Dr B. Pott, personal communication).

The aim of this paper is to explore the barriers to IC and HeV management in private practices prior to September 2010 as perceived by equine veterinarians and allied staff in Queensland, Australia.

Methods

Research protocol

The purpose of this qualitative study was to identify and understand the factors affecting IC and HeV management in veterinary private practices in Queensland, Australia. This study was conducted as an exploratory, descriptive design using semi-structured interviews. This method was chosen in order to gain an in-depth understanding of the perceptions and experiences related to the management of HeV and IC implementation in private practices in Queensland [18-20]. No adequate research tool had been previously developed to conduct such a study in the context of HeV emergence. After consultation with major stakeholders involved in the management of HeV (private equine veterinary practitioners, lecturers in equine medicine and representatives from professional and State government agencies) a series of open-ended interview questions were formulated to explore HeV related risk perceptions as well as barriers to IC and HeV management in equine veterinary practices in Queensland. The interview questions were piloted with one equine veterinarian and questions modified accordingly.

Between December 2009 and September 2010 individual, face-to-face interviews were conducted with 21 veterinary personnel from 14 veterinary practices in rural and urban areas along the eastern coast of Queensland, Australia. Interviews were semi-structured to allow the in-depth exploration of issues relating to barriers to IC and HeV management in the context of their veterinary work as perceived by the participating veterinary staff [20]. This project was conducted with the approval of the James Cook University Human Ethics Committee (permit H3513) and complied with qualitative research guidelines on relevance, appropriateness, transparency and soundness of research methodology (RATS) [21,22].

Recruitment and interview protocols

Participation was voluntary and participants could withdraw from the study at any time. Prospective suitable veterinary practices were identified from public phone directories and their associated advertisements and web links. Potential participants were initially contacted by phone, by the lead interviewer (DM), at which time the purpose and protocol of the study were explained to them by the researcher. Prospective participants were subsequently provided via e-mail with a project information sheet and explanations about what would be required of them at the time of the interview. Some declined to participate without further explanation while others were "too busy" or suspicious of the research process. Upon agreement to participate, a suitable interview date, time and location for each participant were organised. At the time of the interviews, the lead interviewer (DM) provided further information about the project and the study protocol when requested by a participant prior to the signing of the consent form. In particular, many participants were concerned about retaining anonymity and wished to ascertain their responses would remain unidentified. This was assured. Prior to commencing each interview, participants were required to provide socio-demographic and professional profile information such as the type of practice they worked in, their role in the practice, an estimation of percentage of their working time spent providing veterinary services to horses and their experience with HeV outbreaks. Recruitment of new participants ceased when data saturation was reached; i.e., interviews stopped yielding new perspectives. This occurred after interview number 18.

Participants

The target population were veterinary personnel working in private practice in Queensland. The eligibility criteria were: 1) working in private veterinary practice providing veterinary services to either horses exclusively (i.e., equine practice) or to horses as well as to other large and small domestic animals (i.e., mixed practice); 2) working within the known geographic distribution area of HeV in Queensland: the eastern coast between the Far North and the Queensland-New South Wales border [23]. In order to collect a comprehensive range of views within the target population, participants, with different socio-demographic and professional profiles, were purposively selected from regions where HeV outbreaks had occurred (South East; Central; North; and Far North of Queensland). The final study population comprised 21 participants from a total of 14 mixed private veterinary practices. According to the Australia Rural, Remote and Metropolitan Areas (RRMA) classification system nine participants were from areas classified as metropolitan, nine were from rural areas and three were from remote areas [24]. The majority of participants (18) were veterinarians; two were experienced female veterinary nurses and one was a male practice manager who although having no direct involvement with equine patients, worked in a practice with a strong equine component. In most cases, the first point of contact during the recruitment process was the principal veterinarian owner of the practice. More than half the veterinarians interviewed were principal veterinarians (10) of whom only one was female. Interviews with principal veterinarians lasted, on average, longer (75.6 minutes) than interviews with other participants (46 minutes). The remaining eight veterinarians were partners/associates or employees, five of whom were female. Females were on average younger and aged between 31 and 48 years old while males were aged between 28 and 63 years old. This was reflected in the difference of the average number of years since graduation between males (mean = 26.4 yrs, range: 4–40 yrs) and females (mean = 13.1 yrs; range: 4–27 yrs). Excluding the practice manager, on average, females spent proportionally less of their working time than males attending to horse patients (30.4% vs 52.1%). Prior to this study there had only been 13 confirmed outbreaks of HeV with one outbreak occurring during the data collection period [6]. However, more than half of the participants (60%) had dealt with at least one suspected case of equine HeV and over a third (35%) had dealt with at least one confirmed equine HeV case prior to being interviewed. Further details of this study population have been described elsewhere [25-27].

Data collection

For convenience, the majority of interviewees chose to be interviewed in an office at their place of work or in their own homes. The interviews were conducted by the lead author (DM), a female veterinarian with research skills in qualitative interview techniques, who was well aware of the issues under investigation, with a research assistant participating in some interviews. With written consent from each participant, responses were recorded as digital audio files with complementary hand written notes. Participants were asked to share their experiences when dealing with HeV and what, in their opinion, were the barriers to IC and WHS compliance. At the conclusion of each interview, the notes were read back to each participant to give them the opportunity to clarify or amend their responses. Audio files were later transcribed and entered into qualitative data analysis software (NVivo qualitative data analysis software; QSR International Pty Ltd. Version 9, 2010). After each interview, the interviewer reviewed the notes and recorded a number of reflections capturing the context of each interview. Interviews took between 40 and 160 minutes, with an average time of 64 minutes.

Data analysis

Prior to analysis, each participant was identified using a unique alphanumeric code (V* for veterinarians, VN* for veterinary nurses and PM* for practice manager) and a unique alphanumeric veterinary practice code (P*). Thematic analysis was used to analyse the qualitative data [28]. Interview transcripts were analysed with NVivo (QSR International Pty Ltd. Version 9, 2010) for repeating units of meaning and the main themes and sub-themes were conceptualised using inductive thematic analysis [20,28]. This process was repeated on more than one occasion with identified themes discussed and agreed upon by three of the researchers (DM, RS, JK). Two of the researchers were veterinarians and thus were able to review the themes within the context of private veterinary practice and the emergence of HeV and its management.

Results

Data analysis revealed six main themes expressing the participants' responses about the difficulties associated with the implementation of adequate IC and HeV management in private veterinary practices between the first outbreak in 1994 and the time of the interviews (2009–2010) (Table 1).These themes are: the emerging epidemiology of

Table 1 Main themes surrounding the topics of barriers to infection control and Hendra virus management in private veterinary practices identified in Queensland, Australia, between 2009 and 2010, as illustrated by participants' quotes

Themes	Examples of quotes from participants' responses which best illustrate the themes
The emerging epidemiology of the virus	*"When the first case of Hendra came about, it was seen as being rare so we didn't see* [it] *as a problem."* (V3/Pa)
	"It would have been better to have known more about the virus. Where do you draw the line when you don't know enough about the risks and the non-risks?" (V4/Pc)
	"The drive [for IC*] *needs to be continuous…HeV cases are seldom, so it's easy for people to be slack, to back off from infection control."* (V10/Pg)
	"The biggest challenge is how to manage a hospital facility for horses, because the case definition is not clear…Our biggest concern…a horse that shows up without Hendra on the differential list and it [HeV#] *shows up on the list later."* (V16/Pl)
	"This is a disease that is here to stay….so we have to learn to live with it." (V15/Pk)
Risk perception determines risk mitigation	*"Some think that Hendra is only a North Queensland problem and that it wouldn't happen in South Queensland or northern New South Wales."* (V7/Pa)
	"I didn't think a great deal about it [HeV] *because I studied in Victoria and it was presented to us as a disease only found in Queensland."* (V14/Pj)
	"No way in the world would I put a mask or gloves on unless I saw something dramatic."(V13/Pi)
	"You will not get a primary Hendra case with a horse living in a stable." (V1/Pa)
	"At the time [before HeV], *human safety was not being kicked* [by a horse patient], *not being trampled on, avoiding any physical injury…Zoonoses were not a big one on my list."* (V14/Pj)
	"Seeing a mate die I think is enough. Obviously you think of self-preservation. I have a life to live…Dying is a pretty big cost." (V5/Pd)
Risk and risk mitigation communication	*"There were no guidelines in place in regards to what* [protective] *equipment should be worn…there was information on what samples were needed but not how to take them."* (V14/Pj)
	"The trouble with AVA† is that there is only 50% membership…weekends are when the AVA has the workshops and that is when we have a lot of work on here." (V15/Pk)
	"Most vets would receive information through email. Some think it's not enough but some of those don't read their emails." (V1/Pa)
	"They [people at the DPI‡] *are excellent. The DPI is the most authoritative source of knowledge because they have been dealing with the issues and they are responsible for biosecurity."* (V15/Pk)
	"The local DPI were useless, almost burying their heads in the sand. They didn't have enough knowledge, were unwilling to investigate and had a lack of resources and people." (V9/Pf)
	"I contacted Biosecurity Queensland on a Saturday afternoon…They transferred me on the phone 19 times to talk to a vet… they have to realise that private vets work 24/7…This disease is too serious to be ignored…they should have been more responsive. It would have been easier to put the horse in a hole and forget about it!" (V5/Pd)
	"I find great difficulty dealing with owners because it is a power play and ultimately we are responsible for the safety of all involved but some owners don't believe that, which compromises the legal situation. We usually end up with less authority out of concern for the welfare of the animal." (V4/Pc)
	"By the time you get to the horse you are only the 3rd or 4th opinion…A lot of people around here are gung ho who [think they] *know better."* (V5/Pd)
	"Some owners burr at the cost…He [the owner] *said 'if you want to test the horse why don't you pay for it'."* (V14/Pj)
	"[The owner said] *I don't want them tested for Hendra. If they turn up positive they'll have to be put down. My horses are like my children and I wouldn't euthanase my own children."* (V9/Pf)
Education and work culture	*"Students are very well aware of the risks to the point of being scared to do things."* (V7/Pa)
	"These days young vets lack confidence around horses because of their lack of experience through their training and personal life." (V1/Pa)
	"Coming out of Uni the biggest issue was not whether I could follow protocols it was getting the practice of using those protocols." (V17/Pm)
	"[I]*had been inadequately trained* [about HeV] *when studying in Victoria* [another state] *…I didn't realise that interstate* [studies] *did not offer the same information. Some things should not be disregarded in the curriculum because it doesn't happen in that area."* (V14/Pj)
	"Hopefully they [the students] *will go into practice in clinics where they follow best practice."* (V7/Pa)
	"Poor mentorship is a problem. Training is very important. A principal vet can teach a lot to younger vets." (V8/Pe)
	"I think overall we, as vets, were pretty grubby...to get around with blood on your shirt all day that is just what veterinarians did." (V16/Pl)

Table 1 Main themes surrounding the topics of barriers to infection control and Hendra virus management in private veterinary practices identified in Queensland, Australia, between 2009 and 2010, as illustrated by participants' quotes *(Continued)*

	"Old school vets always considered getting infected with a zoonosis as a badge of honour." (V8/Pe)
	"The biggest obstacle is trying to retrain someone who has done something a certain way for 30 odd years." (V13/Pi)
	"The culture needs to change…[but]*…change won't happen overnight. Human medicine was hit in the 1980s* [by HIV[Ω]], *it sparked infection control improvement but it's still not perfect now. The* [veterinary] *profession has to change but this will take time."* (V8/Pe)
Use of Personal Protective Equipment	*"If I am going to be completely honest, a few years ago there would be no way I'd put it* [PPE[◊]] *on."* (V13/Pi)
	"We have always been casual about horses. In cattle you have brucellosis but I have never been worried about catching anything from horses." (3/Pa)
	"The right PPE … was not available at the clinic at the time. PPE was still not considered to be an issue at the time." (V10/Pg)
	"You can read the protocol all you like but until you actually do it and take the gear off under the assumption that you are contaminated it is not an easy thing to do." (V12/Ph)
	"By following the DPI protocol it took us two hours before the animal was finally sedated." (V4/Pc)
	"PPE can be cumbersome…smelling the breath of a horse gives you an idea of what's going on. If you are wearing a mask it makes it difficult." (V11/Pg)
	"The ability to move properly…can be a problem. When you have to deal with horses with fractures you have to move quickly!" (V10/Pg)
	"The biggest obstacle: heat and humidity…When you are wearing the full PPE it can be very hot." (V6/Pa)
	"I hate masks, they press on the bottom of my eyes and I can't see…I won't wear goggles it's too difficult with my glasses." (V5/Pd)
	"Comfort and practicability is an issue for me because one size fits none!!…PPE suits are baggy on me, with a lot of flapping about and this scares horses." (V7/Pa)
	"During the EI[§] campaign I had to vaccinate between 800 and 1000 horses and at each farm I had to put on a new set of PPE so it's not a big issue for me." (V2/Pb)
	"Cost is a big one. You have to pass the cost on. The bill can be a lot dearer than before and if the horse turns out negative, the owner will whinge about the money spent." (V5/Pd)
	"We are lucky in that our clients are used to spending money on their horses." (V12/Ph)
	"It is potentially dangerous…to have two people walk up [to a horse] *looking like spacemen with their clothes rustling and their voices distorted."* (V12/Ph)
	"Vets like me don't want to be seen with over the top PPE…in more rural situations you tend to think you are being a bit of a Wally[silly] *dressed up for minor issues."* (V10/Pg)
	"…You felt silly in front of other colleagues to be wearing all the gear." (V3/Pa)
	"Clients could be a driving force behind it [IC] *because they would start questioning why some vets use PPE and others don't."* (V1/Pa)
Running a private veterinary practice	*"When you have a big backlog of work there is time pressure… your logistics are stretched…many cases end up being emergency cases at the end of the day, which is a recipe for disaster because you start cutting corners and making mistakes."* (V4/Pc)
	"Vets are often busy and to get through a large case load is hard enough, let alone stopping to put protective gear on." (V16/Pl)
	"Cost is an issue …Do you then transfer the cost onto the owner? What if the case turns out negative? How do you justify it?" (VN2/Pe)
	"There would be cases out there that have not been reported because of the cost…I think this puts people at risk. As long as it is hurting the pocket of the clients or the pocket of the vet, cases will go unreported." (V14/Pj)
	"In the hospital system everything is …disposable. If we had to treat everything as disposable our cost would increase… The industry would suffer from it." (V3/Pa)
	"As vets we don't have the luxury of the health system behind us to make [IC] *decisions, we don't have a large buying power… for vets the one size fits all approach doesn't work".* (V8/Pg)
	"You look at the paper trail that they [WHS[¥] authorities] *say you need to have…you would have to employ somebody full time for six months to put it in place."* (V12/Ph)
	"As an employer you can do everything in your power and you can make all the recommendations but it comes down to the individual and if the individual doesn't have Hendra on their mind there is not much you can do." (V14/Pj)

Table 1 Main themes surrounding the topics of barriers to infection control and Hendra virus management in private veterinary practices identified in Queensland, Australia, between 2009 and 2010, as illustrated by participants' quotes *(Continued)*

	"Legally the only way you could send a staff to a property is if on the day the employer went to that property and addressed the risks and said it was safe to work there, because the conditions from yesterday might not apply today." (V9/Pf)
	"More positive cases are going to land in our hospitals…Infection control is imperative but what scares me is the unknown [when HeV is not readily suspected]*."* (V16/Pl)
	"The DPI[‡] *contacted me to do this work and they weren't being flexible about it: they wanted me there and then. This was [8 months ago] …I am still waiting for my money! Next they'd have to pay me up front."* (V5/Pd)
	"Everyone's fear is you'll act to the best of your ability and you'll act in the best interest of everyone involved but later your actions will be audited by someone who has never worked in a vet practice and has no idea of the pressures at play and who will apply the letter of the law and potentially cost you your livelihood." (V12/Ph)
	"I don't talk to local [WHS] *officers anymore because they don't have enough knowledge. This immediately established a low level of credentials with us. Everything after that we see it more as an inconvenience."* (V8/Pe)

*IC: Infection control; #HeV: Hendra virus; †AVA: Australian Veterinary Association; ‡DPI: Department of Primary Industries; ΩHIV: Human Immunodeficiency Virus; ◊PPE: Personal protective equipment; §EI: Equine influenza; ¥WHS: Workplace health and safety.

HeV; risk perception determines risk mitigation; risk and risk mitigation communication; education and work culture; personal protective equipment; and running a private veterinary practice.

Each theme included a number of subthemes that are illustrated in Table 1 by selected quotes from participants' responses. The quotes included in Table 1 were selected as best illustrations of the themes and subthemes identified in this study.

The emerging epidemiology of the virus

Many participants were initially not overly concerned about HeV; the sporadic occurrence of equine cases and the rarity of human cases separated by long periods of time belied the seriousness of the epidemic. When HeV first emerged, participants reported that they and others in the profession failed to recognise the significance of this new zoonosis. Most participants felt that in the first few years of HeV emergence, there was insufficient knowledge about the disease and its epidemiology to adequately assess and therefore manage the risks involved. Nevertheless, when HeV began recurring more regularly, participants started implementing HeV management strategies, although these strategies were not always sustained over time. Another major stumbling block identified by many participants was the difficulty associated with the clinical diagnosis of the disease in horses. As some participants pointed out, the case-definition of HeV is non-specific and there can be substantial variations in clinical presentations which rendered the initiation of a HeV management plan difficult. Furthermore, an asymptomatic horse did not always equate to a healthy uninfected horse as it could be in the late incubation period of the disease during which viral shedding is possible. In 2010, however, most participants agreed that HeV was likely to recur in the future and that they needed to adopt a sustainable HeV management plan.

Risk perception determines risk mitigation

Participants who failed to mitigate the HeV-related risks often perceived the risk of being exposed to HeV to be low. Their risk perceptions were initially based on geographic consideration. This viewpoint echoed that of other participants who recalled that prior to 2010 there was an ongoing belief that occurrence of HeV would be restricted to specific geographic areas outside of which the likelihood of HeV spilling over was low as was the risk of exposure. This belief seemed to be perpetuated outside the initial affected state of Queensland. Participants who had studied or started their career in other states were not overly concerned about HeV.

Hendra virus was generally perceived to be a more significant risk by participants if they initially included it in their differential diagnosis, which in turn determined their HeV management attitudes. However, many participants reported that prior to the last fatal human case in 2009, they did not perceive the HeV-related risk to be high unless the symptomatology of a horse was severe and that they would only have considered taking precautions in extreme clinical cases. Some participants were confident they could rule out HeV, and the related risks, on clinical examination alone despite HeV having a non-specific case definition. Another common belief amongst participants was that HeV could only spillover into horses kept in paddocks and therefore, examining a horse kept in a stable represented a low HeV risk.

Participants also prioritised risk management according to risk likelihood. Because of their experience prior to the emergence of HeV, many participants perceived the risk of contracting an infectious disease in equine practice significantly lower than sustaining a serious injury from a horse. Conversely, the HeV-related infectious risk appeared to be of greater relevance for participants who had had direct dealings with early HeV positive cases or personally knew one of the people who had been infected with HeV. For example, one participant, who had dealings with one of the early outbreaks, became more circumspect when dealing with sick horses; while another participant was reconsidering the viability of managing equine cases after losing a close colleague to HeV.

Risk and risk mitigation communication

At the time this study was conducted, participants were seeking and receiving information about the HeV from government and professional agencies such as the department of primary industries (DPI)/Biosecurity Queensland, the Australian Veterinary Association (AVA) and Equine Veterinarians Australia (EVA). However, not all information was perceived as complete, useful, specific or practical enough in assisting them with HeV management in the field. Additionally, not all information was accessible by all veterinarians. Some modes of information delivery, such as emails, were described as being ineffective in reaching the entirety of its target population; and professional associations could only reach their veterinary membership.

The majority of participants from or around large urban centres were mostly satisfied with the support they received from government agencies in charge of biosecurity. In contrast, participants from rural and remote areas were mostly dissatisfied with the level of support they received from the local representatives of the same government agencies. Government officers from these areas were perceived as lacking capacity, knowledge and experience.

Some participants from rural and remote areas further cautioned that the lack of responsiveness from the government at the local level could lead in some instances to potential cases of HeV going unreported and/or uninvestigated.

Risk and risk mitigation communication also occurred between veterinary staff and horse owners. Some participants found risk communication with horse owners challenging as some clients were not receptive to veterinary directives about HeV-related risks. Many participants thought that the three main reasons for horse owners to refuse veterinary decisions were due to denial of the risk, cost issues and emotional attachment between owners and their animals.

Education and work culture

Australian and overseas educated early career veterinarians who worked in the participating practices were mostly perceived by interviewees as being well informed about IC and HeV related risks. However, a number of participants thought that some undergraduate Australian veterinary students and newly graduated veterinarians lacked experience and confidence in applying IC and animal handling skills. Some participants recalled their own lack of confidence in applying IC principles earlier in their career which they thought was due to insufficient practical experience and variability in veterinary curricula between universities.

Other participants questioned the role of senior private veterinarians overseeing the practical training of veterinary students on extramural placements and early career veterinarians. Professional mentorship was reported as having a pivotal effect on veterinary IC training. In some instances, poor professional mentorship was deemed responsible for undergraduate students and early career veterinarians failing to adopt and develop adequate IC standards.

Participating senior veterinarians thought that their IC attitudes and beliefs about veterinary occupational risks, which were now considered suboptimal, were the norm at the beginning of their career. This enduring work culture was viewed as a major obstacle to IC improvement in veterinary practice as it required a drastic change in the way veterinarians thought, behaved and made decisions. However, most participants, regardless of how long they had worked in private practice, recognised that veterinary IC required amelioration but warned that it would take some time before this occurred.

Use of personal protective equipment (PPE)

A number of participants, who began their career before the emergence of HeV, pointed out that prior to 1994 the use of PPE in equine practice was not a common occurrence. Some thought the lack of experience with zoonotic risk in equine practice led to the belief that the use of PPE for the management of HeV was not critical. By 2010 all participants were using some form of PPE in combination with other IC strategies to mitigate the risk of exposure to HeV and/or other zoonoses. However, some participants still found it difficult to use PPE routinely in equine practice. Participants gave a range of reasons why they thought the use of PPE presented some drawbacks: it sometimes hindered their ability to work efficiently, competently, safely and comfortably; or was deemed unsuitable for reasons of fit. Interestingly, participants who had repeatedly used PPE during the equine influenza outbreaks and vaccination campaigns did not perceive the use of PPE in equine practice to be an issue.

Some participants also thought that the systematic use of PPE had the disadvantage of increasing the running cost of a consultation which affected the veterinary practice as well as the client, although not all participants viewed the added PPE-related cost as a big issue.

A number of participants were also concerned about the way they were perceived by their patients, clients and colleagues when they wore PPE and the effect this would have on their workplace health and safety (WHS) and their professional credibility. Other participants thought that the clients who perceived the use of PPE as positive work practice could be a driving force behind equine veterinary practices more readily adopting the use PPE.

Running a private veterinary practice

Time management was an issue for most veterinarians interviewed who reported that implementing additional IC measures affected work schedule, quality and safety. The extra time spent implementing additional IC measures was also reported to affect consultation fees. Many participants further explained that any additional cost, such as costs related to the management of HeV, needed to be justifiable to clients as it often affected their level of satisfaction with veterinary services provided. Cost was perceived by many participants as a limiting factor to the management of HeV from a client's and a business perspective.

Some participants highlighted the discrepancies that existed between the business models of veterinary practices and public medical hospitals for people. They pointed out that veterinary practices were small businesses operating solely privately unlike medical hospitals and therefore could not be run as sustainably because of cost and logistical considerations.

Many participants were principal veterinarians who had the added responsibility of ensuring that the running of their practice, including the management of potential HeV cases, complied with the WHS legislation. However, many found that compliance was not easily achieved and in some instances hindered the running of the practice. The need to document WHS policies and procedures, training and incidents, for example, was perceived as unwelcomed extra work. The need to ensure the health and safety of staff who were not always receptive to warnings and instruction was viewed as another major challenge to compliance. Some participants thought that the legislation was open to interpretation; thus making it difficult to always comply. Many participants also felt that because compliance was not legally protective they remained vulnerable to unexpected situations. Although, most participants were aware that they could legally refuse to provide veterinary services if they deemed a situation unsafe, some were not afforded this option when being requested to fulfil HeV management duties on behalf of the government without receiving logistic support or compensation for their skilled services. Additionally, some participants thought that scrutiny of veterinary practices by WHS authorities was often inadequate and arbitrary to the detriment of their businesses.

Discussion

Private veterinarians are likely to be the first frontline clinicians to encounter emerging zoonoses; which puts them at a higher occupational risk of exposure to these diseases [1,29]. Many studies, including Australian studies, have shown veterinarians' attitudes and behaviours towards IC and zoonotic risks to be suboptimal; however, most studies have failed to explain why this was so [30-34]. The aim of this study was not to evaluate veterinary IC adequacy but to identify and understand the barriers to IC and zoonotic risk mitigation in private veterinary practices within the context of the emergence of HeV in Queensland, Australia. Participants reported experiencing difficulties implementing IC and HeV management for a number of reasons (Table 1). Many of these issues were interconnected and were in actual fact related to four main barriers to IC and HeV management discussed below: veterinary work culture; private workforce managing biosecurity and public health issues; role of government; and uncertainty about the epidemiology of an emerging disease (Table 2).

Strengths and limitations

Between December 2009 and September 2010, the issues surrounding veterinary IC and HeV management were sensitive topics amongst private veterinarians, as two of their colleagues had died of HeV in the previous two years [6,9-11]. Following these events private equine practices came under a high level of government scrutiny. As a result, prospective participants were reluctant to take part in the study. They were concerned their responses would be misunderstood, misrepresented and/or misused. Those who agreed to participate may have had "stronger views on" or "interest in" veterinary IC and HeV management because they had had experience with HeV or biosecurity and WHS government authorities; or because they were principal veterinarians, owners of their practice. Although data were collected over 10 months, the topics brought to the fore during the interviews were very similar and mostly related to veterinary IC and HeV management issues participants had experienced prior to 2010. Many of the views expressed by participants were corroborated by the findings of other reports about HeV management [35-37]. The chief investigator (RS) and the main interviewer (DM) are both veterinarians who were able to communicate with participants as colleagues who understood the context of their workplace. Consequently, participants were more open about their experiences and beliefs, which made for richer data. However, coding and thematic analysis were pursued without any preconceived construct other than the knowledge the researchers had of veterinary workplaces, allowing an in-depth understanding of the issues raised by participants.

Veterinary work culture

Most participants agreed that, as a whole, the veterinary profession had initially been reluctant to adopt new IC strategies for the management of HeV because it required a significant shift in their work culture. Retrospectively, they felt unprepared to deal with an emerging zoonosis. They all agreed that when HeV first emerged veterinary IC was not optimal and needed improvement.

Table 2 Summary of main barriers to infection control and Hendra virus management in private veterinary practices in Queensland, Australia, up until September 2010

Main issues	*Related barriers*
Work culture	• *Longstanding observance of suboptimal IC practices;*
	• *Veterinarians' perception that zoonotic risks in equine veterinary practice were low;*
	• *Veterinarians' perception that they are more likely to be exposed to injury risks than infectious risks in equine practice;*
	• *Mitigation of injury risks more readily implemented by veterinarians than mitigation of infectious risks in equine practice;*
	• *Inadequate veterinary work habits perpetrated in some instances by poor professional mentorship during extramural undergraduate placement or during early career experiences.*
Role of Government	• *Suboptimal HeV testing pathways*
	• *Slow response from government authorities to the emergence of HeV and to HeV outbreaks*
	• *Suboptimal and conflicting communication of risk and risk mitigation from government authorities to veterinarians*
	• *Inconsistent government support for veterinarians throughout the state, with rural remote areas receiving less skilled technical support*
	• *Difficulties in complying and collaborating with WHS legislation and authorities*
Managing animal and public health issues and a private business	• *The logistical, financial and work time costs of implementing infection control changes within the context of running small private businesses*
	• *Difficulty in interpreting and enforcing WHS regulation*
	• *Mitigation of zoonotic risks interfering with the mitigation of injury risks*
	• *Lack of WHS legal protection when a third party breaches the legislation*
	• *Veterinarians' lack of experience choosing and using some of the PPE recommended*
	• *Inadequate, insufficient and inconsistent training of undergraduate veterinarians about IC and HeV management*
	• *Difficulty in implementing IC behavioural changes amongst veterinary staff*
	• *Difficulty inefficiently communicating with clients about HeV-related risks and risk mitigation recommendations*
Uncertainty about the epidemiology of an emerging disease	• *Slow emergence and sporadic nature of HeV outbreaks*
	• *Slow gathering and dissemination of epidemiological information*
	• *Misinterpretation of epidemiological information*
	• *Non-specific HeV case definition*

In 2010 they were still trying to understand how to best manage HeV. A 2010 government study conducted within the same target population also concluded that IC for the management of HeV still needed amelioration [17]. However, participants cautioned this process would take time. By 2009–2010, all participants had made some improvements to their IC and HeV management strategies; some only recently while others had not been sustained long term. According to the hierarchy of control of health and safety risks which categorises risk mitigation strategies, the changes implemented varied greatly, with some participants implementing only low levels of control (using additional PPE); while others addressed IC issues at a much higher level of control (attending specialised training, developing new standard protocols and policies, seeking new engineered solutions) [38]. A few participants were still sceptical of the appropriateness of the recommended changes.

Successfully changing work culture in human healthcare settings has been described as a lengthy and complex process requiring strong leadership within an organisation [39,40]. The adoption of effective hand hygiene by healthcare workers is a good example. While hand hygiene was recognised in the late 1800s as the simplest and most effective IC measure that could help prevent healthcare associated infections, it remains a practice that is neither consistently nor adequately carried out by healthcare workers despite healthcare systems being strongly supported by government leadership [41]. In comparison, the push for veterinarians to adopt new HeV-related IC measures only dates from the last decade. Veterinarians communicated about HeV risk mitigation within and between practices via an informal professional network; however, most participants felt that government agencies in charge of biosecurity could have provided more leadership and support to the veterinary profession. Instead, the leadership in veterinary IC for the management of HeV was fragmented and vested in each principal veterinarian, the owner of his/her practice.

Private workforce managing biosecurity and public health issues

Maintaining the financial viability and credentials of the veterinary practice, a small privately owned business, was a concern for all principal veterinarians and some senior veterinary employees interviewed. In their view any change in work habits/protocols could affect the business, presumably because of the perception that in private veterinary practice there is a cost ceiling and any additional cost would decrease profit. Profitability of the business is a common concern of veterinarians running private practices of all types [42,43]. The constraints of running a private business significantly influenced participants' decisions about IC, and some found it difficult to balance their *de facto* public health and biosecurity roles while running a private business and complying with their WHS responsibilities. The WHS legislation, for example, was viewed as open to interpretation and difficult to implement in unpredictable circumstances not easily controlled. The difficulties of using some standard biosecurity measures in the field in equine practice are common to the management of other equine infectious diseases [44]. Some participants were aware that they could legally refuse provision of services if they deemed a situation unsafe [45]. However this option was considered as a last resort as it could jeopardise the welfare of animals, translate into loss of immediate income and future income if unsatisfied clients did not return to the practice. Refusing to provide veterinary services was not an option for participants who reported having been requested to fulfil HeV management duties on behalf of the government. For some, the weight of the legal responsibilities reached breaking point when HeV started to emerge, resulting in them choosing to exit equine veterinary practice [25]. So, although fear of dying acted as a significant motivator for some participants to implement lasting IC changes, the complexity of their responsibilities to their patients, clients, colleagues, business and the community deterred them from doing so.

Role of the government

Many participants perceived government authorities' slow response to the emergence of HeV as a sign of unpreparedness to deal with emerging zoonoses, which contributed to the slow uptake of new IC measures for the management of HeV management by private veterinarians. The subsequent increased scrutiny into veterinary practices by biosecurity and WHS government agencies was perceived by most participants as intrusive and an indication that they were regarded as the sole responsible for all HeV management shortcomings until 2010. However, most participants thought the government could have better contributed to the management of HeV outbreaks. An Ombudsman's report about government response to HeV outbreaks concurred with this view [37]: prior to 2009 government agencies in charge of biosecurity failed to develop, finalise and implement their policies for the management of HeV and adequately train their staff accordingly. This was reported to have resulted in the communication of incomplete and conflicting information and poor field support of private veterinarians, despite previous independent reports identifying similar issues for the 2008 and 2009 outbreaks [35,36]. Investigation into the handling of equine influenza, an equine specific emerging disease in Australia in 2007, also showed the importance of risk communication from government to private veterinarians when managing emerging infectious diseases [46]. Many of the recommendations from the various reports about the management of HeV have since been adopted by the relevant government agencies [47]. Since 2010 no veterinary personnel have been infected, although equine cases have increased [6]. This may indicate that the provision of early leadership and committed support by government authorities to the veterinary profession may be key to implement more effective management plans of emerging zoonoses from both a biosecurity and a public health perspective.

Uncertainty about the epidemiology of an emerging disease

The lack of preparedness was a major stumbling block in the early management of HeV by veterinarians and government authorities. The slow pattern of HeV emergence appears to have been a contributing factor in delaying the response of both the private and public sectors in charge of HeV management. The practice of IC for HeV management is a matter of biosecurity to protect animal health, of public health and of occupational health and safety. However, deciding to adopt adequate IC strategies and behaviours when managing HeV cases is a matter of personal health choice. Social scientists have developed various cognitive models to help predict health behaviours by examining a number of cognitive skills: *knowledge, motivation, readiness to change behaviour, expected outcomes, risk perception, perception of peer behaviour and beliefs about peer opinion of targeted behaviour* [48]. When HeV first emerged many of these variables would not have scored highly amongst private veterinarians. Veterinarians have been shown to make evidence-based IC decisions [49]. With HeV outbreaks occurring sporadically up until 2010 (13 self-limiting outbreaks with more than four years between the second and third outbreaks and the third and fourth outbreaks) [6], there were few opportunities to gain epidemiological and clinical knowledge about, or management experience of the disease. The full spectrum of clinical signs in horses, non-specific for the most part, was revealed over decades. As more cases accumulated it became obvious that infected horses could also excrete virus during the incubation period [50]. With such a high clinical variability, equine HeV could only be confirmed by laboratory tests, a process that was not deemed straightforward by all veterinarians [26]. Many participants felt that although they understood the principles of zoonotic risk mitigation, they generally lacked experience dealing with emerging zoonoses in equine practice. Thus, HeV-related risk perception, motivation and readiness for IC behavioural change was low during this time, even though during the first two outbreaks three people became infected, two fatally. Participants' behaviours seemed to have also been influenced by: peer perceptions; beliefs about IC and zoonoses; and a strong professional identity based on the long standing belief that using PPE was a sign of weakness and that acquiring a zoonosis was an achievement not a reflection of malpractice [51]. These beliefs may have been stronger amongst older participants who had graduated longer ago as they are likely to have received less theoretical and practical biosecurity than those who graduate more recently [44].

Veterinarians and government actions and decisions relating to the management of HeV followed the typical stages of behaviour change: *pre-contemplation* (behavioural change seen as not needed); *contemplation* (behavioural change under consideration); *preparation* (for behavioural change); *action* (behavioural change implementation); *maintenance* (of behavioural change); *transcendence* (behavioural change becomes the new behavioural norm); and sometimes relapse (reverting to old behaviours) [52,53]. The progression through these stages is determined by a number of cognitive variables (Figure 1). In the context of the emergence of HeV, there was at first disbelief that HeV would recur or spread to other areas, and as the government did not recommend any particular changes, veterinary IC behaviours remained unchanged. With recurring HeV outbreaks and additional human infections, there was a slow recognition that changes to

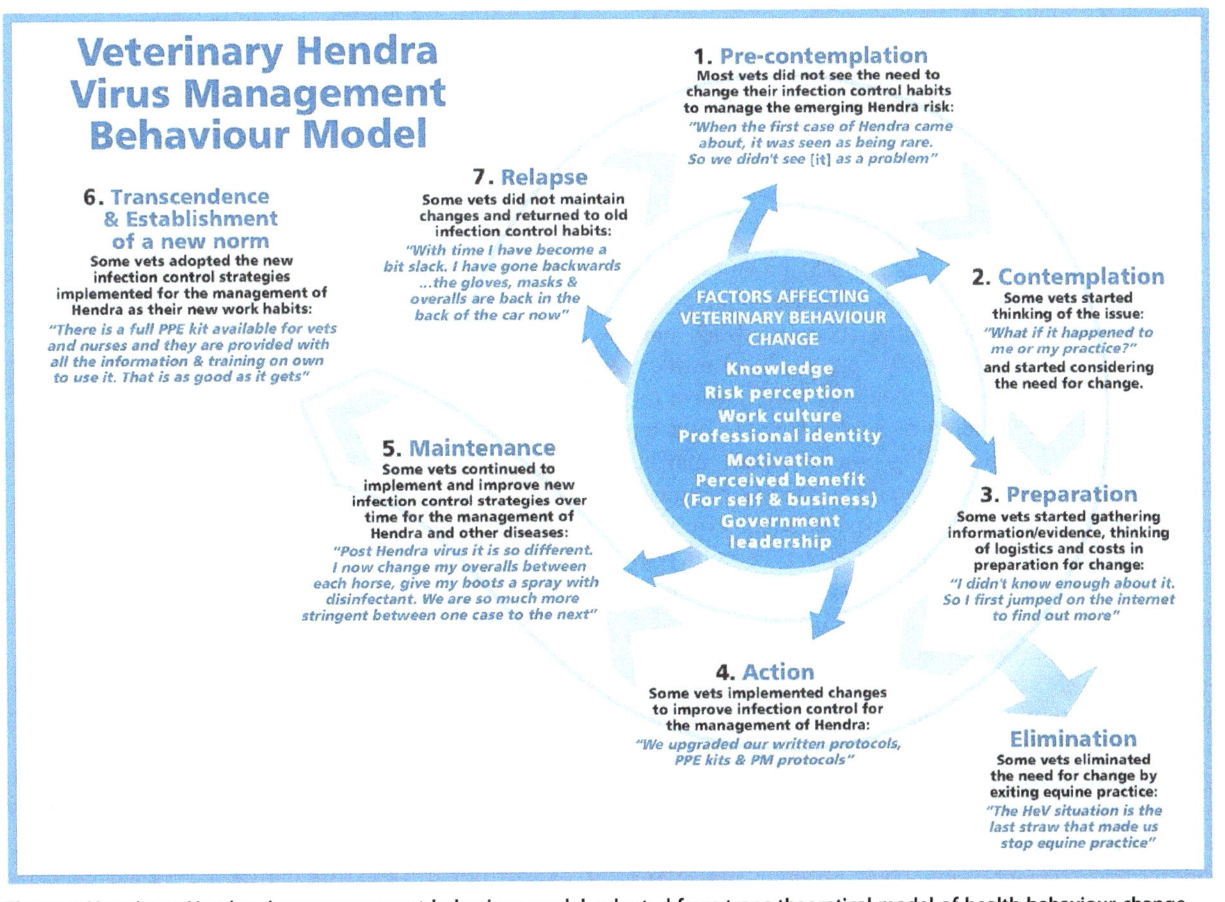

Figure 1 Veterinary Hendra virus management behaviour model, adapted from trans-theoretical model of health behaviour change. Model based on results of a qualitative study investigating barriers to infection control behaviour relevant to Hendra virus management in private veterinary practice in Queensland, Australia, conducted with 21 participants during 2009–2010 [52,53].

veterinary IC were necessary. Some IC changes were made by some veterinarians but these were not always sustained as the required financial and logistic investment could not be justified long-term because of the low frequency of HeV outbreak and the lack of government commitment to a clear HeV management plan. The deaths of two veterinarians in 2008 and 2009 triggered government into finalising their HeV management plan, formulate and widely distribute clear recommendations to private veterinarians and provide more training and field support to equine veterinarians through their emergency response unit. In 2010 all private veterinarians registered in Queensland, received a comprehensive information package from the government. The last three participants to be interviewed for this study had received this package prior to their interview and they were mostly satisfied with this information. Since then there have been no further human infections with HeV even though, in the winter of 2011, there was a marked increase in the number of HeV outbreaks in Queensland and northern New South Wales. Thus, the changes made by the government and the private veterinarians appear to have lowered the risk of human exposure and therefore infection risks for veterinarians and the wider population.

Conclusion

Unlike other zoonoses, which emerged rapidly in human populations causing epidemics (e.g., severe acute respiratory syndrome (SARS), swine influenza (H1N1) in 2009), HeV was slow to emerge, the index cases occurred in horses rather than in humans and HeV did not affect public health on a grand scale. Unlike SARS and swine influenza, HeV is a low-incidence high-consequence pathogen [54]. This type of slow emerging zoonosis, which only affects human health occasionally, comes with its own set of unique challenges. Because they recur infrequently, remain geographically localised or have a limited effect on public health, the health risk they pose to humans may be difficult to assess. However, there is a need to recognise the potential significance of this type of zoonosis earlier and implement risk mitigation measures accordingly. Failing to do so, may put people at risk, in particular professionals such as farmers, zoo and wildlife carers, and veterinarians who may come in contact with an infected animal. However, it would be unrealistic to mobilise the same level of resources used for the management of zoonoses such as SARS or swine influenza. Nevertheless, it may be possible to develop a template framework for the management of slowly emerging zoonoses, which could include: improving veterinary IC and emerging zoonoses management preparedness through education; better communication between government authorities, veterinarians and the public; better recognition of the biosecurity and public health role and services provided by private veterinarians; consultation with private veterinarians when developing zoonoses management plans compatible with running private practices; a clearer definition of the respective roles of government, professional agencies and private veterinarians using officially ratified agreements; and better and equitable government support for the management of emerging zoonoses to all private veterinarians across all affected geographic areas. A closer collaboration and mutual understanding between private veterinarians and government could be the key to improving adaptability of both parties to slowly emerging or infrequent zoonoses.

Abbreviations

HeV: Hendra virus; IC: Infection control; PPE: Personal protective equipment; AVA: Australian veterinary association; EVA: Equine veterinarians Australia; WHS: Workplace health and safety; SARS: Sever acute respiratory syndrome.

Competing interests

The authors declare that they have no competing interests.

Authors' contributions

RS conceived the study and provided support and advice to DM who carried out the study. DM and RS were involved in the drafting and piloting of the research tool. DM recruited participants, conducted interviews, collated and analysed the data. JK assisted in the data analysis as well as the manuscript preparation. DM drafted the initial manuscript which was subsequently reviewed by RS, JK, PB and MN. All authors read and approved the final manuscript.

Acknowledgements

The authors would like to thank all private equine practices and their staff who participated, Dr Jenni Judd who provided initial methodology advice, Jennifer Cox who assisted with interviews and Kylie Halliday who assisted with interview transcription. Funding for this project was provided initially by the Australian Biosecurity Cooperative Research Centre for Emerging Infectious Diseases and subsequently by the Anton Breinl Centre for Public Health and Tropical Medicine.

Author details

[1]College of Public Health, Medical and Veterinary Sciences, James Cook University, Townsville, QLD 4811, Australia. [2]College of Medicine and Dentistry, James Cook University, Townsville, QLD 4811, Australia. [3]Centre for Nursing and Midwifery Research, James Cook University, Townsville, QLD 4811, Australia. [4]Tropical Health Solutions Pty Ltd, Townsville, Queensland 4811, Australia.

References

1. Taylor L, Latham S, Woolhouse M: **Risk factors for human disease emergence.** *Philos Trans R Soc B BiolSci* 2001, **356**(1411):983–989.
2. Murray K, Selleck P, Hooper P, Hyatt A, Gould A, Gleeson L, Westbury H, Hiley L, Selvey L, Rodwell B, Ketterer P: **Amorbillivirus that caused fatal disease in horses and humans.** *Science* 1995, **268**:94–97.
3. Murray K, Rogers R, Selvey L, Selleck P, Hyatt A, Gould A, Gleeson L, Hooper P, Westbury: **A novel morbillivirus pneumonia of horses and its transmission to humans.** *Emerg Infect Dis* 1995, **1**:31–33.
4. Haplin K, Young P, Field H, Mackenzie J: **Isolation of Hendra virus from pteropid bats: a natural reservoir of Hendra virus.** *J Gen Virol* 2000, **81**(8):1927–1932.
5. Haplin K, Hyatt A, Fogarty R, Middleton D, Bingham J, Epstein J, Rahman S, Hughes T, Smith C, Field H, Daszak P, Henipavirus Ecology Research Group: **Pteropid bats are confirmed as the reservoir hosts of henipaviruses: a comprehensive experimental study of virus transmission.** *Am J Trop Med Hyg* 2011, **85**:946–951.

6. Department of Agriculture, Fisheries, and Forestry, Queensland Government: *Hendra virus*. www.daff.qld.gov.au/animal-industries/animal-health-and-diseases/a-z-list/hendra-virus.
7. O'Sullivan J, Allworth A, Paterson D, Snow T, Boots R, Gleeson L, Gould A, Hyatt A, Bradfield J: **Fatal encephalitis due to novel paramyxovirus transmitted from horses.** *Lancet* 1997, **349**:93–95.
8. Hanna J, McBride W, Brookes D, Shield J, Taylor C, Smith I, Craig S, Smith G: **Hendra virus infection in a veterinarian.** *Med J Aust* 2006, **185**:562–564.
9. Playford E, McCall B, Smith G, Slinko V, Allen G, Smith I, Moore F, Taylor C, Kung Y, Field H: **Human Hendra virus encephalitis associated with equine outbreak, Australia 2008.** *Emerg Infect Dis* 2010, **16**:219–223.
10. Field H, Schaaf K, Kung N, Simon C, Waltisbuhl D, Hobert H, Moore F, Middleton D, Crook A, Smith G, Daniels P, Glanville R, Lovell D: **Hendra virus outbreak with novel clinical features, Australia.** *Emerg Infect Dis* 2010, **16**:338–340.
11. Mahalingam S, Herrero L, Playford E, Spann K, Herring B, Rolph M, Middleton D, McCall B, Field H, Wang L: **Hendra virus: an emerging paramyxovirus in Australia.** *Lancet* 2012, **12**:799–807.
12. Symons R: **Re: Canine case of Hendra virus and Hendra virus vaccine.** *Aust Vet J* 2011, **89**(10):N24.
13. Department of Agriculture, Fisheries, and Forestry, Queensland Government: *Guidelines for Veterinarians Handling Potential Hendra Virus Infection in Horses.* http://www.daff.qld.gov.au/__data/assets/pdf_file/0005/126770/2913_-Guidelines-for-veterinarians-handling-potential-Hendra-virus-infection-in-horses-V5.1.pdf.
14. Bossart K, Geisbert T, Feldmann H, Zhu Z, Feldmann F, Geisbert J, Yan L, Feng Y, Brining D, Scott D, Wang Y, Dimitrov A, Callison J, Chan Y, Hickey A, Dimitrov D, Broder C, Rockx B: **A neutralising human monoclonal antibody protects African green monkeys from Hendra virus challenge.** *SciTransl Med* 2011, **3**(105):105ra103.
15. Pallister J, Middleton D, Wang L, Klein R, Haining J, Robinson R, Yamada M, White J, Payne J, Feng Y, Chan Y, Broder C: **A recombinant Hendra virus G glycoprotein-based subunit protects ferrets from lethal Hendra virus challenge.** *Vaccine* 2011, **29**:5623–5630.
16. Pallister J, Middleton D, Broder C, Wang L: **Henipavirus vaccine development.** *J Bioterr Biodef* 2011, **S1**:005. doi:10.4172/2157-2526.S1-005.
17. Workplace Health and Safety Queensland, Department of Justice and Attorney-General, Queensland Government: *Summary Report: Outcomes of an Audit of Hendra Virus Risk Management in the Veterinary Industry.* PN11006 Version 1 2011. http://www.deir.qld.gov.au/workplace/resources/pdfs/outcome-audit-hendra-vet-industry.pdf.
18. Christley R, Perkins E: **Researching hard to reach areas of knowledge: qualitative research in veterinary science.** *Equine Vet J* 2010, **42**(4):285–286.
19. Creswell J, Plano Clark V: *Designing and Conducting Mixed Methods Research.* Los Angeles: Sage Publications; 2010.
20. Minichiello V, Aroni R, Hays T: *In-depth Interviewing: Principles, Techniques, Analysis (3rd edition).* Sydney: Pearson Education Australia; 2008.
21. Clark JP: **How to Peer Review a Qualitative Manuscript.** In *Peer Review in Health Sciences.* Secondth edition. Edited by Godlee F, Jefferson T. London: BMJ Books; 2003:219–235.
22. Biomedical Central: *Qualitative Research Review Guidelines – RATS.* http://www.biomedcentral.com/authors/rats.
23. Field H, De Jong C, Melville D, Smith C, Smith I, Broos A, Kung N, McLaughlin A, Zeddeman A: **Hendra virus infection dynamics in Australian fruit bats.** *PLoS One* 2011, **6**(12):e28678. doi:101371/journal.pone.0028678.
24. Australian Institute of Health and Welfare: *Rural, Regional and Remote Health: A Guide to Remoteness Classifications.* Canberra: AIHW Catalogue No. PHE 53. AIHW; 2004.
25. Mendez D, Judd J, Speare R: **Unexpected result of Hendra virus outbreaks for veterinarians, Queensland, Australia.** *Emerg Infect Dis* 2012, **18**:83–85.
26. Mendez D, Judd J, Speare R: **Testing for Hendra virus: difficulties experienced by veterinarians in Queensland prior to 2011.** *Aust Vet J* 2013, **91**:323–327.
27. Mendez D, Miller K, Judd J, Speare R: **Risk Communication Between Veterinarians and Horse Owners: A key Factor in the Management of Hendra Virus.** *In Online Proceedings of Australian Society for Infectious Diseases, Zoonoses Conference.* Syndey: 2012. www.asid.net.au/documents/item/202.
28. Braun V, Clarke V: **Using thematic analysis in psychology.** *Qual Res Psychol* 2006, **3**(2):77–101.
29. Jackson J, Villarroel A: **A survey of the risk of zoonoses for veterinarians.** *Zoonoses Public Health* 2012, **59**(3):193–201.
30. Van Soest E, Fritschi L: **Occupational health risks in veterinary nursing: an exploratory study.** *Aust Vet J* 2004, **82**(6):346–350.
31. Wright J, Jung S, Holman R, Marano N, McQuiston J: **Infection control and zoonotic disease risks among veterinarians in the United States.** *J Am Vet Med Assoc* 2008, **232**(12):1863–1872.
32. Weese J, Fairies M: **A survey of needle handling practices and needlestick injuries in veterinary technicians.** *Can Vet J* 2009, **50**(12):1278–1282.
33. Leggat P, Smith D, Speare R: **Exposure rate of needlestick and sharps injuries among Australian veterinarians.** *J Occup Med Toxicol* 2009, **4**:25.
34. Dowd K, Taylor M, Toibio J, Hooker C, Dhand N: **Zoonotic disease risk perceptions and infection control practices of Australian veterinarians: call for change in work culture.** *Prev Vet Med* 2013, **111**(1–2):17–24.
35. Perkins N: *Independent Review of Hendra Virus Cases at Redlands and Proserpine in July and August 2008.* Toowoomba: AusVet Animal Health Services; 2008. http://www.tropicalhealthsolutions.com/HeVreports.
36. Perkins N: *Independent Review into Hendra Incident at Cawarral.* Toowomba: AusVet Animal Health Services; 2009. http://www.tropicalhealthsolutions.com/HeVreports.
37. Clarke P: *The Hendra Virus Report. An Investigation into Agency Responses to Hendra Virus Incidents Between January 2006 and December 2009.* Brisbane: Queensland Ombudsman; 2011. http://www.ombudsman.qld.gov.au/Portals/0/docs/Publications/Inv_reports/Hendra/Hendra_Virus_Report_web_V1.pdf.
38. Workplace Health and Safety Queensland, Department of Justice and Attorney-General, Queensland Government: *How to Manage Work Health and Safety Risks, Code of Practice 2011.* [http://www.deir.qld.gov.au/workplace/resources/pdfs/manage-whs-risks-cop-2011.pdf]
39. Rasslan O, Ellingston K, Stricof R, Grant P: **Infection control: accomplishements and priorities from an individual, state, national, and international perspective.** *Am J Infect Control* 2011, **39**:624–627.
40. Lieber S, Mantengoli E, Siant S, Fowler K, Fumagalli C, Bartolozzi D, Magistri L, Niccolini F, Bartoloni A: **The effect of leadership on hand hygiene adherence prior to patient contact in 2 infectious disease units in Tuscany.** *Infect Control Hosp Epidemiol* 2014, **35**(3):313–316.
41. Erasmus V, Daha T, Brug H, Richardus J, Behrendt M, Vos M, Van Beeck E: **Systematic review of studies on compliance with hand hygiene guidelines in hospital care.** *Infect Control Hosp Epidemiol* 2010, **31**(3):283–294.
42. Osborne D, Richardson F: **Model of practice excellence – Budgeting with New Hamburg veterinary clinic.** *Can Vet J* 2006, **47**:923–928.
43. Blach E: **Customer service in equine veterinary medicine.** *Vet Clin Equine* 2009, **25**:421–432.
44. Scheman K, Toribio J, Taylor M, Ward M, Dhand N: **Survey of Australian equine veterinarians evaluating their biosecurity training and perceptions and opinions about the management of the 2007 equine influenza outbreak.** *Aust Vet J* 2014, **92**(4):93–100.
45. Health W, Queensland S: *Department of Justice and Attorney-General.* Queensland Government: Workplace Health and Safety Act; 1995 [https://www.legislation.qld.gov.au/LEGISLTN/ACTS/1995/95AC025.pdf]
46. Schemann K, Firestone S, Taylor M, Toribio J, Ward M, Dhand N: **From the horses's mouth: perceptions of the management of the 2007 equine influenza outbreak in Australia.** *Transbound Emerg Dis* 2012, **59**:503–516.
47. Queensland Government: *Queensland Government's Response to the Ombudsman's Hendra Virus Report.* http://www.parliament.qld.gov.au/documents/tableOffice/TabledPapers/2011/5311T5905.pdf.
48. Whitby M, Pessoa-Silva, McLaws M, Allengranzi B, Sax H, Larson E, Seto W, Donaldson L, Pittet D, Pessoa-Silva A, McLaws M, Allengranzi B, Sax H, Larson E, Seto W, Donaldson L, Pittet D: **Behavioural considerations for hand hygiene practices: the basic building blocks.** *J Hosp Infect* 2007, **65**:1–8.
49. Gunn G, Heffernan C, Hall M, McLeod A, Hovi M: **Measuring and comparing constraints to improved biosecurity amongst GB farmers, veterinarians and auxiliary industries.** *Prev Vet Med* 2008, **84**:310–323.
50. Marsh G, Haining J, Hancock T, Robinson R, Foord A, Barr J, Riddell S, Heine H, White J, Crameri G, Field H, Wang L, Middleton D: **Experimental**

infection of horses with Hendra virus/Australia/Horse/2008/Redlands. *Emerg Infect Dis* 2011, **17**(2):2232–2238.

51. Schnurrenberger P, Grigor K, Walker J, Martin R: **The zoonosis-prone veterinarian.** *J Am Vet Med Assoc* 1978, **173**(4):373–376.
52. Prochaska J, Velicer W, Rossi J, Goldstein M, Marcus B, Rawoski W, Fiore C, Harlow L, Redding C, Rosenbloom D, Rossi S: **Stages of change and decisional balance for 12 problem behaviours.** *Health Psychol* 1994, **13**(1):39–46.
53. Prochaska J, Velicer W: **The transtheoretical model of health behaviour change.** *Am J Health Promot* 1997, **12**(1):38–48.
54. Belay E, Monroe S: **Low-incidence, high-consequence pathogens.** *Emerg Infect Dis* 2014, **20**(2):319–321.

PERMISSIONS

All chapters in this book were first published in VR, by BioMed Central; hereby published with permission under the Creative Commons Attribution License or equivalent. Every chapter published in this book has been scrutinized by our experts. Their significance has been extensively debated. The topics covered herein carry significant findings which will fuel the growth of the discipline. They may even be implemented as practical applications or may be referred to as a beginning point for another development.

The contributors of this book come from diverse backgrounds, making this book a truly international effort. This book will bring forth new frontiers with its revolutionizing research information and detailed analysis of the nascent developments around the world.

We would like to thank all the contributing authors for lending their expertise to make the book truly unique. They have played a crucial role in the development of this book. Without their invaluable contributions this book wouldn't have been possible. They have made vital efforts to compile up to date information on the varied aspects of this subject to make this book a valuable addition to the collection of many professionals and students.

This book was conceptualized with the vision of imparting up-to-date information and advanced data in this field. To ensure the same, a matchless editorial board was set up. Every individual on the board went through rigorous rounds of assessment to prove their worth. After which they invested a large part of their time researching and compiling the most relevant data for our readers.

The editorial board has been involved in producing this book since its inception. They have spent rigorous hours researching and exploring the diverse topics which have resulted in the successful publishing of this book. They have passed on their knowledge of decades through this book. To expedite this challenging task, the publisher supported the team at every step. A small team of assistant editors was also appointed to further simplify the editing procedure and attain best results for the readers.

Apart from the editorial board, the designing team has also invested a significant amount of their time in understanding the subject and creating the most relevant covers. They scrutinized every image to scout for the most suitable representation of the subject and create an appropriate cover for the book.

The publishing team has been an ardent support to the editorial, designing and production team. Their endless efforts to recruit the best for this project, has resulted in the accomplishment of this book. They are a veteran in the field of academics and their pool of knowledge is as vast as their experience in printing. Their expertise and guidance has proved useful at every step. Their uncompromising quality standards have made this book an exceptional effort. Their encouragement from time to time has been an inspiration for everyone.

The publisher and the editorial board hope that this book will prove to be a valuable piece of knowledge for researchers, students, practitioners and scholars across the globe.

LIST OF CONTRIBUTORS

Xiaolong Gao, Xiangyun Hu, Lina Tong, Dandan Liu, Xudong Chang, Haixin Wang, Ruyi Dang, Xinglong Wang, Sa Xiao, Enqi Du and Zengqi Yang
College of Veterinary Medicine, Northwest A & F University, Yangling, Shaanxi Province 712100, P. R. China

J. J. Correia and M. C. Peleteiro
Centro de Investigação Interdisciplinar em Sanidade Animal (CIISA), Faculdade de Medicina Veterinária, Universidade de Lisboa. Av. Da Universidade Técnica, 1300-477 Lisbon, Portugal

F.A. Abade dos Santos
Centro de Investigação Interdisciplinar em Sanidade Animal (CIISA), Faculdade de Medicina Veterinária, Universidade de Lisboa. Av. Da Universidade Técnica, 1300-477 Lisbon, Portugal
Rua Quinta do Pinto N°5 3°D, 2660-067 Loures, Frielas, Portugal

C. Carvalho
Instituto de Ciências Agrárias e Ambientais Mediterrânicas (ICAAM); Instituto de Investigação e Formação Avançada (IIFA), Universidade de Évora. Núcleo da Mitra, 7000 Évora, Portugal

Oliveira Nuno
Sociedade Portuguesa para o Estudo das Aves (SPEA), Av. Columbano Bordalo Pinheiro, 87, 3° Andar, 1070-062 Lisboa, Portugal

M. Henriques, M. Fevereiro and M. D. Duarte
Instituto Nacional de Investigação Agrária e Veterinária (INIAV), Laboratório de Virologia. Av. Da República, Quinta do Marquês, 2780-157 Oeiras, Portugal

V. Milicevic
Virology department, Institute of Veterinary Medicine of Serbia, Vojvode Toze 14, 11000 Belgrade, Serbia

S. Radojicic and M. Valcic
Infectious Animals Diseases and Diseases of Bees, Faculty of Veterinary Medicine, Bulevar oslobodjenja 18, 11000 Belgrade, Serbia

V. Ivovic
Department of Biodiversity, University of Primorska, Faculty of Mathematics, Natural Sciences and Information Technologies, Glagoljaska 8, SI-6000 Koper, Slovenia

V. Radosavljevic
Institute of Veterinary Medicine of Serbia, Vojvode Toze 14, 11000 Belgrade, Serbia

Jessica Coertse and Wanda Markotter
Center for Viral Zoonoses, Department of Medical Virology, School of Medicine, Faculty of Health Sciences, University of Pretoria, Pretoria 0001, South Africa

Kevin le Roux
Allerton Provincial Veterinary Laboratory, Pietermaritzburg, KwaZulu-Natal 3200, South Africa

Daniel Stewart
Department of Agriculture and Environmental Affairs, KwaZulu-Natal Rabies Project, Pietermaritzburg, KwaZulu-Natal, South Africa

Claude T. Sabeta
Agricultural Research Council-Onderstepoort Veterinary Institute (ARC-OVI), Pretoria 0110, South Africa

Louis H. Nel
Department of Microbiology and Plant Pathology, Faculty of Natural and Agricultural Sciences, University of Pretoria, Pretoria 0001, South Africa

Rahul Deb Sarker, Emdadul Haque Chowdhury and Mohammad Rafiqul Islam
Department of Pathology, Bangladesh Agricultural University, Mymensingh, Bangladesh

Mohammad Giasuddin
National Reference Laboratory for Avian Influenza, Bangladesh Livestock Research Institute, Savar, Dhaka, Bangladesh

Qi Chen, Joseph T. Thomas, Luis G. Giménez-Lirola, Ying Zheng, Ganwu Li, Phillip C. Gauger, Darin M. Madson, Drew R. Magstadt and Jianqiang Zhang
Department of Veterinary Diagnostic and Production Animal Medicine, College of Veterinary Medicine, Iowa State University, 1800 Christensen Drive, Ames, IA 50011, USA

Tanja Opriessnig
Department of Veterinary Diagnostic and Production Animal Medicine, College of Veterinary Medicine, Iowa State University, 1800 Christensen Drive, Ames, IA 50011, USA
The Roslin Institute and The Royal (Dick) School of Veterinary Studies, University of Edinburgh, Roslin, Midlothian, Edinburgh EH25 9RG, UK

John M. Hardham and Qinshan Gao
Zoetis, Kalamazoo, MI, USA

Priscilla F. Gerber
The Roslin Institute and The Royal (Dick) School of Veterinary Studies, University of Edinburgh, Roslin, Midlothian, Edinburgh EH25 9RG, UK

Mebrahtu Tedla
Department of Biomedical Sciences, University of Gondar, College of Veterinary Medicine and Animal Sciences, Gondar, Ethiopia

Nega Berhan
Department of Biotechnology, University of Gondar, College of Natural and Computational Sciences, Gondar, Ethiopia

Wassie Molla and Sefinew Alemu
Department of Clinical Studies, University of Gondar, College of Veterinary Medicine and Animal Sciences, Gondar, Ethiopia

Wudu Temesgen
Department of Veterinary Epidemiology and Public Health, University of Gondar, College of Veterinary Medicine and Animal Sciences, Gondar, Ethiopia

A. Malmsten and A.-M. Dalin
Department of Clinical Sciences, Division of Reproduction, Swedish University of Agricultural Sciences, Uppsala, Sweden

E. O. Ågren
Department of Pathology and Wildlife Diseases, National Veterinary Institute, 751 89 Uppsala, Sweden

J. Malmsten
Department of Pathology and Wildlife Diseases, National Veterinary Institute, 751 89 Uppsala, Sweden
Department of Wildlife, Fish, and Environmental studies, Swedish University of Agricultural Sciences, 901 83 Umeå, Sweden

G. Blomqvist, K. Näslund and C. Vernersson
Department of Microbiology, National Veterinary Institute, 751 89 Uppsala, Sweden

S. Hägglund
Department of Pathology and Wildlife Diseases, National Veterinary Institute, 751 89 Uppsala, Sweden

J.-F. Valarcher
Department of Pathology and Wildlife Diseases, National Veterinary Institute, 751 89 Uppsala, Sweden
Department of Clinical Sciences, Host Pathogen Interaction Group, Ruminant medicine, Swedish University of Agricultural Sciences, Uppsala, Sweden

Rui Du and Aidong Qian
College of Animal Science and Technology, Jilin Agricultural University, Changchun 130118, People's Republic of China

Liang Cao, Changzhan Xie and Ningyi Jin
College of Animal Science and Technology, Jilin Agricultural University, Changchun 130118, People's Republic of China
Institute of Military Veterinary, Key Laboratory of Jilin Province for Zoonosis Prevention and Control, Academy of Military Sciences, Changchun 130122, People's Republic of China

Jicheng Han, Wei Wang, Wenchao Sun, Huijun Lu and Mingyao Tian
Institute of Military Veterinary, Key Laboratory of Jilin Province for Zoonosis Prevention and Control, Academy of Military Sciences, Changchun 130122, People's Republic of China

Guanyu Zhao
Institute of Military Veterinary, Key Laboratory of Jilin Province for Zoonosis Prevention and Control, Academy of Military Sciences, Changchun 130122, People's Republic of China
College of Veterinary Medicine, Jilin University, Changchun 130062, People's Republic of China

Min Zheng
Guangxi Center for Animal Disease Control and Prevention, Nanning 530001, People's Republic of China

J. F. Mee
Animal and Bioscience Research Department, AGRIC, Teagasc, Moorepark, Fermoy, Co. Cork, Ireland

Á. B. Collins
Animal and Bioscience Research Department, AGRIC, Teagasc, Moorepark, Fermoy, Co. Cork, Ireland
School of Veterinary Medicine, University College Dublin, Dublin 4, Ireland

M. L. Doherty
School of Veterinary Medicine, University College Dublin, Dublin 4, Ireland

D. Barrett
Sligo RVL, Department of Agriculture, Food and the Marine, Doonally, Co. Sligo, Ireland

M. Larska
Department of Virology, National Veterinary Research Institute, Puławy, Poland

Takehiro Kanda
Department of Animal Hygiene, Joint Facility of Veterinary Medicine, Kagoshima University, Kagoshima, Kagoshima, Japan

Makoto Ozawa and Kyoko Tsukiyama-Kohara
Department of Animal Hygiene, Joint Facility of Veterinary Medicine, Kagoshima University, Kagoshima, Kagoshima, Japan
Transboundary Animal Disease Center, Joint Facility of Veterinary Medicine, Kagoshima University, Kagoshima, Kagoshima, Japan

Qingxia Wu, Hailong Dong, Zhenyu Chang, Suozhu Liu and Hongyun Zhu
Key laboratory of clinical veterinary medicine in Tibet, Tibet Agriculture and Animal Husbandry College, Linzhi 860000, Tibet, People's Republic of China

Jiakui Li
Key laboratory of clinical veterinary medicine in Tibet, Tibet Agriculture and Animal Husbandry College, Linzhi 860000, Tibet, People's Republic of China
College of Veterinary Medicine, Huazhong Agricultural University, Wuhan 430070, People's Republic of China

Hui Zhang, Mujeeb Ur Rehman, Fazul Nabi and Kun Li
College of Veterinary Medicine, Huazhong Agricultural University, Wuhan 430070, People's Republic of China

Khalid Mehmood
College of Veterinary Medicine, Huazhong Agricultural University, Wuhan 430070, People's Republic of China
University College of Veterinary & Animal Sciences, the Islamia University of Bahawalpur, Bahawalpur 63100, Pakistan

Muhammad Tariq Javed
Departmet of Pathology, University of Agriculture, Faisalabad, Pakistan

Erica Spackman, Mary J. Pantin-Jackwood, Darrell R. Kapczynski, David E. Swayne and David L. Suarez
Southeast Poultry Research Laboratory, USDA-Agricultural Research Service, 934 College Station Rd, Athens, GA 30605, USA

Dildar Hussain Kalhoro, Shanshan Gao, Xing Xie, Shan Liang, Su Luo, Yanbing Zhao and Yongjie Liu
College of Veterinary Medicine, Nanjing Agricultural University, Nanjing 210095, China
Montserrat Elemi García-Hernández, José Iván Sánchez-Betancourt, Oscar Rico-Chávez, María E. Trujillo and Rosa Elena Sarmiento-Silva Facultad de Medicina Veterinaria y Zootecnia, Universidad Nacional Autónoma de México, Ciudad de México 04510, México

Mayra Cruz-Rivera
Facultad de Medicina, Universidad Nacional Autónoma de México, 04510 Ciudad de México, México

Arely Vergara-Castañeda
Facultad de Ciencias Químicas, Universidad La Salle, Benjamín Franklin 47, 06140 Ciudad de México, México

Jordan Bjustrom-Kraft, Katie Woodard, Luis Giménez-Lirola, Marisa Rotolo, Jianqiang Zhang, David Baum, Phillip Gauger, Rodger Main and Jeffrey Zimmerman
Department of Veterinary Diagnostic and Production Animal Medicine, College of Veterinary Medicine, Iowa State University, 1850 Christensen Drive, Ames, IA 50011-1134, USA

Chong Wang
Department of Veterinary Diagnostic and Production Animal Medicine, College of Veterinary Medicine, Iowa State University, 1850 Christensen Drive, Ames, IA 50011-1134, USA
Department of Statistics, College of Liberal Arts and Sciences, Iowa State University, Osborn Drive, Ames, IA 50011, USA

Yaxuan Sun
Department of Statistics, College of Liberal Arts and Sciences, Iowa State University, Osborn Drive, Ames, IA 50011, USA

Peter Lasley
Smithfield Hog Production Missouri, 17999 US Highway 65, Princeton, MO 64673, USA

Xiujing Dou, Yang Li, Junlan Han, Weijuan Zhu, Xiaofeng Ren, Na Dong, Xunliang Li and Guangxing Li
Northeast Agricultural University, No. 59 Mucai Street, Xiangfang District, Harbin 150030, China

Dante S. Zarlenga
Animal Parasitic Diseases Laboratory, Agricultural Research Service, United States Department of Agriculture, Building 1180, BARC-East, Beltsville, MD 20705, USA

Zhicheng Liu, Chunhong Zhang, Haiyan Shen, Junying Sun and Jianfeng Zhang
Institute of Animal Health, Guangdong Academy of Agricultural Sciences, Key Laboratory of Livestock Disease Prevention of Guangdong Province, Scientific Observation and Experiment Station of Veterinary Drugs and Diagnostic Techniques of Guangdong Province, Ministry of Agriculture, P. R. China, Guangzhou 510640, Guangdong, China

Mishamo Sulayeman
Faculty of Veterinary Medicine, Hawassa University, Hawassa, Ethiopia

Fufa Dawo and Bedaso Mammo
College of Veterinary Medicine, Addis Ababa University, Debre Zeyit, Ethiopia

Daniel Gizaw and Dereje Shegu
National Animal Health Diagnostics and Investigation Center, Sebeta, Ethiopia

Kayhan Ilbeigi and Sina Aghasharif
Department of Clinical Sciences, Faculty of Veterinary Medicine, Islamic Azad University of Garmsar, Garmsar, Iran

Saied Bokaie
Department of Food Hygiene and Quality Control, Faculty of Veterinary Medicine, University of Tehran, Tehran, Iran

Ricardo J. Soares Magalhães
UQ Spatial Epidemiology Laboratory, School of Veterinary Science, The University of Queensland, Gatton, Australia
Children's Health and Environment Program, Child Health Research Centre, The University of Queensland, Brisbane, Australia

Mohamad Rashtibaf
Iranian Veterinary Organization, Provincial Department of Surveillance and Disease Control, Khorasan Razavi, Islamic Republic of Iran

Ulrika Larsson Pettersson
Department of Pathology and Wildlife Diseases, National Veterinary Institute (SVA), 751 89 Uppsala, Sweden

Aleksija S. Neimanis and Dolores Gavier-Widén
Department of Pathology and Wildlife Diseases, National Veterinary Institute (SVA), 751 89 Uppsala, Sweden
Department of Biomedical Sciences and Veterinary Public Health, Swedish University of Agricultural Sciences (SLU), Uppsala, Sweden

Harri Ahola and Siamak Zohari
Department of Microbiology, National Veterinary Institute (SVA), 751 89 Uppsala, Sweden

Joana Abrantes
CIBIO/InBio, Centro de Investigação em Biodiversidade e Recursos Genéticos, Universidade do Porto, Campus Agrário de Vairão, 4485-661 Vairão, Portugal

Ana M. Lopes
CIBIO/InBio, Centro de Investigação em Biodiversidade e Recursos Genéticos, Universidade do Porto, Campus Agrário de Vairão, 4485-661 Vairão, Portugal
Department of Anatomy and Unit for Multidisciplinary Research in Biomedicine (UMIB), Institute of Biomedical Sciences Abel Salazar (ICBAS), University of Porto, Porto, Portugal

Pedro J. Esteves
CIBIO/InBio, Centro de Investigação em Biodiversidade e Recursos Genéticos, Universidade do Porto, Campus Agrário de Vairão, 4485-661 Vairão, Portugal
Departamento de Biologia, Faculdade de Ciências, Universidade do Porto, R. Campo Alegre s/n, 4169-007 Porto, Portugal
Instituto de Investigação e Formação Avançada em Ciências e Tecnologias da Saúde (CESPU), Gandra, Portugal

S. Bertolini, C. Caruso, C. Maurella, F. Ingravalle, P. L. Acutis, L. Masoero and G. Ru
Istituto Zooprofilattico Sperimentale del Piemonte, Liguria e Valle d'Aosta, Turin, Italy

A. Rosamilia
Istituto Zooprofilattico Sperimentale dell'Abruzzo e del Molise G. Caporale, Teramo, Italy

A. Quasso
Local Health Unit AT, Asti, Italy

M. Pitti
Local Health Unit TO4, Turin, Italy

Index